NURSING RESEARCH

Methods and Critical Appraisal
for Evidence-Based Practice

NURSING RESEARCH

Methods and Critical Appraisal for Evidence-Based Practice

GERI LoBIONDO-WOOD, PhD, RN, FAAN

Associate Professor
University of Texas Health Sciences Center
School of Nursing
Nursing Systems and Technology
Houston, Texas

JUDITH HABER, PhD, APRN, BC, FAAN

Professor and Associate Dean for Graduate Programs
Master's Program and Post-Master's Advanced Certificate Program
College of Nursing
New York University
New York, New York

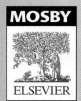

MOSBY

ELSEVIER

MOSBY
ELSEVIER

11830 Westline Industrial Drive
St. Louis, Missouri 63146

NURSING RESEARCH: METHODS AND CRITICAL APPRAISAL FOR
EVIDENCE-BASED PRACTICE
Copyright © 2006, Mosby Inc.

ISBN 0-323-02828-4

Previous editions copyrighted 2002, 1998, 1994, 1990, 1986

ISBN 0-323-02828-4

Acquisitions Editor: Lee Henderson
Senior Developmental Editor: Rae L. Robertson
Developmental Editor: Julie Vitale
Publishing Services Manager: John Rogers
Senior Project Manager: Kathleen L. Teal
Design Direction: Teresa McBryan

Printed in the United States of America
Last digit is the print number: 9   8   7   6   5   4   3   2   1

About the Authors

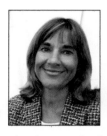

Geri LoBiondo-Wood, PhD, RN, FAAN, is an Associate Professor at the University of Texas Health Science Center at Houston, School of Nursing (UTHSC-Houston). She received her Diploma in nursing at St. Mary's Hospital School of Nursing in Rochester, New York and her Bachelor's and Master's degrees from the University of Rochester and a PhD in Nursing Theory and Research from New York University. Dr. LoBiondo-Wood currently teaches research and theory to undergraduate, graduate, and doctoral students at UTHSC–Houston, School of Nursing. She also holds a joint appointment for the development of evidence-based practice at the MD Anderson Cancer Center in Houston. She has extensive experience guiding nurses and other health care professionals in the development and utilization of research in clinical practice. Dr. LoBiondo-Wood is currently a member of the Editorial Board of *Progress in Transplantation* and a reviewer for *Nursing Research, the Journal of Advanced Nursing,* and *Nephrology Nursing Journal.* Her research and publications focus on chronic illness and the impact of solid organ transplant on child or adult recipients and their families throughout the transplant process.

Dr. LoBiondo-Wood has been active locally and nationally in many professional organizations, including the Southern Nursing Research Society, the Midwest Nursing Research Society, and the North American Transplant Coordinators Organization. She has received local and national awards for teaching and contributions to nursing. In 1997, she received the Distinguished Alumnus Award from New York University, Division of Nursing Alumni Association. In 2001, she was inducted as a Fellow of the American Academy of Nursing.

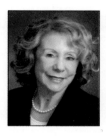

Judith Haber, PhD, APRN, BC, FAAN, is Professor and Associate Dean for Graduate Programs in the College of Nursing at New York University. She received her undergraduate nursing education at Adelphi University in New York and holds a Master's degree in Adult Psychiatric-Mental Health Nursing and a PhD in Nursing Theory and Research from New York University. Judith Haber is internationally recognized as a clinician and educator in psychiatric-mental health nursing. She has extensive clinical experience in psychiatric nursing, having been an advanced practice psychiatric nurse in private practice for over 30 years, specializing in treatment of families coping with the psychosocial sequelae of acute and chronic catastrophic illness. Dr. Haber is currently on the Editorial Board of the *Journal of the American Psychiatric Nurses Association (JAPNA)* and, as a contributing editor, writes a column on policy and politics for this journal. Her areas of research involvement include tool development, particularly in the area of family functioning. She is internationally known for developing the Haber Level of Differentiation of Self Scale. Another program of research addresses physical and psychosocial adjustment to illness, focusing specifically on women with breast cancer and their partners. Based on this research, she and Dr. Carol Hoskins have written and produced an award-winning series of evidence-based psychoeducational videotapes, *Journey to Recovery: For Women with Breast Cancer and Their Partners,* which they are currently testing in a randomized clinical trial funded by the National Cancer Institute.

Dr. Haber has been active locally and nationally in many professional organizations, including the American Nurses Association, American Psychiatric Nurses Association, and the American Academy of Nursing. She has received numerous local, state, and national awards for public policy, clinical practice, and research, including the APNA Psychiatric Nurse of the Year Award in 1998. In 1993, she was inducted as a Fellow of the American Academy of Nursing.

Contributors

Lauren S. Aaronson, PhD, RN, FAAN
Professor
School of Nursing and
Professor Department of Health Policy and
    Management
School of Medicine
University of Kansas
Kansas City, Kansas
Research Vignette

Linda H. Aiken, PhD, RN, FAAN, FRCN
Claire M. Fagin Leadership Professor in Nursing and
    Professor of Sociology and Director of the Center
    of Health Outcomes Policy Research
School of Nursing
University of Pennsylvania
Philadelphia, Pennsylvania
Research Vignette

Susan Bankston, BSN, RN
Emergency Department
Memorial Hermann Hospital
Houston, Texas
Example Glossary

Marlene Z. Cohen, PhD, RN, FAAN
John S. Dunn, Sr., Distinguished Professor in
    Oncology Nursing
Interim Chair
Department of Target Populations
School of Nursing
The University of Texas Health Science Center
Houston, Texas

Professor
Department of Symptom Research
The University of Texas M.D. Anderson Cancer Center
Houston, Texas

Nurse Researcher
Lyndon B. Johnson General Hospital
Houston, Texas
Introduction to Qualitative Research

Betty J. Craft, PhD, RN, CS
Retired, Faculty Emeritus
College of Nursing
University of Nebraska
Omaha, Nebraska
Evaluating Quantitative Research

Margaret Grey, DrPH, RN, FAAN
Dean and Annie Goodrich Professor of Nursing
Yale School of Nursing
Yale University
New Haven, Connecticut
Experimental and Quasiexperimental Designs
Data-Collection Methods
Data Analysis: Descriptive and Inferential

Judith A. Heermann, PhD, RN
Associate Professor
College of Nursing
University of Nebraska

Clinical Nurse Researcher
University of Nebraska Medical Center
Omaha, Nebraska
Evaluating Quantitative Research

Carl Kirton, RN, MA, APRN, BC
Adjunct Faculty
College of Nursing
New York University;

Director, Ambulatory Care and Nurse Practitioner
AIDS Clinic
Mount Sinai Hospital
New York, New York
  Tools for Applying Evidence to Practice

Barbara Krainovich-Miller, EdD, APRN, BC
Clinical Professor
College of Nursing
New York University
New York, New York
  The Research Process: Integrating Evidence-
    Based Practice
  Literature Review
  Critical Thinking Challenges

Patricia R. Liehr, PhD, RN
Professor, Associate Dean for Nursing Research and
    Scholarship
Christine E. Lynn College of Nursing
Florida Atlantic University
Boca Raton, Florida
  Theoretical Framework
  Qualitative Approaches to Research

Marianne T. Marcus, EdD, RN, FAAN
John P. McGovern Professor in Addiction Nursing
    Director, Center for Substance Abuse Education,
    Prevention, and Research
School of Nursing
University of Texas Health Science Center
Houston, Texas
  Qualitative Approaches to Research

Elizabeth Norman, PhD, RN, FAAN
Professor
New York University
New York, New York
  Research Vignette

Glenda L. Smith, DSN, RNC, NNP, APRN, BC, PNP
Associate Professor of Nursing
Department of Nursing
Tuskegee University
Tuskegee, Alabama
  Critical Thinking Challenges

Mary Jane Smith, PhD, RN
Professor and Associate Dean for Graduate Academic
    Affairs
School of Nursing
Robert C. Byrd Health Sciences Center
West Virginia University
Morgantown, West Virginia
  Theoretical Framework

Helen J. Streubert Speziale, EdD, RN
Professor
Nursing Department
College Misercordia
Dallas, Pennsylvania
  Evaluating Qualitative Research

Kristen M. Swanson, PhD, RN, FAAN
Professor and Chair
Department of Family and Child Nursing
University of Washington
School of Nursing
Seattle, Washington
  Research Vignette

Marita G. Titler, PhD, RN, FAAN
Director, Research, Quality, and Outcomes
    Management
Department of Nursing Services and Patient Care
University of Iowa Hospitals and Clinics
Iowa City, Iowa
  Developing an Evidence-Based Practice

Robin Whittemore, PhD, APRN
Associate Research Scientist, Lecturer
School of Nursing
Yale University
New Haven, Connecticut
  Experimental and Quasiexperimental Designs
  Data-Collection Methods
  Data Analysis: Descriptive and Inferential

Reviewers

Denise Coté-Arsenault, PhD, RNC, IBCLC
Associate Professor
State University of New York
University at Buffalo
Buffalo, New York

Jean Anne Jacko, PhD, RN
Associate Professor of Nursing
School of Nursing
Capital University
Columbus, Ohio

Lois W. Lowry, RN, DNSc
East Tennessee State University
Johnson City, Tennessee

Pamela Johnson Rowsey, PhD
University of North Carolina
Chapel Hill, North Carolina

Josephine Ryan, DNSc, RN
Professor Emeritus
University of Massachusetts
Amherst, Massachusetts

Anita S. Tesh, MSN, EdD, RNBC
School of Nursing
University of North Carolina
Greensboro, North Carolina

Pat Trethewey, MSN, NP-C, RN
Department of Nursing
St. Mary's College
Notre Dame, Indiana

Ann B. Tritak, RN, BSN, MA, EdD
Fairleigh Dickinson University
Teaneck, New Jersey

Cynthia J. Weiss, APRN, CNS, P-MH, BC
Academic Associate Professor
School of Nursing
Texas Tech University Health Sciences Center;
Chief Nursing Officer
Lubbock Regional Mental Health and Mental
    Retardation Center
Sunrise Canyon Hospital
Lubbock, Texas

To the Instructor

The foundation of the sixth edition of *Nursing Research: Methods and Critical Appraisal for Evidence-Based Practice* continues to be the belief that nursing research is integral to all levels of nursing education and practice. Over the past 20 years since the first edition of this textbook, we have seen the depth and breadth of nursing research grow, with more nurses conducting and using research evidence to shape clinical practice, education, administration, and public policy.

The Institute of Medicine has challenged all health professionals to provide care based on the best available scientific evidence. This is an exciting challenge to meet. Nurses are using the best available research evidence to influence the nature and direction of health care delivery and document outcomes related to the quality and cost-effectiveness of patient care. As nurses continue to develop a unique body of nursing knowledge through research, decisions about clinical nursing practice will be increasingly evidence-based.

As editors, we believe that all nurses need not only to understand the research process but also to know how to critically read, evaluate, and apply research findings in practice. We realize that understanding research, as a component of evidence-based practice, is a challenge for every student, but we believe that the challenge can be accomplished in a stimulating, lively, and learner-friendly manner.

Consistent with this perspective is a commitment to advancing the paradigm shift to evidence-based practice. Nursing research must be an integral dimension of baccalaureate education, evident not only in the undergraduate nursing research course but also threaded throughout the curriculum. The research role of baccalaureate graduates calls for evidence-based practice competencies; central to this are critical appraisal skills—that is, nurses should be competent research consumers.

Preparing students for this role involves developing their critical thinking and reading skills, thus enhancing their understanding of the research process, their appreciation of the role of the critiquer, and their ability to actually appraise research critically. An undergraduate course in nursing research should develop this basic level of competence, which is an essential requirement if students are to engage in evidence-based clinical decision making and practice. This is in contrast to a graduate-level research course in which the emphasis is on carrying out research, as well as understanding and appraising it.

The primary audience for this textbook remains undergraduate students who are learning the steps of the research process, as well as how to develop clinical questions, critique published research literature, and use research findings to inform evidence-based clinical practice. This book is also a valuable resource for students at the master's and doctoral levels who want a concise review of the basic steps of the research and critiquing processes, as well as the basic tools for evidence-based practice. Furthermore, it is an important resource for practicing nurses who strive to use research evidence as the basis for clinical decision making and development of evidence-based policies, protocols, and standards, rather than rely on tradition, authority, or trial and error. It is also an important resource for nurses who collaborate with nurse-scientists in the conduct of clinical research and evidence-based practice.

Building on the success of the fifth edition, the modified title of the sixth edition, *Nursing Research: Methods and Critical Appraisal for Evidence-Based Practice,* reflects our commitment to introduce evidence-based practice and research principles to baccalaureate students, thereby providing a "cutting-edge," research consumer foundation for their clinical practice. *Nursing Research: Methods and Critical Appraisal for Evidence-Based Practice* prepares nursing students and practicing nurses to become knowledgeable nursing research consumers by the following:

- Addressing the role of the nurse as a research consumer, thereby embedding evidence-based competence in the clinical practice of every baccalaureate graduate.
- Demystifying research, which is sometimes viewed as a complex process.
- Using an evidence-based approach to teaching the fundamentals of the research process.
- Teaching the critical appraisal process in a user-friendly, but logical and systematic, progression.
- Promoting a lively spirit of inquiry that develops critical thinking and critical reading skills, facilitating mastery of the critiquing process.
- Developing information literacy and research consumer competencies that prepare students and nurses to effectively locate and evaluate the best available research evidence.
- Elevating the critiquing process and research consumership to a position of importance comparable to that of producing research. Before students become research producers, they must become knowledgeable research consumers.
- Emphasizing the role of evidence-based practice as the basis for clinical decision making and nursing interventions that support nursing practice, demonstrating quality and cost-effective outcomes of nursing care delivery.
- Presenting numerous examples of recently published research studies that illustrate and highlight each research concept in a manner that brings abstract ideas to life for students new to the research and critiquing process. These examples are a critical link for reinforcement of evidence-based concepts and the related research and critiquing process.
- Showcasing, in **Research Vignettes,** the work of renowned nurse researchers whose careers exemplify the links among research, education, and practice.
- Providing numerous pedagogical chapter features, including **Learning Outcomes, Key Terms, Key Points, Critical Thinking Challenges, Helpful Hints,** new **Evidence-Based Practice Tips, Critical Thinking Decision Paths,** and **Critiquing Criteria,** as well as numerous tables, boxes, and figures.
- Offering a **Companion CD-ROM** with interactive Review Questions that provide chapter-by-chapter review in a format consistent with that of the NCLEX® Examination.
- Providing a **Study Guide** that promotes active learning and assimilation of nursing research content.
- Presenting an **Instructor's Electronic Resource** on CD-ROM, as well as web-based interactive **Evolve** resources, including Critiquing Exercises—six articles with multiple-choice questions for additional practice in reviewing and critiquing—as well as WebLinks and Content Updates.

In the sixth edition of *Nursing Research: Methods and Critical Appraisal for Evidence-Based Practice,* the text is organized into four parts that are preceded by an introductory section and open with an exciting "Research Vignette" by a renowned nurse researcher.

- **Part One, Research Overview,** contains five chapters: Chapter 1, "The Role of Research in Nursing," provides an excellent overview of contemporary roles, approaches, and issues in nursing research. It introduces the importance of the nurse's role as a research consumer and provides a futuristic perspective about research and evidence-based practice principles that shape clinical practice. Chapter 2, "The Research

Process: Integrating Evidence-Based Practice," speaks directly to students by highlighting critical thinking and critical reading concepts and strategies that facilitate student understanding of the research process and its relationship to the critiquing process. The chapter introduces a model rating system for the hierarchy of evidence, and this model is used through the text. The style and content of this chapter are designed to make subsequent chapters more user-friendly. The next three chapters address foundational components of the research process. Chapter 3, "Developing Research Questions and Hypotheses," focuses on how research questions and hypotheses are derived, operationalized in research studies, and critically appraised. Numerous clinical examples that illustrate different types of research questions and hypotheses are used to maximize student understanding. Students are also taught how to develop clinical questions that are used to guide evidence-based inquiry. Chapter 4, "Literature Review," showcases cutting-edge information related research consumer competencies that prepare students and nurses to effectively search, retrieve, manage, and evaluate research studies and their findings. Chapter 5, "Theoretical Framework," addresses the importance of theoretical foundations to the design and evaluation of research studies.

- **Part Two, Processes Related to Qualitative Research,** contains three interrelated qualitative research chapters. Chapter 6, "Introduction to Qualitative Research," provides a framework for understanding qualitative research designs and literature and the contribution of qualitative research to evidence-based practice. Chapter 7, "Qualitative Approaches to Research," presents and illustrates major qualitative designs and methods using examples from the literature as exemplars. This chapter is designed to highlight the questions most appropriately answered using qualitative design and methods. Chapter 8, "Evaluating Qualitative Research," synthesizes essential components of and criteria for critiquing qualitative research reports.

- **Part Three, Processes Related to Quantitative Research,** contains Chapters 9 to 18. These chapters delineate the essential steps of the quantitative research process, with published clinical research studies used to illustrate each step. Links between the steps and their relationship to the total research process are examined. These chapters make the case for linking an evidence-based approach to delineating essential steps of the research process. The steps of the research process and evidence-based concepts are synthesized in Chapter 18.

- **Part Four, Application of Research: Evidence-Based Practice,** contains Chapters 19 and 20. Chapter 19, "Developing an Evidence-Based Practice," provides a dynamic conclusion to this text through its vibrant presentation of how to apply the best available evidence in clinical practice using an evidence-based practice framework. Chapter 20, "Tools for Applying Evidence to Practice," provides a user-friendly, evidence-based toolkit with "real-life" exemplars that capture the totality of implementing high-quality evidence-based nursing care.

Critical thinking is stimulated through the presentation of the potential strengths and weaknesses in each step of the research process. Innovative chapter features such as Critical Thinking Decision Paths, new Evidence-Based Practice Tips, Helpful Hints, and Critical Thinking Challenges enhance critical thinking and promote the development of evidence-based decision-making skills. Consistent with previous editions, each chapter includes a section describing the critiquing process related to the focus of the chapter, as well as Critiquing Criteria that are designed to stimulate a systematic and evaluative approach to reading and understanding qualitative and quantitative research literature. Extensive Internet resources are provided on the accompanying Evolve site that can be used to develop evidence-based knowledge and skills.

The Evolve website that accompanies the sixth edition provides interactive learning activities that promote the development of critical thinking, critical reading, and information literacy skills designed to develop the competencies necessary to produce informed consumers of nursing research. Student resources include Critiquing Exercises, which consist of research articles and corresponding multiple-choice questions that review cross-chapter content to challenge students, as well as a comprehensive list of nursing research WebLinks and important Content Updates. Instructor resources include a passcode-protected website that gives faculty access to all instructor materials online, including the Instructor's Resource Manual, Image Collection, Lecture Slides, and a Test Bank that allows faculty to create exams using the Exam-View test generator program.

The development and refinement of an evidence-based foundation for clinical nursing practice is an essential priority for the future of professional nursing practice. The sixth edition of *Nursing Research: Methods and Critical Appraisal for Evidence-Based Practice* will help students develop a basic level of competence in understanding the steps of the research process that will enable them to critically analyze research studies, judge their merit, and judiciously apply evidence in clinical practice. To the extent that this goal is accomplished, the next generation of nursing professionals will have a cadre of clinicians who derive their practice from theory and research evidence specific to the health care of patients and their families in health and illness.

GERI LOBIONDO-WOOD
Geri.L.Wood@uth.tmc.edu

JUDITH HABER
jh33@nyu.edu

To the Student

We invite you to join us on an exciting nursing research adventure that begins as you turn the first page of the sixth edition of *Nursing Research: Methods and Critical Appraisal for Evidence-Based Practice*. The adventure is one of discovery! You will discover that the nursing research literature sparkles with pride, dedication, and excitement about the research dimension of professional nursing practice. Whether you are a student or a practicing nurse whose goal is to use research evidence as the foundation of your practice, you will discover that nursing research and a commitment to evidence-based practice positions our profession at the forefront of change. You will discover that evidence-based practice is integral to meeting the challenge of providing quality biopsychosocial health care in partnership with patients and their families/significant others, as well as with the communities in which they live. Finally, you will discover the richness in the "Who," "What," "Where," "When," "Why," and "How" of nursing research and evidence-based practice, developing a foundation of knowledge and skills that will equip you for clinical practice and making a significant contribution to quality patient outcomes!

We think you will enjoy reading this text. Your nursing research course will be short but filled with new and challenging learning experiences that will develop your research consumer skills. The sixth edition of *Nursing Research: Methods and Critical Appraisal for Evidence-Based Practice* reflects "cutting-edge" trends for developing competent consumers of nursing research. The four-part organization and special features in this text are designed to help you develop your critical thinking, critical reading, information liter-

acy, and evidence-based clinical decision-making skills, while providing a user-friendly approach to learning that expands your competence to deal with these new and challenging experiences. The companion Study Guide, with its chapter-by-chapter activities, will serve as a self-paced learning tool to reinforce the chapter-by-chapter content of the text. A Companion CD-ROM included with the text includes review questions that help you to reinforce the concepts discussed in the chapters. The accompanying Evolve website offers "summative" review material to help you tie the chapter material together and apply it to six current research articles. An extensive list of applicable WebLinks is also available.

Remember that evidence-based consumer skills are used in every clinical setting and can be applied to every patient population or clinical practice issue. Whether your clinical practice involves primary care or specialty care and provides inpatient or outpatient treatment in a hospital, clinic, or home, you will be challenged to apply your research consumer skills and use nursing research as the foundation for your evidence-based practice. The sixth edition of *Nursing Research: Methods and Critical Appraisal for Evidence-Based Practice* will guide you through this exciting adventure, where you will discover your ability to play a vital role in contributing to the building of an evidence-based professional nursing practice.

GERI LOBIONDO-WOOD
Geri.L.Wood@uth.tmc.edu

JUDITH HABER
jh33@nyu.edu

Acknowledgments

No major undertaking is accomplished alone; there are those who contribute directly and those who contribute indirectly to the success of a project. We acknowledge with deep appreciation and our warmest thanks the help and support of the following people:

- Our students, particularly the nursing students at the University of Texas–Houston Health Science Center School of Nursing and the College of Nursing at New York University, whose interest, lively curiosity, and challenging questions sparked ideas for revisions in the sixth edition.
- Our chapter contributors, whose passion for research, expertise, cooperation, commitment and punctuality, made them a joy to have as colleagues.
- Our vignette contributors, whose willingness to share evidence of their research wisdom made a unique and inspirational contribution to this edition.
- Our foreword contributor, Carol Noll Hoskins, our former research professor and a chapter contributor to the first edition of this text, whose insightful introduction to the sixth edition lends special meaning to this text.

- Our colleagues, who have taken time out of their busy professional lives to offer feedback and constructive criticism that helped us prepare this sixth edition.
- Our editors, Lee Henderson, Julie Vitale, Kathy Teal, Rae Robertson, and Laurie Sparks, for their willingness to listen to yet another creative idea about teaching research in a meaningful way and for their timely help with manuscript preparation and production.
- Our families: Brian Wood, who now is pursuing his own college education, and over the years has sat in on classes, provided commentary, and patiently watched and waited as his mother rewrote each edition, as well as provided love, understanding, and support. Lenny, Andrew, and Abbe and Brett Haber and Laurie, Bob, and Mikey, Benjy and Noah Goldberg for their unending love, faith, understanding, and support throughout what is inevitably a consuming—but exciting—experience.

GERI LOBIONDO-WOOD

JUDITH HABER

Contents

PART I

RESEARCH OVERVIEW

Effects of Workplace Environments for Hospital Nurses on Patient Outcomes

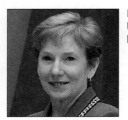

Linda H. Aiken
University of Pennsylvania
Philadelphia, Pennsylvania

My research has been heavily influenced by my clinical practice with heart surgery patients early in my nursing career. I loved the pace and drama of hospitals, the close personal ties with patients and their families, and the miracles of successful surgery. However, I was frustrated by the myriad of organizational impediments to providing excellent nursing care in hospitals. My research has thus been driven by a desire to understand the institutional dynamics that enable or constrain effective clinical care at the bedside, and how these dynamics can be modified to produce both safe and effective care for patients as well as professionally and personally rewarding careers for nurses.

The first step in the development of my program of research was to undertake doctoral education with a strong focus on quantitative methods, while the second step involved the study of sociology because of my interest in complex organizations. My program of research was motivated by my clinical observations of a link between poor workplace environments for nurses and adverse patient outcomes, a link I wanted to explore empirically. I found the research literature of interest to my concerns divided into two separate streams of inquiry: one on factors associated with hospital nurse shortages and one on correlates of hospital outcomes. Some studies suggested an association between hospital organization and patient outcomes, particularly mortality rates. However, the measures of organization in these studies were of macro features of hospitals that, even if associated with outcomes, would be difficult to modify, such as ownership (for example, for-profit, non-profit, public), teaching status, and size. Some of these studies noted in passing an association between variation in nurse to bed ratios and mortality rates, but staffing was treated as a structural characteristic of hospitals primarily of interest as a control variable rather than as a factor of primary interest. There were very few studies of organizational culture, and fewer still that explored how culture influenced processes of care and patient outcomes.

Studying whether and how modifiable features of hospitals are associated with patient outcomes is challenging. The unit of analysis is the organization, thus requiring studies of large numbers of institutions. However, little information is available about organizational and cultural features of nurse practice settings from existing administrative or public use data files, meaning that expensive primary data collection is required. Additionally, the science of measurement of organizational features of clinical care environments has lagged the measurement of attitudes or physiological traits of individuals. Therefore my colleagues and I had to pioneer new methods and measures. We were aided in our search for measures of organizational features of interest by a review of existing measures of nurse job satisfaction that yielded the Nursing Work Index (NWI) developed by Marlene Kramer in her research on magnet hospitals. The items that constituted the NWI had been derived by Kramer from research on professional nurse practice environments. We modified Kramer's NWI using her items not to measure job satisfaction but to determine the presence or absence of organizational features in the nurse practice environment. Building upon research methods in organizational sociology that employed workers as informants of organizational culture, we surveyed nurses, asking them to complete the revised NWI (NWI-R) in relation to their employment setting and provide the name of their employer. Instead of using the NWI as a conventional attitude survey that summarized the perceptions of individual nurses, we aggregated the responses of every nurse working in a particular hospital or hospital unit to a single item on the NWI that yielded an empirical measure of an organizational trait. We used theoretical constructs and factor analysis to create NWI-R subscales measuring different characteristics of the nurse practice environment that previous research had suggested would affect the nursing care process. Examples of these subscales included nurse autonomy, nurse control over resources, nurse-physician relations, and organizational support for nursing practice.

Since it is not feasible to study organizational innovation by randomizing hospitals into treatment and control groups, we looked for natural experiments or targets of opportunity that would enable us to contrast hospitals with different organizational features. An example of a target of opportunity that helped launch our program of research was the identification in 1982 by the American Academy of Nursing of a group of hospitals called magnet hospitals, named for their success in attracting and retaining nurses when other hospitals in their local labor markets experienced shortages. Other investigators had established that these magnet hospitals shared a common set of organizational features that distinguished them from other hospitals. We designed a study to determine whether magnet hospitals also had better patient outcomes. Establishing an appropriate comparison group of hospitals was essential to answering this question. We used a social science analytical technique known as propensity scoring to select 5 hospitals that were most like each magnet hospital, using 12 matching criteria and the full sample of all U.S. acute care hospitals. We showed that magnet hospitals had significantly lower risk-adjusted Medicare mortality than their matched comparisons (Aiken, Smith, and Lake, 1994). This study was the first to show that better nurse practice environments were associated with better patient outcomes, a hallmark of our research program over 15 years. We subsequently studied the natural experiment in hospital innovation motivated by the AIDS epidemic, the targets of opportunity represented by widespread hospital restructuring, and the emergence of the American Nurses Credentialing Magnet Recognition Program to learn more about the effect of nurse practice environments on patient and nurse outcomes.

We began our program of research by recruiting hospitals and then surveying their nurses; this process was expensive and resulted in a potential bias in our samples in favor of innovative hospitals. To overcome these limitations, we perfected a design that employed sampling nurses from licensing organizations at the state level in the United States and at the provincial or national levels in other countries, and aggregated their responses to their employing institution. We could thus study the links between the nurse practice environment and outcomes in large, representative groups of hospitals in a state or country (Aiken, Clarke, Sochalski, and Silber, 2002). This innovation in research design has been central in our latest studies showing that nurse staffing and the nurse practice environment are associated with significant variation in patient mortality, as well as explaining the problems many hospitals experience retaining qualified nurses.

REFERENCES

Aiken LH, Smith HL, and Lake ET: Lower Medicare mortality among a set of hospitals known for good nursing care, *Medical Care* 32(8): 771-787, 1994.

Aiken LH, Clarke SP, Sloane DM, Sochalski J, and Silber JH: Hospital nurse staffing and patient mortality, nurse burnout and job dissatisfaction, *JAMA* 288(16): 1987-1993, 2002.

GERI LOBIONDO-WOOD

JUDITH HABER

The Role of Research in Nursing

KEY TERMS

consumer
critique
evidence-based practice

generalizability
research
theory

LEARNING OUTCOMES

After reading this chapter, the student should be able to do the following:
- State the significance of research to evidence-based nursing practice.
- Identify the role of the consumer of nursing research.
- Discuss the differences in trends in nursing research.
- Describe how research, education, and practice relate to each other.
- Evaluate the nurse's role in the research process as it relates to the nurse's level of educational preparation.
- Identify the future trends in nursing research.
- Formulate the priorities for nursing research in the twenty-first century.

STUDY RESOURCES

Go to your Companion CD for review activities for this chapter.

evolve Go to Evolve at http://evolve.elsevier.com/LoBiondo/ for Weblinks, Content Updates, and additional research articles for practice in reviewing and critiquing.

We invite you to join us on an exciting nursing research adventure that begins as you read the first page of this chapter. The adventure is one of discovery! You will discover that the nursing research literature sparkles with pride, dedication, and excitement about this dimension of professional nursing practice. Whether you are a student or a practicing nurse whose goal is to use **research** as the foundation of your practice, you will discover that nursing research positions our profession at the cutting edge of change. You will also discover that nursing research is integral with meeting the challenge of achieving the goal of providing quality biopsychosocial outcomes in partnership with clients, their families/significant others, and the communities in which they live. Finally, you will discover the cutting edge "Who," "What," "Where," "When," "Why," and "How" of nursing research and developing a foundation of knowledge, evidence-based practice, and competencies that will equip you for twenty-first century clinical practice.

Your nursing research adventure will be filled with new and challenging learning experiences that will develop your research consumer skills. Your critical reading, critical thinking, and clinical decision-making skills will all be expanded as you develop clinical questions, search the research literature, evaluate the research evidence found in the literature, and make decisions about applying the evidence to your practice. For example, you will be encouraged to ask adventurous questions such as the following: What makes this intervention effective with one group of patients with congestive heart failure but not another? What is the effect of computer learning modules on children's self-management of asthma? What research has been conducted in the area of identifying barriers to colon cancer screening in African-American men? What is the quality of the studies done on therapeutic touch? Are the findings from the studies done on pain management ready for use in practice? This chapter will help you begin your nursing research adventure by developing an appreciation of the significance of research in nursing and the research roles of nurses through a historical and futuristic approach.

SIGNIFICANCE OF RESEARCH IN NURSING

Professional nurses are constantly challenged to stay abreast of new information to provide the highest quality of patient care (Barnsteiner and Prevost, 2002; IOM, 2001). Nurses are challenged to expand their "comfort zone" by offering creative approaches to old and new health problems, as well as designing new and innovative programs that truly make a difference in the health status of our citizens. This challenge can best be met by integrating rapidly expanding evidence-based knowledge about biological, behavioral, and environmental influences on health into patient care decisions. Nursing research provides a specialized scientific knowledge base that

empowers the nursing profession to anticipate and meet these constantly shifting challenges and maintain our societal relevance.

You can think of **evidence-based practice** as the collection, interpretation, and integration of valid, important, and applicable patient-reported, clinician-observed, and research-derived evidence. The best available evidence, moderated by patient circumstances and preferences, is applied to improve the quality of clinical judgments and facilitate cost-effective health care (Sackett, Straus, Richardson, Rosenberg, and Haynes, 2000) Knowledge obtained from research evidence is transformed into clinical practice, culminating in nursing practice that is evidence-based. For example, to help you understand the importance of evidence-based practice, think about the study by Koniak-Griffin and colleagues (2003) (see Appendix A), which sought to determine whether there would be any differences in the 2-year postbirth infant health and maternal outcomes for children of adolescent versus adult mothers enrolled in an early intervention program (EIP) of home visitation by public health nurses (PHNs). Samples of Latina and African-American adolescent mothers were followed from pregnancy through 2-years postpartum. They received either preparation for motherhood classes plus intense home visitation by PHNs (EIP) ($n = 56$) or traditional public health nursing care (TPHNC) ($n = 54$). Findings from this randomized clinical trial (RCT) indicate that child health outcomes for the EIP group reflect decreased morbidity as evidenced by a significantly lower number of total days of non–birth-related hospitalization (143 days vs. 211 days) and hospitalization episodes that were sustained over 24 months, including the year following termination of the intervention. Although the rates of adequate infant immunization at 24 months did not differ between the EIP and TPHNC groups, the sample as a whole had an immunization rate that was 81%, higher than that of a comparable state-wide cohort. Maternal outcomes reflect a significant decrease in marijuana use in the EIP group, but an increase in alcohol and tobacco use across both groups, which is consistent with findings from other studies that focus on adolescents as they progress from pregnancy through postpartum. There was a significantly higher rate of achievement of educational outcomes for mothers (e.g., enrolled and attending high school, graduated high school, and attending college) in the EIP group, as well as significantly increased social competence scores that reflect improvements in the ability to manage emotions, communicate, and use social interaction skills more effectively. The EIP mothers also had 15% fewer repeat pregnancies in the following 2 years in comparison to the TPHNC mothers.

These findings provide nurses with outcome data that confirm that EIP programs for adolescent mothers produce clinical outcomes that improve the care for Latina and African-American adolescent mothers and their children as well as decrease the cost of providing care to this patient population through reduction in the number and length of stay of hospitalizations and emergency room visits. Such data support scientifically based clinical decisions about making changes in EIP models rather than adhering to traditional models of public health nursing. Although the data from this research study have definite potential for use in practice, and can contribute to reducing health disparities in minority populations, changes in hospital or public health policy will not and should not occur as a result of one study. Replication of this study is necessary to build an adequate evidence base for implementation in practice, one that has been systematically evaluated over time.

Nurses are required to be accountable for the quality of patient care they deliver. In an era of consumerism during which the quality of health care and high health care costs are being questioned, consumers and employers—the purchasers of health insurance—are asking health professionals to document the effectiveness of their services (Hinshaw, 2000; Melnyk and Fineout-Overholt, 2002; IOM, 2001). Essentially, it is asked, "How do nursing services make a difference?" The message can hardly be more clear;

how consumers and employers perceive the value of nurses' contributions will determine the profession's role in any future delivery system (Cronenwett, 2002; Dykes, 2003; Naylor, 2003; Titler, Cullen, and Ardery, 2002). Public and private sector reimbursement groups, including insurance companies, managed-care organizations, and governmental agencies using capitated and prospective payment systems (e.g., Medicare and Medicaid), are also requiring accountability for services provided. The standards used by the Joint Commission on Accreditation of Healthcare Organizations (JCAHO, 2004) require health care agencies to implement outcomes-management programs that demonstrate the link between quality care and cost-effective patient outcomes.

The need for research skills at all levels of professional nursing is a commonly agreed upon priority (AACN, 1996; AACN, 1998a; ANA, 1997; NONPF, 2002). It is proposed that all nurses share a commitment to the advancement of nursing science by conducting research and using research findings in practice. Scientific investigation promotes accountability, which is one of the hallmarks of the nursing profession and a fundamental concept of the ANA (2002) Code for Nurses. There is a consensus that the research role of the baccalaureate graduate calls for the skills of critical appraisal. That is, the nurse must be a knowledgeable **consumer** of research, one who can **critique** research and use existing standards to determine the merit and readiness of research for use in clinical practice (ANA, 1997; AACN, 1998b). The remainder of this book is devoted to helping you develop that consumer expertise.

RESEARCH: LINKING THEORY, EDUCATION, AND PRACTICE

Research links **theory,** education, and practice. Theoretical formulations supported by research findings is the foundation of theory-based nursing practice. Your educational setting, whether it be a nursing program or health care organization where you are employed, provides an environment in which you, as students, can learn about the research process. In this setting, you can also explore different theories and begin to evaluate them in light of research findings (Larsen et al., 2002).

A classic research study by Naylor and colleagues (1999) addresses the national challenge to: (1) expand the body of nursing science, (2) be socially relevant and interdisciplinary, (3) test the effectiveness of nursing interventions, and (4) provide research experiences for students. Funded by a grant from the National Institute of Nursing Research, the multisite study by Naylor and colleagues (1999) involved 363 patients. Improved patient care and cost savings in terms of reduced admissions, more time between discharge and readmission, and decreased cost of providing health care were the study's outcomes. For example, in this randomized clinical trial (RCT) Medicare reimbursements for health services were about $1.2 million in the control group and $0.6 million in the intervention group with no significant differences between groups on clinical outcome indicators such as functional status, depression, and patient satisfaction. The study further validated earlier studies by Naylor and colleagues that examined the effectiveness of an advanced practice nurse-centered discharge and home follow-up intervention model for elders and others at risk for hospital readmission including very low birth weight babies, women with unplanned cesarean births, high-risk pregnancies, and hysterectomies (Brooten, Naylor, and York, 1995; Naylor et al., 1994; Brooten et al., 2002). The findings related to advanced practice nursing intervention consistently result in improved patient outcomes and reduced health care costs across groups. These findings have had enormous implications not only for nursing practice but also for related health care disciplines, all of which compose the interdisciplinary health care team involved in the care of any and all patient populations. Future research is needed to identify other patient populations who are at high risk during transitions in the health care systems and would particularly benefit from this

type of intervention program (Brooten et al., 2002).

Another study (Plach, Stevens, and Moss, 2004) (Appendix C) examined social role experiences of women living with rheumatoid arthritis (RA). The researchers sought to determine: (1) how women with RA fulfilled their social role expectations as a spouse, mother, worker, and homemaker while contending with RA and (2) what circumstances made these role experiences more positive. Themes descriptive of the experience were characterized by struggling to balance multiple roles while contending with fatigue, pain, and disability imposed by RA.

These themes illustrate how women with a chronic illness experienced the frustration and disappointment associated with role limitations when illness-related symptoms precluded their capacity to meet family expectations and social role norms. Although most women in the study described a tremendous capacity to cope with the symptoms of RA and strive to maintain as much normalcy in their lives as possible, they still experienced guilt and low self-esteem when family expectations exceeded the limitations of their illness. Similar to other research, the findings of this study provide evidence of the deleterious effect a chronic, debilitating illness such as RA can have on the social role activities and psychological health of women. Based on the data from this and other studies, therapeutic nursing actions were suggested that provide family-centered education and counseling to identify evidence-based repatterning strategies that help women with RA, and their families, juggle their illness more effectively with competing family, work, and personal demands.

The preceding examples answer a question that you may have been asking: How will the theory and research content of your course relate to your nursing practice? The data from each study have clearly demonstrated societal and practice implications. The classic study by Naylor et al. (1999) provided data that illustrated an innovative nursing intervention protocol that was cost-effective and maintained high-quality outcomes. In an era of continuing concern about health care costs, evidence supported programs that are cost-effective without compromising quality are essential.

Given the dramatic increase in chronic illness created by advances in technology, a national concern has emerged about the long-term impact that chronic and life-threatening illness has on individuals and families. The study by Plach, Stevens, and Moss (2004) provided important data for understanding the experience of women living with rheumatoid arthritis (see Appendix C). The findings can be used to plan treatment that addresses the specific emotional and physical needs of women with RA; in this way nurses can help engineer the best treatment options so that women with RA can achieve the best physical well-being and still fulfill their various social roles.

At this point in your nursing research adventure, you may be wondering how education in nursing research links theory and practice. The answer is twofold. First, it will provide you with an appreciation and understanding of the research process such that you will become a participant in research activities. Second, it must help you become an intelligent consumer of research. A **consumer** of research uses and applies research in an active manner. It is not necessary to conduct studies to be able to appreciate and use research findings in practice. To be intelligent consumers, nurses must understand the research process and develop the critical evaluation skills needed to judge the merit and relevance of evidence provided by the findings before applying them in practice. This understanding and development will prepare each of you for evidence-based practice, in which there are many research-related activities that rely on your use of excellent research consumer skills.

ROLES OF THE NURSE IN THE RESEARCH PROCESS

There is a research role for every practicing nurse. One of the marks of success in nursing

research is the delineation of research competencies geared for nurses prepared in different types of educational programs (Hinshaw, 2000). In its classic document, *Commission on Nursing Research: Education for Preparation in Nursing Research,* the American Nurses Association (ANA, 1989) identified research competencies related to the specific type of educational program a nurse has completed. Obviously, these competencies will expand over time for nurses committed to lifelong learning.

- Associate degree graduates will demonstrate an awareness of the value or relevance of research in nursing. As registered nurses (RNs), they may help identify problem areas in nursing practice within an established structured format, assist in data-collection activities, and, in conjunction with the professional nurse, appropriately use research findings in practice. This means that as RNs they will participate as team members in evidence-based practice activities, including development and revision or implementation of clinical standards, protocols, and critical paths (see Chapter 20).

- Baccalaureate graduates must be intelligent consumers of research; that is, they must understand each step of the research process and its relationship to every other step. Understanding must be linked with a clear idea about the standards of satisfactory research. This comprehension is necessary when critically reading and understanding research reports, thereby determining the strength and consistency of the evidence in the findings of reported studies. Before considering use of research findings in practice, the nurse discriminates between interesting ideas that require further investigation and findings that have sufficient evidence to support practice. Nurses who are baccalaureate graduates will use these competencies to advance the nursing or interdisciplinary evidence-based practice projects (e.g., developing clinical standards, tracking quality-improvement data, coordinating implementation of a pilot project to test the efficacy of a new wound-care protocol) of workplace committees for which they are members or chairpersons.

- Baccalaureate graduates also have a responsibility to generate clinical questions to identify nursing problems that require investigation and to participate in the implementation of scientific studies. Clinicians often generate research ideas or questions from hunches, gut-level feelings, or observations of patients or nursing care. In the clinical setting, nurse researchers can often lead and direct staff nurses in the systematic investigation of such ideas in an on-site clinical research project. Systematic collection of data about a clinical problem such as this one contributes to evidence-based practice.

- Baccalaureate graduates may also participate in research projects as members of interdisciplinary or intradisciplinary research teams in one or more phases of such a project. For example, a staff nurse may work on a clinical research unit where a particular type of nursing care is part of an established research protocol (e.g., for pain management, prevention of falls, or urinary incontinence). In such a situation, the nurse administers the care according to the format described in the protocol. The nurse may also be involved in collecting and recording data relevant to the administration of and the patient response to the nursing care.

- Baccalaureate graduates must share research findings with colleagues. This may involve developing a presentation for a research or clinical conference on the findings of a study in which you participated, or it may involve sharing with colleagues the findings of a research report that you have critiqued and have found to have merit and potential for application in your practice. In a more formal way, it may involve joining your health care agency's research committee or its quality assurance (QA) or quality improvement (QI) committee, where research study articles,

integrative reviews of the literature, and clinical practice guidelines are evaluated for evidence-based clinical decision making.

- Nurses who have their master's and doctoral degrees must also be sophisticated consumers of research, but they have also been prepared to conduct research as a coinvestigator or a primary investigator.

- At the master's level, nurses are prepared to be active research team members. They can assume the role of clinical expert, collaborating with an experienced researcher in proposal development, data collection, data analysis, and interpretation. Nurses with a master's degree enhance the quality and relevance of nursing research by providing not only clinical expertise about problems but also evidence-based knowledge about the way the clinical services are delivered. They facilitate the investigation of clinical problems by providing a climate that is favorable to conducting research and engaging in evidence-based practice projects. In the capacity of change champions (see Chapter 20), this includes collaborating with others in investigations, promoting the competency of staff nurses as research consumers, and expanding staff nurse involvement in implementing evidence-based practice projects.

- At the master's level, nurses conduct research investigations to monitor the quality of nursing practice in a clinical setting and provide leadership by helping others apply scientific knowledge in nursing practice.

- Doctorally prepared nurses have the most expertise in appraising, designing, and conducting research. They develop theoretical explanations of phenomena relevant to nursing. They develop studies using both qualitative and quantitative methods to discover ways to modify or extend existing knowledge so that it is relevant to nursing.

- Doctorally prepared nurses act as role models and mentors who guide, stimulate, and encourage other nurses who are developing their research skills. They also collaborate and consult with social, educational, and health care institutions or governmental agencies in research endeavors.

- Doctorally prepared nurses disseminate their research findings to the scientific community, clinicians, and—as appropriate—the lay public. Scientific journals, professional conferences, and the news media are among the mechanisms for dissemination (Fitzpatrick, 2000).
- Regardless of educational preparation, all nurses promote ethical principles of research, especially the protection of human subjects. For example, a nurse caring for a patient who is beginning an anti-nausea chemotherapy research protocol would make sure that the patient had signed the informed consent and had all of his or her questions answered by the research team before beginning the protocol. A nurse who saw the patient having an adverse reaction to the medication protocol would know that his or her responsibility would be not to administer another dose before notifying an appropriate member of the research team (see Chapter 13).

The most important implication delineating research activities according to educational preparation is for maintaining a collaborative research relationship within nursing. Not all nurses must or should conduct research, but all nurses must play some part in the research process. Nurses at all educational levels—whether they are consumers or producers of research, or both—need to view the research process as integral to nursing.

HISTORICAL PERSPECTIVE

The history of nursing research comprises many changes and developments. The groundwork for what has blossomed was laid late in the nineteenth century and throughout the twentieth century and continues today. Capturing the essence of the development of nursing research and the works of so many excellent researchers, especially in the 1980s and 1990s, is beyond the scope of this chapter. A review of the many nursing journals available provides further support of the efforts of nursing researchers. Box 1-1 highlights key events that have set the stage for the richness of the current nursing research efforts.

Nineteenth Century—After 1850

In the mid-nineteenth century, nursing as a formal discipline began to take root with the ideas and practices of Florence Nightingale. Her concepts have contributed to and are congruent with the present priorities of nursing research. Promotion of health, prevention of disease, and care of the sick were central ideas of her system. Nightingale believed that the systematic collection and exploration of data were necessary for nursing. Her collection and analysis of data on the health status of British soldiers during the Crimean War led to a variety of health care reforms. Nightingale also noted the need for measuring outcomes of nursing and medical care (Nightingale, 1863), and she had expertise in statistics and epidemiology. Nightingale stated, "Statistics are history in repose, history is statistics in motion" (Keith, 1988).

Twentieth Century—Before 1950

A review of Box 1-1 reflects nursing research in the first half of the twentieth century. Research focused mainly on nursing education, but some patient- and technique-oriented research was evident. The early efforts in nursing education research were made by such leaders as Lavinia Dock (1900), Anne Goodrich (1932), Adelaide Nutting (1912, 1926), Isabel Hampton Robb (1906), Lillian Wald (1915), and Nutting and Dock (1907). These pioneering works consist of documentation gathered for the purpose of reforming nursing education and establishing nursing as a profession.

Clinically oriented research in the early half of the century mainly centered on the morbidity and mortality rates associated with problems such as pneumonia and contaminated milk (Carnegie, 1976). A few of these projects were

BOX 1-1 HISTORICAL PERSPECTIVE

NINETEENTH CENTURY—AFTER 1850

1859
Nightingale's *Notes on Nursing* is published.
1860
Nightingale founds St. Thomas's Hospital School of Nursing in England.
1872
First nursing schools in United States are opened: New England Hospital for Women and Children (Boston) and Women's Hospital (Philadelphia).
1899
International Council of Nurses is organized.

TWENTIETH CENTURY—Before 1950

1900
American Journal of Nursing begins publication.
1909
Nursing programs begin at Columbia University Teacher's College and University of Minnesota.
1912
American Nurses Association is established.
1913
Committee on Public Health Nursing studies infant mortality, blindness, and midwifery and calls for nursing to distinguish its role in disease prevention and health promotion.
1923
Goldmark Report is published (Committee on Nursing and Nursing Education in the United States, 1923).
1924
First nursing doctoral program in education is started at Teacher's College, Columbia University.
1934
Nursing doctoral program is established at New York University.
1948
Nurses for the Future (The Brown Report) is published.

TWENTIETH CENTURY—AFTER 1950

1950
American Nurses Association establishes a Master Plan for Research.
1952
National League for Nursing is established.
Journal of Nursing Research begins publication.
1953
Nursing Outlook begins publication.
Institute of Research and Service in Nursing Education is established at Teacher's College, Columbia University.

1954
ANA Committee on Research and Studies is formed, focusing on patient care improvement and nursing research funds.
1955
American Nurses Foundation is formed as a center for research.
1956
United States Public Health Service begins awarding nursing research grants.
Predoctoral fellowships for nursing research are first awarded.
1957
Western Council on Higher Education in Nursing (WCHEN) sponsors Western Interstate Commission for Higher Education (WICHE) to augment graduate nursing education, especially in nursing research.
1959
National League for Nursing (NLN) Research and Studies Service is established.
1962
American Nurses Association's Blueprint for Nursing Research is issued.
Nurse Scientist Graduate Training Grants Program is initiated.
1963
International Journal of Nursing Studies begins publication.
1966
First Nursing Research Conference of the ANA is held.
1970
Abstract for Action—Lysaught Report is published.
1971
American Nurses Association Council of Nurse Researchers is organized.
1974
ANA Commission on Nursing Research proposes student involvement from various levels in research and a clinical trust for research.
1975
ANA representatives testify at President Gerald Ford's Panel on Biomedical Research.
1976
ANA publishes its report of nursing research trends, *Research in Nursing: Toward a Science of Health Care.*
1978
Research in Nursing and Health begins publication.
Advances in Nursing Science begins publication.

BOX 1-1   HISTORICAL PERSPECTIVE—cont'd

1979
Western Journal of Nursing Research begins
publication.
1980
ANA's Commission on Nursing Research sets
research priorities.
1986
National Center for Nursing Research is
established at the National Institutes of Health.
1987
Scholarly Inquiry for Nursing Practice and *Applied
Nursing Research* begin publication.
1988
Nursing Science Quarterly and *Nursing Scan in
Research* begin publication.
Conference on Research Priorities in Nursing
Science (CORP No. 1) sets research priorities
known as the National Nursing Research
Agenda.

1991
Qualitative Health Research begins publication.
1992
Conference on Research Priorities in Nursing
Science (CORP No. 2) meets to update
research priorities.
1993
National Center for Nursing Research releases
report of a proposed multiyear funding
mechanism to increase the integration of
biological and nursing sciences.
National Center for Nursing Research becomes
the National Institute of Nursing Research
(NINR).
Sigma Theta Tau International publishes *Online
Journal of Knowledge Synthesis.*
1996
ANA establishes the Nursing Information and Data
Set Evaluation Center (NIDSEC).

---

instrumental in the development of patient-care protocols and the employment of nurses in community settings. An experimental project by Wald and Dock conducted in 1902 led to the employment of school nurses in the New York City school system and subsequently in other cities.

The 1920s saw the development and teaching of the earliest nursing research course because of the influence of Isabel M. Stewart (Henderson, 1977). The course introduced students to the scientific method of investigation. Students were encouraged to question all aspects of nursing care and perform experiments; one topic nurses explored was measurement of the oxygen content in an oxygen tent during a patient's bed bath to determine whether the gas dropped below a therapeutic level.

Social change and World War II affected all aspects of nursing, including research. There was an urgent need for more nurses; increased hospital admissions and military needs created a shortage of personnel. After the war, nursing, like the rest of the world, began to reassess itself and its goals. Brown's report in 1948 reemphasized the inconsistencies in educational preparation

and the need to move into the university setting, and included an updated description of nursing practices. An outgrowth of Brown's report were a number of studies on nursing roles, needs, and resources.

Twentieth Century—After 1950

Nursing research blossomed in the 1950s and laid the groundwork for nursing's current level of research skill. Nursing schools at the undergraduate and graduate levels grew in number, and graduate programs were including research courses. The worth and benefit of research were appreciated by nursing leadership and began to filter to all nursing levels.

Thus in the 1960s, research priorities began to be reordered and practice-oriented research was targeted. These priorities were supported by nursing's major organizations. During the 1960s, nurses were attaining educational preparation in research design in order to teach research and conduct their own research courses. Therefore during this time, nurses primarily worked with others from related disciplines (e.g., psychology, education, and sociology) that had the expertise to teach these courses.

During the 1960s, studies on nurses and nursing continued while pioneers in the development of nursing theories and models (e.g., Orlando [1961], Peplau [1952], and Wiedenbach [1964]) called for the development of nursing practice based on theory. The early development of those theories spurred nurses into a more critical level of thinking about nursing practice.

Collaborative efforts in the 1960s on practice-oriented research led to research by Diers and Leonard (1966) and Dumas and Leonard (1963). These studies explored the effects of patient teaching and communication on events such as hospitalization, surgery, and labor. Another classic study, the culmination of 8 years of work by Glaser and Strauss (1965), explored various aspects of thanatology among dying patients and their caretakers.

A review of the nursing research published during the 1960s reveals that clinical studies were beginning to predominate. These studies investigated nursing care issues, such as infection control, alcoholism, and sensory deprivation. Hall (1963) published the results of a 5-year study that looked at alternatives to hospitalization for a select group of elderly clients. This study led to a care facility run entirely by nurses, the Loeb Center in New York City. The rich history of nursing was also recognized during the 1960s when the nursing archives at Boston University's Mugar Library were established.

In 1970 the National Committee for the Study of Nursing and Nursing Education Report, or the Lysaught Report, was published. This report offered conclusions that more practice- and education-oriented research was necessary and that these data must be applied to the improvement of educational organizations and curricula. The call for clinically oriented study was becoming a reality.

The 1970s also saw new growth in the number of master's and doctoral programs for nursing. These programs, along with the ANA, NLN, Sigma Theta Tau, and Western Interstate Council for Higher Education in Nursing, supported nurses not only learning the research process but also producing research that could be used

to enhance care quality. Box 1-1 lists the first year of publication for new journals that promoted the generation of nursing theory and research.

The 1980s were exciting and productive for research in nursing. This period saw extended growth among upper-level programs in nursing, especially at the doctoral level. By 1989, more than 5000 of the doctorally prepared nurses held their doctorate in nursing. Many centers for nursing research developed in educational settings and hospitals. A number of these centers have programs joining education and practice that provide support and guidance for research efforts. Mechanisms for communicating research also increased. Journals and reviews now provide additional forums for communicating research. Most nursing organizations also have research sections that serve to foster the conduct and use of research.

Public Law 99-158, enacted in 1985, allowed for the development of the National Center for Nursing Research (NCNR). Established in 1986, the NCNR provided funding programs focused on studies related to health care outcomes. The efforts of the 1980s were aimed at refining and developing research and the utilization of research findings in clinical practice. The strides in research made in the 1980s suggested that nursing was ready to rise to the societal and professional demands that now confront the discipline.

During the 1990s, nursing research stood on its own through the work of many forward-thinking educators, scholars, and researchers. At the federal level, nursing leaders moved to influence policy and monies for nursing research. In 1993, the National Institutes of Health (NIH) reauthorization bill gave the NCNR institute status. The NCNR then became known as the National Institute of Nursing Research (NINR). At the university level, nursing leaders developed mechanisms for faculty to develop and implement research. Centers of excellence developed in several academic settings, and leaders mentored newer nurse scientists. During the nineties, nurses and nursing students at all levels learned about research, and debates about how and what type of research was appropriate ensued. Donaldson presented an important paper in 1998 entitled "Breakthroughs in Nursing Research" (Donaldson, 1998). In this paper, Donaldson identified "pathfinders" in nursing research who developed research programs in which they, their colleagues, and students worked.

Throughout the nineties and to the present, the original pathfinders and many new pathfinders have conducted research on a wide range of clinical topics, describing phenomena and testing interventions. A review of the many nursing journals shows the growth in the number, quality, and depth of research available for potential use in practice. Tracing nursing's research roots and the conduct of science to improve the health and well-being of individuals, families, and communities shows that nursing has made significant contributions to health care. Nurses are far from finished with their quest to generate and test knowledge, but the nursing leaders of the twentieth century have—by example—paved the way for the next millennium.

FUTURE DIRECTIONS

In the twenty-first century, the continuing explosion of nursing knowledge provides numerous opportunities for nurses to study important research questions and issues in promoting health and ameliorating the side effects of illness and the consequences of treatment, while optimizing the health outcomes of people and their families (Jennings and McClure, 2004). The growing number of nursing doctoral programs both in the United States (now totaling 88) and outside of the United States (now totaling 150), as well as the additional programs that are under development, contribute to preparing a record number of nurse researchers worldwide who are challenged to bring research-based knowledge to life by applying diverse research methods that address the compelling needs of people around the world (Berlin, 2004; http://www.umich.edu/~inden/).

Major shifts in the delivery of health care include the following:
- Emphasis on community-based care
- Emphasis on reducing health disparities
- Focus on health promotion and risk reduction
- Increased severity of illness in inpatient settings
- Increased incidence of chronic illness
- Expanding number of elderly people
- Emphasis on provider accountability through focus on quality and cost outcomes
- Use of technology to serve human needs

Consistent with these trends, nurse researchers are focusing on development of programs of quantitative and qualitative research and clinically based outcome studies, which provide the foundation for evidence-based practice demonstrating how nursing makes a difference in quality and outcomes. Strategies that enhance nurses' focus on outcomes management through evidence-based quality-improvement activities and use of research findings for effective clinical decision making also are being refined and identified as priorities (see Chapter 20). Evidence-based practice guidelines, standards, protocols, and critical pathways will become benchmarks for cost-effective quality clinical practice (O'Neill and Dluhy, 2000; Titler, Cullen, and Ardery, 2002). Box 1-2 highlights NINR research themes for the future (NINR, 2004). Nursing has truly risen to the challenges

BOX 1-2 NINR RESEARCH THEMES FOR THE FUTURE

1. Changing lifestyle behaviors for better health
2. Managing the effects of chronic illness to improve health and quality of life
3. Identifying effective strategies to reduce health disparities
4. Harnessing advanced technologies to serve human needs
5. Enhancing end-of-life experiences for patients and their families

From the NINR: *National Institute of Nursing Research, Mission statement and strategic plan,* Washington, DC, 2004, The Institute.

of developing nursing science with the ultimate goal of improving health care.

Promoting Depth in Nursing Research

Evidence-based practice reflects the characteristics of the research from which it is derived. The quality of research that nursing scientists generate and the information that is provided to guide practice will be the major keys to testing nursing interventions, producing predictable patient outcomes, and improving patient care for our discipline (Melnyk and Fineout-Overholt, 2005). An increasing number of nurses who have expertise in appraising, designing, and conducting research will continue to emerge and provide a "critical mass" of investigators who will be at the forefront of the ongoing development and refinement of our scientific knowledge base for nursing practice.

To maximize use of resources and prevent duplication, researchers must develop intradisciplinary and interdisciplinary networks in similar areas of study across disciplines (O'Neill and Dluhy, 2000; Larson, 2003). Clinical consortia will help delineate common and unique aspects of patient care. Cluster studies, multiple-site investigations, and programs of research will facilitate the accumulation of evidence supporting or negating a theory, thereby contributing to defining nursing practice. The increasing importance of health service research will promote scientific inquiry that will produce knowledge of health care delivery, knowledge that can be used to address issues that cross disciplinary boundaries such as resource utilization and policy making (Aiken, et al, 2003; Beuerhaus, Staiger, and Auerbach 2000).

Depth in nursing science will be evident when replicated. Programs of research that include a series of studies in a similar area of study, each of which builds on prior investigation, both replicating and adding to the questions being studied, will promote depth in nursing science (Whittemore and Grey, 2002). An example of a program of research is provided by the work of Mishel and Clayton (2003), whose research program has blended research, theory, and instrument development. The early studies by Mishel focused on developing and testing "The Uncertainty in Illness Scale," developed from interviews with hospitalized patients. This tool measured several dimensions of uncertainty over the course of an illness; Mishel used it to conduct a series of studies with patients having cancer, lupus, rheumatoid arthritis, or multiple sclerosis, and also with caregivers of Alzheimer's patients. The findings of these studies were used to further refine the conceptualization of uncertainty. As other researchers used the Uncertainty Scales (it has been translated into eight languages and is used throughout the world), it became clear that uncertainty was a negative experience related to anxiety, depression, and reduced optimism. The effects of uncertainty on emotional status were found in many studies with different populations; the findings of all of these studies supported the uncertainty theory. It also became apparent that uncertainty functioned differently in acute versus chronic illness. For example, in chronic illness, where the course of the illness fluctuates over time, uncertainty is a constant companion that can lead to a change in one's orientation to the world and a change in values—it becomes a major life theme. To help people cope with the uncertainty of acute illness, Mishel developed the Uncertainty Management Intervention based on the original theory of uncertainty in illness. The nursing intervention consists of eight to ten weekly telephone interviews that follow a defined protocol that taps into the concerns of the specific target population and determines the nature of the uncertainty and the degree of threat perceived by the patient. Based on the assessment, the intervention is structured to provide information, resources, or management and communication skills. Although the outcomes differ in some ways across patient populations, the Uncertainty Management Intervention helps cancer patients problem-solve, reevaluate their situation as manageable, gain cancer knowledge, improve patient-provider communication, and improve management of treatment side effects. Consistent and replicated findings across studies and sites yield a body of practice-relevant, in-depth knowledge about the effects of nursing interventions on clinical patient outcomes.

The preceding example illustrates the value of replication studies that are built into programs of research that are the hallmark of research careers. Stone, Curran, and Bakken (2002) proposed that the adoption of research findings in practice, with their potential risks and benefits (including the cost of implementation), should be based on a series of replicated studies that provide a body of evidence, thereby increasing how the findings can be generalized. A greater focus on **generalizability** is important if the evolving science is to be considered reliable and usable in developing nursing practice and influencing health policy. As such, in the future replication studies will be more credible and play a crucial role in developing depth in nursing science; the findings of such studies can then be applied in clinical practice through evidence-based practice projects (Fahs, Stewart, and Kalman, 2003).

This example also highlights why research training will increasingly become an essential component of a research career plan whose objective is development of a program of research. A larger cadre of nurse researchers who begin their research career at a young age is important to the development of programs of research like Mishel's. The goal is to increase the longevity of research careers, enhance the discipline's science development, promote mentoring opportunities, prepare the next generation of researchers, and provide leadership in health care for interdisciplinary health care debates.

Nurse researchers will be committed to developing research programs that are supported by public and private sources. They will also subscribe to a lifestyle of periodic education and retraining funded by awards, grants, and fellowships. For example, NINR awards fund predoctoral, postdoctoral, midcareer, and senior scientist programs of study. These programs facilitate growth in the depth and breadth of research expertise and recognize that some researchers need to be retrained as they develop or shift the emphasis of their research, seek to broaden their scientific background, and acquire new research capabilities.

Nursing research is increasingly addressing the biological and behavioral aspects of nursing science, reflecting the discipline's holistic approach to health and illness for individuals and their families. Investigations that reflect state-of-the-art science examine the interface of the biological sciences with the evolving knowledge base of nursing. Nurse researchers will continue to have increased methodological expertise. They are becoming increasingly sophisticated in developing and applying computer technology to the research process (Im and Chee, 2003).

Measurement issues (e.g., development of instruments that accurately measure clinical phenomena) will still be emphasized. The increasing focus on the need to use multiple measures to assess clinical phenomena accurately is also apparent. The development of noninvasive methods to measure physiological parameters of interest in high-technology settings is related to this focus. These methods may be another aspect of using multiple measures to assess particular clinical phenomena. The development of qualitative measures and new qualitative computer analysis packages is also expanding as the qualitative mode of inquiry is now commonly used in research.

Nurse researchers will employ new, more diverse and advanced methods to design research studies and analyze and apply findings. For example, qualitative research methods are now a respected mode of scientific inquiry, contributing to theory development and providing essential descriptive data to direct clinical practice and future research studies. Consider how the findings from both qualitative and quantitative studies conducted by Swanson-Kauffman (1983, 1986a,b; Swanson, 1991) on the experience of miscarriage have lead to the testing of interventions for women who have experienced miscarriage. In her dissertation, Swanson-Kauffman

(1983) studied the experience of miscarriage; from this work and further qualitative study, she developed the middle range theory of caring (Swanson-Kauffman, 1986a,b; Swanson, 1991). She used this theory and her other previous research (Swanson-Kauffman, 1986a,b; Swanson, 1993) to develop an instrument to test the impact of miscarriage on women (Swanson, 1999a). She used this research base to test the effect of caring-based counseling interventions over time on miscarriage impact, self-esteem, and disturbed moods (Swanson, 1999a,b) and then later to test the effect of this intervention on couples' relationships (Swanson et al., 2003). Swanson's work provides a view of the development of a program of research that carefully assesses an area of nursing phenomena and patient care that was not tested in one study but in many studies over time. See Kristen Swanson Vignette on p. 130.

Nurses prepared to direct the conduct of research will head an expanding number of nursing research departments in clinical settings. The nurse researchers who head these centers will involve the nursing staff in identifying nursing-sensitive outcome indicators to use in generating and conducting evidence-based practice projects that critically evaluate existing research data before using it as evidence to guide decisions about changes in clinical practice (Thompson, Cullum, McCaughan, Sheldon, and Raynor, 2004). A commitment to investigating common clinical outcome indicators that link nursing practice strategies with nursing-sensitive outcomes common to acute care or community-based clinical settings nationwide should be promoted. Such a commitment will facilitate the merging of large data sets, the objective of which is to demonstrate how nursing intervention makes a difference (ANA, 1996, 1997; Titler, Cullen, and Ardery, 2002; Ryan, Stone, and Raynor, 2004; Rantz and Connolly, 2004). Many academic centers for nursing research will partner with clinical research department counterparts to develop and implement exciting research-related initiatives that support evidence-based practice.

An International Perspective

The continuing development of a national and international research environment is essential to the nursing profession's mission to establish a global research community (Chang, 2000; Hegyvary, 2004). The opportunities for cross-cultural and cross-national studies of problems of common interest to clinical and health care systems are consistent with this priority (Hinshaw, 2000; Hegyvary, 2004). Challenges associated with developing a global research community include establishing international networks, websites, and databases; understanding different cultural perspectives and adapting the research accordingly; and obtaining funding for international projects (Hinshaw, 2000; Messias, 2001; Evers, 2003).

With the discipline's emphasis on cultural aspects of care and the influence of such factors on practice, increasing international research is a natural futuristic trend. Access to multiple populations as a function of globalization allows the testing of nursing science from various perspectives. Interaction with colleagues from other countries provides a rich context for the generation and dissemination of research (IOM, 2001; Ward, 2003; Dickenson-Hazard, 2004). Evidence supporting the global development of nursing research is provided by the number of measurement tools developed by researchers in the United States that are being translated and validated in the language of the nurse researcher conducting studies in their country of origin (Nahcivan, 2004).

Alliances with international organizations committed to the goal of health for all create natural research partnerships. For example, the World Health Organization (WHO), through the Pan-American Health Organization, has designated that 12 WHO Collaborating Centers for Research and Clinical Training in Nursing be located in American schools and colleges of nursing, a total of 32 worldwide. These centers provide research and clinical training in nursing to colleagues around the globe. The International Council of Nurses (ICN) and conferences sponsored by ANA and other specialty organizations are examples of international nursing-research forums designed to inform nurses of the global breadth of health problems. Such forums will continue to increase, challenging nurse researchers in various regions of the world to form collaborative research relationships in which they share research expertise, educational opportunities, and the ability to conduct research projects of mutual interest, as well as, perhaps, ultimately create an international research agenda (Evers, 2003; Hinshaw, 2000).

Research Priorities

In 2000, the U.S. Department of Health and Human Services published the revised summary report entitled *Healthy People 2010.* The original document *Healthy People 2000,* published in 1992, was a product of 22 expert working groups and nearly 300 national organizations—including nursing—and contained 22 priority areas geared to improving the nation's health. The current document reaffirms these priority areas. The National Research Agenda identifies priorities that are consistent with the goals of this national health agenda. By the year 2010, a cost-effective, community-based health care delivery system that emphasizes primary care and promotes prevention through risk reduction in partnership with members of a culturally diverse society will actualize a high-quality health care vision. One of the objectives, for example, is to "increase the proportion of persons with long-term care needs who have access to the continuum of long-term care services" (U.S. Department of Health and Human Services, 2001). Several nurse researchers, such as Bull, Hansen, and Gross (2000); Naylor and associates (1999, 2003); Phillips and Ayres (1999); and Roberts (1999), have been conducting research, developing theoretical perspectives, and conducting synthesis conferences in the area of maintaining the independence of elders, managing cognitive impairment and depression in the elderly, and providing supportive care environments for the elderly. Widespread use of models

(e.g., the transitional care model for the elderly developed by Naylor and associates [1999, 2003]) could save significant health care dollars and influence policy to improve the quality of care for the elderly.

Reducing health disparities in poor communities and vulnerable populations will be integral to shaping the focus of nursing and other interdisciplinary research agendas. In the United States, evidence exists that minority populations have higher rates of birth defects, infant mortality, cancer, asthma, cardiovascular disease, and diabetes, contributing to increased disability and shorter life expectancy. Reducing these disparities is one of the two umbrella goals of the *Healthy People 2010* initiative (DHHS, 2001). To direct more research toward reducing health disparities, NINR is collaborating with the National Center on Minority Health and Health Disparities (NCMHD) to create eight research center partnerships between schools of nursing with established research programs in health disparities and minority-serving schools of nursing. These partnerships are aimed at expanding the cadre of nurse researchers involved in minority health or health disparities' research, facilitating nurse-scientist collaboration, increasing research projects on health disparities, eliminating health disparities, and enhancing the career development of minority nurse researchers. This perspective will include health promotion and risk reduction research that is population-focused and community-based (e.g., health promotion programs that promote positive health and lifestyle changes for cardiovascular risk reduction and reduction of obesity and diabetes in children, as well as linking interventions and outcomes in smoking cessation and violence reduction programs) (Hinshaw, 2000; Phillips and Grady, 2002; Grady, 2003).

By the year 2010, the population will include a higher proportion of children and elderly who are chronically ill or disabled (Dochterman, et al, 2005). The health problems of mothers and infants will continue to spur concern for dealing effectively with the maternal-infant mortality rate. Individuals of all ages who have sustained life-threatening illnesses will live by means of new life-sustaining technology that will create new demands for self-care, as well as family support that facilitates effective patient management of their conditions. Cancer, heart disease, arthritis, asthma, chronic pulmonary disease, diabetes, and Alzheimer's disease are prevalent during middle age and later life and will command large proportions of the available health care resources. The impact of HIV/AIDS as a chronic illness for men, women, and children will continue to have a significant influence on the health care delivery system. As a wave of national initiatives are launched to improve end-of-life care, the shortage of nurses—as clinicians and investigators—will become a major problem worldwide (WHO, 2001). There will be an increased understanding of mental disorders as a result of psychobiological knowledge advancements and research initiatives. Mental health problems will continue to be a major public health issue. Depression has been cited as the number one health problem worldwide (WHO, 2001). Alcohol and drug abuse will continue to be responsible for significant health care expense. Investigations that address quality of care outcomes related to nursing interventions are a top psychiatric nursing priority for the twenty-first century (President's New Freedom Commission on Mental Health, 2003) as well as nursing contributions to end-of-life research (Matzo and Sherman, 2001).

One of the most exciting research opportunities for nurses focuses on the area of genetics and the human genome, where study prospects range from basic biological to clinical decision-making and behavioral interventions (Williams, Tripp-Reimer, Schutte, and Barnette, 2004; Grady and Collins, 2003) proposed that nurse researchers can make significant contributions to the following:

- Understanding the gene-environment-behavior interface
- Developing and using biological, psychosocial, and neuroimmunological markers
- Participating in biological-psychosocial intervention
- Providing counseling related to genetic health
- Developing and testing cognitive models for decision making regarding genetic factors and genetic therapies
- Investigating new delivery models for health care given the evolving genetic knowledge base
- Addressing related ethical issues and dilemmas

Hinshaw (2000) suggests that nurses will need to play a major role in the area of genetics so that the evolving knowledge base is structured within a "holistic" understanding of the person. Over the next 10 years, many hard questions of cost containment and access to care will be addressed through an interdisciplinary approach and will need to address the related ethical dilemmas. An important emphasis of research studies will be related to clinical and systems' issues and problems and their links to the improvement of patient outcomes (Stone, Curran, and Bakken, 2002; Kohn et al., 1999; IOM, 2001). The preeminent goal of scientific inquiry by nurses will be the ongoing development of knowledge for use in the practice of nursing. This refers to an action agenda that establishes how the quality of patient care is connected to nursing practice and how the interventions of nurses are related to patient satisfaction and important clinical outcomes. For example, the development of evidence-based approaches to reduce medication errors provides a leadership opportunity for nurses to influence solutions for a nationwide interdisciplinary system problem identified by the Institute of Medicine (2001). It also refers to patient care initiatives related to the organization and delivery of nursing care. This type of research, sometimes referred to as health-services research, would include studies that predict the future supply and demand for nursing care (Aiken, et al, 2003; Rogers et al., 2004). Consequently, priority will be given to nursing research that generates knowledge to guide practice in the areas listed in Box 1-2. See Research Vignette by Dr. Linda Aiken on p. 2.

In light of the priority given to clinical research issues, the funding of investigations increasingly emphasizes clinical research projects in relation to populations of interest. For example, the historical exclusion of women from clinical research is well-documented. Men have been the subjects in the major contemporary research studies related to adult health. Minority women have been even more likely to be excluded from research studies; as a result, research data on minority women are extremely scarce. Funding for research related to women's health issues and problems (e.g., infertility, menopause, breast and ovarian cancer, and osteoporosis) has been less than equitable. Given the indisputable nature of this research bias, the Office of Research on Women's Health at the NIH continues to address these historical inequities in research design and allocation of federal resources (Crane, Lefvak, Lewallen, Hu, and Jones, 2004).

Based on a review of literature that focused on the research priorities identified by nine nursing specialties, Hinshaw (2000) identified the top five American nursing research priorities as the following:

1. Quality of care outcomes and their measurement
2. Impact/effectiveness of nursing interventions
3. Symptom assessment and management
4. Health care delivery systems
5. Health promotion/risk reduction

Areas of special research interest delineated by the NINR for 2000 to 2010 (NINR Website, 2004) include the following:

- **Chronic illness experiences**—managing symptoms, avoiding complications of disease and disability, supporting family caregivers, promoting adherence and self-management activities, and promoting healthy behaviors within the context of the chronic condition
- **Cultural and ethnic considerations**—culturally sensitive interventions to decrease health disparities among groups by focusing on health-promotion activities and strategies for managing chronic illness

- **End-of-life/palliative care research**—clinical management of physical and psychological symptoms, communication, ethics and clinical decision making, caregiver support, and care-delivery issues
- **Health promotion and disease prevention research**—initiatives focusing on lifestyle changes and healthy behavior maintenance across the lifespan
- **Implications of genetic advances**—reducing factors that increase risk of disease, issues related to genetic screening, and subsequent gene-therapy techniques
- **Quality of life and quality of care**—initiatives focusing on cost savings for the patient, health care system, and society
- **Symptom management**—of illness and treatment (e.g., pain, cognitive impairment, fatigue, nausea and vomiting, and sleep problems)
- **Telehealth interventions and monitoring**—focus on emerging technologies to promote patient education and treatment

Other types of research investigations (e.g., those using historical, feminist, or case study methods) embody the rich diversity of nursing research methods. The nursing profession must continue to value and promote creativity and diversity in research endeavors at all educational levels as a way of empowering nursing practice for the future. As opportunities are recognized and gaps in science are observed, nurses will engage in the conduct, critique, and utilization of nursing research in ways that publicly demonstrate how nursing care makes a difference.

Nurse researchers will have an increasingly strong voice in shaping public policy. Shaver (2004) states that disciplines such as nursing—because it focuses on treatment of chronic illness, health promotion, independence in health, and care of the acutely ill, all of which are heavily emphasized values for the future—are going to be central to shaping health care policy. Research data providing evidence that supports or refutes the merit of health care needs and programs focusing on these issues will be timely and relevant. Thus nursing and its science base will be strategically placed to shape health policy decisions (Fitzpatrick, 2004).

Because we will continue to live in the "information age," dissemination of nursing research becomes increasingly important. Research findings will continue to be disseminated in professional arenas (e.g., international, national, regional, and local electronic and print publications and conferences), as well as in consultations and staff development programs that are implemented on-site, through Web-based programs or via satellite. Dissemination of research findings in the public sector, however, is an exciting future trend that has already begun. Nurse researchers are increasingly asked to present testimony at governmental hearings and serve on commissions and task forces related to health care. Nurses are increasingly quoted in the media when health care topics are addressed, and their visibility expands significantly. Today nurses and nurse researchers are participating in teleconferences, developing their own home pages for the internet, starring in videos, and appearing in interviews on television and radio and in printed and electronic media (e.g., the internet, newspapers, and magazines). Nurses have their own radio shows and are beginning to have their own television shows. Dissemination of research through the public media provides excellent exposure to thousands of potential viewers, listeners, and readers. Practicing nurses are using technological innovations (e.g., computerized documentation systems and electronic access to databases and literature searches, interactive telecommunication educational offerings, online journals, and research-based practice guidelines) to make the information revolution come of age in research-related clinical practice activities (Carty, 2001; Jenkins and Dunn, 2004). Nursing has a research heritage to be proud of and a challenging and exciting future direction. Both consumers and producers of research will engage in a united effort to provide acknowledgment to research findings that make a difference in the care that is provided and the lives that are touched by our commitment to evidence-based nursing practice.

Critical Thinking Challenges

- How will expanding your computer technology "comfort zone" generate evidence-based practice information that can affect health care?
- What is the assumption underlying ANA's (1989) recommendation that the role of the baccalaureate graduate in the research process is primarily that of a knowledgeable consumer?
- What effects will evidence-based patient outcomes studies have on the practice of nursing?
- Discuss how research will contribute to the development of intradisciplinary and interdisciplinary evidence-based practice networks.

KEY POINTS

- Nursing research provides the basis for expanding the unique body of scientific evidence that forms the foundation of evidence-based nursing practice. Research links education, theory, and practice.
- Nurses become knowledgeable consumers of research through educational processes and practical experience. As consumers of research, nurses must have a basic understanding of the research process and critical appraisal skills that provide a standard for evaluating the strengths and weaknesses of research evidence provided by the findings of research studies before applying them in clinical practice.
- In the first half of the twentieth century, nursing research focused mainly on studies related to nursing education, although some clinical studies related to nursing care were evident.
- Nursing research blossomed in the second half of the twentieth century: graduate programs in nursing expanded; research journals began to emerge; the ANA formed a research committee; and funding for graduate education and nursing research increased dramatically.
- Nurses at all levels of educational preparation have a responsibility to participate in the research process.
- The role of the baccalaureate graduate is to be a knowledgeable consumer of research. Nurses with master's and doctorate degrees must be sophisticated consumers, as well as producers, of research studies.
- A collaborative research relationship within the nursing profession will extend and refine the scientific body of knowledge that provides the grounding for evidence-based practice.
- The future of nursing research will continue to be the extension of the scientific knowledge base for nursing expertise in appraising, designing, and conducting research and will provide leadership in both academic and clinical settings. Collaborative research relationships between education and service will multiply. Cluster research studies and replication of studies will have increased value.
- Research studies will emphasize clinical issues, problems, and outcomes. Priority will be given to research studies that focus on promoting health, diminishing the negative impact of health problems, ensuring care for the health needs of vulnerable groups, and developing cost-effective health care systems.
- Both consumers and producers of research will engage in a collaborative effort to further the growth of nursing research and accomplish the research objectives of the profession.

REFERENCES

Aiken L, Clarke SP, Cheung RB, Sloane DM, and Silber JH: Education levels of hospital nurses and patient mortality, *JAMA* 290: 1617-1623, 2003.

American Association of Colleges of Nursing: *The essentials of master's education for advanced practice nursing*, Washington, DC, 1996, The Association.

American Association of Colleges of Nursing: *Position statement on nursing research*, pp 1-6, Washington, DC, 1998a, The Association; available at http://www.aacn.nche.edu/publications/positions/rscposst.htm.

American Association of Colleges of Nursing: *The Essentials of baccalaureate education for professional nursing practice*, Washington, DC, 1998b, The Association.

American Nurses Association: *Commission on nursing research: education for preparation in nursing research*, Kansas City, Mo, 1989, The Association.

American Nurses Association: *Nursing quality indicators: guide for implementation*, Washington, DC, 1996, The Association.

American Nurses Association: *Implementing nursing's report card*, Washington, DC, 1997, The Association.

American Nurses Association: *Code for nurses with interpretive statements*, Washington, DC, 2002, The Association.

Barnsteiner J, Prevost S: How to implement evidence-based practice: some tried and true pointers, *Reflect Nurs Leadership* 28(2): 18-21, 2002.

Berlin L: Personal communication, August 12, 2004.

Brooten D, Naylor MD, and York R: Effects of nurse specialists' transitional care on patient outcomes and cost: results of five randomized clinical trials, *Am J Managed Care* 1: 35-41, 1995.

Brooten D, Naylor MD, York R, Brown LP, Munro BH, Hollingsworth AO, Cohen S, Finkler S, Deatrick J, and Youngblut JM: Lessons learned from testing the quality cost model of advanced practice nursing (APN) transitional care, *J Nurs Scholarship* 34(4): 369-376, 2002.

Buerhaus P, Staiger D, and Auerbach D: Implications of a rapidly aging registered nurse workforce, *JAMA* 283(22): 2948-2954, 2000.

Bull MJ, Hansen HE, and Gross CR: A professional-patient partnership model of discharge planning with elders hospitalized with heart failure, *Appl Nurs Res* 13(1): 19-28, 2000.

Carnegie E: *Historical perspectives of nursing research,* Boston, 1976, Boston University.

Carty B, editor: *Nursing informatics: education for practice,* New York, 2001, Springer.

Chang WY: Priority setting for nursing research, *West J Nurs Res* 22(2): 119-121, 2000.

Committee on Nursing and Nursing Education in the United States, Josephine Goldmark, Secretary, New York, 1923, Macmillan.

Crane PB, Lefvak S, Lewallen L, Hu J, and Jones E: Inclusion of women in nursing research: 1995-2001, *Nurs Res* 53(4): 237-242.

Cronenwett LR: Research, practice, and policy: issues in evidence based care, *Online J Issues Nurs,* 2002; available at http://www.nursingworld.org/ojin/keynotes/speech_2.htm.

Dickenson-Hazard N: Global health issues and challenges, *J Nurs Scholarship* 36(1): 6-10, 2004.

Diers D, Leonard RC: Interaction analysis in nursing research, *Nurs Res* 15: 225-228, 1966.

Dochterman J, Titler M, Wong J, Reed D, Pettit D, Mattlew-Watson M, Budreau G, Bulechek G, Kraus V, and Kanak M: Describing use of nursing interventions in three groups of patients, *J Nurs Scholarship* 37(1): 57-66, 2005.

Dock LL: What we may expect from the law, *Am J Nurs* 1: 8-12, 1900.

Donaldson SK: Breakthroughs in nursing research, presentation, Proceedings of the 25th Anniversary of the American Academy of Nursing, Acapulco, Mexico, 1998.

Dumas RG, Leonard RC: The effect of nursing on the incidence of postoperative vomiting, *Nurs Res* 12: 12-15, 1963.

Dykes PC: Practice guidelines and measurement: state of the science, *Nurs Outlook* 51(2): 65-69, 2003.

Evers G: Developing nursing science in Europe, *J Nurs Scholarship* 35(1): 9-13, 2003.

Fahs PS, Stewart LL, and Kalman M: A call for replication, *J Nurs Scholarship* 35(1): 67-72, 2003.

Fitzpatrick JJ: A decade of applied nursing research: a new millennium and beyond, *Appl Nurs Res* 13(1): 1, 2000.

Fitzpatrick JJ: Translating clinical research into health policy, *Appl Nurs Res* 17(2): 71, 2004.

Glaser BG, Strauss AL: *Observations series: awareness of dying,* Chicago, 1965, Aldine.

Goodrich A: *The social and ethical significance of nursing: a series of addresses,* New York, 1932, Macmillan.

Grady PA: A NINR initiative to address health disparities, *Nurs Outlook* 51(1): 5, 2003.

Grady PA, Collins FS: Genetics and nursing science; realizing the potential, *Nurs Res* 52(2): 69, 2003.

Hall LE: A center for nursing, *Nurs Outlook* 11: 805-806, 1963.

Hegyvary ST: Working paper on grand challenges in improving global health, *J Nurs Scholarship* 36(2): 96-101, 2004.

Henderson V: We've "come a long way," but what of the direction?, *Nurs Res* 26: 163-164, 1977 (guest editorial).

Hinshaw AS: Nursing knowledge for the 21st century: opportunities and challenges, *J Nurs Scholarship* 32(2): 117-123, 2000.

Im E, Chee W: Issues in internet research, *Nurs Outlook* 51(1): 6-12, 2003.

Institute of Medicine Committee on Quality of Health Care in America: *Crossing the quality chasm: a new health system for the 21st century,* Washington, DC, 2001, National Academy Press.

Jenkins ML, Dunn D: Enhancing web-based health information for consumer education, *Appl Nurs Res* 17(1): 68-70, 2004.

Jennings BM, McClure ML: Strategies to advance health quality, *Nurs Outlook* 52(1): 17-22, 2004.

Joint Commission on Accreditation of Healthcare Organizations: *Accreditation manual for hospitals,* Oakbrook Terrace, Ill, 2004, The Commission.

Keith JM: Florence Nightingale: statistician and consultant epidemiologist, *Int Nurs Rev* 35(5): 147-149, 1988.

Kohn L, Corrigan J, and Donaldson M, editors: *To err is human: building a safer health system*, Washington, DC, 1999, National Academy Press.

Koniak-Griffin D, Verzemnieks IL, Anderson NLR, Brecht M, Lesser J, Kim S, and Turner-Pluta C: Nurse visitation for adolescent mothers: two-year infant health and maternal outcomes, *Nurs Res* 52(2): 127-136, 2003.

Larson E: Minimizing disincentives for collaborative research, *Nurs Outlook* 51(6): 267-271, 2003.

Larson K, Adamsen L, Bjearregaard L, and Madsen, JK: There is no gap 'per se' between theory and practice: research knowledge and clinical knowledge are developed in different contexts and follow their own logic, *Nurs Outlook* 50(5): 204-212, 2002.

Matzo M, Sherman DW, editors: *Palliative care nursing: quality care to the end of life*, New York, 2001, Springer.

Melnyk BM, Fineout-Overholt E: Putting research into practice, *Reflect Nurs Leadership* 28(2): 22-25, 2002.

Melnyk BM, Fineout-Overholt E: *Evidence-based practice in nursing and healthcare*, Philadelphia, 2005, Lippincott Williams & Wilkins.

Messias DKH: Globalization, nursing, and health for all, *J Nurs Scholarship* 33(1): 9-11, 2001.

Mishel MH, Clayton MF: Theories of uncertainty in illness. In Smith MF, Liehr PR, editors: *Middle range theory for nursing*, New York, 2003, Springer.

Nahcivan NO: A Turkish language equivalence of the exercise of self-care agency scale, *West J Nurs Res* 26(7): 813-824, 2004.

National Institute of Nursing Research: *About NINR*, available at www.nih.gov/ninr/a mission.html, August 17, 2004.

National Organization of Nurse Practitioner Faculties: *Nurse practitioner primary care competencies in specialty areas: adult, family, gerontological, pediatric, and women's health*, Rockville, Md, 2002, US Department of Health and Human Services, Health Resources and Services Administration, Bureau of Health Professions, Division of Nursing.

Naylor M: Nursing intervention research and quality of care, *Nurs Res* 52(6): 380-385, 2003.

Naylor M et al.: Comprehensive discharge planning for the hospitalized elderly: a randomized clinical trial, *Ann Int Med* 120: 999-1006, 1994.

Naylor MD et al.: Comprehensive discharge planning and home follow-up of hospitalized elders: a randomized clinical trial, *JAMA* 281(7): 613-620, 1999.

Nightingale F: *Notes on hospitals*, London, 1863, Longman Group.

Nutting MA: *Educational status of nursing (Bull. No. 7)*, Washington, DC, 1912, US Bureau of Education.

Nutting MA: *A second economic basis for schools of nursing and other addresses*, New York, 1926, GP Putnam's Sons.

Nutting MA, Dock LL: *A history of nursing*, vol I-IV, New York, 1907-1912, GP Putnam's Sons.

O'Neill ES and Dluhy NM: Utility of structured care approaches in education and clinical practice, *Nurs Outlook* 48(3): 132-135, 2000.

Orlando IJ: *The dynamic nurse-patient relationship*, New York, 1961, GP Putnam's Sons.

Peplau HE: *Interpersonal relations in nursing: a conceptual frame of reference for psychodynamic nursing*, New York, 1952, GP Putnam's Sons.

Phillips J, Grady PA: Reducing health disparities in the twenty-first century: opportunities for nursing research, *Nurs Outlook* 50(3): 117-120, 2002.

Phillips LR, Ayres M: Supportive and nonsupportive care environments for the elderly. In Hinshaw AS, Feetham SL, Shaver JLF, editors: *Handbook of clinical nursing research*, Thousand Oaks, Calif, 1999, Sage.

Plach SK, Stevens PE, and Moss VA: Social role experiences of women living with rheumatoid arthritis, *J Fam Nurs* 10(1): 33-49, 2004.

President's New Freedom Commission on Mental Health: *Achieving the promise: transforming mental health care in America, final report*; DHHS Pub No. SMA-03-3832, Rockville, Md, 2003.

Rantz MJ, Connolly RP: Measuring nursing care quality and using large data sets in nonacute care settings: state of the science, *Nurs Outlook* 52(1): 23-37, 2004.

Robb IH: *Nursing: its principles and practice for hospitals and private use*, ed 3, Cleveland, 1906, EC Koeckert.

Roberts BI: Activities of daily living: factors related to independence. In Hinshaw AS, Feetham SL, Shaver JLF, editors: *Handbook of clinical nursing research*, Thousand Oaks, Calif, 1999, Sage.

Rogers AAE, Hwang W, Scott LD, Aiken LH, and Dinges DF: The working hours of hospital staff nurses and patient safety, *Health Affairs* 23(4): 202-212, 2004.

Ryan J, Stone RI, and Raynor CR: Using large data sets in long-term care to measure and improve quality, *Nurs Outlook* 52(1): 38-44, 2004.

Sackett DL, Straus S, Richardson S, Rosenberg W, and Haynes RB: *Evidence-based medicine: how to practice and teach EBM,* ed 2, London, UK, 2000, Churchill Livingstone.

Shaver J: Improving the health of communities: the position, *Nurs Outlook* 52: 116-117, 2004.

Sigmon HD, Grady PA, and Amende LM: The National Institute of Nursing Research explores opportunities in genetics research, *Nurs Outlook* 45(5): 215-219, 1997.

Stone PW, Curran CR, and Bakken S: Economic evidence for evidence-based practice, *J Nurs Scholarship* 34(3): 277-282, 2002.

Swanson KM: Empirical development of a middle range theory of caring, *Nurs Res* 40: 161-166, 1991.

Swanson KM: Nursing as informed caring for the well-being of others, *Image: J Nurs Scholarship* 25: 352-357, 1993.

Swanson KM: Effects of caring, measurement, and time on miscarriage impact and women's well being in the first year subsequent to loss, *Nurs Res.* 48(6): 288-298, 1999a.

Swanson KM: Research-based practice with women who have had miscarriages, *Image: J Nurs Scholarship* 31(4): 339-345, 1999b.

Swanson KM, Karmali ZH, Powell SH, and Pulvarmakher F: Miscarriage effects on couples' interpersonal and sexual relationships during the first year after loss: women's perspectives, *Psychosomat Med* 65: 902-910, 2003.

Swanson-Kauffman KM: *The unborn one: the human experience of miscarriage,* Doctoral dissertation, University of Colorado Health Sciences Center, Dissertation Abstracts International 43,AAT8404456, 1983.

Swanson-Kauffman KM: A combined qualitative methodology for nursing research, *Adv Nurs Sci* 8(3): 58-69, 1986a.

Swanson-Kauffman KM: Caring in the instance of unexpected early pregnancy loss, *Top Clin Nurs* 8(2): 37-46, 1986b.

Thompson C, Cullum N, McCaughan D, Sheldon T, and Raynor P: Nurses, information use, and clinical decision making: the real world potential for evidence-based decisions in nursing, *Evidence-Based Nurs* 7(3): 68-72, 2004.

Titler MG, Cullen L, and Ardery G: Evidence-based practice: an administrative perspective, *Reflect Nurs Leadership* 28(2): 26-27,46, 2002.

United States Department of Health and Human Services: *Healthy people 2010,* Washington, DC, 2001, The Department.

United States Public Health Service Office of the Surgeon General: *Mental health: culture, race, and ethnicity: a supplement to mental health: a report to the surgeon general,* Rockville, Md, 2001, Department of Health and Human Services, US Public Health Service.

Wald LD: *House on Henry Street,* New York, 1915, Henry Holt and Co.

Ward LS: Race as a variable in cross-cultural research, *Nurs Outlook* 51(3): 120-125, 2003.

Whittemore R, Grey M: The systematic development of nursing interventions, *J Nurs Scholarship* 34(2): 115-120, 2002.

Wiedenbach E: *Clinical nursing: a helping art,* New York, 1964, Springer.

Williams JK, Tripp-Reimer T, Schutte D, and Barnette J: Advancing genetic nursing knowledge, *Nurs Outlook* 52(3): 73-79, 2004.

World Health Organization: *The World health report 2001—Mental health: new understanding, new hope,* Geneva, 2001, World Health Organization.

FOR FURTHER STUDY

🔘 Go to your Companion CD for review activities for this chapter.

evolve Go to Evolve at http://evolve.elsevier.com/LoBiondo/ for WebLinks, Content Updates, and additional research articles, for practice in reviewing and critiquing.

2

GERI LOBIONDO-WOOD

JUDITH HABER

BARBARA KRAINOVICH-MILLER

The Research Process: Integrating Evidence-Based Practice

KEY TERMS

assumptions	critique	qualitative research
abstract	critiquing criteria	quantitative research
critical reading	evidence-based practice	
critical thinking	levels of evidence	

LEARNING OUTCOMES

After reading this chapter, the student should be able to do the following:

- Identify the steps of quantitative and qualitative research.
- Identify the importance of critical thinking and critical reading for the reading of research articles.
- Identify the steps of critical reading.
- Use the steps of critical reading for reviewing research articles.
- Use identified strategies for critically reading research articles.
- Use identified critical thinking and reading strategies to synthesize critiqued articles.
- Identify components of the levels of evidence.
- Discuss the importance of levels of evidence in relation to being an effective research consumer.
- Identify the format and style of research articles.

STUDY RESOURCES

Go to your Companion CD for review activities for this chapter.

evolve Go to Evolve at http://evolve.elsevier.com/LoBiondo/ for Weblinks, Content Updates, and additional research articles for practice in reviewing and critiquing.

As you venture through this text, you will see the steps of the research process unfold. The steps are systematic and orderly and relate to the development of evidence-based practice. Understanding the step-by-step process that researchers use will help you develop the critiquing skills necessary to judge the soundness of research studies. Throughout the chapters, research terminology pertinent to each step is identified and illustrated with many examples from the research literature. Four published research studies are found in the appendixes and used as examples to illustrate significant points in each chapter. Judging not only the study's soundness but also a study's applicability to practice is key. Before you can judge a study it is important to understand the difference between and among studies. There are many different study designs that you will see as you read through this text and the appendixes. There are standards for critiquing the soundness of each step of a study but also for judging the strength of evidence provided by a study and its application to practice. This chapter provides an overview of types of research studies, critical thinking, critical reading, and critiquing skills. It introduces the overall format of a research article and provides an overview of the subsequent chapters in the book. It also introduces the evidence-based practice levels of evidence model, another tool for helping you evaluate the strength of a research study. These topics are designed to help you read research articles more effectively and with greater understanding, making this book more "user-friendly" as you learn about the research process so that you can practice from a base of evidence and contribute to quality and cost-effective patient outcomes.

TYPES OF RESEARCH: QUALITATIVE AND QUANTITATIVE

Research can be classified into two major categories: qualitative and quantitative. A researcher chooses between these categories based primarily on the question they are asking. That is, a researcher may wish to test a cause and effect situation or to assess if variables are related, or they may wish to discover and understand the meaning about an experience or process. A researcher would choose to conduct a **qualitative research** study if the question to be answered is about understanding the meaning of a human experience such a grief, hope, or loss. The meaning of an experience is based on the view that meaning varies and is subjective. The

context of the experience also plays a role in qualitative research. That is, the experience of loss as a result of a miscarriage would be different than the experience from the loss of a parent. Qualitative research is generally conducted in natural settings and uses data that are words or text rather than numeric in order to describe the experiences being studied. Data are collected from a small number of subjects, allowing an in-depth study of a phenomenon. For example, Plach, Stevens, and Moss (2004, Appendix C) studied in-depth the experience of 20 women who were living with rheumatoid arthritis. Although qualitative research is systematic in its approach, it uses a subjective approach. Data from qualitative studies help nurses to understand experiences or phenomena that affect patients; these data also assist in generating theories that lead clinicians to developing improved care and further research. Highlights of the general steps of qualitative studies and the journal format for a qualitative article are outlined in Table 2-1. Chapters 6 through 8 provide an in-depth view of qualitative research underpinnings, designs, and methods. While qualitative research looks for meaning, **quantitative research** encompasses the study of research questions and/or hypotheses that describe phenomena, test relationships, assess differences, and seek to explain cause and effect interactions between variables and tests for intervention effectiveness. The numeric data in quantitative studies are summarized and analyzed using statistics. Quantitative research techniques are systematic, and the methodology is controlled. Appendixes A, B, and D illustrate examples of different quantitative approaches to answering research questions. Table 2-2 indicates where the step can usually be located in a quantitative research article and where it is discussed in this text. Chapters 3, 4, 5, and 9 through 18 describe processes related to quantitative research. The primary difference is that a qualitative study seeks to interpret meaning and phenomena whereas quantitative research seeks to test a hypothesis or answer research questions based on a framework. Remember as you are reading

TABLE **2-1 Steps of the Research Process and Journal Format—Qualitative Research**

Research Process Steps and/or Format Issues	Usual Location in Journal Heading or Subheading
Identifying the phenomenon	Abstract and/or in introduction
Research question study purpose	Abstract and/or in beginning or end of introduction
Literature review	Introduction and/or discussion
Design	Abstract and/or in introductory section or under method section entitled "Design" or stated in method section
Sample	Method section labeled "Sample" or "Subjects"
Legal-ethical issues	Data-collection or procedure's section or in sample section
Data-collection procedure	Data-collection or procedure's section
Data analysis	Methods section under subhead "Data Analysis" or "Data Analysis and Interpretation"
Results	Stated in separate heading: "Results" or "Findings"
Discussion and recommendation	Combined in separate section: "Discussion" or "Discussion and Implications"
References	At end of article

See Chapters 6, 7, and 8.

research articles that a researcher may vary the steps slightly, depending on the nature of the research problem, but all of the steps should be addressed systematically.

CRITICAL THINKING AND CRITICAL READING SKILLS

As you read a research article, you may be struck by the difference in style or format between a research article and a clinical article. The terms of a research article may be new, and the focus of the content is different. You may also be thinking that the research article is too hard for you to read or that it is too technical and bores you. You may simultaneously wonder, "How will I possibly learn to evaluate (critique) all the steps of a research study, as well as all the terminology? I'm only on Chapter 2. This is not so easy; research is as hard, as everyone says."

Try to reframe these thoughts with "the glass is half-full approach." That is, tell yourself, "Yes I can learn how to read and critique research, and this chapter will provide the strategies for me to learn this skill." Remember that learning occurs with time and help. Reading research articles is difficult and frustrating at first, but the best way

to become a knowledgeable research consumer is to use critical thinking and reading skills when reading research articles. As a student, you are not expected to understand a research article or critique it perfectly the first time. Nor are you expected to develop these skills on your own. An essential objective of this book is to help you acquire critical thinking and reading skills so that you can reach this goal, Remember that becoming a competent critical thinker and reader of research, similar to learning the steps of the research process, takes time and patience.

Critical thinking is the examination of ideas, inferences, assumptions, principles, arguments, conclusions, issues, statements, beliefs, and actions (Elder and Paul, 2004). As applied to critically reading research, this means that you are engaged in the following:

- Systematic, self-directed thinking that exemplifies thinking consistent with the research process
- Thinking that displays a mastery of the criteria for critiquing research
- The art of being able to make one's thinking better (i.e., clearer, more accurate, or more defensible) by clarifying what you do understand and what you do not know

TABLE **2-2** **Steps of the Research Process and Journal Format—Quantitative Research**

Research Process Steps and/or Format Issue	Usual Location in Journal Heading or Subheading	Text Chapter
Research problem	Abstract and/or in introduction (not labeled) or in separate labeled heading: "Problem"	3
Purpose	Abstract and/or in introduction or at end of literature review or theoretical framework section, or labeled as separate heading: "Purpose"	3
Literature review	At end of heading "Introduction" but not labeled as such, or labeled as separate heading: "Literature Review," "Review of the Literature," or "Related Literature"; or not labeled or variables reviewed appear as headings or subheadings	4
Theoretical framework (TF) and/or conceptual framework (CF)	Combined with "Literature Review" or found in separate heading as TF or CF; or each concept or definition used in TF or CF may appear as separate heading or subheading	5
Hypothesis/research questions	Stated or implied near end of introductory section, which may be labeled or found in separate heading or subheading: "Hypothesis" or "Research Questions"; or reported for first time in "Results" section	3
Research design	Stated or implied in abstract or in introduction or under heading: "Methods" or "Methodology"	9, 10, 11
Sample: type and size	"Size" may be stated in abstract, in methods section, or as separate subheading under methods section as "Sample," "Sample/Subjects," or "Participants" "Type" may be implied or stated in any of previous headings described under size	12
Legal-ethical issues	Stated or implied in labeled headings: "Methods," "Procedures," "Sample," or "Subjects"	13
Instruments (measurement tools)	Found in headings labeled "Methods," "Instruments," or "Measures"	14
Validity and reliability	Specifically stated or implied in headings labeled "Methods," "Instruments," "Measures," or "Procedures"	15
Data-collection procedure	Stated in methods section under subheading "Procedure" or "Data Collection," or as separate heading: "Procedure"	14
Data analysis	Stated in methods section under subheading "Procedure" or "Data Analysis"	16
Results	Stated in separate heading: "Results"	16, 17
Discussion of findings and new findings	Combined with results or as separate heading: "Discussion"	17
Implications, limitations, and recommendations	Combined in discussion or presented as separate or combined major headings	17
References	At end of article	2, 4
Communicating research results	Research articles, poster, and paper presentations	1, 2, 19, 20

In other words, being a critical thinker means that you are consciously thinking about your thoughts and what you say, write, read, or do, as well as what others say, write, or do. While thinking about all of this, you are questioning the appropriateness of the content, applying standards or criteria, and seeing how things measure up.

Developing the ability to evaluate research critically requires not only critical thinking skills but also critical reading skills. **Critical reading** is defined as "an active, intellectually engaging process in which the reader participates in an inner dialogue with the writer. Most people read uncritically and so miss some part of what is expressed while distorting other parts . . ." (Paul and Elder, 2001). Critical reading means entering into a point of view other than our own, the point of view of the writer. A critical reader actively looks for **assumptions** or accepted truths, key concepts and ideas, reasons and justifications, supporting examples, parallel experiences, implications and consequences, and any other structural features of the written text, to interpret and assess it accurately and fairly (Paul and Elder, 2003).

Critical thinking and critical reading skills are further developed by learning the research process. You will gradually be able to read an entire research article and reflect on it by identifying assumptions, identifying key concepts, questioning methods, and determining whether the conclusions are based on the study's findings. Once you have obtained this research-critiquing competency, you will be ready to synthesize the findings of multiple research studies to use in developing evidence-based practice. This will be a very exciting and rewarding process for you.

PROCESS OF CRITICAL READING

To read a research study critically, you must have skilled reading, writing, and reasoning abilities. A research study requires several readings. A minimum of three or four readings—or even as many as six readings—is quite common. The first strategy is to keep your research textbook at your side as you read. Using your research text is necessary for you to do the following:

- Identify concepts
- Clarify unfamiliar concepts or terms
- Question assumptions and rationale
- Determine supporting evidence

Critical reading is a process that involves the following levels of understanding:

- Preliminary understanding
- Comprehensive understanding
- Analysis understanding
- Synthesis understanding

Preliminary Understanding: Familiarity: Skimming

Preliminary understanding is gained by scanning an article to familiarize yourself with its content or get a general sense of the material. During the preliminary reading, the title and abstract are read closely, but the content is skimmed. The **abstract,** a brief overview of a study, keys the reader to the main components of the study. The title keys the reader to the main variables of the study. Skimming includes reading the introduction, major headings, one or two sentences under a heading, and the summary or conclusion of the study. Preliminary reading strategies are outlined in Box 2-1.

Using these strategies enables you to identify the article's main theme and use this knowledge in the second step—comprehensive reading. An illustration of how to use a number of these strategies is provided by the example in Box 2-2, which contains an excerpt from the abstract, introduction, literature review, theoretical framework literature, and methods and procedure section of a quantitative study (Koniak-Griffin et al., 2003) (see Appendix A). Note that in this particular article there is both literature review and a theoretical framework section that clearly supports the objectives and purpose of the study. Also note that parts of the text of this section from the article were deleted to offer a number of examples within the text of this chapter.

BOX 2-1 HIGHLIGHTS OF CRITICAL READING PROCESS STRATEGIES

Photocopy the article to be critiqued and make notations directly on the copy.

STRATEGIES FOR PRELIMINARY UNDERSTANDING:

- Keep a research text and a dictionary by your side.
- Review the chapters in the text on various steps of the research process, critiquing criteria, unfamiliar terms, etc.
- List key variables at the top of the photocopy.
- Highlight or underline on the photocopy new terms, unfamiliar vocabulary, and significant sentences.
- Look up the definitions of new terms and write them on the photocopy.
- Review old and new terms before subsequent readings.
- Highlight or underline identified steps of the research process.

STRATEGIES FOR COMPREHENSIVE UNDERSTANDING:

- Identify the main idea or theme of the article; state it in your own words in one or two sentences.
- Continue to clarify terms that may be unclear on subsequent readings.
- Before critiquing the article, make sure you understand the main points of each reported step of the research process that you identified.

STRATEGIES FOR ANALYSIS UNDERSTANDING:

- Using the critiquing criteria determine how well the study meets the criteria for each step of the process.
- Determine which level of evidence fits the study.
- Write cues, relationships of concepts, and questions on the photocopy.
- Ask fellow students to analyze the same study using the same criteria and then compare results.
- Consult faculty members about your evaluation of the study.

STRATEGIES FOR SYNTHESIS UNDERSTANDING:

- Review your notes on the article and determine how each step discussed in the article compares with the critiquing criteria.
- Type a one-page summary in your own words of the reviewed study.
- Cite article references at the top according to APA or another reference style.
- Briefly summarize each reported research step in your own words using the critiquing criteria.
- Briefly describe strengths and weaknesses in your own words.

Comprehensive Understanding: Content in Relation to Context

The purpose of reading a research study for a comprehensive understanding is to understand the researcher's perspective or intent. Perhaps you have been assigned to read a research article on a topic you were interested in, but you found it difficult to understand how the study was actually conducted or what the findings mean. This occurred because you could not read at a comprehension level (i.e., you probably did not know the definitions of terms the researcher used and therefore could not understand the terms in relation to the study's context or even if the terms were used appropriately). For example, when reading the qualitative study of Plach, Stevens, and Moss (2004) (see Appendix C) for comprehension, it is essential to understand

the purpose of qualitative research that uses content analysis. The researchers wanted to investigate insider's views (women with rheumatoid arthritis [RA]) on how fulfilling they found their various social roles while living with RA. These intensive interviews allowed the researchers to develop patterns and themes that exemplified the roles of women living with RA (see Chapters 6 and 7). To simply recall that the major variable of their study was the concept of social role experiences is inadequate. At the comprehension level of reading, you would be able to discuss the variables that emerged relevant to social roles and psychological health for women with RA.

When reading for comprehension, keep your research text and dictionary nearby. Do not hesitate to write cues or keywords on the article. If

BOX 2-2 EXAMPLES OF SKIMMING STRATEGIES AND STUDENT OUTCOMES: INITIAL READING OF STUDY BY KONIAK-GRIFFIN ET AL. (2003) (APPENDIX A)

Introductory paragraphs (no subheading indicated)	Introductory paragraphs Although teen birth rates have declined sharply in recent years (22% from 1991 to 2000) (Martin, et al., 2002), Hispanic and Black adolescents continue to have much higher birth rates than Caucasians. Early child-bearing impacts the nation's health care system, and social and economic functioning; hence, community-based nursing intervention programs are needed to improve health and social outcomes for teen mothers and their children . . . their children have higher rates of morbidity and unintentional injuries leading to emergency room (ER) visits and hospitalizations during their first 5 years of life, as compared to children of adult mothers . . . (pp. 127-128)	Significance of problem and major impact on resources **Gaps in literature
Introductory paragraphs	This article describes research of a randomized clinical trial designed **to determine effects of early intervention program (EIP) provided through home visits by public health nurses (PHNs) to culturally diverse adolescent mothers and their children on infant health and maternal outcomes at 24 months** (p. 128).	COMMENT: Objectives and text described similar purpose of study, but text specifies randomized clinical trial
	Review of Literature	
**Koniak-Griffin et al. have program of research: findings contribute to nursing science	*Notable among nurse home visitation programs that have demonstrated improvement in both maternal and child outcomes is the series of randomized clinical trials by Olds and associates (Olds, et al., 1999). In the first of these studies . . . decreased smoking, improved diet . . . (Olds, 1986). In a second trial, . . . were found to have lower rates of morbidity for selected prenatal health conditions than a comparison group (Kitzman, et al., 1997).* *However, positive effects on birth weights and premature birth rates were not replicated.* *Less comprehensive home visiting programs by PHNs have (a) decreased incidence of low*	Gap in literature **Maybe Literature Review section was shortened; seems like type of synthesis of literature *QUESTION: This third "clinical trial" reviewed does not describe sample or size; was sample culturally diverse? **Hypothesis of study stated at end of Review of Literature

Text from Koniak-Griffin et al. (2003).   *Continued*
KEY:
Single underline = Significance of Problem
Boldface = Purpose(s) of Study
Italics = Literature Review
Dotted underline = Gap in Literature
Double underline = Hypothesis
Dashed underline = Theoretical Framework
Boldface dotted underline = Sample Description

birth weight (LBW) infants (Norbeck, DeJoseph, and Smith, 1996); (b) improved mother-child interactions and maternal educational attainment (Booth et al., 1987); (c) reduced rates of school dropout and repeat pregnancy; weight (LBW) infants (Norbeck, DeJoseph, and and (d) improved immunization rates (**O'Sullivan and Jacobsen, 1992**). *Earlier findings laid important groundwork for the 2-year postbirth outcomes . . . longitudinal study on the effects of a PHN EIP for adolescent mothers.*

Findings revealed that infants in the EIP had significantly fewer total days of birth-related hospitalization and rehospitalization in the first year of life, and higher immunization rates than TPHNC infants (Koniak-Griffin et al., 2000, 2002). It was hypothesized that at 2-years postbirth, participants in the EIP would demonstrate improved infant health and maternal outcomes in comparison to those in the TPHNC group (p. 128).

Theoretical framework (TF)	The construct of social competence was conceived to have two facets: internal and external. The young mother's internal competence (ability to handle her inner world) was proposed to be increased through training in self-management skills, including self-care, life planning and decision making, handling emotions, and coping with stress and depression. At the same time, her external competence (ability to interact effectively with partners, family, peers, and social agencies) was anticipated to improve through training in communication and social skills (pp. 128-129).	**TF: a subheading under literature review **TF: supported by two previous studies Clausen, 1991; Olds, et al., 1999

Methods

Setting and Sample

Adolescents were recruited from referrals to the Community Health Services Division of the County Health Department in San Bernardino, California. They were eligible if they were: (a) 14-19 years of age; (b) at 26 weeks gestation or less; (c) having their first child; and (d) planning to keep the infant . . . Excluded were those dependent on narcotics. . . . Recruitment continued until the sample reached a target number (N = 144) based on power analysis

**Procedure section under Method indicated that adolescents were randomly assigned using computer-based program
**Text indicated n of EIP and TPHNC in separate section under Method
**Randomized clinical trial is evidence Level II; it is Experimental design

Text from Koniak-Griffin et al. (2003).

KEY:

<u>Single underline</u> = Significance of Problem
Boldface = Purpose(s) of Study
Italics = Literature Review
Dotted underline = Gap in Literature
Double underline = Hypothesis
Dashed underline = Theoretical Framework
Boldface dotted underline = Sample Description

BOX 2-2   EXAMPLES OF SKIMMING STRATEGIES AND STUDENT OUTCOMES: INITIAL READING OF STUDY BY KONIAK-GRIFFIN ET AL. (2003) (APPENDIX A)—cont'd

([alpha] = 0.05, power = 0.80, and moderate effect size of approximately 0.47) using pilot data available for a measure of maternal-child interaction. Because of attrition the sample size ($n = 101$) available for analysis of 24-month outcomes, adjusting for unequal n, was adequate to detect a moderate effect size of $d = 0.57$ in group differences on outcomes.

Procedure

After securing written informed consent in accordance with the university Internal Review Board requirements for <u>pregnant minors, adolescents were randomly assigned</u>, using a computer-based program, into the EIP or TPHNC group, based on specific criteria (<u>maternal age, ethnicity, language, gestation age, geographic region of residence</u>).

*QUESTION: What are outcome variables of EIP experimental group and TPHNC control group?

**Procedure section under Method fully described sample; adolescents randomly assigned based on criteria (maternal age, ethnicity, language, gestation age, geographic region of residence): only maternal age and gestation were mentioned in the Setting and Sample section as eligibility criteria

the article still does not make sense after the second reading, ask for assistance. Indicate the unclear areas and write out specific questions. What is or is not highlighted as well as the comments on the copy often help the faculty person to understand your difficulty. Strategies for comprehensive reading are listed in Box 2-1.

HELPFUL H I N T

If you still have difficulty understanding a research study after using the strategies related to skimming and comprehensive reading, make another copy of your "marked up" research article, include your specific questions or area of difficulty, and ask your professor to read it.

Comprehensive understanding is necessary to analyze and synthesize the material. Understanding the author's perspective for the study reflects critical thinking and facilitates the evaluation of the study. The next reading or two allows for analysis and synthesis of the study.

Analysis Understanding: Breaking into Parts

The purpose of reading for analysis is to break the content into parts and understand each aspect of the study. Some of the questions that you can ask yourself as you begin to analyze the research article are as follows:

- Am I confident that I know the specific design type so that I apply the appropriate criteria when critiquing the study?
- Did I capture the main idea or theme of this article in one or two sentences?
- How are the major parts of this article organized in relation to the research process?
- What is the study's purpose?
- How was this study carried out? Can I explain it step by step?
- What are the author's or authors' main conclusions?
- Can I say that I understand the parts of this article and summarize each section in my own words?

In a sense, you are determining how the steps of the research process are presented or organized in the article and what the content related to each step is about. This is also when you begin to critique or evaluate the study by asking and answering the questions related to the research process that was used by the researcher/author. At this point of critical reading, you are ready to begin the critiquing process that will help determine the study's merit.

 HELPFUL HINT

Remember that not all research articles include headings related to each step or component of the research process, but that each step is presented at some point in the article.

The **critique** is the process of objectively and critically evaluating a research report's content for scientific merit and application to practice, theory, and education. It requires some knowledge of the subject matter and knowledge of how to critically read and use critiquing criteria. You will find summarized examples of critiquing criteria for qualitative studies and an example of a qualitative critique in Chapter 8, and summarized critiquing criteria and examples of a quantitative critique in Chapter 18. An in-depth exploration of the criteria for analysis required in quantitative research critiques is given in Chapters 9 through 18. The criteria for qualitative research critiques are presented in Chapters 6, 7, and 8. Chapters 3, 4, and 5 provide general principles for quantitative and qualitative research.

Critiquing criteria are the standards, evaluation guides, or questions used to judge (critique) an article. In analyzing a research report, the reader must evaluate each step of the research process and ask questions about whether each step of the process meets the criteria. For instance, the critiquing criteria in Chapter 4 ask if "the literature review identifies gaps and inconsistencies in the literature about a subject, concept, or problem" and if "all of the concepts and variables are included in the review." These two questions relate to critiquing the research

question and reviewing the literature components of the research process. Box 2-2 shows several places that the researchers identified gaps in the literature, and how the study intended to fill these gaps by conducting a study for the stated objective and purpose (see Appendix A for the complete study). Therefore your answer to these posed questions might be as follows:

> Koniak-Griffin et al. (2003) clearly stated the major gaps in the literature related to the lack of follow-up study of the outcomes of children of Hispanic and Black adolescent mothers. The identified gaps became the studied variables, and their clearly stated aims addressed the gaps in the literature.

This critiquing statement implies that reading for analysis took place. As a beginner, you are not expected to write a critique at the same level as a seasoned researcher who critiques a colleague's work (e.g., as published in the commentary section of the *Western Journal of Nursing Research*). Remember that when you are doing a critique, you are pointing out strengths, as well as weaknesses. Developing critical reading skills at the comprehension level will enable you to successfully complete a critique. The critiquing strategies that facilitate the understanding gained by reading for analysis are listed in Box 2-1.

Synthesis Understanding: Putting Together

Synthesis is the pulling together or combining of parts into a whole. The purpose of reading for synthesis is to pull all the information together to form a new whole, make sense of it, and explain relationships. Although the process of synthesizing the material may be taking place as the reader is analyzing the article, a fourth reading is recommended. It is during this synthesis reading that the understanding and critique of the whole study are put together. In this final step, you decide how well the study meets the critiquing criteria and how useful it is to practice (see Chapters 19 and 20). This is also when you decide how well each step of the research process relates to the previous step. Synthesis can be thought of as looking at a completed jigsaw puzzle. Does it form a comprehensive picture, or is there a piece out of place? What is the level of evidence provided by the study and its findings? In the case of reading several studies for synthesis, the interrelationship of the studies is assessed as is the overall level of evidence and applicability to practice. Reading for synthesis is essential in critiquing research studies. For example, answering the previously posed critiquing questions after reading for synthesis in relation to the Koniak-Griffin, et al. (2003) study (see Appendix A), you would add the following to your critique:

> Koniak-Griffin, et al. (2003) clearly stated the major gaps in the literature related to the needs of children of culturally diverse adolescent mothers. Additionally, an overall strength of this study was how the researchers' literature review and theoretical framework clearly (1) explained variables that impact adolescent mothers and their babies negatively, as well as (2) its use of the theoretical framework of social competence and (3) its application to the development of these components to a long-term intervention program for the adolescent mothers and their babies. They randomly assigned mothers to either an early intervention program (EIP) or the traditional public health nursing care. The researchers compared the impact of the two interventions on several maternal and child outcomes over a 2-year period. This study used previous research and theory to develop a comprehensive program that could be tested and assessed for successful outcomes.

The steps for reading for synthesis and writing a summary critique are outlined in Box 2-1.This type of summary is viewed as the first draft of a final written critique. It teaches brevity, facilitates easy retrieval of data to support the critiquing evaluation, and increases your ability to write a scholarly report. In addition, the ability to synthesize one study prepares you for the task of critiquing several studies on a similar topic and comparing and contrasting the findings (see Chapters 19 and 20).

HELPFUL H I N T

If you have to write a paper on a specific concept or topic that requires you to critique and synthesize the findings from several studies, you might find it useful to create a table of the data. Include the following information: author, date, type of study, design, level of evidence, sample, data analysis, findings, and implications.

PERCEIVED DIFFICULTIES AND STRATEGIES FOR CRITIQUING RESEARCH

The best way to become an intelligent consumer of research is to use critical thinking and reading skills. Box 2-1 presents strategies for reading and evaluating a research report. Remember when reading research articles to keep your text nearby in order to clarify unfamiliar terms, and review the steps of the research process. Read the entire article and reflect on it. Most importantly, draw on previous knowledge, common sense, and the critical thinking skills you already possess.

Another important strategy is to ask questions; remember that questioning is essential to developing critical thinking. Asking faculty members questions and sharing your thoughts about what you are reading is an effective way of developing your skills. Do not hesitate to write or to call a researcher if you have a question about their work. You will be pleasantly surprised by how willing researchers are to discuss your questions.

Throughout the text, you will find special features that will help refine the critical thinking and critical reading skills essential to developing your competence as a research consumer. A Critical Thinking Decision Path related to each step of the research process will sharpen your decision-making skills as you critique research articles. Look for internet resources in chapters that will enhance research consumer activities. Critical Thinking Challenges, which appear at the end of each chapter, are designed to reinforce your critical thinking and critical reading skills in relation to the steps of the research process. Helpful Hints, designed to reinforce your understanding and critical thinking, appear at various points throughout the chapters. Also Evidence-Based Practice Tips, which will help you apply evidence-based practice strategies in your clinical practice, are provided in each chapter.

When you complete your first critique, congratulate yourself; mastering these skills is not easy at the beginning, but we are confident that you can do it. Once you complete a research critique or two, you will be ready to discuss your critique with your fellow students and professor. Best of all, you can look forward to discussing the points of your critique because your critique will be based on objective data, not just personal opinion. As you continue to use and perfect critical analysis skills by critiquing studies, remember that these very skills are an expected clinical competency for delivering evidence-based nursing care.

LEVELS OF EVIDENCE

Along with gaining comfort while reading and critiquing research studies, a final step must be undertaken. The final step of reading and critiquing the research literature is deciding how, when, and if to apply a study or studies to your practice so that your practice is evidence-based. **Evidence-based practice (EBP)** is the careful and judicious use of research literature in making patient care decisions (Sackett et al., 2000). Evidence-based practice allows one to systematically use the best available evidence along with the integration of individual clinical expertise as well as the patient's values and preferences in making clinical decisions. Chapter 19 provides an overview of evidence-based practice, and Chapter 20 conceptually introduces you to the strategies associated with evidence-based practice. When using EBP strategies, the first step is to decide which level of evidence a research article provides. Table 2-3 illustrates a model for determining the levels of evidence (Melnyk and Fineout-Overholt, 2005) that are associated with the design of a study, ranging from systematic reviews of randomized clinical trials (RCTs) (see Chapters 4, 10, and 11) to expert opinions. This model represents a hierarchy for judging the strength of a study's design, which in turn influences the confidence one has in the conclusions the researcher has drawn. Assessing the strength of scientific evidence provides a vehicle to guide nurses in evaluating research studies for their applicability in clinical decision making. Grading the strength of a body of evidence should incor-

TABLE **2-3 Levels of Evidence: Rating System for the Hierarchy of Evidence**

Assessing Level of Evidence	Source of Evidence
Level I	Evidence from systematic review or meta-analysis of all relevant randomized controlled trials (RCTs) or evidence based clinical practice guidelines based on systematic reviews of RCTs
Level II	Evidence obtained from at least one well-designed RCT
Level III	Evidence obtained from well-designed controlled trials without randomization (e.g., quasi-experimental study)
Level IV	Evidence from nonexperimental studies (e.g., case-control and cohort studies)
Level V	Evidence from systematic reviews of descriptive and qualitative studies
Level VI	Evidence from single descriptive or qualitative study
Level VII	Evidence from opinion of authorities and/or reports of expert committees

Modified from Melnyk and Fineout-Overholt, 2005.

porate three domains: quality, quantity, and consistency (AHRQ, 2002):

- **Quality**—the extent to which a study's design, implementation, and analysis minimizes bias (see Chapter 9)
- **Quantity**—the number of studies that have evaluated the research question, including overall sample size across studies (see Chapter 12) as well as the strength of the findings from the data analyses (see Chapter 16)
- **Consistency**—the degree to which studies that have similar and different designs, but investigate the same research question, report similar findings (see Chapters 10, 11, 16, 19, and 20)

The meaningfulness of these levels will become clearer to you as you read Chapters 7, 9, 10, and 11. For example, the Koniak-Griffin et al. (2003) study falls into Level II because of its experimental design while the Plach et al. (2004) study falls into Level VI because of its qualitative design. The level in and of itself does not tell the full worth of a study but is another tool that helps you think about the strengths and weaknesses of a study and the nature of the evidence provided in the findings and conclusions. You will use the level of evidence hierarchy presented in Table 2-3 throughout the book as you develop your research consumer skills, so become familiar with its content.

RESEARCH ARTICLES: FORMAT AND STYLE

Before one considers the reading of research articles, it is important to have a sense of their organization and format. Many journals publish research, either as the sole type of article in the journal or in addition to clinical or theoretical articles. Although many journals have some common features, they also have unique characteristics. All journals have guidelines for manuscript preparation and submission, which are published by each journal. A review of these guidelines will give you an idea of the format of articles that appear in specific journals. It is important to remember that even though each step of the research process is discussed at length in this text, you may find only a short paragraph or a sentence in the research article that gives the details of the step in a specific study. Because of the journal's publishing guidelines, the published study that one reads in a journal is a shortened version of the complete work done by the researcher(s). You will also find that some researchers devote more space in an article to the results, whereas others present a longer discussion of the methods and procedures. In recent years, most authors give more emphasis to the method, results, and discussion of implications than to details of assumptions, hypotheses, or definitions of terms. Decisions about the amount of material presented for each step of the research process are bound by the following:

- A journal's space limitations
- A journal's author guidelines
- The type or nature of the study
- An individual researcher's evaluation of what is the most important component of the study

The following discussion provides a brief overview of each step of the research process and how it might appear in an article. It is important to remember that a quantitative research article will differ from a qualitative research article. The components of qualitative research are discussed in Chapters 6 and 7 and summarized in Chapter 8.

Abstract

An **abstract** is a short comprehensive synopsis or summary of a study at the beginning of an article. An abstract quickly focuses the reader on the main points of a study. A well-presented abstract is accurate, self-contained, concise, specific, nonevaluative, coherent, and readable (American Psychological Association, 2001). Abstracts vary in length from 50 to 250 words. The length and format of an abstract are dictated by the journal's style. Both quantitative and qualitative research studies have abstracts that provide a succinct overview of the study. An example of an abstract can be found at the beginning of the study by Koniak-Griffin and associates (2003) (see Appendix A). Their abstract follows an outline format that highlights the major steps of the study. It partially reads as follows:

"Objective: The purpose of this study was to evaluate the 2-year postbirth infant health and maternal outcomes of an early intervention program (EIP) of home visitation by public health nurses (PHNs)."

Within this example, the authors provide a view of the study variables. The remainder of the abstract provides a synopsis of the background of the study and the methods, results, and conclusions. The studies in Appendixes A through D all have abstracts.

ⓘ HELPFUL HINT

A journal abstract is usually a single paragraph that provides a general reference to the research purpose, research questions, and/or hypotheses and highlights the methodology and results, as well as the implications for practice or future research.

Identification of a Research Purpose/Question

Early in a research article, in a section that may or may not be labeled "Introduction," the researcher presents a picture of the area researched. This is the presentation of the research purpose or question (see Chapter 3). When reading the study by Koniak-Griffin et al. (2003) (Appendix A), the reader can find the basis of the research question early in the report:

"Adolescent mothers and their children may benefit from home visitation, as they often lack the resources needed to maintain health and reduce risks in their lives . . . An important consideration in evaluation of health promotion interventions for adolescent mothers and their children is whether the effects are maintained beyond the treatment period."

Another example can be found in the Plach, Stevens, and Moss (2004) study (Appendix C), as follows:

"In summary, discomforts and progressive disability appear to limit women's ability to carry out social, occupational, and leisure activities in the face of rheumatoid arthritis (RA) and, therefore increase their vulnerability for impaired well-being. Given these morbidity problems, it is important to learn more about women with RA and their experience in social roles so that appropriate and effective interventions might be planned."

Definition of the Purpose

The purpose of the study is defined either at the end of the researcher's initial introduction or at the end of the "Literature Review" or "Conceptual Framework" section. The study's purpose may or may not be labeled as such (see Chapters 3, 4, and 5), or it may be referred to as the study's aim or objective. The studies by Plach et al. (2004, Appendix C) and Van Cleve et al. (2004, Appendix B) have sections entitled "Aims" and "Purposes." Koniak-Griffin et al. (2003) specifically stated their purpose in the abstract, the purpose is also clearly stated at the end of the third introductory paragraph before the "Review of the Literature" section.

The purpose of the Davison et al. (2003, Appendix D) study appears in the abstract in the "Purposes/Objectives" section and is repeated in the article's text under the subhead "Study Purpose and Hypotheses."

Literature Review and Theoretical Framework

Authors of studies and journal articles present the literature review and theoretical framework in different ways. Many research articles merge the "Literature Review" and the "Theoretical Framework." This section includes the main concepts investigated and may be called "Review of the Literature," "Literature Review," "Theoretical Framework," "Related Literature," "Background," or "Conceptual Framework"; or may not be labeled at all (see Chapters 4 and 5). By reviewing Appendixes A through D, the reader will find differences in the headings used. Koniak-Griffin et al. (2003) (Appendix A) have both a "Literature Review" and a "Theoretical Framework" section, Van Cleve et al. (2004) have an unlabeled literature section in the beginning of the article and a section labeled "Theoretical Framework" (Appendix B), and Davison et al. (2003) (Appendix D) have a section labeled "Literature Review" and one labeled "Conceptual Framework." All three studies have literature reviews and use a framework. One style is not better than another; all of the studies in the appendixes contain all the critical elements but present the elements differently.

Hypothesis/Research Question

A study's research questions or hypotheses can also be presented in different ways (see Chapter 3). Research reports in journals often do not have separate headings for reporting the "Hypotheses" or "Research Question." They are often embedded in the "Introduction" or "Background" section or not labeled at all (e.g., as in the studies in the appendixes). If a study uses hypotheses, the researcher may report whether the hypotheses were or were not supported toward the end of the article in the "Results" or "Findings" section. Quantitative research studies have hypotheses or research questions. Qualitative research studies do not have hypotheses but have research questions and purposes. Koniak-Griffin et al. (2003) (Appendix A) and Davison et al. (2003) (Appendix D) have hypotheses. Plach et al. (2004) (Appendix C) and Van Cleve et al. (2004) (Appendix B) have aims and purpose.

Research Design

The type of research design can be found in the abstract, within the purpose statement, or in the introduction to the "Procedures" or "Methods" section, or not stated at all (see Chapters 7, 10, and 11). For example, the four studies in the appendixes identify the design type in the abstract.

One of your first objectives is to determine whether the study is qualitative (see Chapters 6 and 9) or quantitative so that the appropriate criteria are used. Although the rigor of the critiquing criteria addressed do not substantially change, some of the terminology of the questions differs for qualitative and quantitative studies. For instance, in regard to Davison et al. (see Appendix D), you might be asking if the hypotheses were generated from the theoretical framework or literature review and if the design chosen was appropriate and consistent with the study's problem and purpose (see Chapters 9, 10, and 11). With a qualitative study such as that by Plach et al. (see Appendix C), however, you might be asking if the researchers conducted the study consistent with the principles of qualitative research and therefore focused on the identification of the themes of social experience (see Chapters 6 and 7).

Do not get discouraged if you cannot easily determine the design. More often than not, the specific design is not stated or, if an advanced design is used, the details are not spelled out. One of the best strategies is to review the chapters in this text that address designs (Chapters 7, 10, and 11) and to ask your professors for assistance. The following tips will help you determine whether the study you are reading uses a quantitative design:

- Hypotheses are stated or implied (see Chapter 3).
- The terms *control* and *treatment group* appear (see Chapter 10).
- The term *survey, correlational,* or *ex post facto* is used (see Chapter 11).
- The term *random* or *convenience* is mentioned in relation to the sample (see Chapter 12).
- Variables are measured by instruments or scales (see Chapter 14).
- Reliability and validity of instruments are discussed (see Chapter 15).
- Statistical analyses are used (see Chapter 16).

In contrast, generally qualitative studies do not usually focus on "numbers." Some qualitative studies may use standard quantitative terms (e.g., subjects) rather than qualitative terms (e.g., informants). Deciding on the type of qualitative design can be confusing; one of the best strategies is to review this text's chapters on qualitative design (see Chapters 6 and 7), as well as to critique qualitative studies (see Chapter 8). Begin trying to link the study's design with the level of evidence associated with that design as illustrated in Table 2-3. This will give you a context for evaluating the strength and consistency of the findings and their applicability to practice. Reading Chapters 9, 10, and 11 will increase your understanding of how to link the levels of evidence with quantitative designs, and Chapters 6 and 7 will help you do the same with qualitative designs. Although many studies may not specify the particular design used, all studies inform the reader of the specific methodology used, which can help you decide the type of design used to guide the study.

Sampling

The population from which the sample was drawn is discussed in the section entitled "Methods" or "Methodology" under the subheadings of "Subjects" or "Sample" (see Chapter 12). For example, Davison and associates (2004) (Appendix D) discuss the sample under the title "Participants" in the "Methods" section as do Koniak-Griffin et al. (2003) (Appendix A). However, Van Cleve et al. (2004) (Appendix B) present the sample characteristics in a table noted in the "Results" section. Researchers should tell you both the population from which the sample was chosen and the number of subjects that participated in the study, as well as if they had subjects who dropped out of the study. The authors of all of the studies in the appendixes discuss their samples in enough detail so that the reader is quite clear about who the subjects are and how they were selected.

Reliability and Validity

The discussion related to instruments used to measure the variables of a study is usually included in a "Methods" section under the subheading of "Instruments" or "Measures" (see Chapter 14). The researcher usually describes the particular measure (i.e., instrument or scale) used by discussing its reliability and validity (see Chapter 15). Davison et al. (2004) (Appendix D) discuss each of the measures used in their "Methods" section under the subheading "Instruments." The reliability and validity of each measure were presented.

In some cases, researchers do not report on commonly used valid and reliable instruments in an article and may refer you to other references. Ask assistance from your instructor if you are in doubt about the validity or reliability of a study's instruments.

Procedures and Data-Collection Methods

The procedures used to collect data or the step-by-step way that the researcher(s) used the measures (instruments or scales) is generally given under the "Procedures" head (see Chapter 14). In each of the studies in Appendixes A, B, and D, the researchers indicate how they conducted the study in detail under the subheading "Procedure." Notice that the researchers in each study in Appendixes A, B, C, and D also provided information that the studies were approved by an Institutional Review Board (see Chapter 13), thereby ensuring that each meets ethical standards.

Data Analysis/Results

The data-analysis procedures (i.e., the statistical tests used and the results of descriptive and/or inferential tests applied in quantitative studies) are presented in the section labeled "Results" or "Findings" (see Chapters 16 and 17). Although qualitative studies do not use statistical tests, the procedures for analyzing the themes, concepts, and/or observational or print data are usually described in the "Method" or "Data Collection" section and reported in the "Results" or "Findings" section (see Appendix C and Chapters 7 and 8). Plach et al. (2004) (see Appendix C) report the results of their qualitative analysis in the "Results" section of the article.

Koniak-Griffin et al. (2003) (Appendix A) have two separate sections: one that describes the statistical analyses used to analyze the data, labeled "Statistical Analyses," and a second overall "Results" section that breaks down the findings according to the variables studied. In the qualitative study by Plach et al. (2004), the researchers describe the data analysis used in the "Method" section and the results are reported under the heading "Results."

Discussion

The last section of a research study is the "Discussion" section. As you will find when you read Chapters 18 and 19, in this section the researcher(s) tie(s) together all the pieces of the study and give(s) a picture of the study as a whole. The researcher(s) go back to the literature reviewed and discuss how their study is similar to or different from other studies. Researchers may report the results and discussion in one section but usually report their results in separate "Results" and "Discussion" sections (see Appendixes A, B, C, and D). One way is no better than the other. Journal and space limitations determine how these sections will be handled. Any new findings or unexpected findings are usually described in the "Discussion" section.

Recommendations and Implications

In some cases a researcher reports the implications, and limitations based on the findings, for practice and education and recommends future studies in a separate section labeled "Discussion" (see Appendixes A and B); in other cases this appears in several sections labeled with such titles as "Discussion," "Limitations," "Nursing Implications," and "Summary" (see Appendix D). In the qualitative study found in Appendix C, the "Discussion" section presents the overview of the findings and the implications for practice, education, and research. Again, one way is not better than the other—only different.

References

All of the references cited in a research or scholarly article are included at the end of the article. The main purpose of the reference list is to support the material presented by identifying the sources in a manner that allows for easy retrieval by the reader. Journals use various referencing styles to organize references.

Communicating Results

Communicating the results of a study can take the form of a research article, poster, or paper presentation (see Chapters 19 and 20). All are valid ways of providing nurses with the data and the ability to provide high-quality patient care based on research findings. Evidence-based nursing care plans and practice protocols, guidelines, or standards are outcome measures that effectively indicate communicated research.

As you develop critical thinking and reading skills by using the strategies presented in this chapter, you will become more familiar with the research and critiquing processes. Your ability to read and critique research articles will gradually improve. You will be well on your way to becoming a knowledgeable user of research from nursing and other scientific disciplines for application in nursing practice.

Critical Thinking Challenges

- It is claimed that the critical reading of research articles may require a minimum of three or four readings. Is this always the case? What assumptions underlie this claim?
- Why is reading for analysis a necessary stage of the critical reading process before attempting to critique a study?
- To synthesize a research article, what questions must you first be able to answer?
- How would you answer a nursing colleague who stated the following: "Why can't I say in my critique that, based on the findings of this study, the researchers proved their hypotheses?"
- Margaret is a part-time baccalaureate nursing student who works full-time as an RN in an actue care ICU setting and is a full-time mother of two children under the age of 4 years. Discuss both the disadvantages and the advantages of Margaret using the critical reading strategies found in Box 2-1.
- If nurses with a baccalaureate degree are not expected to conduct research, how can nursing students be expected to critique each step of the research process, or an entire study, or several studies? Support either a pro or con position.
- Discuss several strategies that might motivate practicing nurses to critically appraise research articles.
- What level of evidence is presented in the article by Van Cleve and colleagues (2004) (see Appendix B)? Justify your answer.

KEY POINTS

- The best way to develop skill in critiquing research studies is to use critical thinking and reading skills while reading research articles.
- Critical thinking in learning the research process, as well as critiquing, requires disciplined, self-directed thinking.
- Critical thinking and critical reading skills will enable you to question the appropriateness of the content of a research article, apply standards or critiquing criteria to assess the study's scientific merit for use in practice, or consider alternative ways of handling the same topic.
- Critical reading involves active interpretation and objective assessment of an article, looking for key concepts, ideas, and justifications.
- Critical reading requires four stages of understanding: preliminary (skimming), comprehensive, analysis, and synthesis. Each stage includes strategies to increase your critical reading skills.

- Critically reading for preliminary understanding is gained by skimming, or quickly and lightly reading, an article to become familiar with its content or obtain a general sense of the material.
- Critically reading for comprehensive understanding is designed to increase your understanding of the concepts and research terms in relation to the context of the study as a whole.
- Critically reading for analysis understanding is designed to break the content into parts so that each part of the study is understood; the critiquing process begins at this stage.
- Critical reading to reach the goal of synthesis understanding is to combine the parts of a research study into a whole. During this final stage the reader determines how each step relates to all of the steps of the research process, how well the study meets the critiquing criteria, and the usefulness of the study for practice.

- Critiquing is the process of objectively and critically evaluating the strengths and weaknesses of a research article for scientific merit and application to practice, theory, or education; the need for more research on the topic/clinical problem is also addressed at this stage.
- Critiquing criteria are the measures, standards, evaluation guides, or questions used to judge the worth of a research study.
- Each article should be reviewed for level of evidence as a means of judging the application to practice.
- Research articles have different formats and styles depending on journal manuscript requirements and whether they are quantitative or qualitative studies.
- Basic steps of the research process are presented in journal articles in various ways. Detailed examples of such variations can be found in chapters throughout this text.
- Evidence-based practice begins with the careful reading and understanding of each article contributing to the practice of nursing.
- A level of evidence model is a tool for evaluating the strength (quality, quantity, and consistency) of a research study and its findings.

REFERENCES

Agency for Healthcare Research and Quality (AHRQ): Systems to rate the strength of scientific evidence. File inventory, Evidence Report/Technology Assessment No. 47, AHRQ Publication No. 02-E016, Rockville, Md.

Davison BJ, Goldenberg SL, Gleave ME, and Degner LF: Provision of individualized information to men and their partners to facilitate treatment decision making in prostate cancer, *Oncol Nurse Forum* 30: 107-114, 2003.

Elder L, Paul R: *The thinker's guide to the art of strategic thinking,* Dillon Beach, Calif, 2004, Foundation for Critical Thinking.

Koniak-Griffin D, Verzemnieks IL, Anderson NLR, Janna Lesser MB, Kim S, and Turner-Pluta C: Nurse visitation for adolescent mothers: two-year infant health and maternal outcomes, *Nurs Res* 52: 127-135, 2003.

Melnyk BM, Fineout-Overholt E: Making the case for evidence-based practice. In Melnyk BM, Fineout-Overholt E, editors: *Evidence-based practice in nursing and health care,* Philadelphia, 2005, Lippincott Williams & Wilkins.

Paul R, Elder L: *Critical thinking: tools for taking charge of your learning and your life,* Englewood, NJ, 2001, Prentice-Hall.

Paul R, Elder L: *The thinker's guide on how to read a paragraph,* Dillon Beach, Calif, 2003, Foundation for Critical Thinking.

Plach SK, Stevens PE, and Moss VA: Social role experiences of women living with rheumatoid arthritis, *J Fam Nurs* 10: 33-49, 2004.

Sackett DL, Straus SE, Richardson WS, Rosenburg W, and Hayes RB: *Evidence-based medicine: how to practice and teach EBM,* London, 2000, Churchill Livingstone.

Van Cleve L, Bossert E, Beecroft P, Adlard K, Alvarez O, and Savedra MC: The pain experience of children with leukemia during the first year after diagnosis, *Nurs Res* 53: 1-10, 2004.

FOR FURTHER STUDY

Go to your Companion CD for review activities for this chapter.

evolve Go to Evolve at http://evolve.elsevier.com/LoBiondo/ for WebLinks, Content Updates, and additional research articles, for practice in reviewing and critiquing.

3

JUDITH HABER

Developing Research Questions and Hypotheses

KEY TERMS

conceptual definitions
dependent variable
directional hypothesis
hypothesis
independent variable

nondirectional hypothesis
operational definitions
population
purpose
research hypothesis

research question
statistical hypothesis
testability
theory
variables

LEARNING OUTCOMES

After reading this chapter, the student should be able to do the following:

- Describe how the research question and hypothesis relate to the other components of the research process.
- Describe the process of identifying and refining a research question.
- Identify the criteria for determining the significance of a research question.
- Discuss the purpose of developing a clinical question.
- Identify the characteristics of research questions and hypotheses.
- Discuss the appropriate use of the purpose, aim, or objective of a research study.
- Discuss how the purpose, research question, and hypothesis suggest the level of evidence to be obtained from the findings of a research study.
- Describe the advantages and disadvantages of directional and nondirectional hypotheses.
- Compare and contrast the use of statistical vs. research hypotheses.
- Discuss the appropriate use of research questions vs. hypotheses in a research study.
- Discuss the differences between a research question and a clinical question in relation to evidence-based practice.
- Identify the criteria used for critiquing a research question and hypothesis.
- Apply the critiquing criteria to the evaluation of a research question and hypothesis in a research report.

STUDY RESOURCES

Go to your Companion CD for review activities for this chapter.

evolve Go to Evolve at http://evolve.elsevier.com/LoBiondo/ for Weblinks, Content Updates, and additional research articles for practice in reviewing and critiquing.

When nurses ask questions such as, "Why are things done this way?", "I wonder what would happen if . . . ?", "What characteristics are associated with . . . ?", or "What is the effect of . . . on patient outcomes?", they are often well on their way to developing a research question or hypothesis.

Formulating the research question or hypothesis is a key preliminary step in the research process. The **research question** (sometimes called the problem statement) presents the idea that is to be examined in the study and is the foundation of the research study. The **hypothesis** attempts to answer the research question.

Hypotheses can be considered intelligent hunches, guesses, or predictions that help researchers seek the solution or answer the research question. Hypotheses are a vehicle for testing the validity of the theoretical framework assumptions and provide a bridge between **theory** and the real world. In the scientific world, researchers derive hypotheses from theories and subject them to empirical testing. A theory's validity is not directly examined. Instead, it is through the hypotheses that the merit of a theory can be evaluated.

Research consumers often find research questions or hypotheses at the beginning of a research article. However, because of space constraints or stylistic considerations in such publications, they may be embedded in the purpose, aims, goals, or even in the results section of the research report. Nevertheless, it is equally important for both the consumer and the producer of research to understand the importance of research questions and hypotheses as the foundational elements of a research study. This chapter provides a working knowledge of quantitative research questions and hypotheses, as well as the standards for writing them and a set of criteria for evaluating them.

DEVELOPING AND REFINING A RESEARCH QUESTION: THE RESEARCHER'S PERSPECTIVE

A researcher spends a great deal of time refining a research idea into a testable research question. Unfortunately, the evaluator of a research study is not privy to this creative process because it occurs during the study's conceptualization. Although this section will not teach you how to formulate a research question, it is important to provide a glimpse of what the process of developing a research question may be like for a researcher.

As illustrated in Table 3-1, research questions or topics are not pulled from thin air. Research questions should indicate that practical experience, critical appraisal of the scientific literature, or interest in an untested theory has provided the basis for the generation of a research idea. The research question should reflect a refinement of the researcher's initial thinking. The evaluator of a research study should be able to discern that the researcher has done the following:

1. Defined a specific question area
2. Reviewed the relevant scientific literature
3. Examined the question's potential significance to nursing
4. Pragmatically examined the feasibility of studying the research question

Defining the Research Question

Brainstorming with teachers, advisors, or colleagues may provide valuable feedback that helps the researcher focus on a specific research question area. For example, suppose a researcher told a colleague that the area of interest was pain experienced by children with cancer. The colleague may have said, "What is it about the topic that specifically interests you?" Such a conversation may have initiated a chain of thought that resulted in a decision to explore the pain experiences, management strategies, and outcomes of children with cancer (children with leukemia during the first year after diagnosis). Figure 3-1 illustrates how a broad area of interest (pain experiences of children with cancer) was narrowed to a specific research topic (children's pain experience, pain management strategies, and outcomes during the first year after the diagnosis of leukemia).

 EVIDENCE-BASED PRACTICE TIP

A well-developed research question guides a focused search for scientific evidence about assessing, diagnosing, treating, or assisting patients with understanding of their prognosis related to a specific health problem.

Beginning the Literature Review

The databases that are searched (e.g., CINAHL, PsycINFO, MEDLINE, PubMed) for the literature review should reveal a relevant collection of articles that have been critically examined. Concluding sections in such articles, that is, the recommendations and implications for practice, often identify remaining gaps in the literature, the need for replication, or the need for extension of the knowledge base about a particular research focus (see Chapter 4). In the previous example about children's pain experience, man-

TABLE **3-1** **How Practical Experience, Scientific Literature, and Untested Theory Influence the Development of a Research Idea**

Area	Influence	Example
Practical experience	Clinical practice provides a wealth of experience from which research problems can be derived. The nurse may observe the occurrence of a particular event or pattern and become curious about why it occurs, as well as its relationship to other factors in the patient's environment.	Although breast self-examination (BSE) has long been recommended by nurses and other health care providers as a complement to mammography and clinical breast examination, only a small percentage of U.S. women report doing a monthly BSE, and nurses observe that an even smaller percentage of women perform this health-promotion self-care procedure proficiently. Nurses working in a women's health center speculate about the effect of a structured training protocol on improving thoroughness using two dimensions of BSE technique (i.e., depth of palpation and duration of the BSE examination in each of two search patterns [vertical strip and concentric circle]) using biomedical instrumentation (Leight et al., 2000).
Critical appraisal of the scientific literature	The critical appraisal of research studies that appear in journals may indirectly suggest a problem area by stimulating the reader's thinking. The nurse may observe the outcome data from a single study or a group of related studies that provide the basis for developing a pilot study or quality improvement project to determine the effectiveness of this intervention in their own practice setting.	At a staff meeting where cost-effectiveness was being discussed, a nurse reported that she had read an article indicating that comprehensive discharge planning and home follow-up for hospitalized elders at risk for readmission by advanced practice nurses have demonstrated short-term reductions in readmissions of elderly patients. At 24 weeks after discharge, Medicare reimbursements for health services were about $1.2 million in the control group vs. about $0.6 million for the intervention group. There were no significant differences in post-discharge acute care visits, functional status, depression, or patient satisfaction. Another nurse said that other articles on file indicated that this model had been studied using other patient populations (i.e., very low birth weight

Area	Influence	Example
Critical appraisal of the scientific literature–cont'd		babies, women having hysterectomies, and unplanned cesarean births) with similar quality and cost-effectiveness outcomes (**Naylor et al., 1999**). However, another nurse reported reading an integrative review of the literature that highlighted the strengths and weaknesses of nine intervention studies of family caregivers with hospitalized elderly relatives, among them the **Naylor (1999)** study (**Li, Melnyk, and McCann, 2004**). This review cautioned the reader about accepting the conclusions of this group of studies because of weaknesses in sample size, lack of a comparison intervention, lack of consistent involvement of family caregivers, and lack of commonly defined and measured variables. The group agreed that despite the shortcomings of the studies, there was a sufficient body of related research findings to use in defining their own problem focus and would capitalize on the recommendations of the authors.
Gaps in the literature	A research idea may also be suggested by a critical appraisal of the literature that identifies gaps in the literature and suggests areas for future study. Research ideas also can be generated by research reports that suggest the value of replicating a particular study to extend or refine the existing scientific knowledge base.	A nurse who had just begun working at a cancer center in a urological clinic observed that a significant number of men newly diagnosed with prostate cancer were presenting at their surgeon's office for treatment discussions with little or no knowledge of the disease or potential treatment options. Men and their partners indicated that informal sources such as family, friends, and men with prostate cancer were the most frequent source of information. While men with prostate cancer have been shown to prefer to participate in decision making about their treatment, the extent to which partners wish to participate in treatment decisions and the influence they have on final treatment decisions are unknown. Investigators have demonstrated that providing information to men who are newly diagnosed with prostate cancer does result in benefits such as increased participation in treatment decision making, decreased levels of anxiety, and improved communication of illness-related information to family. The benefits of providing information to partners are unknown. The nurse found no controlled research studies that provided individualized information to men newly diagnosed with prostate cancer (and their partners) and the impact of that information on levels of psychological distress (state anxiety and depression) and active involvement in treatment decision making (Davison et al., 2003; Appendix D).

Continued

TABLE **3-1 How Practical Experience, Scientific Literature, and Untested Theory Influence the Development of a Research Idea—cont'd**

Area	Influence	Example
Interest in untested theory	Verification of an untested nursing theory provides a relatively uncharted territory from which research problems can be derived. Inasmuch as theories themselves are not tested, a researcher may consider investigating a particular concept or set of concepts related to a particular nursing theory or a theory from another discipline. The deductive process would be used to generate the research question. The researcher would pose questions such as the following: "If this theory is correct, what kind of behavior will I expect to observe in particular patients and under which conditions?" "If this theory is valid, what kind of supporting evidence will I find?"	Development of theoretical models that are derived from nursing and related literature are conducted to provide empirical support for the accuracy of a particular theoretical model that examines the fit between the hypothesized model and the data. Using a theoretical framework synthesized from the Roy adaptation model (Roy and Andrews, 1999), Murrell-Armstrong's empowerment matrix (Murrell and Meredith, 2000), and Harter's developmental perspective (Harter, 1999), a nurse researcher provided a unique perspective for looking at preadolescents with attention deficit/hyperactivity disorder (ADHD) and designing, implementing, and evaluating a school-based, nurse-facilitated support group for improving the self-worth of preadolescents with ADHD. The significant findings support the role of the school nurse as facilitator of the support group, a role consistent with the Roy adaptation model that indicates that the nurse's role is one of interaction directly with patients. It is also consistent with Harter's developmental perspective on preadolescence, which is posited to be a time when children compare themselves to others, either positively or negatively, with their peers. Consequently, preadolescence is an optimal time to implement self-esteem interventions designed to help adolescents with ADHD. Finally, the significant changes in perception of self-worth, perceptions of social acceptance, athletic competence, and physical appearance validate the Murrell-Armstrong empowerment matrix. Overall, the findings lend support to the use of a school nurse facilitated support group model for preadolescents with ADHD based on three theoretical perspectives (Frame, Kelly, and Bayley, 2003).

agement strategies, and outcomes, the researcher may have conducted a preliminary review of books and journals for theories and research studies on factors apparently critical to pain assessment, management strategies, and outcomes in children with cancer. These factors, termed variables in the language of research, should be potentially relevant, of interest, and measurable.

Possible relevant factors mentioned in the literature begin with an exploration of the relationship between pain perception, intensity, and experience; pain management strategies; and outcomes of effective pain management in children. Other variables, such as demographic characteristics of children and their parents, type of leukemia, and also type of diagnostic and treatment procedures, are also suggested as essential

---

Idea Emerges

Pain experiences of children with cancer

↓

Brainstorming

- What are the dimensions of the pain experience for children with acute lymphocytic leukemia (ALL) (eg. perception, evaluation, response)?
- What pain management strategies are used (eg. medication, play therapy, distraction)?
- How effective are they in alleviating pain (eg. perspective of patient, family, health provider)?
- What are the outcomes of effective pain management (eg. functional status, quality of life, morbidity, health service utilization)?

↓

Literature Review

- Electronic search of CINAHL, MEDLINE, and Evidence-based Nursing using the search terms, children, leukemia, and pain.
- The literature suggests that cancer pain research with children has focused almost exclusively on procedure-related pain with an emphasis on non-pharmacological strategies for managing pain.
- Pain was a presenting symptom at diagnosis with pain intensity ranging from mild to severe.
- Significant lack of knowledge about Latino children and how they experience and report pain.
- Four persisting treatment problems were mucositis, abdominal pain, neuropathic pain, and pain related to infection pain.
- Minimal data on dimensions of pain experience, effective pain management strategies, and outcomes.
- The Symptom Management Model of the University of California School of Nursing could be used to theoretically frame the symptom experience (pain), symptom management (pharmacological and non-pharmacological interventions), and symptom outcome dimensions (quality of life, functional status, and health resource utilization).

↓

Identify Variables

Potential Variables:
- Pain experience
  - Perception
  - Evaluation
  - Response
- Pain management strategies
- Outcomes
  - Functional status
  - Quality of life
  - Morbidity/co-morbidity
  - Health service utilization

↓

Research Question Formulated

What is childrens' pain experience, management strategies, and outcomes during the first year after the diagnosis of acute lymphocytic leukemia (ALL)?

Figure 3-1. Development of a research question.

---

to consider. This information can then be used by the researcher to further define the research question and address a gap in the literature, as well as extend the knowledge base related to the impact of pain management strategies on children's outcomes including quality of life and functional status. At this point the researcher could write the following tentative research question: What are childrens' pain experiences, management strategies, and outcomes during the first year after the diagnosis of acute lymphocytic leukemia (ALL)? Although the research problem is not yet in its final form, readers can envision the interrelatedness of the initial definition of the question area, the literature review, and the refined research question. Readers of research reports examine the end product of this process in the form of a research question and/or hypothesis, so it is important to have an appreciation of how the researcher gets to that point in constructing a study (Van Cleve et al., 2004; see Appendix B).

 HELPFUL H I N T

Reading the literature review or theoretical framework section of a research article helps you trace the development of the implied research question, and/or hypothesis.

Significance

Before proceeding to a final development of the research question, it is crucial that the researcher has examined the question's potential significance to nursing. The research question should have the potential to contribute to and extend the scientific body of nursing knowledge. Guidelines for selecting research questions should meet the following criteria:

- Patients, nurses, the medical community in general, and society will potentially benefit from the knowledge derived from the study.
- The results will be applicable for nursing practice, education, or administration.
- The results will be theoretically relevant.

- The findings will lend support to untested theoretical assumptions, extend or challenge an existing theory, fill a gap in the literature, or clarify a conflict in the literature.
- The findings will potentially provide evidence that supports developing, retraining, or revising nursing practices or policies.

If the research question has not met any of these criteria, it is wise to extensively revise the question or discard it. For example, in the previously cited research question, the significance of the question includes the following facts:

- Children with cancer, including those with leukemia, experience pain from the disease process, diagnostic procedures, and the treatment.
- There is limited knowledge of children reporting pain over time.
- There is a significant lack of knowledge about Latino children and how they experience and report pain.
- There are minimal data on dimensions of the pain experience, effective management strategies, and outcomes.
- This study sought to fill a gap in the related literature by examining the pain experience, management strategies, and outcomes during the first year after the diagnosis of acute leukemia.
- This study sought to extend the knowledge base about this phenomenon, thereby providing a foundation for the development and testing of interventions.

☀ EVIDENCE-BASED PRACTICE TIP

Without a well-developed research question, the researcher may search for wrong, irrelevant, or unnecessary information. This will be a barrier to identifying the potential significance of the study.

Feasibility

The feasibility of a research question must be pragmatically examined. Regardless of how significant or researchable a question may be, pragmatic considerations such as time; availability of subjects, facilities, equipment, and money; experience of the researcher; and any ethical considerations may cause the researcher to decide that the question is inappropriate because it lacks feasibility (see Chapters 6, 9, and 13).

THE FULLY DEVELOPED RESEARCH QUESTION

When a researcher finalizes a research question, the following three characteristics should be evident:

- It clearly identifies the variables under consideration.
- It specifies the population being studied.
- It implies the possibility of empirical testing.

Because each of these elements is crucial to the formulation of a satisfactory research question, the criteria will be discussed in greater detail.

Variables

Researchers call the properties that they study variables. Such properties take on different values. Thus a **variable** is, as the name suggests, something that varies. Properties that differ from each other, such as age, weight, height, religion, and ethnicity, are examples of variables. Researchers attempt to understand how and why differences in one variable relate to differences in another variable. For example, a researcher may be concerned about the variable of pain in postoperative patients. It is a variable because not all postoperative patients have the same amount of pain—or any pain at all. A researcher may also be interested in what other factors can be linked to postoperative pain. There is clinical evidence to suggest that anxiety is associated with pain. Thus anxiety is also a variable, because not all postoperative patients have the same amount of anxiety—or any anxiety at all.

When speaking of variables, the researcher is essentially asking, "Is X related to Y? What is the effect of X on Y? How are X_1 and X_2 related to Y?" The researcher is asking a question about the relationship between one or more independent variables and a dependent variable.*

An **independent variable,** usually symbolized by **X,** is the variable that has the presumed effect on the dependent variable. In experimental research studies, the researcher manipulates the independent variable. For example, a nurse may study how different methods of administering pain medication affect the patient's perception of pain. The researcher may manipulate the independent variable (i.e., the method of administering pain medication) by using nurse- vs. patient-controlled administration of analgesia (see Chapter 10). In nonexperimental research, the independent variable is not manipulated and is assumed to have occurred naturally before or during the study. For example, the researcher may be studying the relationship between the level of anxiety and the perception of pain. The independent variable—the level of anxiety—is not manipulated; it is just presumed to occur and is observed and measured as it naturally happens (see Chapter 11).

The **dependent variable,** represented by **Y,** is often referred to as the consequence or the presumed effect that varies with a change in the independent variable. The dependent variable is not manipulated. It is observed and assumed to vary with changes in the independent variable. Predictions are made from the independent variable to the dependent variable. It is the dependent variable that the researcher is interested in understanding, explaining, or predicting. For example, it might be assumed that the perception of pain (i.e., the dependent variable) will vary with changes in the level of anxiety (i.e., the independent variable). In this case we are trying to explain the perception of pain in relation to the level of anxiety.

Although variability in the dependent variable is assumed to depend on changes in the independent variable, this does not imply that there

is a causal relationship between **X** and **Y** or that changes in variable **X** cause variable **Y** to change. Let us look at an example in which nurses' attitudes toward patients with depression were studied. The researcher discovered that older nurses had a more negative attitude about patients with depression than younger nurses. The researcher did not conclude that the nurses' negative attitudes toward patients with depression were because of their age, but at the same time it is apparent that there is a directional relationship between age and negative attitudes about patients with depression. That is, as the nurses' ages increase, their attitudes about patients with depression become more negative. This example highlights the fact that causal relationships are not necessarily implied by the independent and dependent variables; rather, only a relational statement with possible directionality is proposed. Table 3-2 presents a number of examples to help you learn how to write research questions. Practice substituting other variables for the examples in Table 3-2. You will be surprised at the skill you develop in writing and critiquing research questions with greater ease.

Although one independent and one dependent variable are used in the examples just given, there is no restriction on the number of variables that can be included in a research question. Remember, however, that questions should not be unnecessarily complex or unwieldly, particularly in beginning research efforts. Research questions that include more than one independent or dependent variable may be broken down into subquestions that are more concise.

Finally, it should be noted that variables are not inherently independent or dependent. A variable that is classified as independent in one study may be considered dependent in another study. For example, a nurse may review an article about sexual behaviors that are predictive of risk for HIV/AIDS. In this case, HIV/AIDS is the dependent variable. When another article about the relationship between HIV/AIDS and maternal parenting practices is considered, HIV/AIDS status is the independent variable. Whether a

---

* In cases in which multiple independent or dependent variables are present, subscripts are used to indicate the number of variables under consideration.

TABLE **3-2 Research Question Format**

Type	Format	Example
Quantitative Experimental		
Correlational	Is there a relationship between **X** (independent variable) and **Y** (dependent variable) in the specified population?	Is there a relationship between effectiveness of pain management strategies and quality of life?
Comparative	Is there a difference in **Y** (dependent variable) between people who have **X** characteristic (independent variable) and those who do not have **X** characteristic?	Is there a difference in prevention of osteoporosis in at-risk breast cancer survivors who receive a combination of long-term progressive strength training exercises, alendronate, calcium, and vitamin D compared to those who do not?
Quantitative	Is there a difference in **Y** (dependent variable) between Group A who received **X** (independent variable) and Group B who did not receive **X**?	What is the difference in physical, social, and emotional adjustment in women with breast cancer (and their partners) who have received phase-specific standardized education by video vs. phase-specific telephone counseling?
Qualitative		
Phenomenological	What is/was it like to have **X**?	How do older adults learn to live with early stage dementia?

variable is independent or dependent is a function of the role it plays in a particular study.

Population

The **population** being studied must be specified in the research question. If the scope of the question has been narrowed to a specific focus and the variables have been clearly identified, the nature of the population will be evident to the reader of a research report. For example, a research question may ask, "Is there a relationship between the type of discharge planning for elders hospitalized with heart failure and the caregivers?" This question suggests that the population under consideration includes elders hospitalized for heart failure and their caregivers. It is also implied that some of the elders and their caregivers were involved in a professional-patient partnership model of discharge planning in contrast to other elders who received the typical discharge planning. The researcher or reader will have an initial idea of the composition of the

study population from the outset (see Chapter 12).

 EVIDENCE-BASED PRACTICE TIP

Make sure that the population of interest and setting have been clearly described so that if you were going to replicate the study, you would know exactly who the study population needed to be.

Testability

The research question must imply that it is **testable,** that is, measurable by either qualitative or quantitative methods. For example, the research question "Should postoperative patients control how much pain medication they receive?" is stated incorrectly for a variety of reasons. One reason is that it is not testable; it represents a value statement rather than a research question. A scientific research question must propose a relationship between an independent and a dependent variable and do this in such a way that it indicates that the variables of the relationship can somehow be measured. Many interesting and important clinical questions are not valid research questions because they are not amenable to testing.

The question "Should postoperative patients control how much pain medication they receive?" could be revised from a philosophic question to a research question that implies testability. Two examples of the revised research question might be the following:

- Is there a relationship between patient-controlled analgesia (PCA) vs. nurse-administered analgesia and perception of postoperative pain?
- What is the effect of PCA on pain ratings by postoperative patients?

These examples illustrate the relationship between the variables, identify the independent and dependent variables, and imply the testability of the research question.

Now that the elements of the formal research question have been presented in greater detail, this information can be integrated by formulating a formal research problem about the adaptation of families faced with stressful health care experiences (e.g., their child's need for organ transplantation). Earlier in this chapter, the following unrefined research problem was formulated: What are children's pain experiences, management strategies, and outcomes during the first year after diagnosis of acute lymphocytic leukemia (ALL)? This problem statement was originally derived from a general area of interest—pain experiences of children with cancer. The topic was more specifically defined by delineating a particular problem area—pain experiences, pain management strategies, and outcomes (e.g., functional status, quality of life, morbidity, health service utilization)—during the first year following a diagnosis of leukemia. The problem crystallized further after a preliminary literature review and emerged in the

unrefined form just given. With the four criteria inherent in a satisfactory research question, it is now possible to propose a refined research question, that is, one that specifically states the question and specifies the relationship of the key variables in the study, the population being studied, and the empirical testability of the question. Congruent with these three criteria, the following research question can then be formulated: What are children's pain experiences, management strategies, and outcomes during the first year after diagnosis of acute lymphocytic leukemia (ALL)? (Van Cleve et al., 2004). Table 3-3 identifies the components of this research question as they relate to and are congruent with the three research question criteria.

 HELPFUL H I N T

Remember that research questions are often not explicitly stated. The reader has to infer the research question from the title of the report, the abstract, the introduction, or the purpose.

DEVELOPING AND REFINING A CLINICAL QUESTION: A CONSUMER'S PERSPECTIVE

Practicing nurses, as well as students, are challenged to keep their practice up-to-date by searching for, retrieving, and critiquing research articles that apply to practice issues that are encountered in their clinical setting (Cullum, 2000). They strive to use the current best evidence from research in clinical and health care decisions. Although research consumers are not conducting research studies, their search for information from practice is also converted into focused, structured clinical questions. Using similar criteria related to framing a research question, the focused clinical questions are used as a basis for searching the literature to identify supporting evidence from research. The

TABLE **3-3** **Components of the Research Question and Related Criteria**

Variables	Population	Testability

Independent variable:
  Pain perception
  Pain evaluation
  Pain management strategies
Dependent variable:
  Management effectiveness
  Functional status
	Children diagnosed with acute lymphocytic leukemia (ALL)	Differential effect of pain and management strategies on management effectiveness and functional status

TABLE **3-4** **Consumer Perspective: Elements of a Clinical Question**

Situation	Intervention	Counterintervention	Outcome
People with advanced cancer	Pain diaries	No pain diaries	Increased pain control

significance of the clinical question becomes apparent as the research evidence from the literature is critiqued. The research evidence is used side by side with clinical expertise and the patient's perspective to develop or revise nursing standards, protocols, and policies that are used to plan and implement patient care (Cullum, 2000; Sackett, et al., 2000; Thompson et al., 2004). Issues or questions can arise from multiple clinical and managerial situations. Using the example of pain, albeit from a different perspective, a nurse working in a palliative care setting wondered whether completing pain diaries was a useful thing in the palliative care of patients with advanced cancer. She wondered whether time was being spent developing something that had previously been shown to be useless or even harmful. After all, it is conceivable that monitoring one's pain in a diary actually heightens one's awareness and experience of pain. To focus the nurse's search of the literature, she developed the following question: *Does the use of pain diaries in the palliative care of patients with cancer lead to improved pain control?* Sometimes it is helpful for nurses who develop clinical questions from a consumer perspective to consider three elements

as they frame their focused question: (1) the situation, (2) the intervention, and (3) the outcome:

- The situation is the patient or problem being addressed. This can be a single patient or a group of patients with a particular health problem (palliative care of patients with cancer).
- The intervention is the dimension of health care interest and often asks whether a particular intervention is a useful treatment (pain diaries).
- The outcome addresses the effect of the treatment (intervention) for this patient or patient population in terms of quality and cost (decreased pain perception/low cost). It essentially answers whether the intervention makes a difference for the patient population.

The individual parts of the question are vital pieces of information to remember when it comes to searching for evidence in the literature. One of the easiest ways to do this is to use a table as illustrated in Table 3-4. Examples of clinical questions are highlighted in Box 3-1. Chapter 4 will provide numerous examples of how to effectively search the literature to find answers to

BOX 3-1   EXAMPLES OF CLINICAL QUESTIONS

- Do self-management educational interventions improve lung function, decrease morbidity, and lessen the need for professional health care in children and adolescents with asthma (Handoll et al., 2002)?
- How do women with ovarian cancer experience cancer recurrence (Howell, Fitch, and Deane, 2003)?
- Do personal factors (education and intrinsic religiosity) and contextual factors (extrinsic religiosity and sources of information), either separately or combined, function as moderators in explaining intervention benefits on specific outcomes (level of cancer knowledge, patient-provider communication) (Mishel et al., 2003)?
- In postmenopausal women, does estrogen plus progesterone hormone therapy increase the risk of abnormal mammographic results and diagnosis of breast cancer (Chlebowski et al., 2003)?

- In postmenopausal women, does exercise slow bone loss or have an effect on axial and appendicular bone density (Bonaiuti et al., 2002)?
- Do unfractionated heparin (UH) levels, low molecular weight heparin (LMWH) levels, or physical methods (compression stockings and calf or foot pumps) prevent deep venous thrombosis (DVT) and pulmonary embolism (PE) after surgery for hip fracture in elderly patients (Handoll et al., 2002)?
- Is there a significant difference in the incidence of menopausal hot flashes between conditions of fasting and experimentally sustained (130-140 mg/dl) blood glucose concentrations (Dormire and Reame, 2003)?
- In patients with diabetes and high blood pressure (BP) or high cholesterol, is a nurse-led hypertension or hyperlipidemia clinic more effective than usual care for controlling BP and lipid concentrations (New et al., 2003)?

questions posed by researchers and research consumers.

 EVIDENCE-BASED PRACTICE TIP

You should be formulating clinical questions that arise from your clinical practice. Once you have developed a focused question, you will search the literature for the best available evidence to answer your clinical question.

STUDY PURPOSE, AIMS, OR OBJECTIVES

Once the research question is developed and the literature review is critiqued in terms of the level, strength, and quality of evidence available for the particular research question, the purpose, aims, or objectives of the study become focused so that the researcher can decide whether a hypothesis should be tested or a research question answered.

The **purpose** of the study encompasses the aims or goals the investigator hopes to achieve with the research, not the question to be answered. For example, a nurse working with rehabilitation patients who have bladder dysfunction may be disturbed by the high incidence of urinary tract infections. The nurse may propose the following research question: "What is the optimum frequency of changing urinary drainage bags in patients with bladder dysfunction to reduce the incidence of urinary tract infection?" If this nurse were to design a study, its purpose might be to determine the differential effect of a 1-week and a 4-week urinary drainage bag change schedule on the incidence of urinary tract infections in patients with bladder dysfunction. The purpose communicates more than just the nature of the question. Through the researcher's selection of verbs, the purpose statement suggests the manner in which the researcher sought to study the question and the level of evidence to be obtained through the study findings. Verbs like *discover, explore,* or *describe* suggest an investigation of an infrequently researched topic that might appropriately be guided by research questions rather than hypotheses. In contrast, verb statements indicating that the purpose is to test the effectiveness of an intervention or compare two alternative nursing strategies suggest a study with a better-established knowledge base that is hypothesis testing in nature. The research consumer should be aware that when the purpose of a study is to test the effectiveness of an intervention or compare the effectiveness of two or more interventions, the level of evidence is likely to have more strength and rigor than a study whose purpose is to explore or describe phenomena (see Table 2-3 in Chapter 2). Box 3-2 provides other examples of purpose, aims, and objectives.

 EVIDENCE-BASED PRACTICE TIP

The purpose, aims, or objectives often provide the most information about the intent of the research question and hypotheses and suggest the level of evidence to be obtained from the findings of the study.

DEVELOPING THE RESEARCH HYPOTHESIS

Like the research question, hypotheses are often not stated explicitly in a research article. The evaluator will often find that hypotheses are embedded in the data analysis, results, or discussion section of the research report. It is then up to the reader to discern the nature of the hypotheses being tested. For example, in the study by Van Cleve and colleagues (2004), the hypotheses are embedded in the *Results* section of the article; the reader must interpret that the statement, "The older children (self-report) showed a significant relation between pain intensity and management effectiveness in interviews, indicating that pain decreased as management effectiveness increased," represents the hypothesis that tests the relationship between pain intensity and management effectiveness in children with ALL. In light of that stylistic reality, it is important to be acquainted with the components of hypotheses, how they are developed, and the standards for writing and evaluating them.

Hypotheses flow from the research question, literature review, and theoretical framework. Figure 3-2 illustrates this flow. A **hypothesis** is a statement about the relationship between two or

---

BOX 3-2 EXAMPLES OF PURPOSE STATEMENTS

- The purpose of this study was to examine outcomes of the existing brief psychiatric treatment program (Tucker, Moore, and Luedtke, 2000).
- The aim of this study was to describe the scientific basis of the polydipsia screening tool and evaluate its scientific properties (Reynolds, Schmid, and Broome, 2004).
- The purpose of this study was to test the efficacy of therapeutic back massage (TBM) to reduce stress in spouses of patients with cancer (Goodfellow, 2003).
- The objective of the present study was to explore the role of substance abuse (smoking, alcohol, and drug use) and weight gain of less than 15 pounds during pregnancy as potential mediators of the relation between recent partner abuse and infant

birth weight, and to investigate the role of demographic risk factors as potential moderators for the impact of abuse on birth weight (Kearney et al., 2004).
- The purpose of this study was to determine whether providing individualized information to men (and their partners) who were newly diagnosed with prostate cancer would lower their levels of psychological distress and enable them to be more actively involved in treatment decision making (Davison et al., 2003).
- The purpose of this study was to evaluate the 2-year postbirth infant health and maternal outcomes of an early intervention program (EIP) of home visitation by public health nurses (PHNs) (Koniak-Griffin et al., 2003).

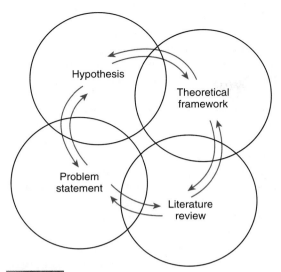

Figure 3-2. Interrelationships of research question, literature review, theoretical framework, and hypothesis.

more variables that suggests an answer to the research question. A hypothesis converts the research question into a declarative statement that predicts an expected outcome. It explains or predicts the relationship or differences between two or more variables in terms of expected results or outcomes of a study.

Each hypothesis represents a unit or subset of the research question. For example, a research question might be the following: "What is the effect of perceived job-related stress on job performance among hospital nurses and the effect of social support from coworkers on job stress, job performance, and the stress-performance relationship (AbuAlRub, 2004)?" This question can be broken down into the following two subquestions:

1. What is the effect of perceived job stress on job performance among hospital nurses?
2. What is the effect of social support from co-workers on job stress, job performance, and the stress-performance relationship?

A hypothesis can then be generated for each unit of the research question (i.e., the subquestions). The hypotheses of the research question already mentioned might be stated in the following way:

- **Hypothesis 1:** Hospital nurses with high social support from co-workers have low perceived job stress.
- **Hypothesis 2:** Nurses with high perceived job stress have low job performance.
- **Hypothesis 3:** Nurses with high social support from co-workers have high job performance.
- **Hypothesis 4:** As perceived job stress increases, nurses with high social support from co-workers will perform better than will nurses with less support.

The critiquer of a research report will want to evaluate whether the hypotheses of the study represent subsets of the main research question as illustrated by the examples just given.

Hypotheses are formulated before the study is actually conducted because they provide direction for the collection, analysis, and interpretation of data. Hypotheses have the following three purposes:

1. To provide a bridge between theory and practice, in this sense, unifying the two domains
2. To be powerful tools for the advancement of knowledge because they enable the researcher to objectively enter new areas of discovery and accumulate evidence
3. To provide direction for any research endeavor by tentatively identifying the anticipated outcome

---

 HELPFUL HINT

When hypotheses are not explicitly stated by the author at the end of the Introduction section or just before the Methods section, they will be embedded or implied in the Results or Discussion section of a research article.

Characteristics

Nurses who are conducting research or critiquing published research studies must have a working knowledge about what constitutes a "good" hypothesis. Such knowledge will enable them to have a standard for evaluating their own work or the work of others. The following discussion about the characteristics of hypotheses presents criteria to be used when formulating or evaluating a hypothesis.

Relationship Statement

The first characteristic of a hypothesis is that it is a declarative statement that identifies the predicted relationship between two or more variables. This implies that there is a systematic relationship between an independent variable and a dependent variable. The direction of the predicted relationship is also specified in this statement. Phrases such as *greater than; less than; positively, negatively,* or *curvilinearly related;* and *difference in* connote the directionality that is proposed in the hypothesis. The following is an example of a directional hypothesis: "The rate of continuous smoking abstinence (dependent variable) at 6 months postpartum, based on self-report and biochemical validation, will be significantly higher in the treatment group (postpartum counseling intervention) than in the control group (independent variable)." The two variables are explicitly identified, and the relational aspect of the prediction is contained in the phrase *significantly higher than.*

The nature of the relationship, either causal or associative, is also implied by the hypothesis. A causal relationship is one in which the researcher can predict that the independent variable (X) causes a change in the dependent variable (Y). In research, it is rare that one is in a firm enough position to take a definitive stand about a cause-and-effect relationship. For example, a researcher might hypothesize that relaxation training would have a significant effect on the physical and psychological health status of patients who have suffered myocardial infarction. It would be difficult for a researcher to predict a strong cause-and-effect relationship, however, because of the multiple intervening variables (e.g., age, medication, and lifestyle changes) that might also influence the subject's health status.

Variables are more commonly related in noncausal ways; that is, the variables are systematically related but in an associative way. This means that there is a systematic movement in the associated values of the two phenomena. For example, there is strong evidence that asbestos exposure is related to lung cancer. It is tempting to state that there is a causal relationship between asbestos exposure and lung cancer. Do not overlook the fact, however, that not all of those exposed to asbestos will have lung cancer and not all of those who have lung cancer have had asbestos exposure. Consequently, it would be scientifically unsound to take a position advocating the presence of a causal relationship between these two variables. Rather, one can say only that there is an associative relationship between the variables of asbestos exposure and lung cancer, a relationship in which there is a strong systematic association between the two phenomena.

Testability

The second characteristic of a hypothesis is its **testability.** This means that the variables of the study must lend themselves to observation, measurement, and analysis. The hypothesis is either supported or not supported after the data have been collected and analyzed. The predicted outcome proposed by the hypothesis will or will not be congruent with the actual outcome when the hypothesis is tested. Hypotheses advance scientific knowledge by confirming or refuting theories.

Hypotheses may fail to meet the criteria of testability because the researcher has not made a prediction about the anticipated outcome, the variables are not observable or measurable, or the hypothesis is couched in terms that are value-laden. Table 3-5 illustrates each of these points and provides a remedy for each problem.

TABLE **3-5 Hypotheses that Fail to Meet Criteria of Testability**

Problematic Hypothesis	Problematic Issue	Revised Hypothesis
Coping is related to adaptation.	No predictive statement about the relationship is made; so the relationship is not verifiable.	Coping is positively related to adaptation.
Patients who receive preoperative instruction have less postoperative emotional stress than patients who do not.	The "postoperative stress" variable must be specifically defined so that it is observable or measurable, or the relationship is not testable.	Patients who attend preoperative education classes have less postoperative stress than have patients who do not attend.
Small-group teaching will be better than individualized teaching for dietary compliance in patients with coronary artery disease (CAD).	"Better than" is a value-laden phrase that is not objective. Moral and ethical questions containing words such as *should, ought, better than,* and *bad for* are not scientifically testable.	Dietary compliance will be greater in patients with CAD receiving diet instruction in small groups than in CAD patients receiving individualized diet instruction.
Nurses' attitudes toward patients with tuberculosis cause changes in the patient's mood state.	Causal relationships are proposed without sufficient evidence.	Nurses' attitudes toward tuberculosis patients will be positively related to the emotional status of the tuberculosis patient.

 HELPFUL H I N T

When a hypothesis is complex (i.e., it contains more than one independent or dependent variable), it is difficult for the findings to indicate unequivocally that the hypothesis is supported or not supported. In such cases, the reader must infer which relationships are significant in the predicted direction from the Findings or Discussion section.

Theory Base

A sound hypothesis is consistent with an existing body of theory and research findings. Whether a hypothesis is arrived at inductively or deductively (see Chapter 5), it must be based on a sound scientific rationale. Readers should be able to identify the flow of ideas from the research idea to the literature review, to the theoretical framework, and through the research question(s) or hypotheses (see Chapters 4 and 5). Table 3-6 illustrates this process in relation to the research question, "What are children's pain experiences, management strategies, and outcomes during the first year after diagnosis of ALL?" (Van Cleve et al., 2004; see Appendix B). In this example, it is clear that there is an explicitly developed, relevant body of scientific data that provide the theoretical grounding for the study. The hypotheses, as stated in Table 3-6, are logically derived from the theoretical framework. The research consumer, however, should be cautioned about assuming that the theory-hypothesis link will always be present.

Wording the Hypothesis

As you read the scientific literature and become more familiar with it, you will observe that there are a variety of ways to word a hypothesis. Regardless of the specific format used to state the hypothesis, the statement should be worded in clear, simple, and concise terms. If this criterion is met, the reader will understand the following:

- The variables of the hypothesis
- The population being studied
- The predicted outcome of the hypothesis

TABLE **3-6** **Flow of Data among Research Question, Literature Review, Theoretical Framework, and Hypotheses**

Question	Literature Review	Theoretical Framework	Hypotheses
What are children's pain experiences, management strategies, and outcomes during the first year after the diagnosis of acute lymphocytic leukemia (ALL)?	1. The literature suggests that cancer pain research with children has focused almost exclusively on procedure-related pain with an emphasis on nonpharmacological strategies for managing pain. 2. Pain was a presenting symptom at diagnosis, with pain intensity ranging from mild to severe. 3. The literature has a significant knowledge deficit about Latino children and how they experience and report pain. 4. Four presenting problems noted in clinical articles were mucositis, abdominal pain, neuropathic pain, and pain related to infection. 5. Minimal data are available on the dimensions of pain experience, effectiveness of management strategies, and outcomes. 6. The Symptom Management Model of the University of California, San Francisco, could be used to theoretically frame the symptom experience, symptom management, and symptom outcome dimensions.	1. The Symptom Management Model with its interrelated dimensions (symptom experience, symptom management strategies, and symptom outcomes) provides direction for evaluating the pain experience of children and adolescents based on their perception over a 1-year time frame. 2. The symptom experience dimension included elements of perception, evaluation, and response. 3. The symptom management strategies dimension included the perspectives of patient, health care provider, family, and health care system. 4. The symptom outcomes dimension included areas such as functional status, quality of life, morbidity/comorbidity, and health service utilization. 5. The aims of the study, based on this model, were to describe children's pain for 1 year after diagnosis, describe pain management strategies used by children and their families, and examine the outcomes of management effectiveness and functional status.	1. Pain intensity will be negatively related to management effectiveness. 2. Functional status will be negatively related to perception of pain intensity.

Information about hypotheses may be further clarified in the *Instruments, Sample,* or *Methods* sections of a research report (see Chapters 12, 14, and 15).

Directional vs. Nondirectional Hypotheses

Hypotheses can be formulated directionally or nondirectionally. A **directional hypothesis** is one that specifies the expected direction of the relationship between the independent and dependent variables. The reader of a directional hypothesis may observe not only the proposal of a relationship but also the nature or direction of that relationship. The following is an example of a directional hypothesis: "At four months following the individualized information counseling session, patients and their partners would report lower levels of state anxiety and depression (Davison et al., 2003; Appendix D)." Examples of directional hypotheses can also be found in examples 2 through 7 in Table 3-7.

Whereas a **nondirectional hypothesis** indicates the existence of a relationship between the variables, it does not specify the anticipated direction of the relationship. The following is an example of a nondirectional hypothesis: "Poor physical and functional health status will be associated with emotional stress in both men and women." Sometimes a research article will have both directional and nondirectional hypotheses for the same study. In the van Servellen study, an example of a directional hypothesis is "women will have higher levels of emotional distress than men" (van Servellen et al., 2002). Other examples of nondirectional hypotheses are illustrated in examples 1 and 8 in Table 3-7.

Nurses who are learning to critique research studies should be aware that both the directional and the nondirectional forms of hypothesis statements are acceptable. They should also be aware that there are definite pros and cons pertaining to each one.

Proponents of the nondirectional hypothesis state that this format is more objective and impartial than the directional hypothesis. It is argued that the directional hypothesis is poten-

tially biased, because the researcher, in stating an anticipated outcome, has demonstrated a commitment to a particular position.

On the other side of the coin, proponents of the directional hypothesis argue that researchers naturally have hunches, guesses, or expectations about the outcome of their research. It is the hunch, the curiosity, or the guess that initially leads them to speculate about the question. The literature review and the conceptual framework provide the theoretical foundation for developing the research question and then deriving the hypothesis. Consequently, it might be said that a deductive hypothesis derived from a theory is most always directional (see Chapter 5). For example, the theory will provide a critical rationale for proposing that relationships between variables will have particular outcomes. When there is no theory or related research to draw on for rationale or when findings in previous research studies are ambivalent, a nondirectional hypothesis may be appropriate. As you read research articles, you will note that directional hypotheses are much more commonly used than nondirectional hypotheses.

In summary, the evaluator of a hypothesis should know that there are several advantages to directional hypotheses, making them appropriate for use in most studies. The advantages are as follows:

- Directional hypotheses indicate to the reader that a theory base has been used to derive the hypotheses and that the phenomena under investigation have been critically examined and interrelated. The reader should realize that nondirectional hypotheses may also be deduced from a theory base. Because of the exploratory nature of many studies using nondirectional hypotheses, however, the theory base may not be as developed.
- They provide the reader with a specific theoretical frame of reference, within which the study is being conducted.
- They suggest to the reader that the researcher is not sitting on a theoretical fence, and as a result, the analyses of data can be accomplished in a statistically more sensitive way.

TABLE **3-7** **Examples of how Hypotheses are Worded**

Hypothesis	Variables*	Hypothesis	Type of Design and Level of Evidence Suggested
1. There will be a difference in fatigue between two groups of caregivers of preterm infants (i.e., two on vs. not on apnea monitors) during three time two periods (i.e., prior to discharge, 1-week two postdischarge, and 1- month postdischarge). OR	IV: Apnea monitor DV: Fatigue OR	Nondirectional, research	Nonexperimental; Level IV
There will be a significant difference in menopausal hot flashes between conditions of fasting and experimentally sustained (130-140 mg/dl) blood glucose concentrations.	IV: Blood glucose concentrations DV: Menopausal hot flashes	Nondirectional research	
2. There will be a positive relationship between phase-specific telephone counseling and emotional adjustment in women with breast cancer and their partners.	IV: Telephone counseling DV: Emotional adjustment	Directional, research	Experimental; Level II
3. There will be a greater decrease in state anxiety scores for patients receiving structured informational videos before abdominal or chest tube removal than for patients receiving standard information.	IV: Preprocedure structured videotape information IV: Standard information DV: State anxiety	Directional, research	Experimental; Level II
4. The incidence and degree of severity of subject discomfort will be less after administration of medications by the Z-track intramuscular injection technique than after administration of medications by the standard intramuscular injection technique.	IV: Z-track intramuscular injection technique IV: Standard intramuscular injection technique DV: Subject discomfort	Directional, research	Experimental; Level II

Hypothesis	Variables	Type	Design
5. Therapeutic back massage (TBM) will reduce the effects of stress experienced by spouses of patients with cancer, as measured by a positive change in mood and a decrease in perceived stress, heart rate, and blood pressure at two postintervention time points compared to a control group of spouses of patients with cancer.	IV: Therapeutic back massage DV: Change in mood DV: Decrease in perceived stress DV: Decreased heart rate DV: Decreased blood pressure	Directional, research	Experimental; Level II
6. Nurses with high social support from co-workers have low perceived job stress.	IV: Social support DV: Perceived job stress	Directional, research.	Nonexperimental; Level IV
7. There will be a positive effect from a social support, boosting intervention on levels of stress, coping, and social support among caregivers of children with HIV/AIDS.	IV: Social support boosting intervention DV: Stress DV: Coping DV: Social support	Directional, research	Experimental; Level II
8. There will be a difference in posttest state anxiety scores in subjects treated with noncontact therapeutic touch than in subjects treated with contact therapeutic touch. OR There will be no significant difference in the duration of patency of a 24-gauge intravenous lock in a neonatal patient when flushed with 0.5 ml of heparinized saline (2 U/ml), standard practice, compared with 0.5 ml of 0.9% normal saline.	IV: Noncontact therapeutic touch IV: Contact therapeutic touch DV: State anxiety OR IV: Heparinized saline IV: Normal saline DV: Duration of patency of intravenous lock	Nondirectional, research OR Nondirectional; null	Experimental; Level II

*Abbreviations: *IV,* independent variable; *DV,* dependent variable.

The important point for the critiquer to keep in mind about the directionality of the hypotheses is whether there is a sound rationale for the choice the researcher has proposed regarding directionality.

Statistical vs. Research Hypotheses

Readers of research reports may observe that a hypothesis is further categorized as either a research or a statistical hypothesis. A **research hypothesis,** also known as a scientific hypothesis, consists of a statement about the expected relationship of the variables. A research hypothesis indicates what the outcome of the study is expected to be. A research hypothesis is also either directional or nondirectional. If the researcher obtains statistically significant findings for a research hypothesis, the hypothesis is supported. For example, in a study exploring the relative effectiveness of one intervention, a patient information program (PIP) for men newly diagnosed with prostate cancer and their partners, Davison and associates (2003) hypothesized that at 4 months following the individualized information counseling sessions, patients and their partners would report lower levels of state anxiety and depression; also, they hypothe-

sized that patients and partners would assume a more active role in medical decision making following the individualized information counseling sessions. The authors reported that after 4 months, all participants reported significantly lower levels of state anxiety and depression. However, the hypothesis that patients and partners would assume a more active role in decision making than originally intended following the provision of individualized information counseling sessions was not supported. As such, one hypothesis is supported and one is not (see Appendix D). The examples in Table 3-7 represent research hypotheses.

A **statistical hypothesis,** also known as a null hypothesis, states that there is no relationship between the independent and dependent variables. The examples in Table 3-8 illustrate statistical hypotheses. If, in the data analysis, a statistically significant relationship emerges between the variables at a specified level of significance, the null hypothesis is rejected. Rejection of the statistical hypothesis is equivalent to acceptance of the research hypothesis. For example, in the study by Swanson (1999), the effects of caring-based counseling, measurement, and time on the integration of loss (i.e.,

TABLE **3-8 Examples of Statistical Hypotheses**

Hypothesis	Variables*	Type of Hypothesis	Type of Design Suggested
Oxygen inhalation by nasal cannula of up to 6 L/min does not affect oral temperature measurement taken with an electronic thermometer.	IV: Oxygen inhalation by nasal cannula DV: Oral temperature	Statistical	Experimental
There will be no difference in the performance accuracy of adult nurse practitioners (ANP) and family nurse practitioners (FNP) in formulating accurate diagnoses and acceptable interventions for suspected cases of domestic violence.	IV: Nurse practitioner (ANP or FNP) category DV: Diagnosis and intervention performance accuracy	Null	Nonexperimental

*Abbreviations: *IV*, independent variable; *DV*, dependent variable.

miscarriage loss) and women's emotional well-being (i.e., moods and self-esteem) were tested using a statistical or null hypothesis. One example of a null hypothesis is, "There will be no difference in miscarriage impact, disturbed moods, or self-esteem at 4 months and 1 year after the loss." Swanson (1999) reported that there were significant differences in patient outcomes in relation to these variables. Because the difference in outcomes was greater than expected by chance, the null hypothesis was rejected (see Chapter 17).

Some researchers refer to the null hypothesis as a statistical contrivance that obscures a straightforward prediction of the outcome. Others state that it is more exact and conservative statistically, and that failure to reject the null hypothesis implies that there is insufficient evidence to support the idea of a real difference. Readers of research reports will note that when hypotheses are stated, research hypotheses are generally used more often than statistical hypotheses because they are more desirable to state the researcher's expectation. Readers then have a more precise idea of the proposed outcome. In any study that involves statistical analysis, the underlying null hypothesis is usually assumed without being explicitly stated.

RELATIONSHIP BETWEEN THE HYPOTHESIS, THE RESEARCH QUESTION, AND THE RESEARCH DESIGN

Regardless of whether the researcher uses a statistical or a research hypothesis, there is a suggested relationship between the hypothesis, the research design of the study, and the level of evidence provided by the results of the study. The type of design, experimental or nonexperimental (see Chapters 10 and 11), will influence the wording of the hypothesis. For example, when an experimental design is used, the research consumer would expect to see hypotheses that reflect relationship statements, such as the following:

- X_1 is more effective than X_2 on Y.
- The effect of X_1 on Y is greater than that of X_2 on Y.
- The incidence of Y will not differ in subjects receiving X_1 and X_2 treatments.
- The incidence of Y will be greater in subjects after X_1 than after X_2.

Such hypotheses indicate that an experimental treatment (i.e., independent variable X) will be used and that two groups of subjects, experimental and control groups, are being used to test whether the difference in the outcome (i.e., dependent variable Y) predicted by the hypothesis actually exists. Hypotheses reflecting experimental designs also test the effect of the experimental treatment (i.e., independent variable X) on the outcome (i.e., dependent variable Y). This would suggest that the strength of the evidence provided by the results would be Level II (experimental design) or Level III (quasiexperimental design).

In contrast, hypotheses related to nonexperimental designs reflect associative relationship statements, such as the following:

- X will be negatively related to Y.
- There will be a positive relationship between X and Y.

This would suggest that the strength of the evidence provided by the results of a study that examined hypotheses with associative relationship statements would be at Level IV (nonexperimental design).

Table 3-8 provides additional examples of this concept. The Critical Thinking Decision Path shown in the following diagram will help you determine the type of hypothesis presented in a study, as well as the study's readiness for a hypothesis-testing design.

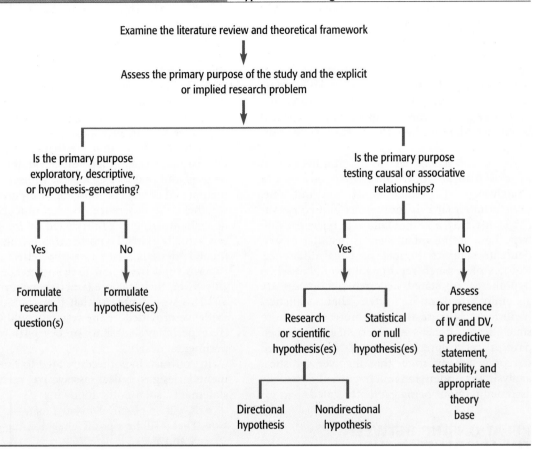

CRITICAL THINKING DECISION PATH   Determining the Type of Hypothesis or Readiness for Hypothesis Testing

Examine the literature review and theoretical framework

Assess the primary purpose of the study and the explicit or implied research problem

Is the primary purpose exploratory, descriptive, or hypothesis-generating?

Yes → Formulate research question(s)

No → Formulate hypothesis(es)

Is the primary purpose testing causal or associative relationships?

Yes → Research or scientific hypothesis(es) / Statistical or null hypothesis(es)

Research or scientific hypothesis(es) → Directional hypothesis / Nondirectional hypothesis

No → Assess for presence of IV and DV, a predictive statement, testability, and appropriate theory base

 EVIDENCE-BASED PRACTICE TIP

Think about the relationship between the wording of the hypothesis, the type of research design suggested, and the level of evidence provided by the findings of a study using each kind of hypothesis. The research consumer may want to consider which type of hypothesis potentially will yield the strongest results applicable to practice.

Research studies do not always contain hypotheses. As you become more familiar with the scientific literature, you will notice that a significant number of research studies that appear in the literature are guided by research questions. Of particular note, exploratory studies usually do not have hypotheses. This is particularly common when there is a dearth of literature or related research studies in a particular area that is of interest to the researcher. The researcher, interested in finding out more about a particular phenomenon, may engage in a fact- or relationship-finding mission, guided only by research questions. The outcome of the exploratory study may be that data about the phenomenon are amassed, so the researcher can then formulate hypotheses for a future study. This is sometimes called a hypothesis-generating study.

A study by McDonald and associates (2000) examined how patients communicate their pain and pain-management needs after surgery. The research question, which includes the following variables, pain (independent variable **X**) and postoperative caregiver pain communication (dependent variable **Y**), illustrates how an investigation designed to generate relationships and fill a gap in the literature was guided by research questions.

- How do postoperative patients communicate their pain and pain-management needs to their health care providers?
- How are demographic variables (e.g., race and gender) related to pain and the communication of pain-management needs to health care providers?

Because there has been little research on the effectiveness of postoperative communication of pain, research questions—rather than hypotheses—are appropriate for this baseline phase of a study. The findings of the study highlighted the importance of effective patient communication of pain as a variable related to effective pain management by health care providers. Reasons for decreased pain communication include the following:

- Not wanting to complain
- Not wanting to take the provider away from other patients
- Avoiding unpleasant analgesic side effects
- Not wanting to take "drugs"

The problems in the communication of pain management identified in this study could be used to design nursing-intervention studies to improve pain communication and the consequent pain relief in postoperative patients.

Qualitative research studies also are guided by research questions rather than hypotheses. The descriptive findings of qualitative studies also can provide the basis for future hypothesis-testing studies. "How do women with ovarian cancer experience cancer recurrence" is an example of a research question from a qualitative study by Howell, Fitch, and Deane (2003) that sought to enrich understanding about how women with ovarian cancer deal with the diagnosis of recurrence, manage treatment-related concerns, and attempt to regain control over their disease (see Chapters 6, 7, and 8).

In other studies, research questions are formulated in addition to hypotheses to answer questions related to ancillary data. Such questions do not directly pertain to the proposed outcomes of the hypotheses. Rather, they may provide additional and sometimes serendipitous findings that enrich the study and provide direction for further study. Sometimes they are the kernels of new or future hypotheses. The evaluator of a research study must determine whether it was appropriate to formulate a research question rather than a hypothesis given the purpose and context of the study. Table 3-2 provides examples of research questions.

 HELPFUL H I N T

Remember that research questions are used to guide all types of research studies, but are most often used in exploratory, descriptive, qualitative, or hypothesis-generating studies.

 EVIDENCE-BASED PRACTICE TIP

The answers to questions generated by qualitative data reflect evidence that may provide the first insights about a phenomenon that has not been previously studied.

The care that the researcher takes when developing the research question or hypothesis is often representative of the overall conceptualization and design of the study. A methodically formulated research question provides the basis for hypothesis development. In a quantitative research study, the remainder of a study revolves around answering the research question or testing the hypothesis. In a qualitative research study, the objective is to answer the research question. This may be a time-consuming, sometimes frustrating endeavor for the researcher, but in the final analysis the product, as evaluated by the consumer, is most often worth the struggle. Because this text focuses on the nurse as a critical consumer of research, the following sections will primarily pertain to the evaluation of research questions and hypotheses in published research reports.

CRITIQUING THE RESEARCH QUESTION

The following Critiquing Criteria box provides several criteria for evaluating the initial phase of the research process—the research question. Because the research question represents the basis for the study, it is usually introduced at the beginning of the research report to indicate the focus and direction of the study to the readers. Readers will then be in a position to evaluate whether the rest of the study logically flows from its foundation—the research question(s). The author will often begin by identifying the background and significance of the issue that led to crystallizing development of the unanswered question. The clinical and scientific background and/or significance will be summarized, and the purpose, aim, or objective of the study is identified. Finally, the research question and any related subquestions will be proposed prior to or following the literature review.

The purpose of the introductory summary of the theoretical and scientific background is to provide the reader with a contextual glimpse of how the author critically thought about the research question's development. The introduction to the research question places the study within an appropriate theoretical framework and sets the stage for the unfolding of the study. This introductory section should also include the significance of the study (i.e., why the investigator is doing the study). For example, the significance may be to solve a problem encountered in the clinical area and thereby improve patient care, to resolve a conflict in the literature regarding a clinical issue, or to provide data supporting an innovative form of nursing intervention that is of equal or better quality and is also cost-effective. In a study by Waltman and colleagues (2003) that tested an intervention for preventing osteoporosis in postmenopausal breast cancer survivors, the significance of the research question was related to the increased risk for osteoporosis faced by this patient population. Moreover, the incidence and treatment of osteoporosis in women with a history of breast cancer have been understudied because frequently researchers exclude women with a history of cancer from studies of osteoporosis.

Sometimes readers find that the research question is not clearly stated at the conclusion of this section. In some cases it is only hinted at, and the reader is challenged to identify the research question under consideration. In other cases the research question is embedded in the introductory text or purpose statement. To some extent, this depends on the style of the journal. Nevertheless, the evaluator must remember that the main research question should be implied if it is not clearly identified in the introductory section—even if the subquestions are not stated or implied.

The reader looks for the presence of three key elements that are described and illustrated in an earlier section of this chapter. They are the following:

- Does the research question express a relationship between two or more variables, or at least between an independent and a dependent variable?
- Does the research question specify the nature of the population being studied?
- Does the research question imply the possibility of empiric testing?

The reader uses these three elements as criteria for judging the soundness of a stated research question. It is likely that if the question is unclear in terms of the variables, the population, and the implications for testability, then the remainder of the study is going to falter. For example, a research study contained introductory material on anxiety in general, anxiety as it relates to the perioperative period, and the potentially beneficial influence of nursing care in relation to anxiety reduction. The author concluded that the purpose of the study was to determine whether selected measures of patient anxiety could be shown to differ when different approaches to nursing care were used during the perioperative period. The author did not go on to state the research question. A restatement of the question might be as follows:

$$(Y_1) \; (X_1, X_2, X_3)$$

What is the difference in patient anxiety level in relation to different approaches to nursing care during the perioperative period?

If this process is clarified at the outset of a research study, all that follows in terms of the design can be logically developed. Readers will have a clear idea of what the report should convey and can knowledgeably evaluate the material that follows. When critically appraising clinical questions, think about the fact that they should be focused and specify the patient or problem being addressed, the intervention, and the outcome for a particular patient population. There should be evidence that the clinical question guided the literature search and suggests the design and level of evidence to be obtained from the study findings.

CRITIQUING THE HYPOTHESIS

As illustrated in the following Critiquing Criteria box, several criteria for critiquing the hypothesis should be used as a standard for evaluating the strengths and weaknesses of hypotheses in a research report.

1. When reading a research study, research consumers may find the hypotheses clearly delineated in a separate hypothesis section of the research article (i.e., after the literature review or theoretical framework section[s]). In many cases the hypotheses are not explicitly stated and are only implied in the *Results* or *Discussion* section of the article. As such, readers must infer the hypotheses from the purpose statement and the type of analysis used. Readers must also be cognizant of this variation and not think that because hypotheses do not appear at the beginning of the article, they do not exist in the particular study. Even when hypotheses are stated at the beginning of an article, they are reexamined in the *Results* or *Discussion* section as the findings are presented and discussed. Readers should expect hypotheses to be appropriately reflected depending on the purpose of the study and format of the article.

2. If a research question was posed at the beginning of the report, the data analysis is designed to answer that question. If a hypothesis or set of hypotheses are presented, the data analysis should directly answer the hypotheses. Its placement in the research report logically follows the literature review, and the theoretical framework, because the hypothesis should reflect the culmination and expression of this conceptual process. It should be consistent with both the literature review and the theoretical framework. The

CRITIQUING CRITERIA   *Developing Research Questions and Hypotheses*

The Research Question

1. Was the research question introduced promptly?
2. Is the research question stated clearly and unambiguously?
3. Does the research question express a relationship between two or more variables or at least between an independent and a dependent variable, implying empirical testability?
4. How does the research question specify the nature of the population being studied?
5. How has the research question been substantiated with adequate experiential and scientific background material?
6. How has the research question been placed within the context of an appropriate theoretical framework?
7. How has the significance of the research question been identified?
8. Have pragmatic issues, such as feasibility, been addressed?
9. How have the purpose, aims, or goals of the study been identified?
10. Are research questions appropriately used (i.e., exploratory, descriptive, or qualitative study or in relation to ancillary data analyses)?

The Clinical Question

1. Does the clinical question specify the patient situation, the intervention, counterintervention, and outcome?

The Hypothesis

1. How does the hypothesis relate to the research problem?
2. Is the hypothesis concisely stated in a declarative form?
3. Are the independent and dependent variables identified in the statement of the hypothesis?
4. How are the variables measurable or potentially measurable?
5. Is each hypothesis specific to one relationship so that each hypothesis can be either supported or not supported?
6. Is the hypothesis stated in such a way that it is testable?
7. Is the hypothesis stated objectively, without value-laden words?
8. Is the direction of the relationship in each hypothesis clearly stated?
9. How is each hypothesis consistent with the literature review?
10. How is the theoretical rationale for the hypothesis made explicit?
11. Given the level of evidence suggested by the research question, hypothesis, and design, what is the potential applicability to practice?

---

flow of this process, as depicted in Table 3-7, should be explicit and apparent to the reader. If this criterion is met, the reader feels reasonably assured that the basis for the hypothesis is theoretically sound.

3. As readers examine the actual hypothesis, several aspects of the statement should be critically appraised:

First, the hypothesis should consist of a declarative statement that objectively and succinctly expresses the relationship between an independent and a dependent variable. In wording a complex vs. a simple hypothesis, there may be more than one independent and dependent variable.

Second, readers can expect that there may be more than one hypothesis, particularly if there is more than one independent and dependent variable. This is a function of the type of study being conducted.

Third, the variables of the hypothesis should be understandable to the reader. In the interest of formulating a succinct hypothesis statement, the complete meaning of the variables is often not apparent. Readers must realize that sometimes a researcher is caught between the "devil and the deep blue sea" on that issue. It may be a choice between having a complete but verbose hypothesis paragraph or having a less complete but concise hypothesis. The solution to this dilemma is for the researcher to have a definition section in the research report. The inclusion of conceptual definitions and operational definitions (see Chapter 5) provides the complete explication of the variables. Other times the conceptual definitions may be embedded in the theoretical framework or the literature review while the operational definitions appear in the methods or instruments section of the research report. The reader is then challenged to evaluate the fit between the conceptual and operational definitions and their relationship to the hypotheses. An excellent example of this process appears in a research article by Koniak-Griffin and colleagues (2003) (Appendix A), who hypothesized the following:

At 2-years postbirth, participants in the early intervention program (EIP) would demonstrate improved infant health and maternal outcomes in comparison to those in the traditional public health nurse care group.

This is an appropriately worded hypothesis. It is not completely clear, however, what the variables "early intervention program (EIP)," "traditional public health nursing care (TPHNC)," "infant health," or "maternal outcomes" imply. The conceptual definitions are implied in the literature review but conceptually defined in the Methods section. The operational definitions, which indicate how the variables will be measured, also appear in the Methods section under Procedure, Measures, and Instruments. It is only upon examination of the conceptual and operational definitions of these variables that their exact nature becomes clear to readers (see Appendix A).

- Early Intervention Program (EIP): "a series of four preparation for motherhood classes focused on behaviors to promote health during pregnancy, parent-child communication, and the transition to motherhood"
- Traditional Public Health Nursing Care (TPHN): "two prenatal home visits (at enrollment and during third trimester) that focused on assessment and counseling related to prenatal health care, self-care, preparation for childbirth, education, and planning as well as well-baby care and immunizations; one postpartum visit within 6 weeks to provide the mother with general information about child care, postpartum recovery, maternal and infant nutrition, home safety, community resources, and family planning
- Infant Health: "hospitalizations (e.g., length in days, number of episodes, diagnoses) and ER visits in the 24 months following birth"
- Maternal Outcomes: "substance use, education, repeat pregnancies, social competence, and quality of mother-child interaction"

After reading all of these sections and subsections of the research article, the context of the variables is now revealed to the evaluator.

Fourth, although a hypothesis can legitimately be nondirectional, it is preferable, and more common, for the researcher to indicate the direction of the relationship between the variables in the hypothesis. Readers will find that when there is a dearth of data available for the literature review (i.e., the researcher has chosen to study a relatively undefined area of interest), the nondirectional hypothesis may be appropriate. There simply may not be enough information available to make a sound judgment about the direction of the proposed relationship. All that could be proposed is that there will be a relationship between two variables. Essentially, readers want to determine the appropriateness of the researcher's choice regarding directionality of the hypothesis.

4. The notion of testability is central to the soundness of a hypothesis. One criterion related to testability is that the hypothesis should be stated in such a way that it can be clearly supported or not supported. Although the previous statement is very important to keep in mind, readers should also understand that ultimately theories or hypotheses are never proven beyond the shadow of a doubt through hypothesis testing. Researchers who claim that their data have "proven" the validity of their hypothesis should be regarded with grave reservation. Readers should realize that, at best, findings that support a hypothesis are considered tentative. If repeated replication of a study yields the same results, more confidence can be placed in the conclusions advanced by the researchers. An important thing to remember about testability is that although hypotheses are more likely to be accepted with increasing evidence, they are ultimately never proven.

Another point about testability for research consumers to consider is that the hypothesis should be objectively stated and devoid of any value-laden words. Value-laden hypotheses are not empirically testable. Quantifiable words such as greater than; less than; decrease; increase; and positively, negatively, and curvilinearly related convey the idea of objectivity and testability. Readers should immediately be suspicious of hypotheses that are not stated objectively.

5. The evaluator of a research study should be cognizant of the fact that how the proposed relationship of the hypothesis is phrased suggests the type of research design that will be appropriate for the study as well as the level of evidence to be derived from the findings. For example, if a hypothesis proposes that treatment X_1 will have a greater effect on Y than treatment X_2, an experimental (Level II evidence) or quasiexperimental design (Level III evidence) is suggested (see Chapter 10). If a hypothesis proposes that there will be a positive relationship between variables X and Y, a nonexperimental design (Level IV evidence) is suggested (see Chapter 11). A review of Table 3-7 provides you with additional examples of hypotheses, the type of research design, and the level of evidence that is suggested by each hypothesis. The reader of a research report should evaluate whether the selected research design is congruent with the hypothesis, and the potential applicability of the evidence to practice. This factor has important implications for the remainder of the study in terms of the appropriateness of sample selection, data collection, data analysis, interpretation of findings, and—ultimately—the conclusions advanced by the researcher.

6. If the research report contains research questions rather than hypotheses, the reader will want to evaluate whether this is appropriate to the study. One criterion for making this decision, as presented earlier in this chapter, is whether the study is of an exploratory, descriptive, or qualitative nature. If it is, then it is appropriate to have research questions rather than hypotheses. Ancillary research questions should be evaluated as to whether they answer additional questions secondary to the hypotheses. Sometimes the substance of an additional research question is more appropriately posed as another hypothesis in that it relates in a major way to the original research problem.

Critical Thinking Challenges

- Do you agree or disagree with the following statement: If a research study published in a journal does not clearly state the research question, then it fails to meet the critiquing criteria for problem statements as presented in this chapter. Justify your answer.
- Is it possible for "level of anxiety" to be the independent variable in one study and the dependent variable in another study? Support your position.
- Is it possible for a research hypothesis not to be theory derived? Support your answer with examples.
- Discuss the difference between a classmate predicting that "students who don't study will not do well on a test" and a research study's hypothesis on the topic. Justify your answer.
- How does the way in which the research question or hypothesis is worded suggest the level of evidence that will be provided by the study findings?

KEY POINTS

- Formulation of the research question and stating the hypothesis are key preliminary steps in the research process.
- The research question is refined through a process that proceeds from the identification of a general idea of interest to the definition of a more specific and circumscribed topic.
- A preliminary literature review reveals related factors that appear critical to the research topic of interest and helps to further define the research question.
- The significance of the research question must be identified in terms of its potential contribution to patients, nurses, the medical community in general, and society. Applicability of the question for nursing practice, as well as its theoretical relevance, must be established. The findings should also have the potential for formulating or altering nursing practices or policies.
- The feasibility of a research question must be examined in light of pragmatic considerations (e.g., time); availability of subjects, money, facilities, and equipment; experience of the researcher; and ethical issues.

- The final research question consists of a statement about the relationship of two or more variables. It clearly identifies the relationship between the independent and dependent variables, specifies the nature of the population being studied, and implies the possibility of empirical testing.
- Focused clinical questions arise from clinical practice and guide the literature search for the best available evidence to answer the clinical question.
- A hypothesis attempts to answer the question posed by the research question. When testing the validity of the theoretical frameworks' assumptions, the hypothesis bridges the theoretical and real worlds.
- A hypothesis is a declarative statement about the relationship between two or more variables that predicts an expected outcome. Characteristics of a hypothesis include a relationship statement, implications regarding testability, and consistency with a defined theory base.
- Hypotheses can be formulated in a directional or a nondirectional manner. Hypotheses can be further categorized as either research or statistical hypotheses.

- Research questions may be used instead of hypotheses in exploratory, descriptive, or qualitative research studies. Research questions may also be formulated in addition to hypotheses to answer questions related to ancillary data.
- The purpose, research question, or hypotheses provides information about the intent of the research question and hypothesis and suggests the level of evidence to be obtained from the study findings.
- The critiquing criteria provide a set of guidelines for evaluating the strengths and weaknesses of the problem statement and hypotheses as they appear in a research report.
- The critiquer assesses the clarity of the research question, as well as the related subquestions, the specificity of the population, and the implications for testability.
- The interrelatedness of the research question, the literature review, the theoretical framework, and the hypotheses should be apparent.
- The appropriateness of the research design suggested by the research question is also evaluated.
- The purpose of the study (i.e., why the researcher is doing the study) should be differentiated from the research question.
- The reader evaluates the wording of the hypothesis in terms of the clarity of the relational statement, its implications for testability, and its congruence with a theory base. The appropriateness of the hypothesis in relation to the type of research design and level of evidence suggested by the design is also examined. In addition, the appropriate use of research questions is evaluated in relation to the type of study conducted.

REFERENCES

AbuAlRub RF: Job stress, job performance and social support among hospital nurses, *J Nurs Scholarship* 36(1): 73-78, 2004.

Bonaiuti D, et al.: Exercise for preventing and treating osteoporosis in postmenopausal women, *Cochrane Database Systematic Review* (3): CD000333 (latest version February 27, 2002), 2002.

Chlebowski RT, et al.: Influence of estrogen plus progestin on breast cancer and mammography in healthy postmenopausal women: the women's health initiative randomized trial, *JAMA* 289: 3243-3253, 2003.

Cullum N: User's guides to the nursing literature: An introduction, *Evidence Based Nurs* 3(2): 71-72.

Davison JB, Goldenberg SL, Gleave ME, and Degner LF: Provision of individualized information to men and their partners to facilitate treatment decision making in prostate cancer, *Oncol Nurs Forum* 30(1): 107-114, 2003.

Dormire S, Reame NE: Menopause hot flash frequency changes in response to experimental manipulation of blood glucose, *Nurs Res* 52(???): 338-342, 2003.

Fleming K: Asking answerable questions, *Evidence Based Nurs* 1998, 1(2), 36-37.

Frame K, Kelly L, and Bayley E: Increasing perceptions of self-worth in preadolescents diagnosed with ADHD, *J Nurs Scholarship* 35(3): 225-229, 2003.

Goodfellow LM: The effects of therapeutic back massage on psychophysiologic variables and immune function in spouses of patients with cancer, *Nurs Res* 52(5): 318-328, 2003.

Handoll HH, et al.: Heparin, low molecular weight heparin and physical methods for preventing deep vein thrombosis and pulmonary embolism following surgery for hip fractures, *Cochrane Database Systematic Review* (4): CD000305 (latest version June 23, 2002), 2002.

Harter S: *The construction of the self: a developmental perspective.* New York, 1999, Guilford.

Howell D, Fitch MI, and Deane KA: Women's experiences with recurrent ovarian cancer, *Cancer Nurs* 26: 10-17, 2003.

Kearney MH, Munro BH, Kelly U, and Hawkins JW: Health behaviors as mediators for the effect of partner abuse on infant birth weight, *Nurs Res* 53(1): 36-45, 2004.

Koniak-Griffin D, Verzemnieks IL, Anderson NL, Brecht ML, Lesser J, Kim S, and Turner-Pluta C: Nurse visitation for adolescent mothers: two year infant and maternal outcomes, *Nurs Res* 52(2): 127-135, 2003.

Leight SB, et al.: The effect of structured training on breast self-examination search behaviors as measured using biomedical instrumentation, *Nurs Res* 49(5): 283-289, 2000.

Li H, Melnyk BM, and McCann R: Review of intervention studies of families with hospitalized elderly relatives, *J Nurs Schol* 36(1): 54-59, 2004.

McDonald DD, et al.: Communicating pain and pain management needs after surgery, *Appl Nurs Res* 13(2): 70-75, 2000.

Mishel MH, et al.: Moderators of an uncertainty management intervention, *Nurs Res* 52(2): 89-97, 2003.

Murrell K, Meredith M: *Empowering employees,* New York, 2000, McGraw-Hill.

Naylor MD, et al: Comprehensive discharge planning and home follow-up of hospitalized elders: a randomized clinical trial, *JAMA* 281(7): 613-620, 1999.

New JP, et al.: Specialist nurse-led intervention to treat and control hypertension and hyperlipidemia in diabetes (SPLINT): a randomized controlled trial, *Diabetes Care* 26: 2250-2255, 2003.

Reynolds SA, Schmid MW, and Broome ME: Polydipsia screening tool, *Arch Psychiatr Nurs* 18(2): 49-59, 2004.

Roy C, Andrews H: *The Roy adaptation model,* ed 2, Stamford, Conn, 1999, Appleton & Lange.

Sackett D, et al.: *Evidence-based medicine: how to practice and teach EBM,* London, 2000, Churchill Livingstone.

Swanson KM: Effects of caring, measurement, and time on miscarriage impact and women's well being in the first year subsequent to loss, *Nurs Res* 48(6): 288-299, 1999.

Thompson C, Cullum N, McCaughan D, Sheldon T, and Raynor P: Nurses, information use, and clinical decision making: the real world potential for evidence-based decisions in nursing, *Evidence-based Nurs* 7(3): 68-72, 2004.

Tucker S, Moore W, and Luedtke C: Outcomes of a brief inpatient treatment program for mood and anxiety disorders, *Outcomes Manage Nursing Pract* 4(3): 117-123, 2000.

Van Cleve L, Bossert E, Beecroft P, Adlard K, Alvarez O, and Savedra MC: The pain experience of children with leukemia during the first year after diagnosis, *Nurs Res* 53(1): 1-10, 2004.

van Servellen G, Aguirre M, Srna L, and Erecht M: Differential predictors of emotional distress in HIV-infected men and women, *West J Nurs Res* 24: 49-72, 2002.

Waltman NL, Twiss JJ, Ott CD, Gross GJ, Lindsay AM, Moore TM, and Berg K: Testing an intervention for preventing osteoporosis in postmenopausal breast cancer survivors, *J Nurs Schol* 35(4): 333-338, 2003.

FOR FURTHER STUDY

Go to your Companion CD for review activities for this chapter.

evolve Go to Evolve at http://evolve.elsevier.com/LoBiondo/ for WebLinks, Content Updates, and additional research articles, for practice in reviewing and critiquing.

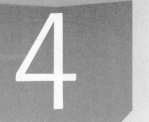

BARBARA KRAINOVICH-MILLER

Literature Review

KEY TERMS

computer databases
conceptual literature
Cumulative Index to Nursing and
    Allied Health Literature (CINAHL)
data-based literature
electronic database
empirical literature
integrative review
internet
literature

MEDLINE
meta-analysis
primary source
print databases
print indexes
qualitative research
qualitative systematic review
quantitative systematic review or
    meta-analysis
quantitative research

refereed, or peer-reviewed, journals
research literature
review of the literature
scholarly literature
scientific literature
secondary source
systematic reviews
theoretical literature
Web browser
World Wide Web (www)

LEARNING OUTCOMES

After reading this chapter, the student should be able to do the following:

- Discuss the relationship of the literature review to nursing theory, research, education, and practice.
- Discuss the purposes of the literature review from the perspective of the research investigator and the research consumer.
- Discuss the use of the literature review for quantitative designs and qualitative approaches.
- Discuss the purpose of reviewing the literature in development of evidence-based practice.
- Differentiate between conceptual (theoretical) and data-based (research) literature.
- Differentiate between primary and secondary sources.
- Compare the advantages and disadvantages of the most commonly used online databases and print database sources for conducting a literature review.
- Identify the characteristics of a relevant literature review.
- Differentiate between a study's literature review and a systematic review.
- Differentiate between a qualitative systematic review and a quantitative systematic review (meta-analysis).
- Critically read, critique, and synthesize conceptual and data-based resources for the development of a literature review.
- Apply critiquing criteria to the evaluation of literature reviews in selected research studies.

STUDY RESOURCES

Go to your Companion CD for review activities for this chapter.

evolve Go to Evolve at http://evolve.elsevier.com/LoBiondo/ for Weblinks, Content Updates, and additional research articles for practice in reviewing and critiquing.

You may wonder why an entire chapter of a research text is devoted to the **review of the literature.** The main reason is because the literature review not only is a key step in the research process but also is used in all steps of the process. A more personal question you might ask is, "Will knowing more about the literature review really help me in my student role or later in my research consumer role as a practicing professional nurse?" The answer is that it most certainly will. The ability to review the literature is a skill essential to your role as a student and your future role as a research consumer (ANA, 2000a).

The **review of the literature** is an organized critique of the important **scholarly literature** that supports a study, and a key step in the research process. The term **scholarly literature** refers to published and unpublished **data-based (research) reports,** as well as **conceptual (theoretical) literature.** A **data-based (research) report or article** is a report of an original research study by the researcher(s) who conducted the study. For example, all the studies in Appendixes A through D are data-based research reports and as such have literature reviews that help to form the basis for each study. Conceptual or theoretical literature can be articles that comprise an author's theory, such as the Lenz et al. Theory of Unpleasant Symptoms (1997); or it can be a discussion of a particular concept, theory, or topic, such as the article by Smith and Liehr (2003) that discusses multiple nursing theories suggested by others. (A review of the literature that reports on the findings of an original published research study would also be considered a secondary source of information on that study.) The differences between a data-based and conceptual article may seem confusing at first. The key to demystifying the difference is determining if the author(s) of the article conducted the study or if the article is the result of an original theory or concept investigated by the author(s).

Figure 4-1 shows the relationship of a review of the literature to theory, research, education,

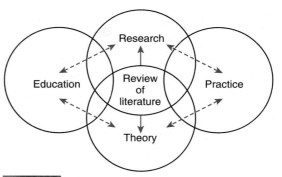

Figure 4-1. Relationship of the review of the literature to theory, research, education, and practice.

and practice. The review of the literature section of a published study often contains both data-based **(research study) literature** and conceptual or theoretical literature, but the entire research article is categorized as data-based literature. The purpose of this chapter is to introduce you to the review of the literature as it is used in research and other evidence-based practice activities. The primary focus of the discussion is on using your critical thinking and reading competencies (see Chapter 2) for developing the necessary skills for critically appraising the literature. This chapter also provides an introduction to systematic reviews, which are a method used to further research and support evidence-based practice. The chapter concludes with methods for retrieving literature and resources for your papers and projects.

REVIEW OF THE LITERATURE

Overall Purpose: Knowledge

The overall purpose of a review of the literature in a research study is to present a strong knowledge base for the conduct of the research project. Before you can critique the literature review in a research study, it is important to understand what purpose the review of the literature serves in a research study. Box 4-1 outlines the overall purposes of a literature review for a research study. The knowledge uncovered from a critical

---

BOX 4-1 OVERALL PURPOSES OF A REVIEW OF LITERATURE

MAJOR GOAL

To develop a strong knowledge base to carry out research and other scholarly educational and clinical practice activities

OBJECTIVES

A review of the literature does the following:
1. Determines what is known and unknown about a subject, concept, or problem
2. Determines gaps, consistencies, and inconsistencies in the literature about a subject, concept, or problem
3. Uncovers research findings that support evidence-based practice
4. Discovers conceptual traditions used to examine problems

5. Uncovers a new practice intervention(s), or gains supporting evidence for current intervention(s), protocols, and policies
6. Promotes evidence-based revision and development of new practice protocols, policies, and projects/activities related to nursing practice
7. Generates useful research questions and hypotheses for nursing
8. Determines an appropriate research design, methodology, and analysis for answering the research question(s) or hypothesis(es) based on an assessment of the strengths and weaknesses of earlier works
9. Determines the need for replication of a study or refinement of a study
10. Synthesizes the strengths and weaknesses and findings of available studies on a topic/problem

---

review of the literature contributes to the development, implementation, and results of a research study.

Research Study: Purpose of the Literature Review

The objectives listed in Box 4-1 reflect the purposes of a literature review for the conduct of quantitative research and most qualitative designs. Critically reading and using the literature for a study is essential to meeting these objectives. The main goal of a literature review is to develop the foundation of a sound study, but it also is used for other scholarly, educational, and clinical practice activities. Table 4-1 summarizes the main focus of the literature review for use in the steps of the research process for quantitative and qualitative designs. Box 4-2 lists the characteristics of a literature review that meet critiquing criteria; these characteristics are discussed throughout the chapter.

Research Consumer: Review of Literature Purposes

Sometimes we want to review the literature to write a paper for a student assignment, to uncover knowledge, or to search for potential

evidence that supports a nursing practice. As a practicing nurse you will be called on to develop evidence-based practice protocols, and conducting a literature review is essential to this practice outcome. Table 4-2 illustrates a few examples of research consumer activities. For example, a student assignment related to the development of an evidence-based practice protocol, practice standard, or policy change would involve retrieving and critically reviewing a number of data-based (research) articles, systematic reviews, and conceptual (theoretical) articles to determine the degree of support found in the literature. A critical review of the literature essentially uncovers data that contribute evidence to support current practice and clinical decision making, as well as for making changes in practice.

Research Conduct and Consumer of Research Purposes: Differences and Similarities

How does the literature review differ when it is used for research purposes vs. consumer of research purposes? The literature review in a research study is used to develop a sound research proposal. In a research study, the literature review includes a critical evaluation of both data-based and conceptual literature related

TABLE **4-1** **Examples of Uses of Literature Review for the Research Process: Quantitative and Qualitative**

Quantitative Process	Qualitative Process

The review of the literature is used for all quantitative research designs.
The review of the literature is defined as a step of the research process. When a research study is written as a proposal or published, the literature review is often written as a separate aspect of the study, even if it is not labeled as such. The actual review of the literature (i.e., the results of the review), however, is used in developing all steps of the research process.
The review of the literature is essential to the following steps of the research process:
  Problem
  Need/significance
  Question/hypothesis(es)
  Theoretical/conceptual framework
  Design/methodology
  Specific instruments (validity and reliability)
  Data-collection method
  Type of analysis
  Discussion of findings (interpretation)
  Implications of findings
  Recommendations based on findings
	The use of the literature review depends on the selected qualitative approach/method, designs/types, and phases. An extensive database is usually not available and conceptual data are somewhat limited, so a qualitative design is used.
	The following examples highlight the predominant use of the literature review for the particular qualitative approach:
	● Phenomenologic: compare findings with information from review of the literature (Tinsley and France, 2004)
	● Grounded theory: constantly compare literature with data being generated (Woodgate and Degner, 2004)
	● Ethnographic: provide framework for study (Glass and Davis, 2004)
	● Case study: conceptual and data-based literature embedded in report (Burger, 2003)
	● Historical: review of literature is source of data (Wall, 2002)
	● Qualitative content analysis: Plach, Stevens, and Moss (2004) (see Appendix C) highlight predominant use of literature review for this particular qualitative "designed as an arm of a large quantitative study" (p. 33)

BOX 4-2 CHARACTERISTICS OF A WRITTEN "RELEVANT" REVIEW OF LITERATURE

Each reviewed source of information reflects critical thinking and scholarly writing and is relevant to the study/topic/project, and the content satisfies the following criteria:
● Purposes of the literature review were met.
● Summary of each data-based or conceptual article is succinct and adequately represents the review source.
● Established criteria for related study designs are used to analyze the study for strengths, weaknesses, or limitations as well as for conflicts or gaps in information that relate directly or indirectly to the area of interest.

● Evidence of synthesis of the critiques of each source of information is presented, that is, putting the parts (i.e., each critique) together to form a new whole or connection link for what is to be studied, replicated, developed, or implemented.
● Review consists of mainly primary sources; there are a sufficient number of data-based sources.
● Summaries/critiques of studies are presented in a logical flow ending with a conclusion or synthesis of the reviewed material that reflects why the study or project could be implemented.

TABLE **4-2 Examples of Uses of the Literature for Research Consumer Purposes: Educational and Practice Settings**

Educational Setting	Clinical/Professional Setting
UNDERGRADUATE STUDENTS	**NURSES IN THE CLINICAL SETTING**
Develop academic scholarly papers (i.e., researching topic, problem, or issue)	Implement research-based nursing interventions and evidence-based practice protocols
Prepare oral presentations or debates of topic, problem, or issue; prepare clinical projects	Develop hospital-specific nursing and/or interdisciplinary protocols or policies related to patient care
GRADUATE STUDENTS (MASTER'S AND DOCTORAL)	Develop, implement, and evaluate hospital-specific quality assurance projects or protocols related to patient outcome data
Develop research proposals	**PROFESSIONAL NURSING**
Develop research- or evidence-based practice protocols and other scholarly projects	*Organizations/Governmental Agencies*
DOCTORALLY PREPARED FACULTY	Develop ANA's major documents (e.g., *Social Policy Statement,* 2003; *Women's Primary Health Care Standards of Clinical Practice,* 1995; *Scope and Standards of Home Health Nursing Practice,* 1999; *Scope and Standards of Practice for Nursing Professional Development,* 2000a; *Scope and Standards of Public Health Nursing Practice,* 2000b; *Scope and Standards of Practice,* 2004).
Develop and revise curricula	
Develop theoretical papers for presentations and/or publication	
Develop research proposals	
Conduct research	
Participate in development of systematic reviews	
Collaborate with practice colleagues in development of evidence-based practice protocols	

to the proposed study. The literature review in a study concludes with a statement relating the proposed study's purpose to the reviewed research. From a broader perspective, the major focus of reviewing the literature as a consumer is to uncover multiple sources of evidence on a given topic. From a student perspective, a critical review of the literature is essential to acquiring knowledge for the development of scholarly papers, presentations, debates, and evidence-based practice projects. Students use data-based and conceptual literature resources to support rationale for nursing interventions written for a nursing diagnosis.

Both types of reviews are similar in that both should be critical, framed in the context of previous data-based and conceptual literature, and pertinent to the objectives presented in Box 4-1. The amount of literature required to be reviewed, however, may differ between a research

proposal and an academic paper or clinical project. Table 4-2 lists a number of research consumer projects conducted in educational and clinical settings.

A critical literature review is central to developing and implementing activities for research consumers. Practice protocols or nursing interventions implemented in a health care setting should be based on a critical review of data-based (research) literature.

LITERATURE REVIEW: UNDERSTANDING THE PERSPECTIVE OF THE RESEARCH INVESTIGATOR

An extensive literature review is essential to all steps of the quantitative research process and to some qualitative designs. From this perspective the review is broad and systematic, as well as in-depth, but not usually exhaustive; it is a critical collection and evaluation of the important published literature in journals, monographs, books, and/or book chapters, as well as unpublished data-based print and computer-accessed materials (e.g., doctoral dissertations and masters' theses), audiovisual materials (e.g., audiotapes and videotapes), and sometimes personal communications (e.g., conference presentations and one-on-one interviews).

From a researcher's perspective the objectives in Box 4-1 direct the questions the researcher asks while reading the literature to determine a useful research question(s) and implementation of a particular study.

As a consumer of research the following brief overview of the use of the literature review in relation to the steps of the quantitative research process will help you to understand the researcher's focus. (Chapters 6, 7, and 8 provide an in-depth presentation related to qualitative research.) A critical review of relevant literature impacts the steps of the quantitative research process as follows:

- *Theoretical or conceptual framework:* A critical literature review reveals conceptual traditions, concepts, and/or theories or conceptual models from nursing and other related fields that can be used to examine problems. This framework presents the context for studying the problem and can be viewed as a map for understanding the relationships between or among the variables in quantitative studies. The literature review provides rationale for the variables and explicates connections or relationships of the individual variables for the theoretical framework of the study. The literature review should demonstrate use of mainly **primary sources;** there are of course exceptions when secondary sources are used. The studies selected for the literature review should offer the strongest and most consistent level of evidence available on the topic.

- *Research question and hypothesis:* The literature review helps to determine what is known and not known; to uncover gaps, consistencies, or inconsistencies; and/or to disclose unanswered questions in the literature about a subject, concept, theory, or problem. The review allows for refinement of research questions and/or hypotheses.

- *Design and method:* The literature review exposes the strengths and weaknesses of the existing evidence in terms of designs and methods of previous research studies and helps the researcher choose an appropriate new, replicated, or refined design, including data-collection method, sample size, valid and reliable instrumentation, effective data analysis method, and appropriate ethical consent forms. Many times it uncovers that the instruments used in various studies lacked adequate validity and reliability, thus jeopardizing study findings as well as identifying the need for instrument refinement or development through research testing. Often, because of space limitations, researchers do not include this information in their journal article.

- *Outcome of the analysis (i.e., findings, discussion, implications, and recommendations):* The literature review is used to accurately interpret and discuss the results/findings of a study. The researcher returns to the literature and uses conceptual and data-based literature to accomplish this goal (see Chapters 17 and 18). For example, Van Cleve et al. (2004) (see Appendix B), in their results related to the pain experience of children with leukemia, noted in their discussion that their findings were confirmed by evidence from previous studies they reviewed. The literature review also helps to develop the implications of the findings for practice, education, and further research. Figure 4-2 relates the literature review to all aspects of the quantitative research process.

PRIMARY AND SECONDARY SOURCES

A credible literature review reflects the use of mainly **primary sources.** Table 4-3 gives the general definition and examples of these sources. Most primary sources are found in published

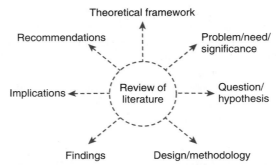

Figure 4-2. Relationship of the review of the literature to the steps of the quantitative research process.

TABLE **4-3 Primary and Secondary Sources**

Primary: Essential	**Secondary: Useful**
This is the person who conducted the study, developed the theory (model), or prepared the scholarly discussion on a concept, topic, or issue of interest (i.e., the original author). Primary sources can be published or unpublished. Data-based examples: An investigator's report of his or her research study (i.e., purpose or aims, questions/hypothesis[es], design/method, sample/setting, findings, results [e.g., articles in Appendixes A through D]) is a primary source of data-based reports; McCloskey Dochterman and Bulechek's (2004) book is a primary source for the data-based nursing intervention classification (NIC) system; Moorhead et al.'s (2004) article is a primary source for the nursing outcomes classification (NOC) system; NANDA's taxonomy of nursing diagnoses (NANDA, 2003) is a primary source of these diagnoses and defining characteristics, many of which have been refined through research studies. Conceptual or theoretical example: A theorist's work reported in the literature by the author in an article, chapter of a book, or a book (Peplau, 1952, 1991) is an example. HINT: Critical evaluation of mainly primary sources is essential to a thorough and relevant review of the literature.	This is someone other than the original author (i.e., the person who conducted the original work—whether it is data-based or conceptual) who writes or presents the author's original work. The material is usually in the form of a summary or critique (i.e., analysis and synthesis) of someone else's scholarly work. Secondary sources can be published or unpublished. Secondary source examples are the following: Response/commentary/critique articles of a research study, a theory/model, or a professional view of an issue; review of literature article published in a refereed scholarly journal; abstracts of a published work written by someone other than the original author; a doctoral dissertation's review of the literature. HINT: Use secondary sources sparingly; however, secondary sources—especially of studies that include a research critique—are a valuable learning tool for a beginning consumer of research.

BOX 4-3   EXAMPLES OF NURSING JOURNALS FOR LITERATURE REVIEWS*

Advances in Nursing Science
American Journal of Critical Care
AORN Journal (Association of Operating Room
    Nurses)
Applied Nursing Research
Archives of Psychiatric Nursing
Cancer Nursing
Clinical Nurse Specialist
Clinical Nursing Research
Evidence Based Nursing
Geriatric Nursing
Heart & Lung
International Journal of Nursing Studies
Issues in Comprehensive Pediatric Nursing
Issues in Mental Health Nursing
Journal of the American Psychiatric Nurses Association
Journal of Advanced Nursing
Journal of Clinical Nursing
Journal of Neonatal Nursing
Journal of Nursing Administration (JONA)
Journal of Nursing Care Quality
Journal of Nursing Education
Journal of Nursing Measurement

Journal of Nursing Scholarship (formerly Image:
    Journal of Nursing Scholarship)
Journal of Obstetric, Gynecologic and Neonatal
    Nursing
Journal of Professional Nursing
Journal of Qualitative Research
Journal of the American Psychiatric Nurses
    Association
Journal of Transcultural Nursing
Nurse Educator
Nursing Diagnosis: The International Journal of
    Nursing Language and Classification (formerly
    Nursing Diagnosis)
Nursing Management
Nursing Outlook
Nursing Research
Nursing Science Quarterly
Oncology Nursing Forum
Pediatric Nursing
Public Health Nursing
Research in Nursing & Health
Scholarly Inquiry for Nursing Practice
Western Journal of Nursing Research

*Main focus: **Peer-reviewed journals**, primary sources of research studies and conceptual articles; sources of some secondary sources (e.g., extensive reviews of literature on a particular concept) and issues, as well as responses or critiques of data-based and conceptual articles; most are **refereed journals**; all can be searched through CINAHL, PubMed, and MEDLINE, as well as other health-related computer and print databases.
Note: Many articles found in these journals are available online.

literature. A **secondary source** often represents a response to or a summary and critique of a theorist's or researcher's work, an in-depth analysis of a topic/issue/problem/concept, or an educational article on a specific practice.

Box 4-3 lists peer-reviewed journals that contain both primary and secondary articles. Table 4-3 highlights the differences between primary and secondary sources. Table 4-4 gives examples of primary and secondary print sources in addition to the data-based articles found in Appendixes A through D. There are two general reasons for use of secondary sources. The first reason is that a primary source is literally unavailable. This is rarely the case in this age of computer searches and interlibrary loans. In addition, most libraries have the ability to copy an article and send or fax it to the person requesting the information. Also, many articles are available today as full-text articles on an electronic database. Another reason to use a secondary source is because it can provide different ways of looking at an issue or problem. Secondary sources can help you develop the ability to see things from another person's point of view, which is an essential aspect of critical reading (Paul and Elder, 2001). Secondary sources should not be overused, however, especially for literature reviews, although they can be very valuable to the beginning consumer of research.

Secondary sources published in refereed journals usually provide a critical evaluation of or a response to a theory or research study.

TABLE **4-4 Conceptual and Data-Based Examples of Primary and Secondary Journal Articles, Books, Chapters in Books, or Documents**

Primary	Secondary
JOURNAL ARTICLE	**JOURNAL COMMENTARY**
Koniak-Griffin D, Verzemnieks IL, Anderson NLR, Janna Lesser MB, Kim S, Turner-Pluta C: Nurse visitation for adolescent mothers: two-year infant health and maternal outcomes, *Nurs Res* 52:127-135, 2003 (Appendix A)	Forbes D: Multisensory stimulation was not better than usual activities for changing cognition, behaviour, and mood in dementia, 2004. Abstract Commentary on Baker R, Holloway J, Holtkamp CCM, Larsson A, Hartman LC, Pearce R et al.: Effects of multi-sensory stimulation for people with dementia, *J Adv Nurs* 43(5):465-477, 2003 (research)
BOOK	**BOOK**
Peplau HE: *Interpersonal relations in nursing: a conceptual frame of reference for psychodynamic nursing,* New York, 1991, Springer (conceptual)	Reed PG, Shearer NC, Nicol LH, editors: *Perspectives on nursing theory,* Philadelphia, 2004, Lippincott Williams & Wilkins
CHAPTER IN A BOOK	**CHAPTER IN A BOOK**
Krainovich-Miller B, Rosedale M: Behavioral health home care. In Shea C et al., editors: *Advanced practice nursing in psychiatric and mental health care,* St Louis, 1999, Mosby	Reed PG: Transforming practice knowledge into nursing knowledge—a revisionist analysis of Peplau. In Reed PG, Shearer NC, Nicol LH, editors: *Perspectives on nursing theory,* pp 485-495, Philadelphia, 2004, Lippincott Williams & Wilkins
DOCUMENTS	**DOCUMENTS**
American Nurses Association: *Scope and standards for nurse administrators,* Washington, DC, 2001a, The Association	Agency for Health Care Research and Quality: *Garlic: effects on cardiovascular risks and disease, protective effects against cancer, and clinical adverse effects,* Rockville, Md, 2000, AHRQ
DOCTORAL DISSERTATION	
Gantt CJ: *Development of the postpartum smoking questionnaire (PPSQ),* Doctoral Dissertation, Research, University of San Diego, 2002 (UMI Order #AAI3062592)	

These sources usually include implications for practice and/or the work's contributions to the development of nursing science. Some issues of the *Western Journal of Nursing Research* contain a critique, entitled "Commentary," that follows a published study; the author of the study is given an opportunity to respond to the critique. The *Annual Review of Nursing Research* (Fitzpatrick, Shandor Miles, and Holditch-Davis, 2003) is another source of critiqued research.

Another secondary source that contains research evidence information presented in a distilled format is the journal *Evidence-Based Nursing*. Strict criteria for the quality and validity of research are applied to reviewed studies, and practicing clinicians assess the strength of evidence and clinical relevance of the best studies. The key details of these essential studies are presented in a succinct, informative abstract with an expert commentary on its clinical application. Secondary sources, especially those mentioned, are an important credible and time-saving measure that can help nurses keep up with the latest evidence for practice. As stressed earlier, to develop research critiquing competencies, research consumers must read primary sources and use standardized critiquing criteria (see Chapters 8 and 18). Consulting faculty, advisors, or librarians about secondary sources is an effective way to secure an appropriate resource.

 HELPFUL H I N T

Remember that a secondary source of a theory or data-based study usually does not include all of the theory's concepts or aspects of a study, and/or definitions may not be fully presented.

If concepts or variables are included in a secondary source's conceptual article, the definitions may be collapsed or paraphrased.

If the purpose, findings, and recommendations are presented in a secondary source, even if it is a literature review, these may be collapsed or paraphrased to such a degree that they no longer represent the researcher's original study.

Perhaps the critique (whether positive or negative) is based on the condensed summary or abstract; as such, it is less useful to the consumer.

Remember, one study on a topic does not prove anything; be cautious when a nurse colleague tells you to change your practice based on the results of one study.

Read a primary data-based study as well as a secondary source critique on the same study; compare your critique with the critique of the secondary source.

SYSTEMATIC REVIEWS

In addition to the literature review within a study and published reviews of the literature that summarize, critique, and synthesize articles while not using systematic methodology, there is another type of literature review called a **systematic review** (SR). A systematic review is a methodology that adheres to explicit and rigorous methods to identify, critically appraise, and synthesize relevant primary/original studies (Mulrow, Cook, and Davidoff, 1997). In general, "systematic reviews differ from other types of (literature) reviews in that they (systematic reviews) adhere to a strict scientific design in order to make them more comprehensive, to minimize the chance of bias, and so ensure their reliability" (*Systematic Reviews,* pp. 3-7). Systematic reviews or evidence summarizations produce the best available objective evidence on a topic (Albanese and Norcini, 2002). However, this type of evidence still must be examined through your evidence-based practice "lens." This means that evidence that you have derived through your critical analysis and synthesis or derived through other researcher's systematic review must be integrated with an individual clinician's expertise and patients' wishes (DiCenso, 2003; Sackett et al., 2000).

The main purpose of SRs is to offer clinicians the best available evidence to make sound clinical judgments for their patients. Systematic reviews are key to developing evidence-based practice protocols. There are two types of systematic reviews: quantitative and qualitative (see the meta-analysis section in Chapter 11). A qualitative systematic review does not use statistical methods to combine the findings. An example of a qualitative SR is found in the studies by Scott et al. (2003); these studies examined interventions for improving communication with children and adolescents about a family member's cancer. Systematic reviews that employ statistical methods to combine the findings of at least two or more studies are usually referred to as meta-analyses or quantitative systematic reviews. An analysis of the Cochrane Reviews, using CINHAL, revealed 10 SRs related to nursing. Of the 10 reviews, 3 were found that used quantitative meta-analyses: cot-nursing versus incubator care for preterm infants (Gray and Flenady,

2001), nursing interventions for smoking cessation (Rice and Stead, 2004), and home care by outreach nursing for chronic obstructive pulmonary disease (COPD) (Smith et al., 2001). The other seven SRs, classified as Cochrane Reviews, used qualitative criteria to judge the studies because there was a lack of sufficient data for quantitative analysis, such as a small number of studies or too many methodological problems (e.g., Mottram, Pitkala, and Lees, 2004; Forster et al., 2000).

Both qualitative and quantitative SRs share the following characteristics:

- Explicit: SRs indicate the question the review will address, the method of retrieving primary sources, the selection process, the critiquing criteria, and the techniques to be used to synthesize the findings.
- Reproducible: The use of explicit criteria enables another researcher to use the criteria and draw the same conclusion.
- Efficient: SRs are an essential information management tool; they condense large amounts of primary/original studies into a manageable objective format.

There are two other terms that you might encounter when retrieving literature that could be confused with traditional literature review. One term is evidence synthesis, which is the term used by the Agency for Healthcare Research and Quality (AHRQ, 2000). It uses basically the same rigorous process as the SR. The other term, integrative review, is similar to an SR but is a broader, sometimes less rigorous, nonquantitative method used to systematically combine results from a body of studies. The review by Li et al. (2004) of nine intervention studies of families with hospitalized elderly relatives is an example of an integrative review. Generally SRs since 1995 have used scientific rigorous methods.

Although a traditional review of the literature is not the same as a systematic review, when you conduct a search of the literature include systematic reviews as often as possible, because they represent the best available evidence on that topic (see section on Level I evidence in Chapter 2). Because this is a growing field, your clinical or research question may not be addressed by systematic reviews, which have more of a medical focus, so it is suggested that you contact Cochrane Field (www.cochrane.org) because they have a wider scope of **systematic review** activities (Forbes and Clark, 2003). For further information on how to conduct systematic reviews, contact the Cochrane Statistical Methods Group at www.cochrane.org. The *British Medical Journal* (BMJ) is another international source of the best available clinical evidence for effective health care that nurses at basic and advanced practice levels should find useful when conducting a review of the literature on a clinical topic. It provides print updates twice a year including a CD, and updates are extended monthly at www.clinicalevidence.com, which is a free internet site (BMJ, June, 2004). Therefore although you may believe that the literature review you wrote for a class assignment was systematically researched and written (and very time-consuming), you should not confuse it with a systematic review.

REVIEW OF THE LITERATURE: RESEARCH CONSUMER PERSPECTIVE

As a consumer of research, you are not expected to write a complete review of the literature on your own. However, you are expected to know how to conduct a literature review and critically evaluate it. Understanding the purpose(s) of a literature review for research and research consumer purposes will enable you to meet beginner goals. In your basic research course, you develop novice competencies in understanding and evaluating research findings that have implications for your practice.

Embedded in the purposes of a literature review is the ability to do the following:

- Efficiently retrieve an adequate amount of scholarly literature using **electronic databases.** Some electronic databases that can be retrieved via the internet are the **Cumulative Index to Nursing and Allied Health Literature (CINAHL), MEDLINE,** and the **Cochrane Data-Base of Systematic Reviews;** a multitude of health information is also available on the Web (Schloman, 2002). Traditional print resources for material not entered into common electronic databases should also be explored.

- Critically evaluate data-based and conceptual material based on accepted critiquing criteria for reviewing the respective literature.
- Synthesize the critically evaluated literature according to your level of educational competence.

The objectives in Box 4-1 are reflections for a beginning consumer of research (see Chapter 1). Table 4-5 presents an overview of the steps for conducting a literature search. In the right-hand column, you will find some useful tips/strategies or rationales for successfully completing these steps. This process is the same whether the purpose is critiquing or writing a literature review; it reflects the cognitive processes and manual techniques of retrieving and critically reviewing literature sources. The remainder of this chapter presents the essential material for accomplishing these goals.

 EVIDENCE-BASED PRACTICE TIP

Formulating a clinical question provides a focus that guides the literature review.

SCHOLARLY LITERATURE

Conceptual and Data-Based Literature: Synonyms and Sources

Synonyms for conceptual and data-based scholarly literature are presented in Table 4-6. The term *theoretical literature* is most often interchanged with **conceptual literature,** while the terms **empirical literature, scientific literature,** or *research literature* are interchanged with *data-based literature.* Table 4-7 presents defini-

tions and examples of conceptual and data-based literature.

The usual sources of conceptual literature are books, chapters of books, and journal articles. The most common sources of data-based literature are journal articles, critique reviews, abstracts published in conference proceedings, professional and governmental reports, and unpublished doctoral dissertations. Data-based and conceptual articles are available online in full-text format. A number of full-text articles are usually available when you conduct your electronic search of databases; if your college/university subscribes to a journal, you can definitely get the article online; if not, it can be requested through an interlibrary loan. An example of a free, peer-reviewed, international online publication that addresses pertinent topics affecting nursing practice, research, and education and the wider health care sector is *The Online Journal of Issues in Nursing (OJIN)* (see http://www. ana.org/ojin/). Both MEDLINE and CINAHL index this journal. The national honor society of nursing Sigma Theta Tau International also has a new online knowledge magazine, *Excellence in Nursing Knowledge* (ENK). The inaugural issue is posted now at www.nursingknowledge.org/enk. Although quarterly summaries will be free, there will be a slight charge for each issue.

 HELPFUL H I N T

The critical reading strategy (see Chapter 2) of scanning an article's abstract is very useful in helping to determine if the article is data-based or conceptual.

 EVIDENCE-BASED PRACTICE TIP

Reading and synthesizing data-based articles and the evidence they provide are essential to implementing evidence-based nursing practice.

TABLE **4-5 Steps and Strategies for Searching for Literature**

Steps of Literature Review	Strategy
Step I: Determine concept/issue/topic/problem **Step II:** Identify variables/terms **Step III:** Conduct computer search using at least two recognized electronic databases	Keep focused on the types of patients/clients you deal with in your work setting. You know what works and does not work in the delivery of nursing care. In your student role, keep focused on the assignment's objective; use the literature to support opinions or develop a concept under discussion.
Step IV: Weed out irrelevant sources before printing	Ask your reference librarian for help, and read the data-based guide books usually found near the computers that are used for student searches; include "research" as one of your variables.
Step V: Organize sources from printout for retrieval	Conduct the search yourself or with the help of your librarian; it is essential to use at least two health-related databases, such as CINAHL, MEDLINE, or PubMed.
Step VI: Retrieve relevant sources	Scan through your search, read the abstracts provided, and mark only those that fit your topic; select "references," as well as "search history" and "full-text articles" if available, prior to printing your search or downloading it to a disk or e-mailing it to yourself.
Step VII: Copy articles, if unable to print directly from database, and/or order through interlibrary loan	Organize by journal type and year and reread the abstracts to determine if the articles chosen are relevant and worth retrieving.
Step VIII: Conduct preliminary reading and weed out irrelevant sources	If an article is available online or in journals or microfiche, scan its abstract before printing or copying it to determine if it is worth your time and money to retrieve it.
Step IX: Critically read each source (summarize and critique each source)	Save yourself time and money; buy a library copying card ahead of time or bring plenty of change so that you avoid wasting time midway to secure change.
Step X: Synthesize critical summaries of each article	Copy the entire article (including the references), making sure that you can clearly read the name of the journal, year, volume number, and pages; this can save you an immense amount of time when you are word-processing your paper.
	Review critical reading strategies (see Chapter 2; e.g., read the abstract at the beginning of the articles; see the example in this chapter).
	Use the critical reading strategies from Chapter 2 (e.g., use a standardized critiquing tool), take time to word-process each summary (no more than 1 page long), include the references in APA style at the top or bottom of each abstract, and staple the copied article to the back of the summary.
	Decide how you will present your synthesis of the reviewed articles (e.g., chronologically or according to type: data-based or conceptual) and word-process the synthesized material and a reference list.

Examples of Theoretical Material

Some conceptual or theoretical articles do not use the term *conceptual* in the title, yet on close review these articles are actually extensive literature reviews of both conceptual and data-based articles on a specific concept or variable; they are usually not exhaustive reviews. You may see the terms literature review and review of the literature used interchangeably; integrative review is also used, but many literature review articles do not employ the broad criteria of an integrative review previously discussed.

Moorhead, Johnson, and Maas (2004) conducted a literature review of both data-based and conceptual articles related to the effect of nursing research on diagnostic specific outcomes. Greenway's (2004) conceptual article on using the ventrogluteal site for intramuscular (IM) injection reviewed 21 data-based and conceptual articles from the UK, United States, and Canada. This review included Beyea and Nicoll's (1996) classic literature review related to the administration of IM injections, which reviewed over 90 studies related to IM injections from the 1920s to 1995. Greenway stated that the purpose of this literature review was to change nursing's common practice of using the dorsogluteal site for IM injections to the evidence-based ventrogluteal site.

Another example of a literature review is the review by Fisher (2004) on health disparities and the mentally retarded. Although search strategies to retrieve both conceptual and data-based articles between 1992 to 2002 were specified, specific critiquing criteria of 33 of the 54 data-based studies retrieved were not identified.

Do not assume that because an article's abstract uses terms such as *purpose, organizing framework, findings,* and *conclusions* that it is a research study. For example, these terms were used in the abstract of the conceptual article by Ferguson (2004) that examined the concepts of external validity and generalizability related to research findings.

TABLE 4-6 **Literature Review Synonyms**

Conceptual Literature	Data-Based Literature
Theoretical literature	Empirical literature
Scholarly nonresearch literature	Scientific literature
Scholarly literature	Research literature
Soft vs. hard science	Scholarly research literature
Literature review article	Research study
Analysis article	Concept analysis (as methodology)
Integrative review	Study

TABLE 4-7 **Types of Information Sources for a Review of Literature***

Conceptual Literature	Data-Based Literature
Published articles; documents; chapters in books; or books discussing theories, conceptual frameworks, conceptual models, concept(s), constructs, or theorems	Published quantitative and qualitative studies, including concept analysis and/or methodology studies on a concept and meta-analyses; material found in journals, monographs, or books that are directly or indirectly related to problem of interest
Literature reviews of a concept that includes both conceptual and data-based critiques	Unpublished studies: masters' theses and doctoral dissertations
Proceedings and audiotapes and videotapes from scholarly conferences containing abstracts of a conceptual paper or entire conceptual presentation	Unpublished research abstracts or entire studies from print, audio, online; proceedings of conferences, compendiums, professional organizations' home pages, or listservs (see library/computer activities section in text)
Web-based online articles and information from professional organizations and state and federal agencies	

*Many of the examples given are or will be available online.

The differences between data-based and conceptual articles will become clear to you as you learn about the various types of quantitative and qualitative designs and become more familiar with the fact that some research journals include theoretical articles, as well as research articles.

As a rule of thumb, even if a research study does not obtain significant findings, it is still considered a data-based article. Also, conceptual articles do not use terminology such as _design, sample, experimental and control group, or methodology_ as headings. When in doubt, ask your reference librarian or a faculty member to help you. Asking for clarification is a true sign of a critical thinker (Paul and Elder, 2001).

Data-Based Material

Nursing has an ever-growing body of data-based or research literature that focuses on testing various concepts, theories, or models, as well as a variety of variables related to the practice of nursing. Data-based articles are _primary sources._ For example, there are studies that tested components of Peplau's theory of "interpersonal relations in nursing" (Peplau, 1952, 1991), such as the work of Forchuk and colleagues (Forchuk, 1993, 1994; Forchuk and Voorberg, 1991; Forchuk et al., 2000) and the work of Peden (1993, 1996, 1998).

The following are data-based articles found in the appendixes of this book that focus on various aspects of patient problems and nursing interventions:

- The randomized control trial of Koniak-Griffin et al. (2003) examined the rates of morbidity, unintentional injuries, and hospitalizations of children of adolescent mothers (see Appendix A).
- The longitudinal descriptive by Van Cleve et al. (2004) evaluated the pain experience, management interventions, and outcomes of children with acute leukemia (see Appendix B).

- The study by Plach, Stevens, and Moss (2004) was a qualitative content analysis of the social role experiences of women living with rheumatoid arthritis (see Appendix C).
- Davison et al. (2003) performed a quasiexperimental study to determine how providing individualized information to men (and their partners) suffering from prostate cancer facilitated treatment decision making (see Appendix D).

Data-based articles may specifically indicate in their title that a study was conducted, but more often they do not. There are several ways to determine if an article is data-based. First, read the title and look for keywords that suggest testing (e.g., effect, relationship, evaluation, exploration, cross-sectional, or longitudinal). Next, see which journal published the article. There are a number of journals that predominantly publish research articles (e.g., _Nursing Research, Applied Nursing Research, Journal of Nursing Scholarship,_ and _Research in Nursing and Health_). The only way to determine if an article is actually a research study is to read the abstract and the article itself. A review of the abstracts of the studies that appear in Appendixes A, B, C, and D indicates that all of the articles are original reports of completed studies. Another helpful tip that will enable you to implement an evidence-based practice is to include "research" as one of your electronic search strategies (see the section of this chapter on conducting electronic searches). If you are still unclear from reading the abstract or scanning the article, review the criteria for evaluating a qualitative study (see Chapter 8) and a quantitative study (see Chapter 18).

Refereed Journals

A major portion of most literature reviews consists of journal articles. Journals are a ready source of the latest information on almost any conceivable subject. Unfortunately, books and texts—despite the inclusion of multiple data-based sources—take much longer to publish than journals. Therefore journals are the preferred mode of communicating the latest theory or results of a research study. As a beginning consumer of research, you should use **refereed or peer-reviewed journals** as your first source of primary scholarly literature. A refereed journal has a panel of external and internal reviewers (i.e., peer-reviewed) or editors who review submitted manuscripts for possible publication. The external reviewers are drawn from a pool of nurse scholars who are experts in various fields. In most cases these reviews are "blind"; that is, the manuscript (i.e., research study or conceptual article) to be reviewed does not include the name of the author(s). The review panels use a set of scholarly criteria to judge whether a manuscript is worthy of publication; these criteria are similar to those used to judge the strengths and weaknesses of a study (see Chapters 8 and 18). The credibility of the reported research or conceptual article is enhanced through this peer-review process.

For example, Cochrane Systematic Reviews published Nixon et al.'s (2004) systematic review on aerobic exercise interventions for adults living with HIV/AIDS. Studies between 1991 and 2002 were reviewed; some were rejected based on exclusion criteria. If you were conducting a literature review on this same topic, you would include their systematic review as well as studies not retrieved for their review; i.e., your search would cover 2002 through 2005.

CONDUCTING A SEARCH AS A CONSUMER OF RESEARCH

In your student role, when you are preparing an academic paper you read the required course materials as well as additional literature retrieved from the library. Students often state, "I know how to do research." Perhaps you have thought the same thing because you "researched" a topic for a paper in the library. In this situation, however, it would be more accurate for you to say that you have been "searching" the literature to uncover data-based and conceptual information to prepare an academic term paper on a certain topic.

Although reviewing the literature for research purposes and research consumer activities requires the same critical thinking and reading skills, a literature review for a research proposal is usually much more extensive and comprehensive, and the critiquing process is more in-depth. From an academic standpoint, requirements for a literature review for a particular assignment differ depending on the level and type of course, as well as the specific objective of the assignment. These factors determine whether a student's literature search requires a minor, selected, or cursory review (i.e., a limited review or a major or extensive review). Regardless, discovering knowledge is the goal of any search; therefore a consumer of research must know how to search the literature. Reference librarians are excellent people to ask about various sources of scholarly literature. If you are unfamiliar with the process of conducting a scholarly computer search, your reference librarian can certainly help.

TYPES OF RESOURCES

Internet: Online Electronic Databases

Before the 1980s, a search was usually done by hand using **print indexes** or **print databases.** This was a tedious and time-consuming process. Print indexes are actually a small portion of what is available electronically because the electronic format has virtually unlimited space. The print indexes, however, are useful for finding sources that have not been entered into electronic databases. Electronic databases specify which years are covered. **Electronic databases** are used to find journal sources (periodicals) of data-based and conceptual articles on a variety of topics (e.g., doctoral dissertations), as well as the publications of professional organizations and various governmental agencies.

Most college/university libraries have an electronic card catalogue such as BobCat to find books, journals (titles only), videos and other media items, scripts, monographs, conference proceedings, masters' theses, dissertations, archival materials, and more. Card catalogues are rarely used except for dates not entered into electronic sources, which are most often accessed via the Web for online direct use. Box 4-4 lists examples of the more commonly used electronic databases. Your college/university most likely enables you to access such databases from your residence whether on campus or not. The most relevant and frequently used source for nursing literature remains the **Cumulative Index to Nursing and Allied Health Literature (CINHAL)** (print versions were known as the "Red Books"). Print versions cover all nursing and related literature from 1956 to the present. These electronic databases include sources from whatever date the particular database added an electronic version; each electronic database usually indicates the starting date of entries. For example, the electronic CINAHL database contains sources from 1982 to the present, whereas the print index covers 1956 to the present. Print resources are still necessary if a search requires materials not entered into an electronic database before a certain year.

You are probably familiar with accessing a **Web browser** (e.g., Netscape Communicator or Internet Explorer) to do searches for music or other entities and using search engines such as Google to find information or articles. However, "surfing" the Web is not a good use of your time for scholarly literature searches. Table 4-8 indicates sources of free online information. Review it carefully to determine if it is a good source of primary data-based studies. Note that it includes government Web sites such as http://www.hrsa.gov/ or http://www.nih.gov/, which are sources of health information, and some clinical guidelines based on systematic reviews of the literature, but most Web sites are not a primary source of data-based reports. Less common and less used sources of scholarly material are audiotapes, videotapes, personal communications (e.g., letters or telephone or in-person interviews), unpublished doctoral dissertations, and masters' theses.

Most searches using electronic databases have under the citation the option of including the abstract, complete reference, OVID full text, and remote link. When possible print the full text, which of course will include the abstract as well as the complete references. If the text is not avail-

able, then choose the option *complete reference,* which will include the abstract. Reading the abstract (see Chapter 2) is critical to determining if you need to retrieve the article through another mechanism.

Using at least two electronic health-related databases such as CINAHL and MEDLINE (see Box 4-4) is recommended.

💡 HELPFUL H I N T

Make an appointment with your educational institution's reference librarian so you can take advantage of his/her expertise in accessing electronic databases.

When you are doing your electronic search, make sure you have an empty/formatted disk so you can download your search and not take up unnecessary room on your computer's hard drive; or e-mail your search to yourself.

Take the time to set up your home/dorm computer for electronic library access.

If the full text of an article is unavailable through your electronic search, choose the option complete reference so you can read the abstract to determine if the article is data-based.

Performing a Computer Search

Why a Computer Search?

Perhaps you are still not convinced that computer searches are the best way to acquire information for a review of the literature. Maybe you have gone to the library, taken out a few of the latest journals, and tried to find a few related articles. This is an understandable temptation, especially if your assignment only requires you to use five articles. Try to think about it once again from another perspective and ask yourself the following question: "Is this the most appropriate and efficient way to find out what is the latest and strongest research on a topic that impacts patient care?" If you take the time to learn how to do a sound electronic search, you will have the essential competency needed for your career in nursing. The Critical Thinking Decision Path illustrated in the diagram below will help you avoid the pitfall of missing important studies because you the chose hands-on strategy of looking at the index of the most recent journals. Box 4-5 presents the advantages of using at least two electronic databases (CINAHL and MEDLINE).

BOX **4-4** COMMON DATABASES

I. COMMON PRINT DATABASES

INDEXES

Cumulative Index to Nursing and Allied Health Literature (CINAHL)
- Initially called Cumulative Index to Nursing Literature
- Print version known as the "Red Books"
- Electronic version available as part of the OVID online service

Index Medicus (IM)
- Published by the National Library of Medicine in the United States
- Includes literature from medicine, allied health, biophysical sciences, humanities, veterinary medicine, and nursing from 1960 to the present
- The electronic version, MEDLINE, covers 1966 to the present and is available on the Web via OVID or PubMed

Psychological Abstracts
- Electronic version, PsychINFO, is available via the Web

International Nursing Index (INI)
- Quarterly publication of American Journal of Nursing Company in cooperation with National Library of Medicine
- Includes over 200 journals of all languages, includes nursing publications in nonnursing journals

Nursing Studies Index
- Developed by Virginia Henderson

Hospital and Health Administration Index (HHAI)
- Formerly known as Hospital Literature Index (HLI)
- Published in 1945 by the American Hospital Association in cooperation with the National Library of Medicine (NLM)
- Included over 700 journals and related journals from the IM
- Main focus is hospital administration and delivery of care

Current Index to Journals in Education (CIJE)
- An electronic version, Educational Resources Information Center (ERIC) is available on the Web

CARD CATALOGUES
List books, monographs, theses, dissertations, audiovisuals, and conference proceedings

ABSTRACT REVIEWS
Dissertation Abstracts International, Masters' Abstracts, Nursing Abstracts, Psychological Abstracts, and Sociological Abstracts

II. COMMON ELECTRONIC DATABASES

INDEXES

Cumulative Index to Nursing and Allied Health Literature (CINAHL)
- Includes all nursing-related data-based and conceptual articles
- Electronic version available as part of the OVID online service
- Initially called Cumulative Index to Nursing Literature

MEDLINE
- Published by the National Library of Medicine in the United States
- Includes literature from medicine, allied health, biophysical sciences, humanities, veterinary medicine, and nursing from 1960 to the present
- Covers 1966 to the present and is available on the Web via OVID or PubMed

Current Index to Journals in Education (CIJE)
- First published in 1969 in cooperation with the
- An electronic version, Educational Resources Information Center (ERIC)is available on the Web

BOBCAT
Reference old card catalogues
List books, monographs, theses, dissertations, audiovisuals, and conference proceedings

ABSTRACT REVIEWS
Dissertation Abstracts International, Masters' Abstracts, Nursing Abstracts, Psychological Abstracts, and Sociological Abstracts

TABLE **4-8** **Selected Examples of Websites and Outcomes for Literature Searches**

Site	Sources	Outcomes for Literature Review
Online Journal of Issues in Nursing: site can be linked from *www.ana.org* and visa-versa; online journal owned by Kent University College of Nursing and published in partnership with the American Nurses Association's (ANA) *Nursing World*	Service offered without charge; simply join by entering your e-mail address; site will keep you posted of new articles; peer-reviewed electronic journal providing a free forum of discussion of issues in nursing	Limited for scholarly review of data-based literature when used as only source; limited to literature published in *Online Journal of Issues in Nursing;* articles from this site's journals can be printed; interesting site for beginning students of nursing (especially in courses in issues and trends) or for practicing nurses; able to link to nursing's professional nursing association (ANA); journal can be accessed via CINAHL
Sigma Theta Tau International (STTI), honor society of nursing: *www.nursingsociety.org*	Visits and updates on news and activities of the society; three online research sources available through links to Virginia Henderson International Library: *Registry of Nursing Research (RNR), Journal of Knowledge Synthesis for Nursing (OJKSN),* and *Nursing Knowledge Indexes*	For a fee, online literature search via MEDLINE can be requested (see Box 4-6 for advantages of CINAHL with MEDLINE); limited for scholarly review of data-based literature if used as the only search tool; OJKSN literature limited to studies published in STTI online journal; RNR contains over 11,000 English language international nursing studies, which are not peer-reviewed
National Institute of Nursing Research: *www.nih.gov/ninr*	Promotes science for nursing practice, funding for nursing and interdisciplinary research, and nurse scientist training programs; provides links to many nursing organizations and search sites; excellent site for graduate students	Although able to link to CRISP (Computer Retrieval of Information on Scientific Projects) and PubMed (National Library of Medicine's search service), which accesses literature via MEDLINE and PreMEDLINE and other related material from online journals, this is a LIMITED site for the beginning consumer of research for conducting scholarly review of nursing data-based literature because MEDLINE alone does not include all nursing literature; searching CINAHL and MEDLINE on your own would be your first choice; useful site for graduate students in addition to CINAHL and MEDLINE and a third database related to topic
Graduate Research in Nursing: *www.graduateresearch.com*	Online journal and search site; provides other opportunities to join listserv groups, employment opportunities, and practice products; subscribe using e-mail address; graduate students might find it worth exploring	Limited site for the beginning consumer of research for scholarly electronic data-based searches; valuable site for graduate students for networking; potential source of additional data-based material not found in CINAHL and MEDLINE; provides links to other professional organizations and information sites

TABLE 4-8 **Selected Examples of Websites and Outcomes for Literature Searches—cont'd**

Site	Sources	Outcomes for Literature Review
Midwest Nursing Research Society (MNRS): *www.mnrs.org*	Web page: site/members share information on nursing research, funding, and its organization; links to other nursing sites as well as related health care sites	Limited site for the beginning consumer of research for scholarly electronic data-based searches; graduate students may seek research grant information (see Box 4-6)
Clinical Evidence: *www.clinicalevidence.org*	Fee-based subscription from British Medical Journal Publishing Group; online full-text compendium of summaries of current knowledge on clinical conditions based on literature sources and reviews; updated and expanded every 6 months; each issue peer-reviewed by a renowned group of international experts	Costly for individuals to subscribe; determine if your institution's (work or school) library is a subscriber; instead choose CINAHL, MEDLINE, and another electronic database to retrieve systematic reviews (see Box 4-6)
Agency for Health Research and Quality (formerly Agency for Health Care Policy and Research): *www.ahrq.gov*	AHRQ supported development of 19 evidenced-based practice guidelines (1992-1996) (AHCP&R); Guideline Clearinghouse for improvement of health outcomes	Free source of primary sources of clinical guidelines; only four clinical practice guidelines can be printed; latest research activities, newest evidence-based guidelines, and previous clinical practice guidelines developed when it was known as AHCPR; important source of latest government documents for both consumers and conductors of research; these government guidelines are not available through CINAHL and other electronic databases
Cochrane Library (*www.cochrane.org*) includes Cochrane Database of Systematic Reviews (COCH), Database of Abstracts of Reviews of Effectiveness, Cochrane Controlled Trials Register, Cochrane Methodology Register, Health Technology Assessment database (HTA), and NHS Economic Evaluation Database (NHS EED), considered a database rather than a website	Electronic publication designed to supply high-quality evidence to inform people providing and receiving care, and those responsible for research, teaching, funding, and administration at all levels	Abstracts of Cochrane Reviews are available without charge and can be browsed or searched; uses many databases in its reviews including CINAHL and MEDLINE; some are primary sources (e.g., systematic reviews/meta-analyses); others (if commentaries of single studies) are a secondary source; important source for clinical evidence but limited as a provider of primary documents for literature reviews; as of Oct 2004, total of 254 reviews

CRITICAL THINKING DECISION PATH Consumer of Research Literature Review

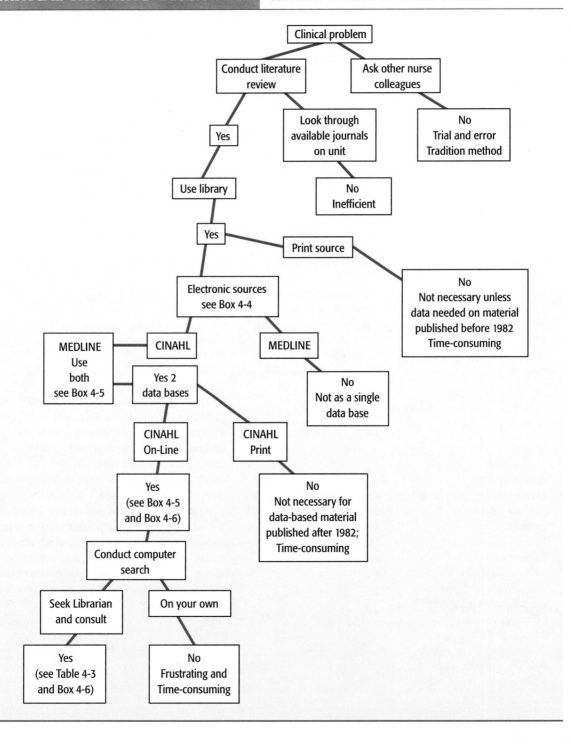

4-5 ADVANTAGES OF USING MULTIPLE ONLINE FEE-BASED DATABASES: CINAHL AND MEDLINE FOR NURSE CONSUMERS OF RESEARCH*

QUICK

Online information can be instantly accessed, especially if you have an LAN/cable connection (as opposed to a modem/telephone connection). Internet access depends on a number of factors (e.g., the server may be "down" or the number of users can affect your ability to access the information [i.e., the number of users slows down access]). As a student in a university or college, access is free via your library.

MULTIPLE DATABASES INCREASE ACCESS TO MULTIPLE SOURCES

Using multiple databases allows you to cover a broad scope of sources. CINAHL accesses more than 900,000 records from 1982 to the present (e.g., journals, books, chapters in books, abstracts, software, audiovisual, index articles from 1777 journals; download full text from 33 journals online). MEDLINE is the National Library of Medicine's database of indexed journal citations and abstracts and now covers nearly 4500 journals published in the United States and more than 70 other countries. Available for online searching since 1971, MEDLINE includes references to articles indexed from 1966 to the present. New citations are added weekly.

ALLOWS KEYWORD SEARCHING

Synonyms and related terms are considered; you can use the thesaurus for each database. For data-based literature include the terms *systematic reviews and meta-analysis.* Keep refining your search by combining terms with Boolean connectors (e.g., *and, or,* and *not*). CINAHL uses ANA-approved taxonomy terms (*NANDA, NIC, NOC, OMAHA System,* and *HHC*).

SOURCE OF ABSTRACTS AND SOME FULL-TEXT ARTICLES AVAILABLE IMPORTANT SOURCES OF DATA-BASED LITERATURE

There is access to clinical trials, meta-analyses, systematic reviews, methodologies, conceptual frameworks, and variables. All research instruments are identified.

FREQUENT UPDATES

These updates are updated monthly or weekly.

DOCUMENT RETRIEVAL

Documents can be retrieved via e-mail, downloaded to disk, and/or delivered via fax or mail for CINAHL direct and PubMed.

SAVES TIME AND INCREASES CREDIBILTY OF SERACH

*Access time and all features are not available with print index. (From CINAHL Information Systems: *Recent statistics for the CINAHL database,* Glendale, Calif, 2004, CINAHL Information Systems. Retrieved 1/10/2004 from www.cinahl.com./prodsvcs.cinahldb.htm and the National Library of Medicine. PubMed information from www.ncbi.nlm.nih.gov/PubMed/.)

 HELPFUL HINT

Use both CINAHL and MEDLINE electronic databases; it will facilitate all steps of critically reviewing the literature, especially steps III, IV, and V (see Table 4-5).

 EVIDENCE-BASED PRACTICE TIP

Reading SRs, if available, on your clinical question/topic will enhance your ability to implement evidence-based nursing practice because they generally offer the strongest and most consistent level of evidence.

How Far Back Must the Search Go?

Students often ask questions such as the following: "How many articles do I need?" "How much is enough?" "How far back in the literature do I need to go?" When conducting a search, you should use basically the same rigorous process of the SR well as variables (i.e., keywords) and other factors (e.g., "research," "abstract," or "full text"), or you may end up with hundreds or thousands of citations. Retrieving too many citations is usually a sign that there was something wrong with your search technique. Each electronic database offers an explanation of each feature; it is worth your time to click on each icon and explore the explanations offered because this will increase your confidence.

A general timeline for most academic or evidenced-based practice papers/projects is to go back in the literature at least 3 years, but preferably 5 years, although some research projects may warrant going back 10 or more years. Extensive literature reviews on particular topics or a concept clarification methodology study helps you to limit the length of your search.

As you scroll through and mark the citations you wish to include in your downloaded or printed search, make sure you review all the fields of the citation manager. In addition to indicating which citations you want and choosing which fields to search (e.g., citation plus abstract or ASCII full text [if available]), there is an opportunity to indicate if you want the "search history" included. It is always a good idea to include this information. It is especially helpful if your instructor suggests that some citations were missed, because then you can replicate your search and together figure out what variable(s) you missed so that you do not make the same error again. This is also your opportunity to indicate if you want to e-mail the search to yourself.

 HELPFUL HINT

Ask your instructor for an assignment if you are in doubt how far back you need to conduct your search.

If you come across a systematic review on your specific clinical topic, scan it to see what years the review covers; then begin your search from the last year forward to the present.

What Do I Need to Know?

Each database usually has a specific search guide that provides information on the organization of the entries and the terminology used. Table 4-9 presents a list of electronic databases you might choose from. The following suggestions and strategies incorporate general search strategies, as well as those related to CINAHL and MEDLINE. Finding the right variables/concepts/terms to "plug in" as keywords for a computer search is an important aspect of conducting a search. Both databases are very user-friendly with regard to this aspect of your search; they have "explode" features (i.e., you can search multiple headings with a single command). Another feature of this program is its mapping capability. If the term you use is not

TABLE **4-9 Online Databases: Examples of Fee-Based Databases**

Electronic Database	Sources: Data-Based and Conceptual Literature
CINAHL (Cumulative Index to Nursing and Allied Health Literature) • 1982 to present • Available as part of OVID online service	Citations of articles in journals from nursing and allied health fields (e.g., medical technology, health care administration) and publications of the ANA, NLN, AACN, professional organizations, and doctoral dissertations
MEDLINE (medical literature analysis and retrieval system online) • 1966 to present • Available as part of OVID online service • On the Web via PubMed search service retrieval system online)	Produced by National Library of Medicine; citations and some abstracts to articles on health-related topics for over 3600 biomedical and nursing journals; search service provides access to over 11 million citations in MEDLINE and PreMEDLINE and other related databases, with links to participating online journals
PsychINFO	Covers professional and academic literature in psychology and related disciplines; worldwide coverage of over 1300 journals in 20 languages; books and chapters in books in English

BOX 4-6 TIPS: USING CINAHL AND MEDLINE ONLINE VIA OVID

Connect to your library's electronic databases via your internet server. Choose "Health sciences related database" or determine which general category houses CINAHL on the menu. Then hit "Enter."

An alphabetical list of databases usually appears. Scroll down to "CINAHL." In the next column, the source of the database is indicated (e.g., on the Web); place your cursor on this term and hit "Enter."

The "Choose a database" menu will appear. You can either choose one database or choose the tab that indicates that you can choose more than one database. It is recommended that you use at least two databases. Chose "Select more than one database to search."

Once the next menu pops up, mark each of the databases you wish to search (e.g., CINAHL [1982 to present] and MEDLINE [1997 to present]).

The top of your next screen will indicate that you are using CINAHL and MEDLINE databases. It asks you to type in the keyword or phrase for your search history. Do not hesitate to explore the various icons that appear at the top of the menu. You can search by author, title, or particular journal. Another useful icon is the "?" or "Help" icon.

Type in your keyword or phrase (e.g., "nursing intervention and depression"). Do not use complete sentences. (Ask your librarian for the manual guide for each database or use feature in the database.)

Each word is searched separately, and "hits" (i.e., a set of corresponding items) are created for each word.

Before choosing "Perform search," make sure you mark "Save search history," limit the years of publication according to the objectives of your assignment, and indicate if you are limiting it to "Research" and/or "Abstracts" or "Full text available."

See the results in Table 4-10 that use the terms *treatment* and *depression:* 12,216 citations were retrieved. This first history did not "limit," as was suggested here. Before performing the search, the program may ask you to limit your search by providing various keywords or phrases for you to mark either "focus" or "explode" (i.e., narrowing or broadening your search).

Add additional variables to narrow your search (e.g., "nursing research"). Marking any additional limitations by typing in the "Keyword" box "#1" and "nursing research" and marking the appropriate "limit to" categories resulted in 9 studies.

Using the Boolean connector "and" between each of the above words you wish to use plus additional variables narrows your search. Using the Boolean "or" broadens your search.

Boolean connectors save time because you do not have to retype each search word.

Once the search results appear and you determine that they are manageable, you can decide whether to review them on screen, print them, save them to disk, or e-mail them to yourself (i.e., in the NYU, Bobst Library, CINAHL, MEDLINE, OVID Search).

---

exactly the same as it is in the database, the program maps or connects you to the term nearest to what you typed in (CINAHL, 2004). Both databases have assigned index terms known in CINAHL as medical headings and in MEDLINE as MeSH; it is important to combine index terms. You should expect to do a number of search histories. This may sound like it will take a great deal of time, but it does not. Once you type in your keywords and choose "perform

search," the results come up almost instantly. If you are still having difficulty, do not hesitate to ask your reference librarian.

Box 4-6 offers a quick overview of how user-friendly these two databases can be; it provides a number of tips that literally walk you through the steps of a search. Implementing an evidence-based nursing practice requires developing efficient electronic search skills. This particular protocol is based on using CINAHL and

MEDLINE. Of course the specifics may differ in your institution, but there are more similarities than differences. The example given in Table 4-10 indicates the number of citations retrieved using two databases at once, CINAHL and MEDLINE. After choosing the tab on the menu entitled "choose more than one database," the keywords "anxiety disorders" and "treatment" were entered and limited to the years 1996 to 2004; then the search was performed. As indicated in Table 4-10, the first search (#1) revealed 18,255 citations, which is a very good indication that you did not narrow your keywords sufficiently. This is far too many citations to scroll through. In addition to the number of citations retrieved, the first few citations usually appear. In this example, the first few were found in the CINAHL database. In the next search (#2), the keywords were combined (e.g., "depression and treatment" and "nursing intervention and adults"). Search #3 was limited to the years 1999 to 2004 and yielded 12,216 citations. Table 4-10 indicates that the next search history (indicated #4 in Table 4-10) revealed a more useful number of retrievals (9). Using the Boolean connector "and" with "nursing" along with checking "research" resulted in 14 research citations for search #2 (see the explanation of the Boolean connector "and" in Box 4-6). Although none were full-text, at this point you can easily read through the abstracts to determine if the articles should be retrieved through library retrieval, i.e., very quickly if your library subscribes to the journal or through interlibrary loan. Having

TABLE **4-10 Example of CINAHL, MEDLINE, OVID Search**

STEP 1: INITIAL TRY			
#	**Search History**	**Results**	**Display**
1	(depression and treatment).mp. [mp = ti, sh, ab, it, ot, rw]	18,255	Display
0 Saved Searches	0 Saved Search History	0 Deleted Searches	0 Removed Duplicates

ENTER KEYWORD OR PHRASE

	Perform Search		
Limit to:			
Abstracts	Consumer Health Journals	English Language	
Full-Text Available	Review Articles Human	Latest Update	Research
Publication Year			
	↓	↑	

Ask a Librarian

STEP 2: SECOND TRY			
#	**Search History**	**Results**	**Display**
2	Limit 14 to research (limit not valid in OVID, MEDLINE(R); records were retained)	16,874	Display
3	Limit 15 to years 1999-2004	12,216	Display
4	Limit 16 to nursing research.mp. [mp = ti, sh, ab, it, ot, rw]	9	Display

Modified from CINAHL, MEDLINE, OVID search.

a copy of each article will allow you to organize them for priority critical reading.

This was a manageable number to review on screen by quickly reading over the abstracts and marking some for print retrieval. Do not forget to mark off the appropriate circles in the "citation," "fields," "citation format," and "action" columns, as well as to check off the box "include search history" before printing your search. The "complete reference" option should be checked in the "fields" column; although this makes for a long print job, you will often come across some classic document or one that was not entered in the computer database because it was published before 1982. If you intend to download your search to a 3.5? microdisk, make sure you include this option. When you upload it on your PC, you will be able to retrieve all of your references, as well as the references of each entry, into your word processing program. Think how much time you will save! Your reference list will be typed, and you will only have to edit the material according to the style, such as APA, required by your instructor.

You can also use two other techniques that use the thesaurus to "focus" (narrow) or "explode" (broaden) your search. "Focus" limits the search to articles that contain the subject heading you identified while "exploding" permits you to search related subject headings with a single command.

How Do I Complete the Search?

Now the truly important aspect of the search begins: your critical reading of the retrieved materials. Critically reading scholarly material, especially data-based articles, requires several readings and the use of critiquing criteria (see Chapters 2, 8, and 18). Do not be discouraged if all of the retrieved articles are not as useful as you first thought; this happens to the most experienced reviewer of literature. If most of the articles are not useful, be prepared to do another search, but discuss the variables you will use next time with your instructor and/or the reference librarian, and you may very well want to add

a third database. In the previous example of interventions with adults diagnosed with anxiety, the third database of choice may be PsychINFO (see Table 4-9). Remind yourself how quickly you will be able to do it, now that you are experienced.

 HELPFUL H I N T

Read the abstract carefully (review the discussion on critical reading strategies in Chapter 2) to determine if it is a data-based article.

It is also a good idea to review the references of your articles; if any seem relevant, you can retrieve them.

LITERATURE REVIEW FORMAT: WHAT TO EXPECT

Becoming familiar with the format of the literature review helps research consumers use critiquing criteria to evaluate the review. To decide which style you will use so that your review is presented in a logical and organized manner, you must consider the following:

- The research question/topic
- The number of retrieved sources reviewed
- The number and type of data-based vs. conceptual materials

Some reviews are written according to the variables being studied and presented chronologically under each variable. Others present the material chronologically with subcategories or variables discussed within each time period. Still others present the variables and include subcategories related to the study's type or designs or related variables.

An example of a literature review, although brief, that is logically presented according to the variables under study was completed by Davison et al. (2003) (see Appendix D). The researchers stated that their study was to "determine if providing individualized information to men who are newly diagnosed with prostate cancer and their partners would lower their levels of psychological distress and enable them to become more active participants in treatment decision making" (p. 107). The authors did not label the first two introductory paragraphs as a review of the literature, but literature related to the problem under study, including those studies later presented in more detail in the section labeled "Literature Review," was presented. They concluded that "the benefits of providing information [related to prostate cancer] to partners are unknown" (p. 108). The next section of the paper was labeled "Literature Review" and presented several studies that explored various variables related to men with prostate cancer. The next section labeled "Conceptual Framework" presented a summary of Lazarus Transaction Model of Stress and Coping, which "provided a framework to explain how men and their partners cope with stress and uncertainty of a prostate diagnosis" (p. 108).

In contrast to the styles of previous quantitative studies, the literature reviews of qualitative studies are usually handled in a different manner (see Chapters 6, 7, and 8). There is often little known about the topic under study, or the very nature of the qualitative design dictates that a review of the literature be conducted after the study is completed; then the researchers compare the literature review with their findings. In some cases, the reviewed literature is used during the analysis process.

 EVIDENCE-BASED PRACTICE TIP

Sort the research articles you retrieve according to the levels of evidence model in Chapter 2. Remember that articles that are systematic reviews, especially meta-analyses, generally provide the strongest and most consistent evidence to include in a literature review.

CRITIQUING GUIDE   *Review of the Literature*

As you analyze (critique) a scholarly report, you must use appropriate criteria. If you are reading a research study, it must be evaluated in terms of each step of the research process. The characteristics of a relevant review of the literature (see Box 4-2) and the purposes of the review of the literature (see Box 4-1) provide the framework for developing the evaluation criteria for a literature review. Difficulties that research consumers might have regarding this task and related strategies are presented after a discussion of the critiquing criteria. For a more in-depth discussion of critiquing criteria, see Chapters 8 and 18.

Critiquing the literature review of data-based or conceptual reports is a challenging task for seasoned consumers of research so do not be surprised if you feel a little intimidated by the prospect of critiquing the published research of doctorally educated researchers. Critiquing criteria have been developed for all aspects of the quantitative research process, for various quantitative designs and qualitative approaches, and for research consumer projects for educational and clinical settings. Critiquing criteria for the review of the literature are usually presented from the quantitative research process perspective. Because the focus of this book is on the baccalaureate nurse in the research consumer role, the critiquing criteria for the literature review incorporate this frame of reference. The processes used in qualitative studies are specifically presented in Chapter 8, and Chapter 18 presents an overview of evaluating quantitative research studies. The important issue for the reader is to determine the overall value of the data-based or conceptual report. Does the review of the literature permeate the report? Does the review of the literature contribute to the significance of the report in relation to nursing theory, research, education, or practice (see Figure 4-1)? The overall question to be answered is, "Does the review of the literature uncover knowledge?" This question is based on the overall purpose of a review of the literature, which is to uncover knowledge (see Box 4-1). The major goal turns into the question, "Did the review of the literature provide a strong knowledge base to carry out the reported research or scholarly educational or clinical practice setting project?" The critiquing criteria box shown below provides questions for the consumer of research to ask about literature review. Whenever possible, read both qualitative and quantitative (meta-analysis) systematic reviews of a clinical question. Remember that although these are a form of research, they also represent a body of research that has been critiqued (analyzed) and summarized through synthesis to represent the best available evidence on a particular clinical problem.

Questions related to the logical presentation of the reviewed articles are somewhat more challenging for beginning consumers of research. The more you read scholarly articles, the easier this question is to answer. At times, the type of question being asked in relation to the particular concept lends itself to presenting the reviewed studies chronologically (i.e., perhaps beginning with early or landmark data-based or conceptual literature).

Questions must be asked about whether each explanation of a step of the research process met or did not meet these guidelines (criteria). For instance, Box 4-1 illustrates the overall purposes of a literature review. The second objective listed states that the review of the literature is to determine gaps, consistencies, and inconsistencies in the literature about a subject, concept, or problem. The critiquing criteria box shown on the following page summarizes general critiquing criteria for a review of the literature. Other sets of critiquing criteria may phrase these questions differently or more broadly. For instance, questions may be the following: "Does the literature search seem adequate?" "Does the report demonstrate scholarly writing?" These may seem to be difficult questions for you to

1. What gaps or inconsistencies in knowledge does the literature review uncover?
2. How does the review reflect critical thinking?
3. Are all of the relevant concepts and variables included in the review?
4. Does the summary of each reviewed study reflect the essential components of the study design (e.g., in a quantitative design: type and size of sample, instruments, validity, and reliability; in a qualitative design: does it indicate the type [e.g., phenomenologic])?
5. Does the critique of each reviewed study include strengths, weaknesses, or limitations of the design; conflicts; and gaps or inconsistencies in information related to the area of interest?
6. Are both conceptual and data-based literature included?
7. Are primary sources mainly used?
8. Is there a written summary synthesis of the reviewed scholarly literature?
9. Does the synthesis summary follow a logical sequence that leads the reader to reason(s) why the particular research or nonresearch project is needed?
10. Does the organization of the reviewed studies (e.g., chronologically, according to concepts/variables, or by type/design/level of study) flow logically, enhancing the reader's ability to evaluate the need for the particular research or nonresearch project?
11. Does the literature review follow the purpose(s) of the study or nonresearch project?

answer; one place to begin, however, is by determining whether the source is a refereed journal. It is fairly reasonable to assume that a scholarly refereed journal publishes manuscripts that are adequately searched, use mainly primary sources, and are written in a scholarly manner. This does not mean, however, that every study reported in a refereed journal will meet all of the critiquing criteria for a literature review and other components of the study in an equal manner. Because of style differences and space constraints, each citation summarized is often very brief, or related citations may be summarized as a group and lack a critique. You still must answer the critiquing questions. Consultation with a faculty advisor may be necessary to develop skill in answering this question.

A literature review in a research article should reflect a synthesis or putting together of the main points or value of all the sources reviewed in relation to the study's research question (see Box 4-1). The relationship between and among these studies must be explained. The synthesis of a written review of the literature usually appears at the end of the review section before the research question or hypothesis reporting section. If not labeled as such, it is usually evident in the last paragraph of the introduction and/or the end of the review of the literature.

Critiquing a review of the literature is an acquired skill. Continued reading and rereading as well as seeking advice from faculty is essential to developing critiquing skills. Synthesizing the

body of literature you have critiqued is even more challenging; in fact, in this era of evidence-based practice, usually teams of researchers conduct systematic reviews (SRs). These specialized teams can critique reviews and synthesize literature that meet the proper criteria to be included in the review. If you are not familiar with SRs, take this opportunity to read both a meta-analysis (quantitative systematic review) and a qualitative metasynthesis (a qualitative type of systematic review) (Jensen and Allen, 1996; Melnyk and Fineout-Overholt, 2005). Critiquing the literature will help you transfer new knowledge from your synthesis of research findings into practice. This process is vital to the "survival and growth of the nursing profession and is essential to evidence-based practice" (Pravikoff and Donaldson, 2001; http://www.nursingworld.org/ojin/topic11/tpc11_6c.htm).

HELPFUL HINT

Use standardized critiquing criteria (see Chapter 2) to evaluate your body of data-based articles; this represents your analysis of the literature.

Making a table to represent the components of your study and filling in your evaluation will help you see the big picture of your analysis.

Synthesizing the results of your analysis means that you try and determine what was similar or different among and between these studies related to your topic/clinical question and then draw a conclusion.

Critical Thinking Challenges

- How is it possible that the review of the literature can be both an individual step of the research process and a research component used in each of the steps of the process? Support your answer with specific examples.
- How does a researcher justify using both conceptual and data-based literature in a literature review and would you, for research consumer purposes (e.g., developing an academic scholarly paper), use the same types of literature?
- A classmate in your research class tells you that she has access to the internet and can do all of her searches from home. What essential questions do you need to ask her to determine if reliable database sources can be accessed?
- An acute care agency's nursing research committee is developing an evidence-based practice protocol for patient-controlled analgesia (PCA). One suggestion is to use the AHCPR's *Pain Guidelines* (1992) and another is to conduct a search and critically appraise the literature from the past 5 years on pain control. How would you settle the question; which one of these suggestions will most effectively contribute to the goal of an evidenced-based protocol?

KEY POINTS

- The review of the literature is defined as a broad, comprehensive, in-depth, systematic critique and synthesis of scholarly publications, unpublished scholarly print and online materials, audiovisual materials, and personal communications.
- The review of the literature is used for development of research studies, as well as other consumer of research activities such as development of evidence-based practice protocols and scholarly conceptual papers for publication.
- The main objectives for the consumer of research in relation to conducting and writing a literature review are to acquire the ability to do the following: (1) conduct an appropriate electronic data-based and/or print data-based search on a topic; (2) efficiently retrieve a sufficient amount of scholarly materials for a literature review in relation to the topic and scope of project; (3) critically evaluate (i.e., critique) data-based and conceptual material based on accepted critiquing criteria; (4) critically evaluate published reviews of the literature based on accepted standardized critiquing criteria; and (5) synthesize the findings of the critique materials for relevance to the purpose of the selected scholarly project.

- Primary data-based and conceptual resources are essential for literature reviews.
- Secondary sources, such as commentaries on data-based articles from peer-reviewed journals, are part of a learning strategy for developing critical critiquing skills.
- It is more efficient to use electronic rather than print databases for retrieving scholarly materials.
- Strategies for efficiently retrieving scholarly literature for nursing include consulting the reference librarian and using at least two electronic sources (e.g., CINAHL and MEDLINE).
- Literature reviews are usually organized according to variables, as well as chronologically.
- Critiquing criteria for scholarly literature reflect the purposes and characteristics of a relevant literature review and are presented in the form of questions.
- Read systematic reviews (meta-analyses and meta-syntheses) whenever possible; they represent the best available evidence on a clinical topic.
- Critiquing and synthesizing a number of data-based articles, including systematic reviews, is essential to implementing evidence-based nursing practice.

REFERENCES

Agency for Healthcare Research and Quality: Garlic: effects on cardiovascular risks and disease, protective effects against cancer, and clinical adverse effects. Evidence Report/Technology Assessment No. 20, 2000 (AHRQ 01-E023), Rockville, Md, 2000, The Agency.

Albanese M, Norcini J: Systematic reviews: what are they and why should we care, *Adv Health Sci Educ* 7(2): 147-151, 2002.

American Nurses Association (ANA): *Women's primary health care: protocols for practice,* Washington, DC, 1995, American Nurses Publishing.

American Nurses Association (ANA): *Scope and standards of home health nursing practice,* Washington, DC, 1999, American Nurses Publishing.

American Nurses Association (ANA): *Scope and standards of practice for nursing professional development,* Washington, DC, 2000a, American Nurses Publishing.

American Nurses Association (ANA): *Scope and standards of public health nursing practice,* Washington, DC, 2000b, American Nurses Publishing.

American Nurses Association (ANA): *Nursing's social policy statement,* ed 2, Washington, DC, 2003, American Nurses Publishing.

American Nurses Association (ANA): *Scope and standards of practice,* Washington, DC, 2004, American Nurses Publishing.

Beyea SC, Nicoll LH: Administering IM injections the right way, *Am J Nurs* 96(1): 34-35, 1996.

BMJ: *Clinical evidence concise,* London, June 2004, BMJ.

Burger S: Case study of organizational and community health changes under New Jersey state welfare reform. *Policy, Politics, & Nursing Practice,* 4(2): 153-160, 2003.

CINAHL: Home page, 2004, CINAHL Information Systems, www.cinahl.com.

Davison BJ, Goldenberg SL, Gleave ME, and Degner LF: Provision of individualized information to men and their partners to facilitate treatment decision making in prostate cancer, *Oncol Nurs Forum* 30: 107-114, 2003 (Appendix D).

DiCenso A: Leadership perspectives. Evidence-based nursing practice: how to get there from here, *Can J Nurs Leader* 16(4): 20-26, 2003.

Ferguson L: External validity, generalizability, and knowledge utilization, *J Nurs Scholarship* 36(1): 16-22, 2004.

Fisher K: Health disparities and mental retardation, *J Nurs Scholarship* 26(1): 48-53, 2004.

Fitzpatrick JJ, Shandor Miles M, and Holditch-Davis D, editors: *Annual review of nursing research, vol 21, Research on child health and pediatric issues,* New York, 2003, Springer.

Forbes D: Multisensory stimulation was not better than usual activities for changing cognition, behaviour, and mood in dementia, 2004. Abstract commentary on Baker R, Holloway J, Holtkamp CCM, Larsson A, Hartman LC, Pearce R et al.: Effects of multi-sensory stimulation for people with dementia, *J Adv Nurs* 43(5): 465-477, 2003.

Forbes D, Clark K: The Cochrane library can answer your nursing care effectiveness questions, *CJNR* 35(3): 19-25, 2003.

Forchuk C, Hildegard E, and Peplau HE: *Interpersonal nursing theory,* Newbury Park, Calif, 1993, Sage.

Forchuk C: The orientation phase of the nurse-client relationship: testing Peplau's theory, *J Adv Nurs Pract* 20: 532-537, 1994.

Forchuk C, Voorberg N: Evaluating a community mental health program, *Can J Nurs Admin* 4(6): 16-20, 1991.

Forchuk C et al.: The developing nurse-client relationship: nurses' perspectives, *J Am Psychiatr Nurs Assoc* 6(1): 3-10, 2000.

Forster A, Smith J, Young J, Knapp P, House A, and Wright J: Information provision for stroke patients and their caregivers, *Cochrane Library (Oxford)(ID #CD001919)* 6(1): 3-10, 2000.

Gantt CJ: *Development of the postpartum smoking questionnaire (PPSQ),* Doctoral Dissertation, University of San Diego (UMI Order #AAI3062592), 2002.

Glass N, Davis K: Reconceptualizing vulnerability: deconstruction and reconstruction as a postmodern feminist analytical research method, *Adv Nurs Sci* 27(2): 82-92, 2004.

Gray PH, Flenady V: Cot-nursing versus incubator care for preterm infants, *Cochrane Library (Oxford)(ID #CD003062),* 2001, Issue 2 CD003062.

Greenway K: Using the ventrogluteal site for intramuscular injection, *Nurs Stand* 18(25): 39-42, 2004.

Jensen LA, Allen MN: Meta-synthesis of qualitative findings, *Qual Health Res* 6: 553-560. 1996.

Koniak-Griffin D, Verzemnieks IL, Anderson NLR, Janna Lesser MB, Kim S, and Turner-Pluta C: Nurse visitation for adolescent mothers: two-year infant health and maternal outcomes, *Nurs Res* 52: 127-135, 2003 (Appendix A).

Krainovich-Miller B, Rosedale M: Behavioral health home care. In Shea C et al., editors: *Advanced practice nursing in psychiatric and mental health care,* St Louis, 1999, Mosby.

Lenz ER, Pugh LC, Milligan RA, Gift A, and Suppe F: The middle range theory of unpleasant symptoms: an update, *Advanc Nurs Sci* 19(3): 14-27, 1997.

Li H, Mazurek Melnyk B, and McCann R: Review of intervention studies of families with hospitalized elderly relatives, *J Nurs Scholarship* 36(1): 54-59, 2004.

McCloskey Dochterman J, and Bulechek GM, editors: *Nursing interventions classification (NIC),* ed 4, St Louis, 2004, Mosby/Elsevier Science.

Melnyk BM, Fineout-Overholt E: *Evidence-based practice in nursing and healthcare: a guide to best practice,* Philadelphia, 2005, Lippincott Williams & Wilkins.

Moorhead S, Johnson M, and Maas M, editors: *Iowa outcomes project: nursing outcomes classification (NOC),* ed 3, St Louis, 2004, Mosby/Elsevier Science.

Mottram P, Pitkala K, and Lees C: Institutional versus at-home long term care for functionally dependent older people, *Cochrane Library (Oxford)(ID #CD003542),* 2004.

Mulrow CD, Cook DJ, and Davidoff F: Systematic reviews: critical links in the great chain of evidence, *Ann Intern Med* 126: 389-391, 1997.

Nixon S, O'Brien K, Glazier RH, and Tynan AM: Aerobic exercise interventions for adults living with HIV/AIDS: systematic review 3, *Cochrane Library (Oxford),* 2004, Issue 4 CD004248.

North American Nursing Diagnosis Association International (NANDA): *Nursing diagnoses: definitions and classification 2003-2004,* Philadelphia, 2003, NANDA.

Paul R, Elder L: *Critical thinking: tools for taking charge of your learning and your life,* Englewood, NJ, 2001, Prentice-Hall.

Peden AR: Recovering in depressed women: research with Peplau's theory, *Nurs Sci Q* 6(3): 140-146, 1993.

Peden AR: Recovering from depression: a one-year follow-up, *J Psychiatr Ment Health Nurs* 3: 289-295, 1996.

Peden AR: Evolution of an intervention—the use of Peplau's process of practice-based theory development, *J Psychiatr Ment Health Nurs* 5(3): 173-178, 1998.

Peplau HE: *Interpersonal relations in nursing: a conceptual frame of reference for psychodynamic nursing,* New York, 1952, Putnam and Sons.

Peplau HE: *Interpersonal relations in nursing: a conceptual frame of reference for psychodynamic nursing,* New York, 1991, Springer.

Plach SK, Stevens PE, and Moss VA: Social role experiences of women living with rheumatoid arthritis, *J Fam Nurs* 10: 33-49, 2004 (Appendix C).

Pravikoff D, Donaldson N: The online journal of clinical innovations, *Online J Issues Nurs* 5(1), 2001, www.nursingworld.org/ojin/topic11/tpc11_6c.htm.

Redman RW, Lenburg CB, and Hinton Walker P: Competency assessment: methods for development and implementation in nursing education, Online J Issues Nurs, September 30, 1999, http://www.nursingworld.org/ ojin/topic10/tpc10_3.htm.

Reed PG: Transforming practice knowledge into nursing knowledge—A revisionist analysis of Peplau. In Reed PG, Shearer NC, Nicol LH, editors: *Perspectives on nursing theory,* pp 485-495, Philadelphia, 2004, Lippincott Williams & Wilkins.

Reed PG, Shearer NC, and Nicol LH, editors: *Perspectives on nursing theory,* Philadelphia, 2004, Lippincott Williams & Wilkins.

Rice VH, Stead LF: Nursing interventions for smoking cessation. Cochrane tobacco addiction group, *Cochrane database of systematic reviews 3,* Oxford, 2004, The Cochrane.

Sackett DL, Straus SE, Rochardson WS, Rosenberg W, and Haynes RB: *Evidenced-based medicine: how to teach and practice EBM,* ed 2, Edinburgh, UK, 2000, Churchill Livingston.

Schloman B: Information resources column: quality of health information on the Web: where are we now, *Online J Issues Nurs,* December 16, 2002; available at http://nursingworld.org/oji.

Scott JT, Prictor MJ, Harmsen M, Broom A, Entwistle V, Sowden A, and Watt I: Interventions for improving communication with children and adolescents about a family member's cancer, The Cochrane Database of Systematic Reviews 2003, Issue 4. Art. No.:CD004511. DOI: 10.1002/14652858.CD004511.

Smith B, Appleton S, Adams R, Southcott A, and Ruffin R: Home care by outreach nursing for chronic obstructive pulmonary disease. The Cochrane Database of Systematic Reviews 2001, Issue 3. Art. No.: CD000994. DOI: 10.1002/14651858. CD000994.

Smith MJ, Liehr PR, editors: *Middle range theory for nursing,* New York, 2003, Springer.

Tinsley C, France NEM: The trajectory of the registered nurse's exodus from the profession: a phenomenological study of the lived experience of oppression, *Int J Hum Caring* 8(1): 8-12, 2004.

Van Cleve L, Bossert E, Beecroft P, Adlard K, Alvarez O, and Savedra MC: The pain experience of children with leukemia during the first year after diagnosis, *Nurs Res* 53: 1-10, 2004 (Appendix B).

Wall BM: The pin-striped habit: balancing charity and business in Catholic hospitals, 1865-1915, *Nurs Res* 51(1): 50-58, 2002.

Woodgate RL and Degner LF: Cancer symptom transition periods of children and families, *J Adv Nurs* 46(4): 358-368, 2004.

FOR FURTHER STUDY

Go to your Companion CD for review activities for this chapter.

evolve Go to Evolve at http://evolve.elsevier.com/LoBiondo/ for WebLinks, Content Updates, and additional research articles, for practice in reviewing and critiquing.

5

PATRICIA LIEHR
MARY JANE SMITH

Theoretical Framework

KEY TERMS

concept
conceptual definition
conceptual framework
deductive reasoning
empirical

grand theory
hypothesis
inductive reasoning
microrange theory
midrange theory

model
operational definition
theoretical framework
theory

LEARNING OUTCOMES

After reading this chapter, the student should be able to do the following:

- Compare inductive and deductive reasoning.
- Differentiate between conceptual and theoretical frameworks.
- Identify the purpose and nature of conceptual and theoretical frameworks.
- Describe how a framework guides research.
- Differentiate between conceptual and operational definitions.
- Describe the relationship between theory and research and practice.
- Discuss levels of abstraction related to frameworks guiding research.
- Differentiate among grand, midrange, and microrange theories in nursing.
- Describe the points of critical appraisal used to evaluate the appropriateness, cohesiveness, and consistency of a framework guiding research.

STUDY RESOURCES

Go to your Companion CD for review activities for this chapter.

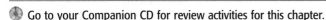 Go to Evolve at http://evolve.elsevier.com/LoBiondo/ for Weblinks, Content Updates, and additional research articles for practice in reviewing and critiquing.

As an introduction to frameworks for research, put yourself in the shoes of Kate and thoughtfully listen to her story by attending to the message it brings to the practicing nurse who wishes to critique, understand, and do research.

Kate works in a coronary care unit (CCU). She has worked in this unit for nearly 3 years since she graduated with a baccalaureate degree in nursing. She has become more comfortable with her job and now believes that she can readily manage whatever comes her way with regard to the complexities of patient care in the CCU. Recently she has been observing the pattern of blood pressure (BP) changes when health care providers enter a patient's room. This observation began when Kate noticed that one of her patients, a 62-year-old African-American woman who had continuous arterial monitoring, had dramatic increases in BP, as much as 100%, each time the health care team made rounds in the CCU. Furthermore, this elevated BP persisted after the team left the patient's room and slowly decreased to pre-round levels within the following hour. Conversely, when the nurse manager visited this same patient on her usual daily rounds, the patient engaged calmly in conversation and usually had lower BP by the time the nurse manager moved on to the next patient. Kate thought about what was happening and adjusted her work so that she could closely observe the details of this phenomenon over several days.

Team rounds were led by the attending cardiologist and included nurses, pharmacists, social workers, medical students, and nursing students. The nurse manager's visit occurred one-on-one. During team rounds, the patient was discussed and occasionally she was asked to respond to a question about her history of heart disease or her current experience of chest discomfort. Participants took turns listening to her heart, and students responded to questions related to her case. During the nurse manager's visit, the patient had solely the nurse's attention. Kate noticed that the nurse manager was especially attentive to the patient's experience. In fact, the nurse usually sat and spent time talking to the patient about how her day was going, what she was thinking about while lying in bed, and what feelings were surfacing as she began to consider how life would be when she returned home.

Kate decided to talk to the nurse manager about her observation. The nurse manager, Alison, was pleased that Kate had noticed these BP changes associated with interaction. She told Kate that she, too, had noticed these changes during her 8-year experience of working in the CCU, leading her to consider the theory entitled *attentively embracing story* (Liehr and Smith, 2000; Smith and Liehr, 2003), which seemed applicable to the observation. Alison had learned the theory as a first-year master's student, and she was applying it in practice and beginning plans to use the theory to guide her thesis research. *Attentively embracing story* proposes that intentional nurse-client dialogue, which engages the human story, enables connecting with self-in-relation to create ease (Figure 5-1). As depicted by the theory model, the central concept of the theory is intentional dialogue, which is what Kate had first observed when she noticed Alison interacting with the patient. Alison was fully attentive to the patient, following the patient's lead and pursuing what mattered most to the patient. Alison seemed to get a lot of information from the patient in a short time, and the patient seemed willing to share things she was not willing to share with other people.

According to the theory, each of the three concepts—intentional dialogue, connecting with self-in-relation, and creating ease—is intricately connected. Therefore when Kate observed intentional dialogue, she also observed connecting with self-in-relation as the patient reflected on her experience in the moment, and creating ease, when she saw lowered BP as the nurse manager left the room.

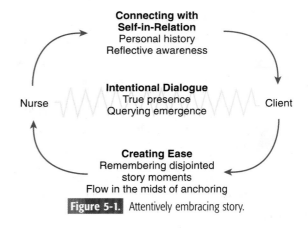

Figure 5-1. Attentively embracing story.

TABLE **5-1 Issues Affecting BP Change and Related Research Questions**

Issues	Research Questions
Number of people in patient's room	Is there a difference in BP for patients in CCU when interacting with one person as compared to interacting with two people or a group of three or more people?
Involvement of patient	For the patient in CCU, what is the relationship between BP and the amount of time spent listening to the health care team's discussion of personal qualities during routine rounds?
	What is the effect of nurse-patient intentional dialogue on BP within the hour after the dialogue?
Continuing effect of experience on routine BP over next hour	What is the BP pattern of patients in CCU from the beginning of health care rounds until 1 hour after the completion of rounds?
Content of dialogue	What is the relationship between issues discussed during intentional dialogue and BP?
Meaning of experience for patient	What is the patient experience of being the object of routine health care rounds?
	What is the patient experience of sharing personal matters with a nurse while in the CCU?

Abbreviations: BP, blood pressure; CCU, coronary care unit.

Alison and Kate shared an understanding that there was a relationship between patient-health care provider interaction and BP. They discussed several possible issues that might be affecting this relationship. They identified research questions related to each issue (Table 5-1). You may be able to think of other issues that could generate a research question contributing to understanding the relationship between patient-health care provider interaction and BP. The list developed by Kate and Alison only serves as a reflection of the complexity of the relationship. The list highlights the fact that the relationship cannot be understood with one study, but a series of studies may enhance understanding and offer suggestions for change. For instance, a thorough understanding may lead to testing different approaches for conducting team rounds.

PRACTICE-THEORY-RESEARCH LINKS

Several important aspects of frameworks for research are embedded in the story of Kate and Alison. First, it is important for the reader to notice the links among practice, theory, and research. Each is intricately connected with the

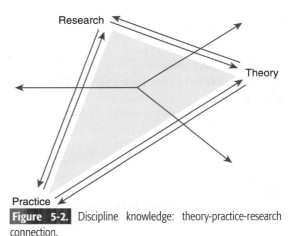

Figure 5-2. Discipline knowledge: theory-practice-research connection.

other to create the knowledge base for the discipline of nursing (Figure 5-2). **Theory** is a set of interrelated concepts that provides a systematic view of a phenomenon. Theory guides practice and research; practice enables testing of theory and generates questions for research; research contributes to theory-building and establishing practice guidelines. Therefore what is learned through practice, theory, and research interweaves to create the knowledge fabric of the discipline of nursing. From this perspective, each reader is in the process of contributing to the knowledge base of the discipline. For instance, if you are practicing, you can use focused observation (Liehr, 1992), just as Kate did, to consider the nuances of situations that matter to patient health. Kate noticed the change in BP occurring with interaction and systematically began to pay close attention to the effect of varying interactions. This inductive process often generates the questions that are most cogent for enhancing patient well-being.

APPROACHES TO SCIENCE

Another major theme of the story of Kate and Alison can be found in each nurse's way of approaching the phenomenon of the relationship between health care provider-patient interaction and BP. Each nurse was using a different approach for looking at the situation, but both were systematically evaluating what was observed. This is the essence of science—systematic collection, analysis, and interpretation of data. Kate was using **inductive reasoning,** a process of starting with details of experience and moving to a general picture. Inductive reasoning involves the observation of a particular set of instances that belong to and can be identified as part of a larger set. Alison told Kate that she, also, had started with inductive reasoning and now was using **deductive reasoning,** a process of starting with the general picture, in this case the theory of *attentively embracing story,* and moving to a specific direction for practice and research. Deductive reasoning uses two or more related concepts that when combined enable suggestion of relationships between the concepts. Inductive reasoning and deductive reasoning are basic to frameworks for research. Inductive reasoning is the pattern of "figuring out what's there" from the details of the nursing practice experience. Inductive reasoning is the foundation for most qualitative inquiry (see Chapters 6, 7, and 8). Research questions related to the issue of the meaning of experience for the patient (see Table 5-1) can be addressed with the inductive reasoning of qualitative inquiry. Deductive rea-

soning begins with a structure that guides one's searching for "what's there." All but the last two research questions listed in Table 5-1 would be addressed with the deductive reasoning of quantitative inquiry.

Given Alison's use of deductive reasoning guided by the theory of *attentively embracing story,* it can be assumed that she has read and critiqued the literature on theoretical frameworks and has chosen *attentively embracing story* to guide her master's thesis research. In order for Kate to move on in her thinking about research to study the way changes in blood pressure are related to health care provider-patient interaction, she needs to become well versed on the importance of theoretical frameworks. As she reads the literature and reviews research studies, she will critique the theoretical frameworks guiding those studies. In critiquing existing frameworks, she will develop the knowledge and understanding needed to choose an appropriate framework for research. As an initial step, Kate is reading this chapter, recognizing that she is critiquing nursing research.

 HELPFUL H I N T

Investigators may not always provide a detailed explicit statement of the observation(s) that led them to their conclusion(s) when using inductive reasoning; likewise, you will not always find a clear picture of the structure guiding the study when deductive reasoning has been used.

FRAMEWORKS AS STRUCTURE FOR RESEARCH

Whether evaluating a qualitative or a quantitative study, it is wise to look for the framework that guided the study. Generally, when the researcher is using qualitative inquiry and inductive reasoning methods, the critical reader will find the framework at the end of the manuscript in the discussion section (see Chapters 6, 7, and 8), and the reader should be aware that the framework may be implicitly suggested rather than explicitly diagrammed. From the findings of the study, the researcher builds either an implicit or an explicit structure for moving forward. In Appendix C of this book, Plach, Stevens, and Moss (2004) report findings from a study of women living with rheumatoid arthritis for at least 3 years. The researchers were interested in understanding what made social roles fulfilling for these participants. They found that the women: (1) struggled to balance roles while managing their arthritis symptoms and (2) were able to unburden social role obligations as they aged, finding meaning and strength in their daily lives. Although these findings are not organized into a model by the researchers, there is an implicit structure that provides an evidence base for practice. For instance, the findings support family-centered education, which would incorporate discussion about "realistic and flexible role expectations and modifications" (Plach, Stevens, and Moss, 2004, p. 45). In contrast, the qualitative work of Calvin (2004), which was undertaken to understand the process of making end-of-life decisions for people with end-stage renal disease, culminates in a diagrammed model of the "Theory of Self-Preservation." The model connects the three major concepts of the theory: knowing the odds; defining individuality; and personal preservation. Calvin (2004) used the grounded theory method (see Chapter 7) as compared to the content analysis method used by Plach and colleagues (2004), accounting for the explicit presentation of a model as part of the findings. Both studies used an inductive approach, moving from the detailed stories of participants to a general structure for understanding that could be modeled.

A **model** is a symbolic representation of a set of concepts that is created to depict relationships. Figure 5-1 is the model of *attentively embracing story*. It represents the nurse-client connection through the rhythmic symbol labeled *intentional dialogue*. The model depicts the process by connecting the concepts of nurse-client dialogue with linking arrows. This model could be the basis for deductive reasoning. An example of a deductive question that could be derived from the model is as follows:

> "What is the difference in salivary cortisol (an indicator of ease) for cancer patients who engage with participants (connecting with self-in-relation) in a nurse-led (intentional dialogue) cancer support group?"

 HELPFUL H I N T

When an investigator has used a deductive approach, the theoretical framework should be described to substantiate how the research question emerged.

When the researcher uses quantitative inquiry and deductive reasoning methods, the critical reader will find the framework at the beginning of the paper before a discussion of study methods. In the study of pain experience of children with leukemia (Van Cleve et al., 2004) in Appendix B, the Symptom Management model of the University of California, San Francisco, was used to guide the study plan. This model depicts a structure for the concepts of the Symptom Management theory. The three major concepts of the theory—symptom experience, symptom management strategies, and symptom outcomes (Van Cleve et al., 2004)—are defined for this study using pain as the symptom. The researchers identify instruments to measure each concept of the theory. The findings of the study provide evidence guiding pain management intervention for Caucasian and Latino children and adolescents. The researchers used deductive reasoning to move from the Symptom Management model to the instruments that were used to measure each concept in the model. This example shows how the theoretical framework guides the selection of instruments to measure the concepts. Symptom Management theory is at the middle range of abstraction, neither too comprehensive nor too narrow, allowing the researcher to readily move from the conceptual to the empirical level of the ladder of abstraction.

The Ladder of Abstraction

The ladder of abstraction is a way for the reader to gain perspective when reading and thinking

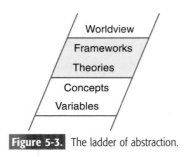

Figure 5-3. The ladder of abstraction.

about frameworks for research. When critiquing the framework of a study, imagine a ladder (Figure 5-3). The highest level on the ladder includes beliefs and assumptions, what is sometimes called the worldview of the researcher. Although the worldview is not always explicitly stated in a manuscript, it is there. In the study (see Appendix D) on individualized information for men and their partners to facilitate treatment decision making in prostate cancer (Davison et al., 2004), the researchers note a commonly held belief that "patients with cancer should be involved in making informed treatment choices" (p. 107). The study was planned because there is evidence that men who present for treatment of prostate cancer know little about the disease or treatment options (Davison et al., 2004). Davison and colleagues (2004) cite the Lazarus Transaction Model of Stress and Coping as a guide for their study, noting that the developers of this model identify information-seeking "as the most frequent method individuals use to cope with and maintain control over a stressful life event" (p. 109). Information is conceptualized as an approach to gain cognitive control from the perspective of the Lazarus model. The study hypotheses addressed how desired information affected stress for patients and their partners dealing with prostate cancer. The researchers used the Lazarus model to logically structure their study, and they provided detail linking this model to the interventions and outcome measures selected for their research. This linking of

the Lazarus model to interventions and outcomes is an example of how theory guides research.

 HELPFUL H I N T

The word "model" is often used interchangeably with "theory." For instance, the Lazarus Transaction Model of Stress and Coping is also referred to as the Lazarus Transaction Theory of Stress and Coping.

This "middle of the ladder" position of frameworks, theories, and concepts moves to a lower rung where **empirical** factors are located. Empirical factors refer to those things that can be observed through the senses and include the variables measured and described in quantitative research studies and the story that is described in qualitative studies. Table 5-2 outlines the concepts and conceptual definitions and the accompanying variables with their operational definitions from the Van Cleve et al. (2004, Appendix B) and the Davison et al. study (2004, Appendix D). For instance, in the Davison et al. study (2004), one dimension of the intervention was a survey questionnaire from the patient information program (PIP), which was designed to assess the individual information needs of men newly diagnosed with prostate cancer. This survey questionnaire brought the concept of cognitive control to the empirical level of the ladder of abstraction. The Spielberger State Anxiety Inventory was one instrument used to bring the concept of stress to the empirical level of the ladder. Thus cognitive control and stress were concepts operationalized using the survey questionnaire of the PIP and the Spielberger State Anxiety Inventory, respectively.

A **conceptual definition** is much like a dictionary definition, conveying the general meaning of the concept. However, the conceptual definition goes beyond the general language meaning found in the dictionary by defining the concept as it is rooted in the theoretical literature. The **operational definition** specifies how the concept will be measured, that is, what instruments will be used to capture the concept. The language of the operational definition is closer to the ground, on the lowest step of the ladder of abstraction.

TABLE 5-2 **Concepts and Variables: Conceptual and Operational Definitions**

Concept	Conceptual Definition	Variable	Operational Definition
Pain experience (Van Cleve et al., 2004)	Symptom experience dimension included elements of perception, evaluation, and response	Pain	Poker chip tool, preschool body outline, adolescent pediatric pain tool
		Pain management	Perception of management effectiveness
		Pain response	Functional status II
Individualized information and decision making (Davison et al., 2003)	Information and decision preferences based on Lazarus Transaction Model of Stress and Coping with focus on cognitive appraisal	Individualized information	Patient information program
Psychological distress	Feeling at the moment	Psychological distress	Spielberger State Anxiety Inventory and Center for Epidemiological Studies depression scale

 HELPFUL H I N T

Some reports of research embed conceptual definitions in the literature review. It is wise for the reader to seek and find the conceptual definitions so that the logical fit between the conceptual and operational definitions can be determined.

The Middle of the Ladder: Frameworks, Theories, and Concepts

It is important to consider the middle of the ladder of abstraction where concepts, theories, and frameworks are located. Pretend to look at the middle section through a magnifying glass so that what is located there can be distinguished and clarified. Concepts, theories, and frameworks can be compared to each other from the perspective of abstraction, with concepts being the lowest on the ladder and frameworks the highest. However, some concepts are closer to the ground than others. The same is true for theories and frameworks. For instance, the concept of pain relief is closer to the ground than the concept of caring. The idea of varying levels of abstraction within the middle of the ladder is emphasized in the section addressing theories, but it has relevance for concepts and frameworks as well.

Concepts

A **concept** is an image or symbolic representation of an abstract idea. Chinn and Kramer (1999) define a concept as a "complex mental formulation of experience." Concepts are the major components of theory and convey the abstract ideas within a theory. In this chapter, you have been introduced to several concepts, such as cognitive control, female social roles, and symptom management. Each concept creates a mental image that is explained further through the conceptual definition. For instance, pain is a concept whose mental image means something based on experience. The experiential meaning of the concept of pain is different for the child who has just fallen off a bike, for the elderly person with

rheumatoid arthritis, and for the doctorally prepared nurse who is studying pain mechanisms
using an animal model. These definitions and
associated images of the concept of pain incorporate different experiential and knowledge
components, all with the same label—pain.
Therefore it is important to know the meaning
of the concept for the person. In the case of the
reader, it is important to know the meaning that
the researcher gives to the concepts in a research
study.

Theories

A theory is a set of interrelated concepts that
structure a systematic view of phenomena for the
purpose of explaining or predicting. A theory is
like a blueprint, a guide for modeling a structure.
A blueprint depicts the elements of a structure
and the relation of each element to the other,
just as a theory depicts both the concepts
that compose it and how they are related. Chinn
and Kramer (1999) define a theory as an "expression of knowledge . . . a creative and rigorous
structuring of ideas that project a tentative, purposeful, and systematic view of phenomena."
Theories are located on the ladder of abstraction
relative to their scope. An often-used label in
nursing is "grand theory," which suggests a broad
scope, covering major areas of importance to the
discipline. Grand theories arose at a time when
nursing was addressing its nature, mission, and
goals (Im and Meleis, 1999), so it is historically
important. However, its significance extends
beyond history to have implications for guiding
the discipline today and in the future. For the
purpose of introducing the reader to theory as a
framework for nursing research, grand theory,
midrange theory, and microrange theory are discussed. As is suggested by the names of these
theory categories, grand theories are highest and
microrange theories are lowest in the level of
abstraction.

Grand Theory   Theories unique to nursing help
the discipline define how it is different from
other disciplines. Nursing theories reflect
particular views of person, health, environment,
and other concepts that contribute to the development of a body of knowledge specific to
nursing's concerns. **Grand theories** are all-
inclusive conceptual structures that tend to
include views on person, health, and environment to create a perspective of nursing. This
most abstract level of theory has established a
knowledge base for the discipline and is critical
for further knowledge development in the discipline.

The grand theories of several well-known
nursing theorists have served as a basis for
practice and research. Among these theories are
Rogers' (1990, 1992) science of unitary human
beings, Orem's (1995) theory of self-care deficit,
Newman's theory of health as expanding consciousness (1997), Roy's adaptation theory
(1991), Leininger's culture care diversity and uni-
versality theory (1996), King's goal attainment
theory (1997), and Parse's theory of human
becoming (1997). Each of these grand theories
addresses phenomena of concern to nursing
from a different perspective. For example, Rogers
views the person and the environment as energy
fields coextensive with the universe. Therefore
she recognizes the person-environment unity as
a mutual process. In contrast, King (1997) distinguishes the personal system from the interpersonal and social systems, focusing on the
interaction among systems and the interaction of
the systems with the environment. For King,
person and environment are interacting as
separate entities. This is different from the
person-environment mutual process described
by Rogers.

If a researcher uses Roger's theory to guide
plans for a study, the research question will
reflect different values than if the researcher had
used the theory by King. The researcher using
Roger's theory might study the relationship of
therapeutic touch to other phenomena that
reflect a valuing for energy fields and pattern
appreciation, whereas the researcher using King's
theory might study outcomes related to nurse-
patient–shared goals or other phenomena related

to interacting systems. It is important for the reader to realize that one grand theory is not better than another. Rather, these varying perspectives allow the nurse researcher to select a framework for research that facilitates movement of concepts of interest down the ladder of abstraction to the empirical level, where they can be measured as study variables. What is most important about the use of theoretical frameworks for research is the logical connection of the theory to the research question and the study design.

Midrange Theory   **Midrange theory** is a focused conceptual structure that synthesizes practice-research into ideas central to the discipline. Merton (1968), who has been the original source for much of nursing's description of midrange theory, says that midrange theories lie between everyday working hypotheses and all-inclusive grand theories. The reader might notice that Merton's view of the "middle" allows for a great deal of space between grand theories and hypotheses. This expansive view of the "middle" has been noted, and efforts have been made to more clearly articulate the middle and to distinguish the characteristics of midrange theory. In a 10-year review of nursing literature using specific criteria, Liehr and Smith (1999) identified 22 midrange theories. Following the suggestion of

Lenz (1996), they considered the scope of the 22 midrange theories and grouped them into high-middle, middle-middle, and low-middle categories using the theory names (Table 5-3). The reader will recognize that the groupings move from a higher to a lower level of abstraction. Because midrange theories are lower in level of abstraction than grand theories, they offer a more direct application to research and practice. As the level of abstraction decreases, translation into practice and research simplifies. In their conclusion, Liehr and Smith (1999) recommend that nurses thoughtfully construct midrange theory, weaving practice and research threads to create a whole fabric that is meaningful for the discipline. Hamric, Spross, and Hanson (2000) in their text on advanced nursing practice call midrange theories to the attention of advanced practice nurses:

> "Middle-range theories address the experiences of particular patient populations or a cohort of people who are dealing with a particular health or illness issue . . . Because middle range theories are more specific in what they explain, practitioners often find them more directly applicable. . . ."

The theory of attentively embracing story, introduced at the beginning of this chapter, is a midrange theory. The theory, which was

TABLE **5-3** **Middle Range Theory by Level of Abstraction**

High-Middle	Middle-Middle	Low-Middle
Caring	Uncertainty in illness	Hazardous secrets and reluctantly taking charge
Facilitating growth and development	Unpleasant symptoms	Affiliated individuation as a mediator of stress
Interpersonal perceptual awareness	Chronic sorrow	Women's anger
Self-transcendence	Peaceful end of life	Nurse-midwifery care
Resilience	Negotiating partnerships	Acute pain management
Psychological adaptation	Cultural brokering	Balance between analgesia and side effects
	Nurse-expressed empathy and patient distress	Homelessness-helplessness
		Individualized music intervention for agitation
		Chronotherapeutic intervention for postsurgical pain

From Liehr P and Smith MJ: Middle range theory: spinning research and practice to create knowledge for the new millennium, *Adv Nurs Sci* 21(4):81–91, 1999.

generated from nursing practice and research experience (Smith and Liehr, 2003), provides a structure for engaging patients to share what is important about a health challenge they are facing.

 EVIDENCE-BASED PRACTICE TIPS

Evidence to guide practice comes from research findings that flow from a theoretical framework.

Since middle range theories come from practice, they offer a more translatable guide for structuring an evidence base than do grand theories.

Microrange Theory **Microrange theory** is a linking of concrete concepts into a statement that can be examined in practice and research. Higgins and Moore (2000) distinguish two levels of microrange theory, one at a higher level of abstraction than the other. They suggest that microrange theories at the higher level of abstraction are closely related to midrange theories, composed of a limited number of concepts and applicable to a narrow issue or event (Higgins and Moore, 2000). The low-middle theory in Table 5-3 may fit this category. Hypotheses are an example of low abstraction microrange theories. The reader will recall that a hypothesis is a best guess or prediction about what one expects to find. Chinn and Kramer (1999) define a **hypothesis** as a "tentative statement of relationship between two or more variables that can be empirically tested." Higgins and Moore (2000) emphasize the value of microrange theory, noting that the "particularistic approach is invaluable for scientists and practitioners as they work to describe, organize and test their ideas."

As you read this text, you could articulate a microrange theory at the level of a hypothesis. At the beginning of this chapter, Kate formulated a hypothesis about the relationship between patient-health care provider interaction and blood pressure. Although Kate did not label her idea as a hypothesis, it was a best guess based on observation. If you would take a minute to think about it, some experience from nursing practice that has provoked confusion could be stated as a hypothesis. A mismatch between what is known or commonly accepted as fact and what one experiences creates a hypothesis-generating moment. Every nurse experiences such moments. Cultivating hypothesis-generating moments requires noticing them, focusing observation to untangle details, and allowing time for creative thinking and dialogue (Liehr, 1992), leading to possibilities for creating low-level microrange theory, or hypotheses.

 HELPFUL HINT

The reader of research will find conflicting views regarding levels and placement of theory. While one author labels a particular theory "grand," another author will label the same theory "midrange." The reader can evaluate the theory and assign its level from the ladder of abstraction. If a theory is at the more concrete level on the ladder, then it falls into microtheory.

Frameworks for Research

The Critical Thinking Decision Path takes the reader through the thinking of a researcher who is about to begin doing research. It is reasonable for the reader to expect to find some but not all of the phases of decision making addressed in a research manuscript. Beginning with the view of the world, the highest rung on the ladder of abstraction (see illustration on the following page), the researcher is inclined to approach a research problem from a perspective of inductive or deductive reasoning. If the researcher pursues an inductive reasoning approach, he or she generally will not present a framework before beginning discussion of the methods. This is not to say that literature will not be reviewed before introducing methods. Authors may provide an

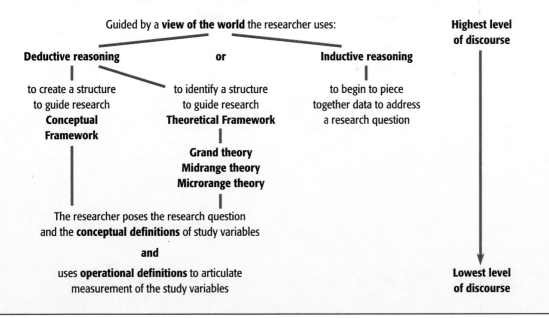

CRITICAL THINKING DECISION PATH   Choosing a Theoretical Path

Guided by a **view of the world** the researcher uses:

Highest level of discourse

Deductive reasoning   **or**   **Inductive reasoning**

to create a structure   to identify a structure   to begin to piece
to guide research   to guide research   together data to address
Conceptual   **Theoretical Framework**   a research question
Framework

Grand theory
Midrange theory
Microrange theory

The researcher poses the research question
and the **conceptual definitions** of study variables

and

uses **operational definitions** to articulate
measurement of the study variables

Lowest level of discourse

---

overview of a literature base documenting the need to do the study, but they will not provide a framework for the study because an inductive approach demands that they begin where their participants are rather than beginning with a framework. Their intent is to be free of the structures that may limit what they learn and to be open to the experience of the person who is living through the experience they are studying.

Conversely, if the researcher's view of the world is guided by deductive reasoning, he or she must choose between a conceptual or a theoretical framework. The reader will notice when reading the theory literature that these terms are used interchangeably (Chinn and Kramer, 1999). However, in the case presented in the Critical Thinking Decision Path, each term is being distinguished from the other on the basis of

whether the researcher is creating the structure or whether the structure has already been created by someone else. Generally, each of these terms refers to a structure that will provide guidance for research. A **conceptual framework** is a structure of concepts and/or theories pulled together as a map for the study. A **theoretical framework** is a structure of concepts that exists in the literature, a ready-made map for the study.

To better understand these differences, refer to the study by Koniak-Griffin et al. (2004) in Appendix C. The authors propose an early home visit intervention for adolescent moms. They base the intervention on a conceptual framework of social competence, constructed with reference to literature about factors affecting maternal and child health outcomes. Although the authors do not create a figure that models the ideas composing social competence, the figure can be inferred from their description, which provides a logical structure for their study. This logical structure is a conceptual framework as defined in the Critical Thinking Decision Path. In contrast, the research team led by Van Cleve (see Appendix B) uses a theoretical framework to guide its research, the Symptom Management Model developed by the University of California, San Francisco. This model is a tested midrange theory offering guidance for nursing practice and research. Instead of creating a structure, Van Cleve and colleagues (2004) used a theoretical framework that already existed in the literature.

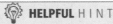 **HELPFUL** H I N T

When researchers use conceptual frameworks to guide their studies, you can expect to find a system of ideas, synthesized for the purpose of organizing thinking and providing study direction.

From the perspective of the Critical Thinking Decision Path, theoretical frameworks can incorporate grand, midrange, or microrange theories. Whether the researcher is using a conceptual or theoretical framework, conceptual and then operational definitions will emerge from the framework. The decision path moves down the ladder of abstraction from the philosophical to the empirical level, tracking thinking from the most abstract to the least abstract for the purposes of planning a research study and accruing evidence to guide nursing practice and research.

CRITIQUING GUIDE *Framework*

The framework for research provides guidance for the researcher as study questions are fine-tuned, methods for measuring variables are selected, and analyses are planned. Once data are collected and analyzed, the framework is used as a base of comparison. Did the findings coincide with the framework? If there were discrepancies, is there a way to explain them using the framework? The reader of research needs to know how to critically appraise a framework for research (see following Critiquing Criteria box).

The first question posed is whether a framework is presented. Sometimes a structure may be guiding the research, but a diagrammed model is not included in the manuscript. The reader must then look for the study structure in the narrative description of the study concepts. When the framework is identified, it is important to consider its relevance for nursing. The framework does not have to be one created by a nurse, but the importance of its content for nursing should be clear. The question of how the framework depicts a structure congruent with nursing should be addressed. For instance, although the Lazarus Transaction Model of Stress and Coping was not created by a nurse, it is clearly related to nursing practice when working with people facing stress. Sometimes frameworks from very different disciplines, such as physics or art, may be relevant. It is the responsibility of the author to clearly articulate the meaning of the framework for the study and to link the framework to nursing.

Once the meaning and applicability to nursing are articulated, the reader will be able to determine whether the framework is appropriate to guide the research. For instance, if a researcher is studying students' responses to the stress of being in the clinical setting for the first time and presents a framework of stress related to recovery from chronic illness, this is a blatant mismatch, which generally will not occur. However, subtle versions of mismatch will occur. Therefore the reader will want to look closely at the framework to determine if it is "on target" and the "best fit" for the research question and proposed study design.

Next, focus on the concepts being studied. Does the reader know which concepts are being studied and how they are defined and translated into measurable variables? Is there literature to support the choice of concepts? Concepts should clearly reflect the area of study; for example, using the general concept of anger when longstanding anger or hostility is more appropriate to

the research focus creates difficulties in defining variables and determining methods of measurement. These issues have to do with the logical consistency between the framework, the concepts being studied, and the methods of measurement.

Throughout the entire critiquing process, from view of the world to operational definitions, the reader is evaluating fit. Finally, the reader will expect to find a discussion of the findings as they relate to the model. This final point enables evaluation of the framework for use in further research. It may suggest necessary changes to enhance the relevance of the framework for continuing study, and thus serves to let others know where one will go from here.

Evaluating frameworks for research requires skill that can only be acquired through repeated critique and discussion with others who have critiqued the same manuscript. The novice reader of research must be patient as these skills are developed. With continuing education and a broader knowledge of potential frameworks, one builds a repertoire of knowledge to judge the foundation of a research study, the framework for research.

CRITIQUING CRITERIA   *Theoretical Framework*
1. Is the framework for research clearly identified?
2. Is the framework consistent with a nursing perspective?
3. Is the framework appropriate to guide research on the subject of interest?
4. Are the concepts and variables clearly and appropriately defined?
5. Was sufficient literature presented to support study of the selected concepts?
6. Is there a logical consistent link between the framework, the concepts being studied, and the methods of measurement?
7. Are the study findings examined in relationship to the framework?

Critical Thinking Challenges

- You are taking an elective course in advanced pathophysiology. The professor compares the knowledge of various disciplines and states that nursing is an example of a nonscientific discipline. She supports this assertion by citing that nursing's knowledge has been generated with unstructured methods such as intuition, trial and error, tradition, and authority. What assumptions has this professor made? Would you defend or support her positions?
- Nurse researchers claim that a theoretical framework is essential for systematically identifying the relationship between the chosen variables. If this is true, why do non-nursing researchers forego the use of theoretical frameworks in their studies? If there is no theoretical framework, does this affect the level of evidence? Explain your answer.
- How would a consumer of research employ computer databases to verify instruments used for measuring operational definitions?
- How would you argue against the following statement: "As a beginning consumer of research it is ridiculous to expect me to determine if a researcher's study has an appropriate theoretical framework; I've only had Nursing Theory 101."
- Is it possible for a research study's theoretical framework and variables to be the same?

KEY POINTS

- The scientific approaches used to generate nursing knowledge reflect both inductive and deductive reasoning.
- The interaction among theory, practice, and research is central to knowledge development in the discipline of nursing.
- Conceptual frameworks are created by the researcher, whereas theoretical frameworks are identified in the literature.
- The use of a framework for research is important as a guide to systematically identify concepts and to link appropriate study variables with each concept.
- Conceptual and operational definitions are critical to the evolution of a study whether or not they are explicitly stated in a manuscript.
- In developing or selecting a framework for research, knowledge may be acquired from other disciplines or directly from nursing. In either case, that knowledge is used to answer specific nursing questions.

- Theory is distinguished by its scope. Grand theories are broadest in scope and at the highest level of abstraction, and microrange theories are most narrow in scope and at the lowest level of abstraction; midrange theories are in the middle.
- Midrange theories are at a level of abstraction that enhances their usefulness for guiding practice and research.
- In critiquing a framework for research, it is important that one examine the logical consistent link among the framework, the concepts for study, and the methods of measurement.

REFERENCES

Calvin A: Hemodialysis patients and end-of-life decisions: a theory of personal preservation, *J Adv Nurs* 46(5): 558-566, 2004.

Chinn PL, Kramer MK: *Theory and nursing: a systematic approach*, ed 5, St Louis, 1999, Mosby.

Davison BJ, Goldenberg SL, Gleave ME, and Degner LF: Provision of individualized information to men and their partners to facilitate treatment decision making in prostate cancer, *Oncol Nurs Forum* 30(1): 107-114, 2004.

Hamric AB, Spross JA, and Hanson CM: *Advanced nursing practice,* Philadelphia, 2000, WB Saunders.

Higgins PA, Moore SM: Levels of theoretical thinking in nursing, *Nurs Outlook* 48(4): 179-183, 2000.

Im E, Meleis AI: Situation-specific theories: philosophical roots, properties and approach, *Adv Nurs Sci* 22(2): 11-24, 1999.

King IM: King's theory of goal attainment in practice, *Nurs Sci Q* 10(4): 180-185, 1997.

Koniak-Griffin D, Verzemnieks IL, Anderson NLR, Brecht ML, Lesser J, Kim S, and Turner-Pluta C: Nursing visitation for adolescent mothers: two-year infant health and maternal outcomes, *Nurs Res* 52(2): 127-135, 2004.

Leininger MM: Culture care theory, *Nurs Sci Q* 9(2): 71-78, 1996.

Lenz E: Middle range theory—role in research and practice. In *Proceedings of the sixth Rosemary Ellis Scholar's Retreat: nursing science implications for the 21st century,* Cleveland, Ohio, 1996, Frances Payne Bolton School of Nursing, Case Western Reserve University.

Liehr P: Prelude to research, *Nurs Sci Q* 5(3): 102-103, 1992.

Liehr P, Smith MJ: Middle range theory: spinning research and practice to create knowledge for the new millennium, *Adv Nurs Sci* 21(4): 81-91, 1999.

Liehr P, Smith MJ: Using story to guide nursing practice, *Int J Hum Caring* 4(2): 13-18, 2000.

Merton RK: *Social theory and social structure,* New York, 1968, Free Press.

Newman MA: Evolution of the theory of health as expanding consciousness, *Nurs Sci Q* 10(1): 22-25, 1997.

Orem DE: *Nursing: concepts of practice,* ed 5, St Louis, 1995, Mosby.

Parse RR: Transforming research and practice with the human becoming theory, *Nurs Sci Q* 10(4): 171-174, 1997.

Plach SK, Stevens PE, and Moss VA: Social role experiences of women living with rheumatoid arthritis, *J Fam Nurs* 10(1): 33-49, 2004.

Rogers ME: Nursing: science of unitary, irreducible human beings: update 1990. In Barrerr E, editor: *Visions of Rogers' science-based nursing,* New York, 1990, National League for Nursing.

Rogers ME: Nightingale's notes on nursing: prelude to the 21st century. In Rogers ME: *Notes on nursing: what it is and what it is not,* commemorative ed, Philadelphia, 1992, Lippincott.

Roy C, Andrews HA: *The Roy adaptation model: the definitive statement,* Norwalk, 1991, Appleton & Lange.

Smith MJ and Liehr P: *Middle range theory for nursing,* New York, 2003, Springer.

Van Cleve L, Bossert E, Beecroft P, Adlard K, Alvarez O, and Savedra MC: The pain experience of children with leukemia during the first year after diagnosis, *Nurs Res* 53(1): 1-10, 2004.

FOR FURTHER STUDY

🌐 Go to your Companion CD for review activities for this chapter.

evolve Go to Evolve at http://evolve.elsevier.com/LoBiondo/ for WebLinks, Content Updates, and additional research articles, for practice in reviewing and critiquing.

PART II

PROCESSES RELATED TO QUALITATIVE RESEARCH

RESEARCH VIGNETTE
Kristen M. Swanson

Program of Research on Miscarriage and Caring

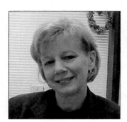

Kristen M. Swanson, RN, PhD, FAAN
University of Washington, Seattle, Washington

The first few years of being a nurse I did things in twos: two years in practice, two years to get my masters in cardiac nursing, two years teaching medical surgical nursing, and two years of course work toward my PhD in psychosocial nursing. Then I became a mother. Five weeks later I found myself sitting in a mothers' support group holding my infant son and listening to an obstetrician talking about spontaneous abortion. He lectured on the diagnosis, prognosis, treatment, and management of unexpected, unintended disruption of pregnancy prior to the point of expected fetal viability. When he finished, the women around me began to talk about what it had felt like to miscarry their babies. Two things happened that night: I looked down at my son and with a chill realized, "My God, I could have lost him!" Until that moment it had honestly never occurred to me. I was 29 years old and naively believed that if I worked hard enough, studied hard enough, or prayed hard enough, I could accomplish whatever I set my mind to. The reality of the fragility of life profoundly touched me. The second thing that happened that night was that I thought about the 1980 ANA Social Policy statement that staked nursing's domain as the diagnosis and treatment of human responses to actual or potential health problems. That evening I became aware that while the obstetrician focused on the diagnosis and treatment of the actual or potential problems of spontaneously aborting, the women were living the human response to miscarriage of a beloved baby. Their very language was different. That night pretty much set my research program in motion.

As a doctoral student of Dr. Jean Watson and Dr. Jody Glittenberg, I had been fully exposed to the importance of context in making meaning of life events and the role of caring in supporting human healing. My philosophy of science and nursing theory courses exposed me to the limits of postpositivist empiricism when trying to understand human experiences. Yet, consistent with many nursing doctoral programs at that time (1980–1983), the research courses focused solely on quantitative methodologies. When it came time to do my dissertation, I found myself in quite a quandary. My question begged an interpretive approach, yet my skills in qualitative methods were lacking. Naively I set out to do my own self-study. I drew inspiration about the importance of phenomenological interpretation of lived experiences from the writings of Giorgi (1970), figured out how to conduct open-ended interviews by reading about Spradley's ethnographic interviewing techniques (1979), and learned how to compare and contrast text data by reading Glaser and Strauss's classic text (1967) on grounded theory. My friend John Seidel showed me how to use a qualitative data management mainframe computer program he was developing. Hence I ended up weaving together a patchwork set of methods that facilitated my ability to analyze the rich stories shared by the 20 women who explained to me what it was like to miscarry and what caring meant in that context. There were three outcomes of that dissertation study: (1) the human experience of miscarriage model; (2) a model of caring in the context of miscarriage; and (3) reinforcement for John Seidel that set new directions for his fledgling computer program that went on to become "The Ethnograph" (available through http://www.qualisresearch.com/). In retrospect, I believe the methodology I used at that time might best be described as a descriptive phenomenology.

Subsequently, I completed two more phenomenological investigations of caring (see Swanson-Kauffman, 1986a, 1986b; and Swanson, 1990, 1991, 1993). I then combined these three studies and developed the caring theory that I later tested through two randomized trials. The caring theory was also further validated through an in-depth review of 130 data-based publications on caring that I did during my sabbatical in 1996. Through that intensive review of the literature, I found approximately 60 studies that focused on caring as a way of practicing. In reviewing those studies, I found tremendous evidence of convergence across many different qualitative studies of nurse caring and was able to draw links between the discoveries of others and my own propositions about what constitutes caring. I never set out to be a nurse theorist. I really just wanted to understand how to care for women in a manner that helped them resolve their losses. Nonetheless, the caring theory I developed has taken on a life of its own, and there are now hospitals that use it as a practice model, schools that use it as a curriculum model, and other investigators who have explored and tested its relevance to their research populations of interest.

My dissertation led me to an exciting and rewarding program of research. It has included instrument development, model testing, and randomized trials. In 1999 I published the results of an NINR-funded Solomon four-group randomized trial of the longitudinal effects of treatment (caring-based counseling) and measurement (early versus delayed) on women's healing during the first year after miscarriage (Swanson, 1999a,b). That study was the first randomized trial to demonstrate treatment effectiveness in assisting women to resolve miscarriage. Briefly, there was evidence that compared to controls (no treatment beyond usual obstetrical care), women who received three 1-hour caring-based nurse counseling sessions in the first 3 months after miscarrying experienced less depression, anger, and overall disturbed moods during the first year after miscarriage.

Based on the findings from that first intervention study, I was invited by Evergreen Hospital and Medical Center in Kirkland, Washington, to set up a couples' miscarriage support group. My colleagues and I based the support group on the miscarriage model and trained group leaders to implement the caring theory. After helping to run several groups myself, I witnessed the healing power of working with couples versus women alone. In addition, in a secondary analysis of data from the first intervention study, we discovered that approximately one third of women claimed to be both interpersonally and sexually more distant from their mates 1 year after miscarriage (Swanson et al., 2003). Hence our current study focuses on couples. It is an NINR-funded randomized trial of three caring-based interventions against a control condition (no treatment). Our goal is to see if we can make a difference for women and their male mates after miscarriage. Outcome variables include his and her mental health and grief responses and the quality of their overall couple relationship. The interventions we are testing include: (1) nurse caring (three 1-hour nurse counseling sessions; (2) self-caring (three videotape and workbook modules mailed to couples for completion at home); (3) combined caring (one nurse counseling session plus three videotape and workbook modules). At 1 year, after completion of their outcome measures, the control group is mailed a complimentary set of the videotape and workbook modules. All interventions, based on the caring theory and miscarriage model, are delivered on the same time schedule and are scheduled to be completed by 11 weeks after enrollment (couples can enroll up to 12 weeks postmiscarriage). We are gathering outcome data at 1, 6, 16, and 52 weeks postenrollment and hope to enroll 340 couples. There have many exciting and interesting components to this study. For the first time ever, I am studying men's responses. Whereas there have been other investigators who have described men's responses to miscarriage, the intended size of this sample and the fact that it includes men in a randomized treatment protocol truly make this a unique study of how miscarriage takes its toll.

I do love my work. Because my research is practice-based, I still have hands-on experience in nursing. It is hard to believe that a research program born of curiosity has become a lifelong passion. I never cease to be amazed at how much there is to be learned about the ways in which men and women experience loss of pregnancy, and how grateful couples are that someone is studying their experience. I, in turn, am eternally grateful that couples trust us enough to allow us to witness their very personal transition through loss and healing.

REFERENCES

Giorgi A: *Psychology as a human science,* New York, 1970, Harper & Row.

Glaser BG, Strauss AL: *The discovery of grounded theory: strategies for qualitative research,* New York, 1967, Aldine.

Spradley JP: *The ethnographic interview,* New York, 1979, Holt, Rinehart, and Winston.

Swanson KM: Providing care in the NICU: sometimes an act of love, *Adv Nurs Sci* 13(1):60-73, 1990.

Swanson KM: Empirical development of a middle range theory of caring, *Nurs Res* 40(3):161-166, 1991.

Swanson KM: Nursing as informed caring for the well-being of others, *Image* 25(4):352-357, 1993.

Swanson KM: The effects of caring, measurement, and time on miscarriage impact and women's well-being in the first year subsequent to loss, *Nurs Res* 48(6):288-298, 1999a.

Swanson KM: Research-based practice with women who have had miscarriages, *Image* 31(4):339-345, 1999b.

Swanson KM, Karmali Z, Powell S, Pulvermahker F: Miscarriage effects on interpersonal and sexual relationships during the first year after loss: women's perceptions, *J Psychosomat Med* 65(5):902-910, 2003.

Swanson-Kauffman KM: *The unborn one: a profile of the human experience of miscarriage,* University of Colorado unpublished doctoral dissertation, 1983.

Swanson-Kauffman KM: A combined qualitative methodology for nursing research, *Adv Nurs Sci* 8(3):58-69, 1986a.

Swanson-Kauffman KM: Caring in the instance of unexpected early pregnancy loss, *Top Clin Nurs* 8(2):37-46, 1986b.

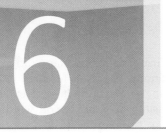

MARLENE ZICHI COHEN

Introduction to Qualitative Research

KEY TERMS

case studies
context
empirical analytical
epistemology
ethnographic research
ethnographies

grounded theory
naturalistic research
ontology
paradigm
phenomenological research
philosophical beliefs

qualitative research
text
triangulation
worldview

LEARNING OUTCOMES

After reading this chapter, the student should be able to do the following:

1
- Define key concepts in the philosophy of science.
- Identify assumptions underlying the positivist or postpositivist view (positivism) and the constructivist view (constructivism) of research.
- Identify assumptions underlying quantitative (empirical analytical) and qualitative methods of grounded theory, case study, ethnographic, and phenomenological approaches to research.
- Identify the links between qualitative research and evidence-based practice.

STUDY RESOURCES

Go to your Companion CD for review activities for this chapter.

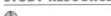 Go to Evolve at http://evolve.elsevier.com/LoBiondo/ for Weblinks, Content Updates, and additional research articles for practice in reviewing and critiquing.

Qualitative research is an important term to understand because it is a broad label that includes many approaches. The word implies a focus on qualities of a process or entity and meanings that are not experimentally examined or measured in terms of quantity, amount, frequency, or intensity. Qualitative research can mean the analysis of open-ended questions that respondents are asked to write on a survey. It also can refer to what is thought of as naturalistic research, a general label for qualitative research methods that involve the researcher going to a natural setting, that is, to where the phenomenon being studied is taking place. Qualitative research includes many methods: grounded theory, case study, ethnography, phenomenology, and many others. These methods share both similarities and differences. Because all methods involve data that are text rather than numbers, all include some means of doing content analysis on the text. **Text** means data are in a textual form, that is, narrative or words written from interviews that were recorded and then transcribed, or notes written from observations of the researcher. However, the methods differ in the philosophical bases upon which they are built and in purpose and outcome. This chapter addresses the philosophies underlying the qualitative research methods most commonly used by nurses.

The first question nurse researchers must answer when they decide to begin research is what approach they will use. Beginning is never easy and requires many forms of preparation. Beginning research is like beginning a marriage. With luck, both are worth the time and trouble, and what you learn about yourself along the way is often the most important part of the process. In research, as in marriage, having a wonderful partner with whom to share the process is both useful and helpful. This partner will make the journey more fun and their presence will make it a better and richer experience. Nursing research, like nursing itself, concerns many different and complex phenomena. Good research is seldom simple, and therefore conducting research alone is seldom feasible. As a nurse you will be in an ideal position to identify practice problems. When these problems require research solutions, if you find a team to help solve them, both your patients and your nursing practice will be the better for it.

So, as you begin your research "marriage," how might you choose among the many different qualitative research methods? Of course, the first lesson learned in research classes is that the research design should match the question being asked. Another important consideration is the philosophy that underlies a research method and how it matches the objectives of the study. Both are addressed in this chapter. Understanding the philosophy upon which research is based also is important in evaluating research as a consumer and user of research in your nursing practice.

Figure 6-1 illustrates one of the reasons your research "marriage" might lead you to select a qualitative method. As this cartoon shows, Garfield is putting on glasses, and the scene changes as he realizes the glasses belong to Picasso. This is the goal of qualitative methods: to be able to see the world in the same way as those men and women undergoing the experience.

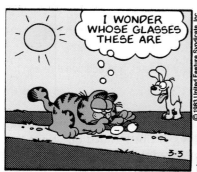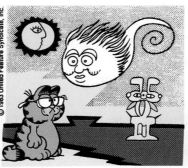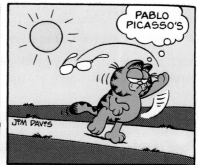

Figure 6-1. Shifting perspectives: seeing the world as others see it. (GARFIELD ©1983 Paws, Inc. Reprinted with permission of UNIVERSAL PRESS SYNDICATE. All rights reserved.)

THE NATURE OF KNOWLEDGE

Of course, qualitative research is not the only way to obtain answers to questions. When you have clinical questions, there are many forms of knowledge that can provide answers to consider while guiding your practice. You are taught rituals and traditions in nursing. We also learn from experts who have experience and wisdom to share. We learn from other disciplines, which is why nursing students take courses in chemistry, philosophy, psychology, and other fields. We also learn from our intuition and sometimes know what to do from trial and error, although this is not a very efficient way to solve problems. We also learn from scientific problem solving.

Science is an important way to learn, and the knowledge from research is an important guide to be used in nursing practice. Knowledge from scientific reasoning or research is less vulnerable to individual skill level. On a good day what you do by "instinct" or naturally may be effective, but on a day when you are tired or have just experienced an upsetting event your performance may be adversely affected. If what we do is based on sound and logically derived research, we will do the same thing when we are tired or distracted as when we are more alert.

We sometimes learn in research that what we believe is helpful and what we have learned from experts may not in fact be helpful to a particular group of patients. An example of this is the now outmoded practice that experts taught for many years of not providing patients with informa-tion. Early nursing research provided evidence that clearly showed that providing patients with information of various types did improve their health in many ways (Johnson et al., 1997).

Questions philosophers deal with include the following: What is truth? How do we know what we know? What is real? What counts for me as evidence? What is good (of value)? What is ethical or right conduct?" The answers to these basic questions are important guides to our nursing practice as they shape how we see the world and our roles in it. How we provide nursing care and how we conduct research differ depending on how we answer these questions.

PHILOSOPHIES OF RESEARCH

Every specialized field uses characteristic language to communicate important features of the work that are not as pertinent to those outside that field. Learning a new language is part of what students do in nursing school and part of what researchers do when they learn research methods and skills. Each research method and all philosophies of science have a special language that you will encounter as you read. A few words are important to clarify so you can read the literature with a good understanding.

The word science comes from a word meaning "knowledge," and the word philosophy comes from one meaning "wisdom" (Oxford University Press, 2004). All research is based on **philosophical beliefs** about the world, also called a **worldview** or **paradigm. Paradigm** is from a Greek word meaning "pattern." Thomas Kuhn (1962) first applied this word to science to describe the way people in society think about the world.

Although those who conduct qualitative research are more likely to explicitly describe their beliefs and assumptions, all research is based on beliefs. Therefore it is important to know and comprehend these beliefs in order to understand and use research findings. These views are not right or wrong, but rather they represent different ways of viewing the world that may be more or less useful, depending on the goals of the research. Table 6–1 compares two paradigms that are the basis for research. Constructivism is the basis for *naturalistic* (qualitative) **research**, while positivism, and more recently postpositivism, is the basis of *empirical analytical* (quantitative) research. These paradigms can be thought of as extremes. That is, research approaches fall along a continuum, with these extremes at either end. Later in this chapter, five research approaches are discussed in the order they would fall along this continuum.

TABLE **6-1** **Basic Beliefs of Research Paradigms**

	Constructivist Paradigm	**Positivist or Postpositivist Paradigm**
Epistemology	"Truth" determined by the individual or cultural group Subjectivism valued	Truth sought via replicable observation Objectivism valued
Ontology	Multiple realities exist, influenced by culture and environment	"Real reality" exists "out there" Driven by natural laws
Context	Emphasized, value placed on rich details of context in which phenomenon occurs Time and place are important	Minimized, value placed on generalizability across contexts
Inquiry aims	Description (narrative), understanding, transformation, reconstruction	Description (statistical), explanation; prediction and control
Values	Included, add to understanding of phenomenon	Excluded, detract from inquiry aim
Voice of researcher	Active participant	Neutral observer
Methodology	Dialogic, transformative	Experimental, controlled

Adapted from Lincoln Y, Guba E: Paradigmatic controversies, contradictions, and emerging confluences. In Denzin NK, Lincoln YS, editors: *Handbook of qualitative research,* ed 2, Thousand Oaks, Calif, 2000, Sage.

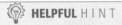 **HELPFUL** H I N T

All research is based on a paradigm, but this is seldom specifically stated in a research report.

The philosophical language in Table 6-1 needs to be clarified. **Epistemology** involves what we know, that is, what is "truth." The origins, nature, and limits of knowledge are included. It concerns why and how we know some things and what constitutes our knowing. **Ontology** (from the Greek *onto,* meaning "to be") is the science or study of being or existence and its relation to nonexistence. Existentialists and phenomenologists discuss Being and non-Being or Nothingness as categories. Ontology deals with what is real (versus fiction or appearance), what is the nature of reality, or matter. Whereas in the positivist view one reality exists and we seek to learn the laws of nature, in the constructivist view reality is constructed differently by different people. For example, what is real and important to patients may be unnoticed by nurses. **Context** is where something occurs. Context can include physical settings such as the hospital or home or less concrete "environments" such as the context

cultural understandings and beliefs bring to an experience. The *aims of inquiry,* or the goals of the research, also vary with the paradigm. The *researchers' role* or *voice* and how their *values* are viewed and *methodology* used also vary with different paradigms.

The "constructivist paradigm" is the basis of most qualitative research (see Chapters 7 and 8), and the "positivist or contemporary empiricist paradigm" is the basis of most empirical analytical or quantitative research (see Chapters 9 through 19). An example from oncology research may make it clear that some types of research are more congruent with the "positivist paradigm" than the "constructivist paradigm" and vice versa. Consider the example of chemotherapy for cancer. When studying the efficacy of a drug for the treatment of cancer, it seems quite logical that experimental research should be used. This approach, based on the positivist paradigm, is guided by the ontological view that there is one reality, that is, that all people will respond in the same way to this drug. Of course, it is also true that responses to drugs may vary by age, gender, ethnicity, and genetic characteristics, for example, but those features can be considered by doing research that includes persons of diverse ethnicity and both genders and by assessing the effect of the drugs by group. Epistemology leads to seeking truth in an objective, replicable way: that is, the way the drug is prepared and provided to people will be the same for each person, and other researchers in other parts of the world would do the research in the same way. In this framework the emphasis is on studying parts, so the focus might be on the responses of tumor cells rather than the whole person. The context is not central in this research, which is why researchers would expect to find the same response to drugs in different parts of the world.

The goal of quantitative or empirical research is to control or cure the cancer and predict the outcome for patients, which is that the cancer would be eliminated or at least its growth slowed. The goal of research guided by the positivist view is to statistically describe, explain, predict, and, finally, to control the cancer. In the positivist view, the basis of most quantitative research, researchers are neutral observers. That means that researchers do not have a vested interest in showing that one drug is better than another drug. Values are thought to detract from the inquiry. If someone who owned a company producing the drug ran a study, concerns would be raised about whether a profit motive was involved in how the research was done. Of course, values are always a part of what we do— we would not study something we did not believe is important or that we value. The goal is to keep the values as separate from the research as possible.

However, when we are interested in what it means to people to have cancer or cancer treatment, a qualitative study is more appropriate. Qualitative studies, based on the constructivist paradigm, are guided by the ontological view that there are multiple realities. The meaning of cancer will likely be different for a young mother than for a grandmother. The meaning of cancer also may be different in the United States than in Japan. Epistemology includes the view that truth varies and is subjective. Context is important, and description is the goal. When seeking to understand patients' experiences of a treatment, we would expect that what is important, and "true," for one person may not be for another. Some of the differences may result from context. The experience may well vary according to where the person is treated and various features of the person such as age, gender, and ethnicity, for example. Having cancer may well be different for someone whose parent died a painful death from cancer than for someone who knew people whose cancer was cured. The values of all involved are acknowledged. Researchers work to be sure their values do not cloud their view and prevent them from understanding how others view experiences. What is valued and important also helps us understand experiences. Qualitative research is conducted in a dialogue or interview with the participant, who is seen as an active part of the research. In fact, while research is done with "subjects" in the positivist view, these people would more likely be called "informants" or "participants" to recognize their active role in the constructivist paradigm. The research results would be useful in describing, understanding, and leading to a way to transform or change situations.

 HELPFUL H I N T

Values are involved in all research. It is important, however, that they not influence the results of the research.

Another way of thinking about these views and linking them to research is illustrated in the Critical Thinking Decision Path. This decision algorithm illustrates that beliefs lead to different questions, which lead to selecting different research approaches. Different research methods have different assumptions that are consistent with that method but more specific than these global worldviews. These beliefs and approaches lead to different research activities, as is illustrated in the critical thinking path in the illustration below.

CRITICAL THINKING DECISION PATH   Selecting a Research Process

If your beliefs are:

Researcher beliefs	Humans are biopsychosocial beings, known by their biological, psychological, and social characteristics.	or	Humans are complex beings who attribute unique meaning to their life situations. They are known by their personal expressions.
	Truth is objective reality that can be experienced with the senses and measured by the researcher.		Truth is the subjective expression of reality as perceived by the participant and shared with the researcher. Truth is context laden.

then you'll ask questions, such as:

Example questions	What is the difference in blood pressure and heart rate for adolescents who are angry compared to those who are not angry?	or	What is the structure of the lived experience of anger for adolescents?

and select approaches:

Approaches	**Quantitative/deductive**	or	**Qualitative/inductive**

leading to research activities:

Research activities	Researcher selects a representative (of population) sample and determines size before collecting data.	or	Researcher selects participants who are experiencing the phenomenon of interest and collects data until saturation is reached.
	Researcher uses an extensive approach to collect data.		Researcher uses an intensive approach to collect data.
	Questionnaires and measurement devices are preferably administered in one setting by an unbiased individual to control for extraneous variables.		Researcher conducts interviews and participant or nonparticipant observation in environments where participants usually spend their time. Researcher bias is acknowledged and set aside.
	Primarily deductive analysis is used, generating a numerical summary that allows the researcher to reject or accept the null hypothesis.		Primarily inductive analysis is used, leading to a narrative summary, which synthesizes participant information, creating a description of human experience.

Continuum of research and methods

Paradigm: —————————————————————————→ Constructivism
Positivism ——————————————————————————→
Post positivism ————————————————————————→ Critical theory

Research tradition:
Quantitative research   /   grounded theory   /   case study   /   ethnographic   /   phenomenological
(Empirical analytical)

Approach to research:
Falsify hypotheses ——————— generate theory ——————— describe ——————— describe and interpret

Figure 6-2.   Continuum of philosophical foundations and qualitative research methods.

This chapter provides an overview of the five research traditions commonly used in qualitative nursing research. These traditions are the quantitative methods or empirical analytical research and the qualitative approaches of grounded theory, case study, ethnographic, and phenomenological research. Each of these is discussed as shown in Figure 6-2, and they are based on views that move along a continuum from the positivist view to the constructivist view.

Quantitative/Empirical Analytical Research

Empirical analytical is a general label for quantitative research approaches that test hypotheses. These methods are discussed in detail in Part III. In this chapter about the philosophical foundations of qualitative research, it is important to note that although all research is based on philosophy, researchers who use quantitative approaches are less aware of, or at least often make less explicit, the philosophy underlying the research. The philosophical basis, positivism or postpositivism, is the basis or research focused on testing hypotheses that are derived from theories or conceptual frameworks. The goal is to support the research hypothesis, and therefore reject the null hypothesis with the data from the study (see Chapter 16). In addition to the positivist view beliefs already discussed, other assumptions underlie contemporary empiricism in nursing (Im and Meleis, 1999) (Box 6-1).

The remainder of this chapter focuses on four qualitative research methods and their

BOX 6-1   ASSUMPTIONS OF CONTEMPORARY EMPIRICISM

1. The world is to some extent predictable. While no universal laws drive health, reasonable predictions are possible.
2. The purpose of research is to develop the basis for nursing care. Careful scientific strategies give results that can be corroborated.
3. Human responses to health and illness can be identified, measured, and understood.
4. Explanation results from linking observable with unobservable processes.

philosophical foundations. The methods are described in the order they appear on the continuum in Figure 6-2.

   EVIDENCE-BASED PRACTICE TIP

Qualitative researchers use more flexible procedures than quantitative researchers. While collecting data for a project, they consider all the experiences that may occur.

Grounded Theory

Grounded theory is a research method designed to inductively develop a theory based on observations of selected people. In an example of a grounded theory study, homeless adolescents were interviewed about what helped them to remain healthy and how they took care of themselves. A theory was developed concerning what constitutes "taking care of oneself in a high-risk environment." The theory included three categories: becoming aware of oneself, staying alive with limited resources, and handling one's own health (Rew, 2003). Grounded theory moves along the philosophical continuum from the positivist view toward the constructivist view (see Figure 6-2). It is a method based on the sociological tradition of the Chicago School of Symbolic Interactionism. Glaser and Strauss (1967) developed the method of grounded theory, which has changed over time, but three major premises continue to underlie grounded theory research (Box 6-2).

The purpose of grounded theory, as the name implies, is to generate a theory from data. Qualitative data are gathered through interviews and observation. Analysis generates substantive codes that are clustered into categories. Propositions about the relationships among and between the categories create a conceptual framework, which guides further data collection. Additional data thought likely to answer generated hypotheses are collected until all categories are "saturated," meaning no new information is generated (see Chapter 7). The goal of generating a theory implies that laws drive at least some portion of reality. The truth is sought from relevant groups, for example, those who are dying. The context is very important, as was shown in a classic work by Glaser and Strauss (1965). They noted that at the time of their research Americans were unwilling to talk openly about the process of dying, American physicians were unwilling to disclose impending death to patients, and nurses were not expected to make these disclosures. This lack of communication led Glaser and Strauss (1965) to their study of the problem of awareness of dying. They described various types of awareness contexts, problems of awareness, and practical uses of awareness theory. Their early fieldwork led to hypotheses and the gathering of additional data, and the framework was refined with further analysis until they formed a systematic substantive theory.

Case Study

Case study as a research method involves an in-depth description of essential dimensions and processes of the phenomenon being studied. Case study research has been given several definitions and can be thought of as the collection of detailed, relatively unstructured information from several sources, usually including the reports of those being studied.

Case studies can be used in a variety of ways, including as a way to present data gathered with another method, as a teaching device, or as a research method. Hammersley (1989) linked case studies to the Chicago School of Sociology, where the grounded theory was developed. Case studies have been used in various disciplines, including nursing, political science, sociology, business, social work, economics, and psychology.

Nurses have a long and continuing tradition of using case studies for teaching and learning about patients (e.g., Parsons, 1911). Nightingale (1969) stressed the importance of coming to know patients and of basing practice on experience. She noted that knowing how to provide care "must entirely depend upon an inquiry into all the conditions in which the patient lives." In case studies, these details are described, and lessons that can be learned from the particular patient are made clear. Persons who have had an

---

BOX 6-2   MAJOR PREMISES OF GROUNDED THEORY

1. Humans act toward objects on the basis of the meaning those objects have for them. Meaning is in, and cannot be separated from, the context or from the consequences of the meanings in a particular setting.
2. Social meanings arise from social interactions with others over time and are embedded socially, historically, culturally, and contextually. The focus of grounded theory is therefore social interactions.
3. People use interpretive processes to handle and change meanings in dealing with their situations.

experience can provide insights that are both valuable and unavailable to those who have not had the experience. Obtaining these descriptions with the use of case studies can serve a variety of functions: sensitization to make practitioners and researchers aware of patients' experiences; conceptualization to make clear the concepts included in an experience or general label; policy decision making; and theory building by identifying hypotheses for testing with further research (Cohen and Saunders, 1996).

The *American Journal of Nursing* features case studies regularly. When this feature was added, the editor noted that case studies are a way of providing in-depth, evidence-based discussion of clinical topics along with practical information and guidelines for improving practice (Mason, 2000). Case studies allow us to understand complex phenomena about which little is known. They can be exploratory and descriptive, or explanatory, involving one case or multiple cases.

When used as research, case studies have the following characteristics:

- Investigate contemporary phenomena within real life context
- Used when boundaries between the phenomenon and context are unclear
- Used when there are more features of interest (or variables) than "data points"
- Use multiple sources of evidence and converge or triangulate data, both quantitative and qualitative
- Use data collection and analysis guided by theory

Examples of recently published case studies illustrate the features of case studies and several uses to which they can be applied. A description of the postoperative course of a patient was used to illustrate the signs and symptoms of alcohol withdrawal, which was contrasted with delirium tremens (Smith-Alnimer and Watford, 2004). Another example used a case study of a patient with a variety of symptoms and an illness that progressed rapidly. Because establishing a diagnosis was difficult, her case was presented with responses from expert clinicians who discussed the important features that were clearer in retrospect (Bliss, Flanders, and Saint, 2004).

Ethnographic Research

Anthropologists developed **ethnographic research,** a tradition viewed as beginning with the British anthropologist Bronislaw Malinowski, who was influenced by Rivers, a physician-anthropologist-psychologist (Stocking, 1983). Scotch (1963) first described medical anthropology as the field of research that focuses on health and illness within a cultural system. Nurses conduct medical ethnographies (Roper and Shapira, 2000). Although early work was done on "foreign" cultures, nurses now often do focused ethnographies, which are the study of distinct problems within a specific context among a small group of people or the study of a groups' social construction and understanding of a health or illness experience (Roper and Shapira, 2000).

Ethnographies describe cognitive models or patterns of behavior of people within a culture. They seek to understand another way of life from the "native's" perspective.

The following values underlie ethnography:

- Culture is fundamental to ethnographic studies. Culture includes behavioral/materialist and cognitive perspectives. The behavioral/materialist perspective sees culture as observed through a group's patterns of behavior and customs, their way of life, and what they produce. In the cognitive perspective, culture consists of beliefs, knowledge, and ideas people use as they live. Culture is the structure of meaning through which we shape experiences.
- Understanding culture requires a holistic perspective that captures the breadth of beliefs, knowledge, and activities of the group being studied.
- Context is important for an understanding of a culture. Understanding context requires intensive face-to-face contact over an extended time. People are studied where they live, in their natural settings, or where an experience occurs, such as in a hospital or in a community setting.

- The aim of ethnographies is to combine the emic perspective—the insider's view of the world—with the etic perspective—the view the researcher (outsider) brings—to develop a scientific generalization about different societies. That is, generalizations are drawn from special examples or details from participant observation.

An example of ethnographic work that has been useful to nurses is the idea of explanatory models. This idea was mostly developed by cognitive anthropologists, especially Kleinman and associates (Kleinman, 1980). Explanatory models use an interactive approach, emphasizing variations between patients' and practitioners' models of illness. They offer evidence through explanations of sickness and treatment, guide choices among available therapies and therapists, and give social meaning to the experience of sickness. These cognitive models vary over time and in response to a particular illness episode. Fair (2003) recently used this idea to explore women's explanatory models of rheumatoid arthritis (RA) and the congruence of these models with professional models and the professionally recommended treatment of RA. The evidence provided by this information can guide selection of nursing interventions with those who need treatment for RA, and illustrated the importance of understanding patients' explanatory models, because those who had different models than their providers would switch providers, not take their medications, or quit conventional medical therapies altogether.

Phenomenological Research

Phenomenological research is used to answer questions of meaning. This method is most useful when the task is to understand an experience as those having the experience understand it. Phenomenological research is an important method with which to begin accumulating evidence when little is known about a particular topic, when studying a new topic, or when studying a topic from a fresh perspective.

Phenomenological research is based on phenomenological philosophy, which has changed over time and with philosophers. Various and differing phenomenological methods exist, including eidetic phenomenology, which is descriptive and based on Husserl's philosophy; Heideggerian phenomenology, which is interpretive and based on Heidegger's philosophy; and hermeneutical phenomenology, which is both descriptive and interpretive and is based on the Dutch phenomenologists (Cohen, Kahn, and Steeves, 2000).

There are five important concepts or values in phenomenological research (Cohen, Kahn, and Steeves, 2000):

1. Phenomenological research was developed to understand meanings. The goal was to develop a rigorous science in the service of humanity. This science seeks to go to the roots or foundations of a topic to be clear about what the basic concepts are and what they mean.
2. Phenomenology was based on a critique of positivism, or the positivist view, which was seen as inappropriate to the study of some human concerns. Carefully considering representative examples was the test of knowledge.
3. The object of study is the life-world (*Lebenswelt*), or lived experience, not contrived situations. That is, as Husserl said, we go to the things themselves. We are concerned with the appearance of things (phenomena) rather than the things themselves (noumena). For example, think about a desk in a classroom. There is a real physical object, the noumena, which we all see. If that were not the case, we would bump into the desk every time we passed it. In addition, there is your view of that desk, the phenomena, which changes as you move in the room. If you sit at the desk, you only see the top of it. However, as you move away you can see the desk's legs, for example. Nurses are often interested in various aspects of peoples'

experiences or views of health, illness, and treatment.

4. Intersubjectivity, the belief that others share a common world with us, is an important tenet in phenomenology. Although phenomena differ, they also share similarities based on the similarities in people. The most fundamental of those similarities is that we all have a body in space and time. That is, our physical bodies and historical sense lead to similarities in how we experience phenomena.

5. The phenomenological reduction, also called bracketing, is more important in some phenomenological approaches than in others. It is the statement that researchers must be aware of and examine their prejudices or values. The term bracketing comes from the mathematical metaphor of putting "brackets" around our beliefs so they can be put aside and we can "see" the experience as the person having it sees it rather than as it changes as filtered through our prejudices.

An example of a phenomenological study was one conducted with persons with advanced cancer who had been referred to a palliative care service because, although they did not report experiencing pain, they had a variety of other symptoms. These symptoms were found to improve when the patients took pain medications. When they were asked to describe their experience, it became clear that there were similarities and differences among these persons that helped to explain why they did not report pain (Cohen et al., 2004). Understanding these experiences provides evidence that can assist nurses to provide comprehensive care to whole persons, rather than focusing only on fragmented tasks that need to be accomplished in providing nursing care. While assessing pain by asking patients to rate their pain on a 0 to 10 scale is a useful beginning, it is clearly only a beginning to pain assessment. Our goal is to come to understand the world as the person who has had the experience sees it. We shift our perspective to see the world as patients see it—something that is central to providing competent nursing care to meet patient needs.

Matching Research Goals with Research Philosophy

Some researchers have written about "qualitative" and "quantitative" research as incompatible approaches. The value of one over the other has been argued. However, others have recognized that different research methods accomplish different goals and offer different types and levels of evidence that enhance practice. They advocate using the method appropriate to the research question and combining methods when this best suits the research goals. Understanding the philosophy underlying each method can help researchers use the method that best meets the intended purpose and can guide the reader to use the research findings in appropriate ways. In the example regarding chemotherapy used at the beginning of this chapter, when studying the effectiveness of a drug for cancer, it would be foolish to ignore measuring changes in tumor size. It would be equally foolish to ignore what patients tell us is important to them when taking this drug when we want to understand what it means to them. Because meanings may well determine needs that can be met with nursing interventions, such as the need for information or the need to talk about fear of death, this evidence is vital to guide effective nursing practice.

Triangulation in Qualitative Research

Triangulation is a term used in surveying and navigation to describe a technique whereby two known or visible points are used to plot the location of a third point. Triangulation in research refers to combining different methods, theories, data sources (including data collected from different sites or at different times), or investigators to converge on a single construct. The idea is that looking at a single question through multiple "glasses" will give a more complete understanding of the issue being studied. This work can accomplish several purposes: triangulating or converging the findings, elaborating on results, using one method to inform another, discovering contradictions or paradoxes, and extending the breadth of a study. Triangulation provides an opportunity to increase the strength and consistency of evidence provided by the use of both qualitative and quantitative research methods.

Some have argued against combining qualitative and quantitative approaches because they are based on different paradigms. While this is true, triangulation can add different insights to the question being examined. Because most important questions in nursing are complex, this combination can be useful to answer questions important to nursing practice. Combining methods adds depth and breadth to the results. It does not, however, bring us to an "objective" truth.

The study of aging was noted as an example of when triangulation is needed (Inui, 2003). The determinants of aging are multiple and interact in complex ways, requiring both holistic and reductionistic approaches to understand successful aging. This point was illustrated by aspects of aging that can be best understood with qualitative data, such as the quality of "resilience," and those that require quantitative data, such as income and falls, for example.

Combining methods can be accomplished in several ways. Both qualitative and quantitative measures can be used simultaneously during data collection, and the results can then be "triangulated" or put together. Researchers also sometimes conduct a qualitative study and follow it with a quantitative one, or the reverse: they first conduct a quantitative study and then a qualitative one. Some examples will help to clarify these approaches.

Triangulation is illustrated in a study that is currently being conducted, which involves various forms of triangulation (Cohen, 2005, in press). A team of investigators are studying symptoms of persons having blood and marrow transplantation (BMT). In addition, multiple data sources and methods are being combined. Data were collected with phenomenological interviews and also with quality of life and symptom assessment instruments. Data analysis has shown that these different views of the experience of BMT and the symptoms people experience provide a more complete understanding that will be useful evidence to use in developing more effective symptom management interventions to improve both symptoms and quality of life. Data are analyzed with appropriate techniques (phenomenological data are analyzed with phenomenological techniques, and statistical analysis is conducted on quantitative measures), and then results are combined. One example is combining qualitative data with symptom measurements to better understand why some people with the same disease and treatment experience more severe symptoms than others.

Another way qualitative methods have been used in triangulation is to conduct a qualitative study and then use the findings to conduct a quantitative study. An example of this is a study that involved interviewing 16 people who have renal failure about their beliefs about hemodialysis (Krespi et al., 2004). They used the findings from their research to develop a questionnaire, which was completed by 156 patients. The reverse has also been done, where findings from a quantitative study have led the researchers to conduct a qualitative study. This is illustrated in the article in Appendix C by Plach, Stevens, and Moss (2004). They found in a quantitative study that, contrary to what is in the literature, women with rheumatoid arthritis (RA) had positive social role experiences. This led the authors to conduct a qualitative study, interviewing a subset of 20 women who provided data in the quantitative study. The results of the qualitative study, reported in Appendix C, help to better understand the circumstances that best facilitated positive social roles, and thus more completely describe the topic.

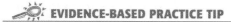

EVIDENCE-BASED PRACTICE TIP

When using results from studies that have used triangulation, it is important to know the strengths and weaknesses of the various designs used as well as how the designs were used to answer the specific questions in each study.

Evidence-Based Practice

Randomized clinical trials and other types of intervention studies traditionally have been the major focus of evidence-based practice as exemplified by the systematic reviews conducted by the Cochrane Collaboration. Typically, the selection of studies to be included in systematic reviews is guided by levels of evidence models that focus on the effectiveness of interventions according to their strength and consistency of their predictive power. Given that the levels of evidence models are hierarchical in nature, which perpetuates intervention studies as the "gold standard" of research design, the value of qualitative studies and the evidence offered by their results have remained unclear. Qualitative studies historically have been ranked lower in a hierarchy of evidence, along with descriptive, evaluative, and case studies, as weaker forms of research designs (see Chapter 2). The same linear application does not seem to fit with the multiple purposes, designs, and methods of qualitative research.

Because nursing is a practice discipline, the most important purpose of nursing research is to put research findings to use. Levels of evidence include qualitative or case studies and systematically obtained evaluation data as sources of evidence to use in practice (see Chapter 2). Yet qualitative methods are the best way to start to answer questions that have not been addressed or when a new perspective is needed in practice. The answers to questions provided by qualitative data reflect important evidence that may offer the first systematic insights about a phenomenon and the setting in which it occurs. Broadening evidence models to beyond a narrow hierarchical perspective is work that has already begun as work groups consider how qualitative evidence can be evaluated and included more in systematic reviews (Pearson, 2002; Powers, 2005). This promises to be an important contribution to expanding the evidence base nurses use for clinical decision making.

As one example, Kearney (2001) developed a useful typology of levels and applications of qualitative research findings. She described and illustrated four modes of clinical application: (1) insight/empathy, (2) assessment, (3) anticipatory guidance, and (4) coaching. A review of what authors said about the usefulness of, or implications of, their qualitative research in oncology found that they focused on two broad uses of the research (Cohen, Kahn, and Steeves, 2002). The first and most common use was to describe implications for future research. The second use of qualitative research evidence for practice was determining ways to change how caregivers and patients talk to each other as well as how patients talk to other patients or caregivers talk to caregivers. This use included six subcategories that were illustrated in the review paper with selected quotes from the papers reviewed. These subcategories were as follows: (1) caregivers talking to each other; (2) patients talking to each other and to family members; (3) caregivers listening to patients and families talk to them; (4) assessment talk; (5) caregivers talking to patients and families; and (6) talking programs and plans.

In addition to these uses of qualitative research, attention has also been focused on what has been called meta-synthesis or meta-study of qualitative research (Paterson et al., 2001). This involves examining reports of qualitative research, interpreting the results to reveal similarities and differences, and creating new knowledge. An example of a meta-synthesis was one that reviewed studies that sought to understand nonvocal mechanically ventilated patients' experiences with communication (Carroll, 2004). Reviews of this kind are useful and important to show clinicians how they can use findings from qualitative research in their practice.

Remember, the definition of evidence-based practice has three components: clinically relevant evidence, clinical expertise, and patient preferences. Qualitative research does not test interventions but does require the researcher to apply their clinical expertise to the choice of the research question and study design as well as gaining a solid understanding of the patient's experience. Though qualitative research uses different methodologies and has different goals, it is important to explore how and when to use the evidence provided by findings of qualitative studies in practice.

 EVIDENCE-BASED PRACTICE TIP

Qualitative research findings can be used in many ways, including improving ways clinicians communicate with patients and with each other.

CRITIQUING GUIDE *Foundation of Qualitative Research*

A final example illustrates the differences in the methods discussed in this chapter and provides you with the beginning skills of how to critique qualitative research. The information in this chapter coupled with the information presented in Chapter 7 will provide the underpinnings of critical analysis of qualitative research (see Critiquing Criteria box). Consider the question of nursing students learning how to conduct research. The empirical analytical approach (quantitative research) might be used in an experiment to see if one teaching method led to better learning outcomes than another. The students' knowledge might be tested, the teaching conducted, and then a posttest of knowledge given. Scores on these tests would be analyzed statistically to see if the different methods produced a difference in the results.

The grounded theorist would be interested in the process, and, for this example, would consider the process of learning research. The researcher might attend the class to see what occurs and then interview students to ask them to describe how their learning changed over time. They might be asked to describe becoming researchers or becoming more knowledgeable about research. The goal would be to describe the stages or process of this learning.

A case study could be written about a particular research class to provide a detailed description of the class or perhaps a particular individual in the class. The case would then be used to explicate what is important in this setting.

Ethnographers would consider the class as a culture and could join to observe and interview students. Questions would be directed at the students' values, behaviors, and beliefs in learning research. The goal would be to understand and describe the group members' shared meanings.

Phenomenologists would be interested in the meaning of the students' experiences. They would get at this by asking students to describe learning research, that is, to give concrete specific examples. The goal would be to understand and describe the meaning of this experience for the students.

Many other research methods exist. Although it is important to be aware of the basis of the research methods used, it is most important that the method chosen is the one that will provide the best approach to answering the question being asked. Some research methods, such as focus groups developed from marketing research, are not explicitly based on philosophy, but they have been useful as a method of collecting data to answer nursing research questions. An example of focus group research was a study conducted with groups of African-American women to explore their beliefs, attitudes, and practices related to breast cancer screening (Phillips, Cohen, and Moses, 1999). This approach was chosen because little qualitative research related to breast cancer screening had been conducted with African-American women. This area is important to study because African-American women have lower survival rates and a higher incidence of breast cancer detected at a later stage than other groups. Therefore this type of information is needed to develop interventions to increase screening in a way that will take into account cultural factors.

A helpful metaphor about the need to use a variety of research methods was used by Seymour Kety, a key figure in the development of biological research in psychiatry, who was the scientific director to the U.S. National Institute of Mental Health (NIMH) for many years. He invited readers to think about a civilization whose inhabitants, although very intelligent, had never seen a book (Kety, 1960). On discovering a library, they set up a scientific institute for studying books, which included anatomists, physical chemists, molecular biologists, behavioral scientists, and psychoanalysts. Each discipline discovered important facts, such as the structure of cellulose and the frequency of collections of letters of varying length. However, the meaning of a "book" continued to escape them. As he put it: "We do not always get closer to the truth as we slice and homogenize and isolate." He argued that a truer picture of a topic under study would emerge only from research by a variety of disciplines and techniques, each with its own virtues and particular limitations. Qualitative research methods could be added to understand how books are used by different groups and the meaning of books for individuals, for example.

This idea can serve as summary of an important point of this chapter. It is not that one research method is better than another, but rather that there are a variety of methods, based on different worldviews. Considering the vast amount of knowledge needed to accomplish the important and complex work of nursing, we need to guide our practice with knowledge from both nonscientific and scientific realms and, within science, from a wide variety of methods.

CRITIQUING CRITERIA *Foundations of Qualitative Research*

1. Is the philosophical basis of the research method consistent with the study's purpose?
2. Are the researchers' values apparent and influencing the research or the results of the study?
3. Is the phenomenon focused on human experience within a natural setting?

Critical Thinking Challenges

- Explain the difference between research that uses a "perceived paradigm" as opposed to a "received paradigm" as the basis of the respective study.
- Discuss how a researcher's values could influence the results of a study. Include an example in your answer.
- If a grounded theory research study developed a theory, for example, on why certain cultural groups do not use pain medication, why is it necessary to test it with empirical methods?
- Can the metaphor "We do not always get closer to the truth as we slice and homogenize and isolate [it]" be applied to both qualitative and quantitative methods? Justify your answer.
- What is the value of qualitative research in evidence-based practice? Give an example.

KEY POINTS

- All research is based on philosophical beliefs or a paradigm.
- Paradigms are useful or not useful in reaching research goals, but are not correct or incorrect.
- Values should be kept as separate as possible from the conduct of research.
- Grounded theory is based on Symbolic Interactionism and is focused on processes or social interactions.
- Case studies are based on the Chicago School of Sociology and are ways to study complex real life situations.
- Ethnographical research, developed by anthropologists, is used to understand cultures.
- Phenomenological research, based on phenomenological philosophy, is designed to understand the meaning of a lived experience.

REFERENCES

Bliss SJ, Flanders SA, and Saint S: A pain in the neck, *N Engl J Med* 350(10): 1037-1042, 2004.

Carroll S: Nonvocal ventilated patients' perceptions of being understood, *West J Nurs Res* 24(4): 454-471, 2004.

Cohen MZ: Symptom management in blood and marrow transplantation, Grant RO1 NR05188, funded by the National Institutes of Health, Bethesda, Md, National Institute of Nursing Research, in press.

Cohen MZ, Kahn D, and Steeves R: *Hermeneutic phenomenological research: a practical guide for nurse researchers,* Thousand Oaks, Calif, 2000, Sage.

Cohen MZ, Kahn D, and Steeves R: Making use of qualitative research, *West J Nurs Res* 24(4): 454-471, 2002.

Cohen MZ, Saunders J: Using qualitative research in advanced practice, *Adv Pract Nurs Q* 2(3): 8-13, 1996.

Cohen MZ, Williams L, Knight P, Snider J, Hanzik K, and Fisch M: Symptom masquerade: Understanding the meaning of symptoms, *Support Care Cancer* 12: 184-190, 2004.

Fair BS: Contrasts in patients' and providers' explanations of rheumatoid arthritis, *J Nurs Scholarship* 35(4): 339-344, 2003.

Glaser B, Strauss A: *Awareness of dying,* Chicago, 1965, Aldine De Gruyter.

Glaser B, Strauss A: *The discovery of grounded theory: strategies for qualitative research,* New York, 1967, Aldine De Gruyter.

Hammersley M: *The dilemma of qualitative research,* Routledge, London, 1989, Herbert Blumer and the Chicago Tradition.

Im EO, Meleis AI: Situation-specific theories: philosophical roots, properties, and approach, *Adv Nurs Sci* 22(2): 11-24, 1999.

Inui T: The need for an integrated biopsychosocial approach to research on successful aging, *Ann Int Med* 139: 391-394, 2003.

Johnson J et al: *Self-regulation theory: applying theory to your practice,* Pittsburgh, 1997, Oncology Nursing Press.

Kearney MH: Levels and applications of qualitative research evidence, *Res Nurs Health* 24(2): 145-153, 2001.

Kety S: A biologist examines mind and behavior, *Science* 132(3443): 1861-1870, 1960.

Kleinman A: *Patients and healers in the context of culture,* Berkeley, 1980, University of California Press.

Krespi R, Bone M, Ahmad R, Worthington B, and Salmon P: Haemodialysis patients' beliefs about renal failure and its treatment, *Patient Educ Couns* 53: 189-196, 2004.

Kuhn T: *The structure of scientific revolutions,* Chicago, 1962, The University of Chicago Press.

Lincoln Y, Guba E: Paradigmatic controversies, contradictions, and emerging confluences. In Denzin NK, Lincoln YS, editors: *Handbook of qualitative research,* ed 2, Thousand Oaks, Calif, 2000, Sage.

Mason D: On centennials and millennia, *Am J Nurs* 100(1): 7, 2000 (editorial).

Melnyk BM, Fineout-Overholt E: *Evidence based practice in nursing and healthcare,* Philadelphia, Lippincott, Williams & Wilkins, 2005.

Nightingale F: *Notes on nursing: what it is and what it is not,* New York, 1969, Dover.

Oxford University Press: Oxford English dictionary (online), Retrieved September 3, 2004, from http://dictionary.oed.com.

Parsons S: The case method of teaching nursing, *Am J Nurs* 11(11): 1009-1011, 1911.

Paterson B, Thorne S, Canam C, and Jillings C: *Meta-study of qualitative research: A practical guide to meta-analysis and meta-synthesis,* Thousand Oaks, Calif, 2001, Sage.

Pearson A: Nursing takes the lead: Redefining what counts as evidence in Australian health care, *Reflect Nurs Leader* 28(4): 18-21, 2002.

Phillips JM, Cohen MZ, and Moses G: Breast cancer screening and African-American women: fear, fatalism, and silence, *Oncol Nurs Forum* 26(3): 561-571, 1999.

Plach SK, Stevens PE, and Moss VA: Social role experiences of women living with rheumatoid arthritis, *J Fam Nurs* 10(1): 33-49, 2004.

Powers BA: Critically appraising qualitative evidence. In Melnyk BM, Fineout-Overholt E, editors: *Evidence-based practice in nursing and healthcare,* pp 127-162, Philadelphia, 2005, Lippincott Williams & Wilkins.

Rew L: A theory of taking care of oneself grounded in experiences of homeless youth, *Nurs Res* 52(4): 234-241, 2003.

Roper J, Shapira J: *Ethnography in nursing research,* Thousand Oaks, Calif, 2000, Sage.

Scotch N: Medical anthropology, *Biennial Rev Anthropol* 3: 30-68, 1963.

Smith-Alnimer M, Watford M: Alcohol withdrawal and delirium tremens, *Am J Nurs* 104(5): 72a-75g, 2004.

Stocking G: *Observers observed: essays on ethnographic fieldwork,* Madison, 1983, University of Wisconsin Press.

FOR FURTHER STUDY

Go to your Companion CD for review activities for this chapter.

evolve Go to Evolve at http://evolve.elsevier.com/LoBiondo/ for WebLinks, Content Updates, and additional research articles, for practice in reviewing and critiquing.

7

PATRICIA R. LIEHR
GERI LOBIONDO-WOOD

Qualitative Approaches to Research

KEY TERMS

auditability
bracketing
case study method
community-based participatory
   research
constant comparative method
credibility
culture
data saturation
domains
emic view

ethnographic method
etic view
evidence
external criticism
fittingness
grounded theory method
historical research method
instrumental case study
internal criticism
intrinsic case study
key informants

life context
lived experience
metasynthesis
phenomenological method
primary sources
qualitative research
secondary sources
theoretical sampling
triangulation

LEARNING OUTCOMES

After reading this chapter, the student should be able to do the following:

- Identify connections between worldview, research question, and research method.
- Recognize the use of qualitative research for nursing.
- Identify the processes of phenomenological, grounded theory, ethnographic, and case study methods.
- Recognize appropriate use of historical methods.
- Recognize appropriate use of community-based participatory research methods.
- Discuss significant issues that arise in conducting qualitative research in relation to such topics as ethics, criteria for judging scientific rigor, combination of research methods, and use of computers to assist data management.
- Discuss qualitative research as a source of evidence for clinical decision making.
- Apply the critiquing criteria to evaluate a report of qualitative research.

STUDY RESOURCES

Go to your Companion CD for review activities for this chapter.

evolve Go to Evolve at http://evolve.elsevier.com/LoBiondo/ for Weblinks, Content Updates, and additional research articles for practice in reviewing and critiquing.

Nursing is a body of knowledge that provides the foundation for practice and research. It is both a science and an art. **Qualitative research** combines the scientific and artistic natures of nursing to enhance understanding of the human health experience. It is a general term encompassing a variety of philosophic underpinnings and research methods. According to Denzin and Lincoln (2000), "qualitative researchers study things in their natural settings, attempting to make sense of, or interpret, phenomena in terms of the meanings people bring to them." Naturalistic settings are ones that people live in every day. So, the researcher doing qualitative research goes wherever the participants are—in their homes, schools, communities, and sometimes in the hospital or an outpatient setting.

This chapter focuses on four commonly used qualitative research methods: phenomenology, grounded theory, ethnography, and case study Historical research as well as a newer methodology—community-based participatory research are also presented. Each of these methods, although distinct from the others, shares characteristics that identify it as a method within the qualitative research approach. In the previous chapter, Cohen located these qualitative methods along a continuum ranging from the "received" to the "perceived" view paradigm. She emphasized the importance of one's paradigmatic perspective, sometimes called a worldview. Embedded in one's worldview are beliefs that guide the choice of an issue for research study and the creation of a research study question. For instance, if your view fits best with the received paradigm, it is likely that you believe in the composite nature of humans, allowing isolation of body systems for accurate measurement purposes. If you hold this perspective, you will pose a research question to be addressed by an empiric/analytic method. If, on the other hand, your view fits best with the perceived paradigm, it is likely that you believe in the unitary nature of human life—that humans are intricately connected to each other and their environment. If

you hold this perspective, you will most often pose a research question that can be best addressed with a qualitative method.

It is important to understand that one research method is not better than another; one is not good while another is excellent and yet another poor. The only judgment of excellence has to do with the fit between one's worldview, the research question, and the research method. If there is congruence between worldview, question, and method, then the researcher has made an excellent choice of method. For instance, if a researcher's worldview comes from the received view paradigm, and a question about the effect of slow stroke back massage on blood pressure is posed, there is a good fit between the worldview and the research question. Massage is an intervention that can be manipulated by the researcher, and blood pressure is an outcome variable that can be measured. When researchers study the effects of an intervention on an outcome variable, they generally use empiric/analytic methods, grounded in the received worldview.

Hierarchies of research evidence (see Chapter 2) traditionally categorize evidence from weakest to strongest, with an emphasis on support for the effectiveness of interventions. That this perspective tends to dominate the evidence-based practice literature makes the merit of qualitative studies seem unclear. The previous chapter, Chapter 6, suggests that different research methods provide different types and levels of evidence, all of which inform practice. Although evidence provided by qualitative studies seems to rank lower in the hierarchy of evidence presented in Chapter 2, that is, Levels V and VI, you as a research consumer should consider that qualitative methods are the best way to start to answer clinical and research questions about which little is known or when a new perspective is needed in practice. Sandelowski (2004) notes that the use of hierarchies assumes that randomized clinical trials are the gold standard and thereby devalue qualitative research. Qualitative research has increased and thrived over the years. Thousands of reports of well-conducted qualitative studies exist on topics such as the following: (a) personal and cultural constructions of disease, prevention, treatment, and risk; (b) living with disease and managing the physical, psychological, and social effects of multiple diseases and their treatment; (c) decision-making experiences with beginning and end-of-life, as well as assistive and life-extending, technological interventions; and (d) contextual factors favoring and mitigating against quality care, health promotion, prevention of disease, and reduction of health disparities (Sandelowski, 2004). The answers provided by qualitative data reflect important evidence that may provide valuable insights about a particular phenomenon, patient population, or clinical situation.

In this chapter, you are invited to look through the lens of the perceived view to learn about phenomenological, grounded theory, ethnographic, historical research and community-based participatory research, and case study methods. You are encouraged to change glasses as each method is introduced—to imagine how it would be to study an issue of interest from the perspective of each of these methods. No matter which method a researcher uses, there is a demand to embrace the wholeness of humans, focusing on the human experience in natural settings. The researcher using these methods believes that each unique human being attributes meaning to their experience, and experience evolves from life context. **Life context** is the matrix of human-human-environment relationships emerging over the course of day-to-day living. So, one person's experience of pain is distinct from another's and can be known by the individual's subjective description of it. The researcher interested in studying the lived experience of pain for the adolescent with rheumatoid arthritis will spend time in the adolescent's natural settings, such as the home and school. Effort will be directed to uncover the meaning of pain as it extends beyond the facts of the number of medications taken or a rating on a reliable and valid scale. These methods are grounded in the belief that factual objective data do not capture the human experience. Rather, the meaning of the adolescent's pain emerges within the context of personal history, current relationships, and future plans as the adolescent lives daily life in dynamic interaction with environment.

The researcher using qualitative methods begins collecting bits of information and piecing them together, building a mosaic or a picture of the human experience being studied. As with a mosaic, when one steps away from the work, the whole picture emerges. This whole picture transcends the bits and pieces and cannot be known from any one bit or piece. In presenting study findings, the researcher strives to capture the human experience and present it so that others can understand it. Often, findings are shared as a summary story that becomes the evidence generated by the data.

QUALITATIVE APPROACH AND NURSING SCIENCE

Qualitative research is particularly well suited to study the human experience of health, a central concern of nursing science. Because qualitative methods focus on the whole of human experience and the meaning ascribed by individuals living the experience, these methods extend understanding of health beyond traditionally measured units of **evidence** to include the complexity of the human health experience as it is occurring in everyday living. In fact, Fawcett et al. (2001) note that evidence must extend beyond the current emphasis on quantitative research and randomized clinical trials to the kinds of evidence also generated by ethical theories, personal theories, and aesthetic theories. Surely, the evidence provided by qualitative studies that consider the unique perspectives, concerns, preferences, and expectations each patient brings to a clinical encounter offers in-depth understanding of human experience and the contexts in which they occur. This closeness to what is "real" and "everyday" evidence promises guidance for nursing practice; it is also important for instrument and theory development (Figure 7-1). Three examples are cited to

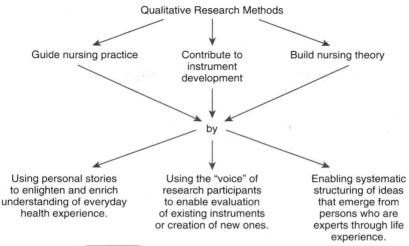

Figure 7-1. Qualitative approach and nursing science.

emphasize the capacity of qualitative methods and the evidence generated by its findings to (1) guide nursing practice, (2) contribute to instrument development, and (3) develop nursing theory.

Qualitative Research Guiding Practice

In a study of caring for dying patients who have air hunger (dyspnea), Tarzian (2000) suggests that "understanding is the first step toward a more consistent and informed response by health care providers to dying patients who suffer from air hunger, and to their family members who witness their distress." Because of the ethical and practical problems of studying dying patients enduring air hunger, Tarzian (2000) studied the experiences of nurses caring for these patients and how family members that witnessed air hunger were affected. Twelve nurses and two family members participated. Family members' descriptions were used to enhance what was shared by the nurses.

An interpretive phenomenological method was used to analyze the data. Tarzian (2000) identified three major themes related to caring for dying patients who have air hunger: patient's panic-stricken appearance, surrendering and sharing control, and fine-tuning dying. The first theme highlights the interactive patient-nurse

relationship. Nurses described their own unsettled feelings when confronting a dying patient struggling to breathe. The second theme continues to emphasize the interactive nurse-patient relationship, describing the balance of surrendering and controlling as choices are made to ease discomfort. The final theme, fine-tuning dying, provides the substance of guidance for practice. Within this theme, the author synthesizes a caring direction: (1) attend to both patient and family needs for comfort; (2) plan ahead to decide what will be done when air hunger episodes occur; (3) prepare patients and family ahead of time so that they know what to expect; (4) be prepared to deal with barriers, such as the failure of physicians to order or the failure of nurses to provide comfort-inducing medication.

In this study the author has provided a description of the human experience of air hunger in the dying patient that becomes the evidence from which the author has derived guidance for health care providers. The importance of the interactive nurse-patient/family relationship during the suffering of the dying patient surfaces as implicit guidance in addition to the explicit direction emerging from the third theme; that is, the ability of the nurse to "be with" the patient and family is a critical dimension in the stories shared by nurses and family members. The consumer of nursing research reading this study can use the evidence to plan care for dying patients suffering from air hunger. The information enables thoughtful consideration of the challenges to be encountered in this nursing situation. When thinking about evidence-based research, it is important to answer the question of how qualitative research also evolves to support evidence-based research.

Qualitative Research Contributing to Instrument Development

As part of a larger study evaluating the reliability and validity of the adolescent version of the Cook-Medley Hostility Scale, Liehr and associates (2000) used qualitative analysis to assess the content validity of the scale. The scale had been tested and used often with adults, but there was little information about the adolescent version of the scale, and all the available information had been collected with Anglo-American children and adolescents.

A total of 57 male and female African-American, Anglo-American, and Mexican-American adolescents were studied. Each adolescent was asked to recall a time when he/she felt angry and to share it with the data collector in as much detail as possible. Remembered circumstances that provoked anger were ones that were likely to be accompanied by hostile attitudes. Data were analyzed using a content analysis procedure outlined by Waltz, Strickland, and Lenz (1991).

Five themes were synthesized to capture the adolescents' descriptions of circumstances that made them angry: aggression, unfulfilled personal expectations, mistrust/lying, criticism of effort, and rejection. These five themes were used to evaluate the comprehensiveness of the 23-item hostility scale. The researchers were interested in whether the hostility scale addressed all the themes presented by the adolescents. Eight hostility scale items were linked with mistrust/ lying, four with rejection, three with aggression, and only one each with unfulfilled personal expectations and criticism of effort. To improve the

comprehensiveness of the scale's content and therefore improve content validity, the authors suggest adding an additional four items: two to tap unfulfilled personal expectations and two to tap criticism of effort. This would result in a minimum of three hostility items for each anger/hostility theme. In this instance, evidence provided by qualitative research was used to strengthen an existing instrument, making it more relevant to the population for whom it was intended.

Qualitative Research Contributing to Theory Building

As a consumer of nursing research, you will notice that the qualitative method most readily linked with theory building is the grounded theory method. Schreiber, Stern, and Wilson (2000) studied depression in 12 black West-Indian Canadian women. They asked participants the following question: "What is it like to go through depression as a black West-Indian Canadian?" In addition to interviews, participant observation occurred, in keeping with the grounded theory method. The authors emphasize that this experience was heavily influenced by major contexts: visible minority status in a Eurocentric society, social stigma of depression imposed by their own cultural group, gender expectations within their cultural group, and Christian upbringing.

"The goal of the women was to be able to manage their depression with grace and to live up to the cultural imperative to be strong." Being strong was the foremost social process used by these women in managing their depression. Being strong included the subprocesses of "dwelling on it," "diverting myself," and "regaining my composure." Dwelling on it referred to the women's recognition that suffering and struggle were integral with being a woman and there was little they could do about it. As a way of dwelling on it, the authors describe patterns of separating from others; gaining a sense of competence by showing compassion when confronted with insensitive behavior; and recognizing the depression for what it was, which enabled them to divert themselves. Diverting self, the second subprocess, was the beginning of efforts to manage depression. These efforts included seeking God's comfort or professional help, socializing, exercising, and thinking positively. The author's suggest that diverting self led to the third subprocess, regaining composure. Regaining composure was characterized by "recognizing God's strength within" and moving on with everyday living.

These central subprocesses of being strong were enhanced by the willingness of some women to consider other ways to manage their depression. The authors labeled this willing effort "trying new approaches." They emphasize the challenging nature of new approaches for women embedded in the black West-Indian Canadian cultural context. The authors provide a model of "being strong," depicting the relationships between subprocesses and contexts. The evidence generated by this qualitative study enabled creation of the structure of "being strong," which contributes to nursing's knowledge base and offers guidance for further research and practice.

 EVIDENCE-BASED PRACTICE TIP

Qualitative research provides guidance for practice through stories, as compared to quantitative research that provides guidance through numbers.

QUALITATIVE RESEARCH METHODS

Thus far an overview of the qualitative research approach has been presented, attending to the importance of evidence offered by qualitative research for nursing science. An effort has been made to highlight how choice of a qualitative approach is reflective of one's worldview and research question and how qualitative methods contribute to guiding practice, testing instruments, and building theory. These topics provide a foundation for examining the qualitative methods discussed in this chapter. The Critical Thinking Decision Path shown below introduces the consumer of nursing research to a process for recognizing differing qualitative methods by distinguishing areas of interest for each method and noting how the research question

CRITICAL THINKING DECISION PATH   Selecting a Qualitative Research Method

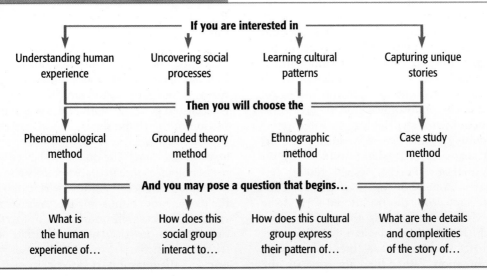

might be introduced for each distinct method. The phenomenological, grounded theory, ethnographic, case study, and historical and community-based participatory research methods are described in detail for the consumer of nursing research.

Parse, Coyne, and Smith (1985) suggested that research methods, whether quantitative or qualitative, include the following five basic elements:

1. Identifying the phenomenon
2. Structuring the study
3. Gathering the data
4. Analyzing the data
5. Describing the findings

Each qualitative method is defined, followed by a discussion of these five basic elements. The factors that distinguish the methods are highlighted, and research examples are presented, providing critiquing direction for the beginning research consumer.

Phenomenological Method

The **phenomenological method** is a process of learning and constructing the meaning of human experience through intensive dialogue with persons who are living the experience. The researcher's goal is to understand the meaning of the experience as it is lived by the participant. Meaning is pursued through a dialogic process, which extends beyond a simple interview and requires thoughtful presence on the part of the researcher. In the previous chapter, Cohen introduced the traditional philosophical bases, which provide a foundation for phenomenological research. Each philosopher-guided (Husserl's eidetic phenomenology; Heidegger's interpretive phenomenology; Dutch hermeneutical phenomenology) base directs slight differences in research methods. Further, Caelli (2000) has distinguished American forms of phenomenological research from the traditional forms. She suggests that nursing tends to use American forms, which focus on understanding the reality of experience for *the person* as they engage with the phenomenon, rather than focusing on the more objective *phenomenon itself,* as is the case

in traditional forms of phenomenological research. Whatever the form of phenomenological research, the consumer of nursing research will find the researcher asking a question about the lived experience.

Identifying the Phenomenon

Because the focus of the phenomenological method is the **lived experience,** the researcher is likely to choose this method when studying some dimension of day-to-day existence for a particular group of people. For instance, the nurse may be interested in the experience of anger for people who have heart disease or the experience of success for baccalaureate nursing students. Chiu (2000) studied the lived experience of spirituality for Taiwanese women with breast cancer, and Burton (2000) studied the experience of living with stroke. Each of these authors used the phenomenological method to explore dimensions of health as it was lived day-to-day. Philips, Cohen, and Tarzian (2001) studied African-American women's experience with breast cancer screening. The researchers used the hermeneutical phenomenological method. Their research report is used to guide understanding of the phenomenological method.

Structuring the Study

For the purpose of describing structuring, the following topics are addressed: the research question, the researcher's perspective, and sample selection. The issue of human subjects' protection has been suggested as a dimension of structuring (Parse, Coyne, and Smith, 1985); this issue is discussed generally with ethics in a subsequent section of the chapter.

Research Question   The question that guides phenomenological research always asks about some human experience. It guides the researcher to ask the participant about some past or present experience. The research question is not exactly the same as the question used to initiate dialogue with the participant, but often the research question and the question used to begin dialogue are very similar. For instance, Orne and associates

(2000) posed the following research question: What is the lived experience of being employed but medically uninsured? The statement that introduced their research dialogue with participants was: "Please describe for me as thoroughly as you can, what it is like to be working without medical insurance." It is important that the question used to begin dialogue be understandable for the participant. The research question used by Philips, Cohen, and Tarzian (2001) was as follows: What is the meaning of breast cancer screening for African-American women? The statements used to encourage dialogue included requests for descriptions about the last time participants did a breast exam, their last mammography, and their last professional breast exam. Participants were encouraged to elaborate based on what was shared in these descriptions.

 HELPFUL H I N T

Although the research question may not always be explicitly reported, it may be identified by evaluating the study's purpose or the question/statement posed to the participants.

Researcher's Perspective When using the phenomenological method, the researcher's perspective is **bracketed.** That is, the researcher identifies personal biases about the phenomenon of interest to clarify how personal experience and beliefs may color what is heard and reported. The researcher is expected to set aside personal biases—to bracket them—when engaged with the participants. By becoming aware of personal biases, the researcher is more likely to be able to pursue issues of importance as introduced by the participant, rather than leading the participant to issues the researcher deems important.

In the previous chapter, Cohen suggested that **bracketing** was more important for some phenomenological methods than others. However, the researcher using phenomenological methods always uses some strategy to identify personal biases and hold them in abeyance while querying the participant. The reader may find it difficult

to identify bracketing strategies because they are seldom explicitly identified in a research manuscript. Sometimes, the researcher's worldview or assumptions provide insight into biases that have been considered and bracketed. In the paper by Philips, Cohen, and Tarzian (2001), the authors let the reader know that they were interested in gaining a better understanding of the meaning of breast cancer screening for African-American women; Philips and associates felt that understanding would lead to more effective approaches to increase breast cancer screening and ultimately improve survival. From the perspective of bracketing, their expectation was held in abeyance as they came to understand the meaning of the experience as described by the persons living it.

Sample Selection The reader of a report of a phenomenological study will find that the selected sample either is living the experience the researcher is querying or has lived the experience in their past. Because phenomenologists believe that each individual's history is a dimension of the present, a past experience exists in the present moment. Even when a participant is describing an experience occurring in the present, remembered information is being gathered. The participants in the study by Philips and associates (2001) were 8 low-income and 16 middle-income African-American women without a known history of breast cancer. The ages ranged from 45 to 81 years with a mean age of 52 years. Women over age 40 were recruited because of the recommendations to have a baseline mammogram by age 40. These women were describing remembered experiences related to performing a breast exam by themselves and having a breast exam performed by a professional.

Data Gathering

Written or oral data may be collected when using the phenomenological method. The researcher may pose the query in writing and ask for a written response or may schedule a time to interview the participant and tape-record the interaction. In either case, the researcher may return to ask for clarification of written or tape-recorded transcripts. To some extent, the particular data-collection procedure is guided by the choice of a specific analysis technique. Different analysis techniques require different numbers of interviews. Data saturation usually guides decisions regarding how many interviews are enough. **Data saturation** is the situation of "having heard the themes before." The researcher knows that saturation has been reached when the ideas surfacing in the dialogue are ones previously heard from other participants. Philips, Cohen, and Tarzian (2001) collected data from 23 participants using open-ended interviews. The reader could assume that data saturation had occurred by the time 23 interviews were completed.

Data Analysis

Several techniques are available for data analysis when using the phenomenological method. For detailed information about specific techniques, the reader is referred to original sources (Colaizzi, 1978; Giorgi, Fischer, and Murray, 1975; Spiegelberg, 1976; van Kaam, 1969). Although the techniques are slightly different from each other, there is a general pattern of moving from the participant's description to the researcher's synthesis of all participants' descriptions. The steps generally include the following:

1. Thorough reading and sensitive reading of presence with the entire transcription of the participant's description
2. Identification of shifts in participant thought, resulting in division of the transcription into thought segments
3. Specification of significant phrases in each thought segment, using the participant's words
4. Distillation of each significant phrase to express the central meaning of the segment in the researcher's words
5. Grouping together of segments that contain similar central meanings for each participant
6. Preliminary synthesis of grouped segments for each participant with a focus on the essence of the phenomenon being studied

7. Final synthesis of the essences that have surfaced in all participants' descriptions, resulting in an exhaustive description of the lived experience

Philips, Cohen, and Tarzian (2001) analyzed data using a hermeneutic phenomenological method (van Manen, 1990; Cohen, Kahn, and Steeves, 2000). Interviews were audiotaped and transcribed verbatim. Subjects were interviewed twice, and during the second interview subjects were given the transcripts of the first interview and asked to clarify and verify information for completeness and accuracy. Transcripts were read and reread by the researchers and also by a researcher who was not present during the interviews, allowing for questions regarding the interviews and for discussion of the interview techniques so that techniques could be refined before the second session with the participant. Themes and passages were compared for all participants. These methods allowed the researchers to synthesize descriptions and develop themes based on the words of the participants.

Describing the Findings

When using the phenomenological method, the nurse researcher provides the research consumer with a path of information leading from the research question, through samples of participant's words and researcher's interpretation, leading to the final synthesis that elaborates the lived experience as a narrative. When reading the report of a phenomenological study, the reader will find that detailed descriptive language is used to convey the complex meaning of the lived experience that offers the evidence for this qualitative method. Philips, Cohen, and Tarzian (2001) provide quotes from participants to support their findings. They synthesized three themes that described women's experience of screening for breast cancer: caring for body, self, and spirit; relationship with others, reminding them that they are not alone; and spreading the word about breast cancer survival. Direct participant quotes enable the reader to evaluate the connection between what the participant said and how the researcher labeled what was said.

EVIDENCE-BASED PRACTICE TIP

Phenomenological research is an important approach for accumulating evidence when studying a new topic about which little is known.

Grounded Theory Method

The **grounded theory method** is an inductive approach involving a systematic set of procedures to arrive at theory about basic social processes. The emergent theory is based on observations and perceptions of the social scene and evolves during data collection and analysis as a product of the actual research process (Strauss and Corbin, 1994). The grounded theory method is used to construct theory where no theory exists or in situations where existing theory fails to provide evidence to explain a set of circumstances. According to Denzin (1998), grounded theory is the qualitative perspective most widely used by social scientists today, largely because it sets forth clearly defined steps for the researcher.

Developed originally as a sociologist's tool to investigate interactions in social settings (Glaser and Strauss, 1967), the grounded theory method is not bound to that discipline. Investigators from different disciplines may study the same phenomenon from varying perspectives (Denzin and Lincoln, 1998; Strauss and Corbin, 1994, 1997). As an example, in an area of study such as chronic illness, a nurse might be interested in coping patterns within families, a psychologist in personal adjustment, and a sociologist in group behavior in health care settings. Theory generated by each discipline will reflect the discipline and serve it in explaining the phenomenon of interest to the discipline (Liehr and Marcus, 2002). In grounded theory, usefulness stems from the transferability of theories from one study to another situation, making the key objective the development of more formal theories that are faithful to the cases from which they were derived (Sandelowski, 2004).

Identifying the Phenomenon

Researchers typically use the grounded theory method when they are interested in social processes from the perspective of human interactions, or "patterns of action and interaction between and among various types of social units" (Denzin and Lincoln, 1998). The basic social process is sometimes expressed as a *gerund*, indicating change across time as social reality is negotiated. For example, O'Brien, Evans, and White-McDonald (2002) studied how women cope when they are hospitalized with severe nausea and vomiting during pregnancy. Calvin (2004) studied end-of-life decisions for people on hemodialysis, culminating in ideas about "knowing the odds," "defining individuality," and "personal preservation." Calvin's study will be used as an example of the grounded theory method.

Structuring the Study

Research Question   Research questions appropriate for the **grounded theory** method are those that address basic social processes. They tend to ask about social processes that shape human behavior. In a grounded theory study, the research question can be a statement or a broad question that permits in-depth explanation of the phenomenon. For example, the reader will recognize Calvin's question implied in the study aim: to explore end-of-life treatment decisions among hemodialysis patients.

Researcher's Perspective   In a grounded theory study, the researcher brings some knowledge of the literature to the study, but the consumer will notice that an exhaustive literature review is not done. This allows theory to emerge directly from data and to reflect the contextual values that are integral to the social processes being studied. In this way, the theory product that emerges is "grounded in" the data.

Sample Selection Sample selection involves choosing participants who are experiencing the circumstance and selecting events and incidents related to the social process under investigation. Calvin (2004) recruited participants from three hemodialysis units. The average time since beginning dialysis treatment for the sample of 20 patients was 5.5 years.

Data Gathering

In the grounded theory method, the consumer will find that data are collected through interviews and through skilled observations of individuals interacting in a social setting. Interviews are audiotaped and then transcribed, and observations are recorded as field notes. Open-ended questions are used initially to identify concepts for further focus. Calvin (2004) interviewed patients during their dialysis treatments, beginning with a discussion about advanced directives. Additional questions included (Calvin, 2004, p. 560):

- What have been your experiences with end-of-life treatment?
- How did you come to your decisions about end-of-life treatment?
- How do you think it is all going to end up?

The interview questions changed as data were collected, focusing on emerging processes central to making end-of-life decisions. For instance, questions about hoping, living in the present, and taking chances were eventually included in the interviews (Calvin, 2004). Detailed field notes about the interview content and observations were written immediately after the interview was completed.

Data Analysis

A major feature of the grounded theory method is that data collection and analysis occur simultaneously. The process requires systematic, detailed record-keeping using field notes and transcribed interview tapes. Hunches about emerging patterns in the data are noted in memos, and the researcher directs activities in the field by pursuing these hunches. This tech-

nique, called **theoretical sampling,** is used to select experiences that will help the researcher test ideas and gather complete information about developing concepts. The researcher begins by noting indicators or actual events, actions, or words in the data. Concepts, or abstractions, are developed from the indicators (Charmaz, 2000; Strauss, 1987).

The initial analytical process is called open *coding* (Strauss, 1987). Data are examined carefully line by line, broken down into discrete parts, and compared for similarities and differences (Strauss and Corbin, 1990). Data are compared with other data continuously as they are acquired during research. This is a process called the **constant comparative method.** Codes in the data are clustered to form categories. The categories are expanded and developed or they are collapsed into one another. Theory is constructed through this systematic process. As a result, data collection, analysis, and theory generation have a direct reciprocal relationship (Charmaz, 2000; Strauss and Corbin, 1990). Calvin (2004) began by analyzing the first 12 interviews using the constant comparative method. The last eight interviews were more focused with the intent of refining the categories, which emerged during the initial analysis.

 HELPFUL H I N T

In a report of research using the grounded theory method, the consumer can expect to find a diagrammed model of a theory that synthesizes the researcher's findings in a systematic way.

Describing the Findings

Grounded theory studies are reported in sufficient detail to provide the reader with the steps in the process, the logic of the method, and the theory that has emerged. Reports of grounded theory studies use descriptive language and diagrams of the process as evidence to ensure that the theory reported in the findings remains connected to the data. Calvin presents a theory of personal preservation that models the relationship between knowing the odds, defining individuality, and personal preservation. She describes the theory of personal preservation as an "interactive paradox of being responsible and taking chances" (Calvin, 2004, p. 561). Each of the three central theory ideas—knowing the odds, defining individuality, and personal preservation—is described in detail and logically linked to the words of the participants.

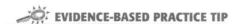 **EVIDENCE-BASED PRACTICE TIP**

When thinking about the evidence generated by the grounded theory method, consider whether the theory is useful in explaining, interpreting, or predicting the study phenomenon of interest.

Ethnographic Method

Derived from the Greek term *ethnos,* meaning people, race, or cultural group, the **ethnographic method** focuses on scientific description and interpretation of cultural or social groups and systems (Creswell, 1998). The reader should know that the goal of the ethnographer is to understand the natives' view of their world or the **emic view.** The emic (insiders') view is contrasted to the **etic** (outsiders') **view** obtained when the researcher uses quantitative analyses of behavior. The ethnographic approach requires that the researcher enter the world of the study participants to watch what happens, listen to what is said, ask questions, and collect whatever data are available. The term *ethnography* is used to mean both the research technique and the product of that technique, the study itself (Creswell, 1998; Tedlock, 2000). Vidick and Lyman (1998) trace the history of ethnography, with roots in the disciplines of sociology and anthropology, as a method born out of the need to understand "other" and "self." Nurses use the method to study cultural variations in health and

patient groups as subcultures within larger social contexts (Liehr and Marcus, 2002).

Identifying the Phenomenon

The phenomenon under investigation in an ethnographic study varies in scope from a long-term study of a very complex culture, such as that of the Aborigines (Mead, 1949), to a shorter-term study of a phenomenon within subunits of cultures. Kleinman (1992) notes the clinical utility of ethnography in describing the "local world" of groups of patients who are experiencing a particular phenomenon, such as suffering. The local worlds of patients have cultural, political, economical, institutional, and social-relational dimensions in much the same way as larger complex societies. A study of cross-cultural relationships between nurses and Filipino-Canadian patients is used as an example to introduce the reader to ethnography (Pasco, Morse, and Olson, 2004).

Structuring the Study

Research Question   When reviewing the report of ethnographic research, notice that questions are asked about lifeways or particular patterns of behavior within the social context of a culture or subculture. **Culture** is viewed as the system of knowledge and linguistic expressions used by social groups that allows the researcher to interpret or make sense of the world (Aamodt, 1991). Ethnographic nursing studies address questions that concern how cultural knowledge, norms, values, and other contextual variables influence one's health experience. The research question of Pasco, Morse, and Olson (2004) is implied in their purpose statement and can be stated as follows: "What are the culturally embedded values that implicitly guide Filipino Canadian patients' interactions in developing nurse-patient relationships?" Other possible ethnographic questions include the following: "What does comforting mean in Hispanic families?" "What is the meaning of health care for migrant workers?" "What are patient and nurse roles like in intensive care units?" This last question does not imply "culture" in the same way as a question about Hispanic families or migrant workers. However, it fits a broader definition of culture, where a particular social context is conceptualized as a culture. In this case, intensive care units are seen as a culture appropriate for ethnographic study.

Researcher's Perspective   When using the ethnographic method, the researcher's perspective is that of an interpreter entering an alien world and attempting to make sense of that world from the insider's point of view (Agar, 1986). Like phenomenologists and grounded theorists, ethnographers make their own beliefs explicit and *bracket,* or set aside, their personal biases as they seek to understand the worldview of others.

Sample Selection   The ethnographer selects a cultural group that is living the phenomenon under investigation. The researcher gathers information from general informants and from key informants. **Key informants** are individuals who have special knowledge, status, or communication skills and who are willing to teach the ethnographer about the phenomenon (Creswell, 1998). Pasco, Morse, and Olson (2004), who selected participants through purposive sampling, spent time with 23 Filipino-Canadian patients who were hospitalized for a range of health problems and had been living in Canada for a minimum of 5 years. These people were recruited because they were uniquely capable of sharing cultural perspectives of interest to the researchers.

 HELPFUL HINT

Managing personal bias is an expectation of researchers using all the methods discussed in this chapter.

Data Gathering

Ethnographic data gathering involves participant observation or immersion in the setting, inter-

views of informants, and interpretation by the researcher of cultural patterns (Crabtree and Miller, 1992). According to Boyle (1991), ethnographic research in nursing, as in other disciplines, always involves "face-to-face interviewing, with data collection and analysis taking place in the natural setting." Thus fieldwork is a major focus of the method. Other techniques may include obtaining life histories and collecting material items reflective of the culture. Photographs and films of the informants in their world can be used as data sources. Spradley (1979) identified three categories of questions for ethnographic inquiry: descriptive, or broad, open-ended questions; structural, or in-depth, questions that expand and verify the unit of analysis; and contrast questions, or ones that further clarify and provide criteria for exclusion. Data gathering techniques for the study of Filipino-Canadian patients began with a request for participants to tell the researcher about their hospital experience. "Follow-up interviews were more structured with questions validating and extending analytic notes" (Pasco, Morse, and Olson, 2004, p. 241). Many participants spoke both English and Filipino during their interviews.

Data Analysis

As with the grounded theory method, data are collected and analyzed simultaneously. Data analysis proceeds through several levels as the researcher looks for the meaning of cultural symbols in the informant's language. Analysis begins with a search for **domains** or symbolic categories that include smaller categories. Language is analyzed for semantic relationships, and structural questions are formulated to expand and verify data. Analysis proceeds through increasing levels of complexity until the data, grounded in the informant's reality and synthesized by the researcher, lead to hypothetical propositions about the cultural phenomenon under investigation. The reader is encouraged to consult Creswell (1998) for a detailed description of the ethnographic analysis process. Pasco,

Morse, and Olson (2004) provide little detail about their analysis process except to state that initial categories of data were used to direct follow-up interviews, moving toward a model depicting types of nurse-patient relationships and levels of interaction.

Describing the Findings

Ethnographic studies yield large quantities of data that reflect a wide array of evidence amassed as field notes of observations, interview transcriptions, and sometimes other artifacts such as photographs. Charmaz (2000) provided guidelines for ethnographic writing that are an excellent framework for the consumer of nursing research wishing to critique descriptions of ethnographic studies. The five techniques recommended in Charmaz' guidelines are: pulling the reader in, recreating experiential mood, adding surprise, reconstructing ethnographic experience, and creating closure for the study. When critiquing, be aware that the report of findings usually provides examples from data, thorough descriptions of the analytical process, and statements of the hypothetical propositions and their relationship to the ethnographer's frame of reference. Evidence provided by complete ethnographies may be published as monographs. Pasco, Morse, and Olson (2004) developed a taxonomy diagrammed as a matrix of levels of progressive nurse-patient interaction (formality, adjustment, acceptance, mutual comfort, oneness) and characteristics of interaction (nature of interaction, patients' needs, patients' feelings, patients' trust, patients' response to nursing care). Their final product also included a glossary of Filipino terms that identified words pertinent to patient-nurse interaction. For instance, *hindi ibang tao* means "one of us" and *ibang tao* means "not one of us", critical ideas for nurse-patient interaction with this group of Filipino-Canadian participants. The evidence provided by the ethnographic information in this study can be used as a guide to providing culturally competent care with this patient population.

 EVIDENCE-BASED PRACTICE TIP

Evidence generated by ethnographic studies will answer questions about how cultural knowledge, norms, values, and other contextual variables influence the health experience of a particular patient population in a specific setting.

Case Study

Case study research, which is rooted in sociology, is currently described slightly differently by Yin, Stake, Merriam, and Creswell, major thinkers who write about this method (Aita and McIlvain, 1999). For the purposes of introducing the nurse consumer to this research method, Stake's view is emphasized. **Case study** is about studying the peculiarities and the commonalities of a specific case—familiar ground for practicing nurses. Stake (2000) notes that case study is not a methodological choice, but rather a choice of what to study. Case study can include quantitative and/or qualitative data, but it is defined by its focus on uncovering an individual case. Stake (2000) distinguishes intrinsic from instrumental case study. **Intrinsic case study** is undertaken to have a better understanding of the case—nothing more or nothing less. "The researcher at least temporarily subordinates other curiosities so that the stories of those 'living the case' will be teased out" (Stake, 2000). **Instrumental case study** is defined as research that is done when the researcher is pursuing insight into an issue or wants to challenge some generalization.

Spear (2004) conducted a study using a naturalistic, qualitative intrinsic case study approach with the intention of pursuing insight. Two adolescent mothers who participated in a previously completed study on teenage pregnancy participated in a follow-up study approximately 18 months after they gave birth. The follow-up interviews occurred in their homes, and the researcher interviewed them about their lives after giving birth. Spear (2004) provides a picture of the young mothers' experiences, noting that the case study approach was chosen because it illustrates a "holistic and lifelike picture of the participant's experience" (p. 121). Both young women expressed satisfaction with being a mother and changed perspectives about motherhood now that they were living with the day-to-day challenges. Spear drew conclusions using these data and the data from her original study to guide practice and future research.

Identifying the Phenomenon

Although some definitions of case study demand that the focus of research be contemporary, Stake's (1995, 2000) defining criterion of attention to the single case broadens the scope of phenomenon for study. By a single case, Stake is designating a focus on an individual, a family, a community, an organization—some complex phenomenon that demands close scrutiny for understanding. Spear chose the teenage mom as a focus for case study research, gathering data from two individuals.

Structuring the Study

Research Question The research question for a case study is one that provokes the curiosity of the researcher. Stake (2000) suggests that research questions be developed around issues that serve as a foundation to uncover complexity and pursue understanding. Although researchers pose questions to begin discussion, the initial questions are never all-inclusive. Rather, the researcher uses an iterative process of "growing questions" in the field. That is, as data are collected to address these questions, other questions will emerge to guide the researcher down another path in the process of untangling the complex story. Therefore research questions evolve over time and recreate themselves in case study research. Spear's (2004) longitudinal approach enabled a question examining change over time

from being pregnant to being a mom. Her opening statement to the participants was: "Tell me about how you are doing since you had your baby."

Researcher's Perspective When the researcher begins with questions developed around suspected issues of importance, the perspective of the researcher is reflected in the questions; this is sometimes referred to as an etic perspective. As the researcher begins engaging the phenomenon of interest, the story unfolds and leads the way, shifting from an etic (researcher) to an emic (story) perspective (Stake, 2000). The reader may recognize a shift from etic to emic perspective when stories spin off of the original questions posed by the researcher.

Sample Selection This is one of the areas where scholars in the field present differing views, ranging from only choosing the most common cases to only choosing the most unusual cases (Aita and McIlvain,1999). Stake (2000) advocates selecting cases that may offer the best opportunities for learning. For instance, if there are several heart transplant patients the researcher may study, practical factors will influence who offers the best opportunity for learning. Persons who live in the area and can be easily visited at home or in the medical center would be a better choice than someone living in another country. The researcher may want to choose someone who has an actively participating family, since most transplant patients exist in a family setting. No choice is perfect when selecting a case. There is much to learn about any one individual, situation, or organization when doing case study research, regardless of the contextual factors influencing the unit of analysis. Spear (2004) had eight participants in her first study, and she attempted to recruit all eight for this case study follow-up. Six of the participants were unavailable for varying reasons, such as moving, having a miscarriage, and not wishing to continue participation.

Data Gathering

Data are gathered using interview, observation, document review, and any other methods that accumulate evidence that enables understanding of the complexity of the case. The researcher will do what is needed to get a sense of the environment and the relationships that provide the context for the case. Stake (1995) advocates development of a data-gathering plan to guide the progress of the study from definition of the case through decisions regarding reporting. The consumer of research may find little explicit information about data gathering in the report of research.

Data Analysis/Describing Findings

Data analysis is closely tied to data gathering and description of findings as the case study story is generated. "Qualitative case study is characterized by researchers spending extended time, on site, personally in contact with activities and operations of the case, reflecting, revising meanings of what is going on" (Stake, 2000). Reflecting and revising meanings are the work of the case study researcher, who has recorded data, searched for patterns, linked data from multiple sources, and arrived at preliminary thoughts regarding the meaning of collected data. This reflective dynamic evolution is the iterative process of creating the case study story that can be thought of as the evidence. The reader of a qualitative case study will have difficulty determining how data analysis was conducted because the research report generally does not list research activities. Findings are embedded in the following: (1) a chronological development of the case; (2) the researcher's story of coming to know the case; (3) the one-by-one description of case dimensions; and (4) vignettes that highlight case qualities (Stake, 1995). Spear (2004) does not describe analysis in detail but reports that participants had the following: regrets about loss, but hopes about the future; shifting relationships, some mended and some broken; and decisions about how to proceed with previous patterns of fighting behavior.

 EVIDENCE-BASED PRACTICE TIP

Case studies are a way of providing in-depth evidence-based discussion of clinical topics that can be used to guide practice.

Historical Research

The **historical research method** is a systematic approach for understanding the past through collection, organization, and critical appraisal of facts. One of the goals of the researcher using historical methodology is to shed light on the past so that it can guide the present and the future. Nursing's attention to historical methodology was initiated by Teresa E. Christy. Christy elaborated the method (1975) and the need (1981) for historical research long before most nurse scholars accepted it as a legitimate research method. More recently, Lusk (1997) summarized important information for the nurse interested in understanding historical research. She provided guidance for choosing a topic, acquiring data, addressing ethical issues, analyzing data, and reporting findings.

When critiquing a study that used the historical method, expect to find the research question embedded in the phenomenon to be studied. The question is stated implicitly rather than explicitly. Data sources provide the sample for historical research. The more clearly a researcher delineates the historical event being studied, the more specifically data sources can be identified. Data may include written or video documents, interviews with persons who witnessed the event, photographs, and any other artifacts that shed light on the subject. Sometimes pivotal information cannot be retrieved and must be eliminated from the list of possible sources. To determine which data sources were used when reviewing a published study, the reader will look at the reference list. Sources of data may be primary or secondary. **Primary sources** are eyewitness accounts provided by varying sorts of communication appropriate to the time. **Secondary** sources provide a view of the phenomenon from another's perspective rather than a first-hand account.

Validity of documents is established by external criticism; reliability is established by internal criticism. **External criticism** judges the authenticity of the data source. The researcher seeks to ensure that the data source is what it seems to be. For instance, if the researcher is reviewing a handwritten letter of Florence Nightingale, some of the validity issues are the following:

- Are the ink, paper, and wax seal on the envelope representative of Nightingale's time?
- Is the wax seal one that Nightingale used in other authentic data sources?
- Is the writing truly Nightingale's?

Only if the data source passes the test of external criticism does the researcher begin internal criticism. **Internal criticism** concerns the reliability of information within the document (Christy, 1975). To judge reliability, the researcher must become familiar with the time in which the data emerged. A sense of the context and language of the time is essential to understanding a document. The meaning of a word in one era may not be equivalent to the meaning in another era. Knowing the language, customs, and habits of the historical period is critical for judging reliability. The researcher assumes that a primary source provides a more reliable account than a secondary source (Christy, 1975). The further a source moves from providing an eyewitness account, the more questionable is its reliability. The researcher using historical methods attempts to establish fact, probability, or possibility (Box 7-1). Keeling (2004) conducted a historical study describing the inception and proliferation of coronary care units in the United States in the 1960s and analyzed the role of nurses within these units. After analysis of historical data, Keeling argued that there were artificial and blurred boundaries between nursing and medicine when nurses assumed the technological skills of cardiac monitoring in the early cardiac units.

BOX 7-1 ESTABLISHING FACT, PROBABILITY, AND POSSIBILITY WITH THE HISTORICAL METHOD

FACT

Two independent primary sources that agree with each other

or

One independent primary source that receives critical evaluation and one independent secondary source that is in agreement and relieves critical evaluation and no substantive conflicting data

PROBABILITY

One primary source that receives critical evaluation and no substantive conflicting data

or

Two primary sources that disagree about particular points

POSSIBILITY

One primary source that provides information but is not adequate to receive critical evaluation

or

Only secondary or tertiary sources

Modified from Christy TE: The methodology of historical research: a brief introduction, *Image: J Nurs Scholarship* 24(3):189-192, 1975.

 HELPFUL H I N T

When critiquing the historical method, do not expect to find a report of data analysis but simply a description of findings synthesized into a continuous narrative.

 EVIDENCE-BASED PRACTICE TIP

The presentation of a historical study should be logical, consistent, and easy to follow.

Community-Based Participatory Research

Community-based participatory research (CBPR) is a method that systematically accesses the voice of a community to plan context-appropriate action. CBPR "provides an alternative to traditional research approaches that assume a phenomenon may be separated from its context for purposes of study . . . CBPR recognizes the importance of involving members of a study population as active and equal participants, in all phases of the research project, if the research process is to be a means of facilitating change" (Holkup et al., 2004, p. 162). Change or action is the intended "end-product" of CBPR and Action Research is a term related to CBPR. Some scholars would consider CBPR a sort of Action Research and would group both Action Research and CBPR within the tradition of critical science (Fontana, 2004). In his book entitled *Action Research,* Stringer (1999) distilled the research process into three phases: *look, think, act.* In the *look* phase Stringer (1999) talks about "building the picture" by getting to know stakeholders so that the problem is defined on their terms and the problem definition is reflective of the community context. The *think* phase addresses interpretation and analysis of what was learned in the *look* phase, where the researcher is charged with connecting the ideas of the stakeholders so that they provide evidence that is understandable to the community group (Stringer, 1999). Finally, in the *act* phase Stringer (1999) advocates for planning, implementing, and evaluating, based on information collected and interpreted in the other phases of research.

Marcus, a nurse researcher, and her community and university colleagues report a study of CBPR to prevent substance use and HIV/AIDS in African-American adolescents (Marcus et al., 2004). The research team used Stringer's phases of look, think, and act to frame their study within an African-American church community in Southwest United States. In the *look* phase university research team members and church leaders formed a coalition, which met to consider the existing community situation and to evaluate the effectiveness of services already provided by the church to address substance use and HIV/AIDS in the adolescent congregation. Weekly meetings were convened to discuss evidence provided by relevant literature and apply the literature to the community situation. The coalition's *look* indicated that community youth could benefit from attention to substance use and HIV/AIDS prevention and the best course of action may be to begin with one community church, realizing that follow-up work could expand to the larger metropolitan community. In the *think* phase the coalition continued its work by analyzing and interpreting what was learned in the first phase of the research process. Analysis and interpretation were simultaneously connected with discussion of what could be done, and the collaborators initiated plans for Project BRIDGE to take African-American adolescents to a new level of understanding about everyday decisions that could seriously affect their health. Project BRIDGE integrated a faith component into structured programs supporting wise choices to reduce substance use and HIV/AIDS exposure. As plans for Project BRIDGE were formulated, the coalition was already moving into the *action* phase of research based on the strength of evidence generated in the previous phases. In the action phase Project BRIDGE was delivered to sixth, seventh, and eighth graders within the structure of the community church environment. The church-university coalition members participated in all components of delivery and continued to meet to evaluate ongoing development, effectiveness, need for adjustment, and outcomes. Project BRIDGE is one example of CBPR that involved community members as equal participants in all phases of research to engage in context-appropriate action for affecting substance use and HIV/AIDS prevention in African-American youth.

ISSUES IN QUALITATIVE RESEARCH

Ethics

Inherent in all research is the demand for the protection of human subjects. This demand exists for both quantitative and qualitative research approaches. Human subjects' protection as applicable to the quantitative approach is discussed in Chapter 13. These basic tenets hold true for the qualitative approach. However, several characteristics of qualitative methodologies outlined in Table 7-1 generate unique concerns and necessitate an expanded view of protecting human subjects.

Naturalistic Setting

The central concern that arises when research is conducted in naturalistic settings focuses on the need to gain consent. The need to acquire informed consent is a basic researcher responsibility, but it is not always easy in naturalistic settings. For instance, when research methods include observing groups of people interacting over time, the complexity of gaining consent is apparent. These complexities generate controversy and debate among qualitative researchers. The balance between respect for human participants and efforts to collect meaningful data must be continuously negotiated. The reader should look for information that the researcher has addressed this issue of balance by recording attention to human participant protection.

Emergent Nature of Design

The emergent nature of the research design emphasizes the need for ongoing negotiation of consent with the participant. In the course of a study, situations change and what was agreeable at the beginning may become intrusive. Sometimes, as data collection proceeds and new information emerges, the study shifts direction in a way that is not acceptable to the participant. For instance, if the researcher were present in a family's home during a time that marital discord arose, the family may choose to renegotiate the consent. From another perspective, Morse (1998) discusses the increasing involvement of participants in the research process, sometimes resulting in their request to have their name published in the findings or be included as a coauthor. If the participant originally signed a consent form

TABLE **7-1** **Characteristics of Qualitative Research Generating Ethical Concerns**

Characteristics	Ethical Concerns
Naturalistic setting	Some researchers using methods that rely on participant observation may believe that consent is not always possible or necessary.
Emergent nature of design	Planning for questioning and observation emerges over the time of the study. Thus it is difficult to inform the participant precisely of all potential threats before he or she agrees to participate.
Researcher-participant interaction	Relationships developed between the researcher and participant may blur the focus of the interaction.
Researcher as instrument	The researcher is the study instrument, collecting data and interpreting the participant's reality.

and then chose an active identified role, Morse (1998) suggests that the participant then sign a "release for publication" form. The underlying nature of this discussion is that the emergent qualitative research process demands ongoing negotiating of researcher-participant relationships, including the consent relationship. The opportunity to renegotiate consent establishes a relationship of trust and respect characteristic of the ethical conduct of research.

Researcher-Participant Interaction

The nature of the researcher-participant interaction over time introduces the possibility that the research experience becomes a therapeutic one. It is a case of research becoming practice. There are basic differences between the intent of the nurse when conducting research or engaging in practice (Smith and Liehr, 2003). In practice, the nurse has caring-healing intentions. In research, the nurse intends to "get the picture" from the perspective of the participant. "Getting the picture" may be a therapeutic experience for the participant. Sometimes, talking to a caring listener about things that matter energizes healing, even though it was not intended. From an ethical perspective, the qualitative researcher is promising only to listen and to encourage the other's story. If this experience is therapeutic for the participant, it becomes an unplanned benefit of the research.

Researcher as Instrument

The responsibility to remain true to the data requires that the researcher acknowledge any personal bias, interpreting findings in a way that accurately reflects the participant's reality. This is a serious ethical obligation. To accomplish this, the researcher may return to the subjects at critical interpretive points and ask for clarification or validation.

Credibility, Auditability, and Fittingness

Quantitative studies are concerned with reliability and validity of instruments, as well as internal and external validity criteria, as measures of scientific rigor (see the Critical Thinking Decision Path), but these are not appropriate for qualitative work. The rigor of qualitative methodology is judged by unique criteria appropriate to the research approach. Credibility, auditability, and fittingness were scientific criteria proposed for qualitative research studies by Guba and Lincoln in 1981. Although these criteria were proposed two decades ago, they still capture the rigorous spirit of qualitative inquiry and persist as reasonable criteria for evaluation. The meanings of **credibility, auditability,** and **fittingness** are briefly explained in Table 7-2.

Triangulation . . . Or Is It Crystallization?

Triangulation has become a "buzzword" in qualitative research over the past several years. There is discussion of theoretical triangulation (Kushner and Morrow, 2003), conceptual triangulation (Dabbs et al., 2004), and method triangulation, which is generally described as the collection of different kinds of data about a single complex phenomenon to bring clarity to the phenomenon that cannot be achieved with only one method. Triangulation provides an opportunity to more fully address the complex nature of the human experience. When referring to methods, **triangulation** can be defined as the expansion of research methods in a single study or multiple studies to enhance diversity, enrich understanding, and accomplish specific goals. Richardson (2000) has suggested that the triangle be replaced by the crystal as a more appropriate metaphor for the multimethod approach. Although there is support for the use of multiple research methods, controversies still exist about the appropriateness of combining qualitative and quantitative research approaches and even about combining multiple qualitative methods in one study (Barbour, 1998). It will not take the serious reader of nursing research very long to figure out that approaches and methods are being combined to contribute to theory building, guide practice, and facilitate instrument development. Table 7-3 synthesizes three manuscripts reporting multimethod analyses. The table notes

TABLE **7-2 Criteria for Judging Scientific Rigor: Credibility, Auditability, Fittingness**

Criteria	Criteria Characteristics
Credibility	Truth of findings as judged by participants and others within the discipline. For instance, you may find the researcher returning to the participants to share interpretation of findings and query accuracy from the perspective of the persons living the experience.
Auditabililty	Accountability as judged by the adequacy of information leading the reader from the research question and raw data through various steps of analysis to the interpretation of findings. For instance, you should be able to follow the reasoning of the researcher step-by-step through explicit examples of data, interpretations, and syntheses.
Fittingness	Faithfulness to everyday reality of the participants, described in enough detail so that others in the discipline can evaluate importance for their own practice, research, and theory development. For instance, you will know enough about the human experience being reported that you can decide whether it "rings true" and is useful for guiding your practice.

the conceptual focus of the work, the study purposes, and whether the manuscript suggests implications for theory, practice, and instrument development.

From the perspective of crystallization, Swanson's work is most complete (see Table 7-3) because she has addressed implications for practice, instrument development, and theory building focused on the issue of caring for women who have had a miscarriage. Her research program has included an initial theory building phase (studies 1 and 2), an instrument development phase (studies 3, 4, and 5), and a phase of testing a practice intervention (study 6). Swanson (1999) used the phenomenological method for studies 1 and 2 and quantitative methods for each of her other studies. In no study (Table 7-3) does she use more than one method, but her use of multimethods during the course of research program development can be likened to examining different facets of one crystal—in this case, the experience of miscarriage. The crystallization process has contributed to theory building, nursing practice, and instrument development. Her practice contribution is highlighted by a case exemplar (Swanson, 1999), which synthesizes her years of work with women living through the life experience of miscarrying their baby. See Kristen Swanson Vignette on p. 128.

Both Hunter and Chandler (1999) and Liehr and colleagues (2000) reported pilot studies that include qualitative findings. Each study indicates plans for further investigation, based on the qualitative findings. Hunter and Chandler's study (1999) combined qualitative (phenomenological method, using focus groups, interview, and written stories) and quantitative (Wagnild and Young's resiliency scale) methods to address their twofold study purpose (see Table 7-3). Data from the quantitative methods provided a different perspective than the one emerging from the qualitative methods—like differing facets of a crystal. The authors synthesize these differing perspectives in a model, entitled "Continuum of resilience in adolescents." They pose questions for further study related to (1) the health-promoting potential of resilience and (2) the likelihood of capturing adolescent resilience with a single paper and pencil measure.

The study reported by Liehr and associates (2000) (see Table 7-3) has a narrow focus. The purpose of the study was focused on instrument development. Within a quantitative context of reliability and validity testing, these researchers used a qualitative method (content analysis of adolescents' remembered descriptions of a time they experienced feeling angry) to evaluate the content validity of the adolescent version of the Cook-Medley Hostility Scale. The researchers

TABLE 7-3 **Research Using Multimethod Approaches**

Author/Date	Conceptual Focus	Multimethod Approach	Study Purpose	Theory Building Implications	Practice Implications	Instrument Development Implications
KM Swanson, 1999	Miscarriage and caring	Six studies, each using one method	**Study 1:** Define common themes for women who had recently miscarried	Yes	Yes	
			Study 2: Describe the human experience of miscarriage and describe the meaning of caring	Yes	Yes	
			Study 3: Use descriptive data to create a survey instrument based on women's experience of miscarriage	Yes		Yes
			Study 4: Evaluate the relevance of the survey items to create miscarriage scale	Yes		Yes
			Study 5: Assess reliability and validity of the miscarriage scale	Yes		Yes
			Study 6: Test the effects of caring, measurement, and time on women's well-being in the first year after miscarriage	Yes	Yes	Yes
AJ Hunter and GE Chandler 1999	Adolescent resilience	One study using multimethods	Pilot study to explore the meaning of resilience for adolescents, and evaluate a resilience instrument	Yes	Yes	Yes
P Liehr et al., 2000	Adolescent hostility	One study using multimethods	Pilot study to test the reliability and validity of the adolescent version of the Cook-Medley Hostility scale with multiethnic sample			Yes

note that the findings from this pilot study have led to changes in the scale for use in ongoing research.

These three manuscripts (see Table 7-3) present a range of approaches for combining methods in research studies, but the combining-methods picture is broader and growing. Although certain kinds of questions may be answered effectively by combining qualitative and quantitative methods in a single study, this does not necessarily make the findings and related evidence stronger. In fact, if a researcher inappropriately uses mixed methods, a study could be weaker and less credible. As a research consumer, you need to determine what led the researcher to choose a triangulated approach and whether this was an appropriate choice. You are encouraged to follow the ongoing debate about combining methods as nurse researchers strive to determine which research combinations promise enhanced understanding of human complexity and substantial contribution to nursing science.

☀ EVIDENCE-BASED PRACTICE TIP

- Triangulation offers an opportunity for researchers to increase the strength and consistency of evidence provided by the use of both qualitative and quantitative research methods.
- The combination of stories with numbers (qualitative and quantitative research approaches) through use of triangulation may provide the most complete picture of the phenomenon being studied and therefore the best evidence for guiding practice.

Computer Management of Qualitative Data

At the completion of data collection, the qualitative researcher is faced with volumes of data requiring sorting, coding, and synthesizing. The researcher may use one of many computer programs available to assist with the task of data

management. Meadows and Dodendorf (1999) categorize computer programs into three types:

- Code and retrieve, which assist in organizing and grouping data
- Theory builders, which move to a different level of data organization by connecting themes and categories
- Conceptual network builders, which incorporate graphics with theory building capabilities

Unlike computer programs used with quantitative data, these programs do not actually analyze data. Data analysis and interpretation remain largely the task of the researcher. However, orderly organization and grouping of data make the job of analysis and interpretation much easier for the researcher.

Synthesizing Qualitative Evidence: Metasynthesis

It has become important to qualitative researchers to synthesize critical masses of qualitative findings. Qualitative **metasynthesis** is a type of systematic review applied to qualitative research. Unlike quantitative research, which uses statistical approaches to aggregate or average data using meta-analysis (see Chapter 11). **Metasynthesis** integrates qualitative research findings on a topic and is based on comparative analysis and interpretative synthesis of qualitative research findings that seeks to retain the essence and unique contribution of each study (Sandelowski and Barroso, 2003). Essentially, metasynthesis provides a way for researchers to build up a critical mass of qualitative research evidence that is relevant to clinical practice (Melnyk and Finout-Overholt, 2005). Sandelowski (2004) cautions that the use of qualitative metasynthesis is laudable and necessary but requires researchers who use metasynthesis methods to clearly understand qualitative methodologies as well as the nuances of the various qualitative methods. It will be interesting for research consumers to follow the progress of researchers who seek to develop criteria for appraising a set of qualitative studies and using those criteria to guide the incorporation of these studies into systematic literature reviews.

Although general criteria for critiquing qualitative research are proposed in the following Critiquing Criteria box, each qualitative method has unique characteristics that influence what the research consumer may expect in the published research report. The criteria for critiquing are formatted to evaluate the selection of the phenomenon, the structure of the study, data gathering, data analysis, and description of the findings. Each question of the criteria focuses on factors discussed throughout the chapter. Critiquing qualitative research is a useful activity for learning the nuances of this research approach. As a research consumer, you are encouraged to identify a qualitative study of interest and apply the criteria for critiquing. Keep in mind that qualitative methods are the best way to start to answer clinical and/or research questions that previously have not been addressed in research studies or which do not lend themselves to a quantitative approach. The answers provided by qualitative data reflect important evidence that may provide the first insights about a patient population or clinical phenomenon.

In summary, the term "qualitative research approach" is an overriding description of multiple methods with distinct origins and procedures. In spite of distinctions, each method shares a common nature that guides data collection from the perspective of the participants to create a story that synthesizes disparate pieces of data into a comprehensible whole that provides evidence and promises direction for building nursing knowledge.

CRITIQUING CRITERIA   *Qualitative Approaches*

Identifying the Phenomenon
1. Is the phenomenon focused on human experience within a natural setting?
2. Is the phenomenon relevant to nursing and/or health?

Structuring the Study

Research Question
3. Does the question specify a distinct process to be studied?
4. Does the question identify the context (participant group/place) of the process that will be studied?
5. Does the choice of a specific qualitative method fit with the research question?

Researcher's Perspective
6. Are the biases of the researcher reported?
7. Do the researchers provide a structure of ideas that reflect their beliefs?

Sample Selection
8. Is it clear that the selected sample is living the phenomenon of interest?

Data Gathering
9. Are data sources and methods for gathering data specified?
10. Is there evidence that participant consent is an integral part of the data gathering process?

Data Analysis
11. Can the dimensions of data analysis be identified and logically followed?
12. Does the researcher paint a clear picture of the participant's reality?
13. Is there evidence that the researcher's interpretation captured the participant's meaning?
14. Have other professionals confirmed the researcher's interpretation?

Describing the Findings
15. Are examples provided to guide the reader from the raw data to the researcher's synthesis?
16. Does the researcher link the findings to existing theory or literature, or is a new theory generated?

Critical Thinking Challenges

- Discuss how the qualitative researcher knows when "data saturation" has occurred. Offer explanations from your life experiences that are similar to the experience of data saturation.
- How would you answer your classmate in research class who insists that it is impossible for researchers to "bracket" their personal biases about the phenomenon they are going to study? Use examples from your own clinical experience in your response.
- You are asked to defend why qualitative studies do not include hypotheses. Include in your argument whether or not you think qualitative studies merit the same evidence recognition as true experimental studies.
- Do you think that it would be legitimate qualitative research to conduct an interview using an internet chat room? Justify your position and address ethical considerations.
- Of what value is the level of evidence provided by the findings of qualitative research studies?

KEY POINTS

- Qualitative research is the investigation of human experiences in naturalistic settings, pursuing meanings that inform theory, practice, instrument development, and further research.
- Qualitative research studies are guided by research questions.
- Data saturation occurs when the information being shared with the researcher becomes repetitive.
- Qualitative research methods include five basic elements: identifying the phenomenon, structuring the study, gathering the data, analyzing the data, and describing the findings.
- The phenomenological method is a process of learning and constructing the meaning of human experience through intensive dialogue with persons who are living the experience.
- The grounded theory method is an inductive approach that implements a systematic set of procedures to arrive at theory about basic social processes.
- The ethnographic method focuses on scientific descriptions of cultural groups.
- The case study method focuses on a selected phenomenon over a short or long time period to provide an in-depth description of its essential dimensions and processes.

- The historical research method is the systematic compilation of data and the critical presentation, evaluation, and interpretation of facts regarding people, events, and occurrences of the past.
- Community-based participatory research is a method that systematically accesses the voice of a community to plan context-appropriate action.
- Ethical issues in qualitative research involve issues related to the naturalistic setting, emergent nature of the design, researcher-participant interaction, and researcher as instrument.
- Credibility, auditability, and fittingness are criteria for judging the scientific rigor of a qualitative research study.
- Triangulation has shifted from a strategy for combining research methods to assess accuracy to expansion of research methods in a single study or multiple studies to enhance diversity, enrich understanding, and accomplish specific goals. A better term may be crystallization.
- Multimethod approaches to research are controversial but promising.
- Qualitative research data can be managed through the use of computers, but the researcher must interpret the data.

REFERENCES

Aamodt AA: Ethnography and epistemology: generating nursing knowledge. In Morse JM, editor: *Qualitative nursing research: a contemporary dialogue,* Newbury Park, Calif, 1991, Sage.

Agar MH: *Speaking of ethnography,* Beverly Hills, Calif, 1986, Sage.

Aita VA, McIlvain HE: An armchair adventure in case study research. In Crabtree B and Miller WL, editors: *Doing qualitative research,* ed 2, Thousand Oaks, Calif, 1999, Sage.

Barbour RS: Mixing qualitative methods: quality assurance or qualitative quagmire?, *Qual Health Res* 8(3): 352-361, 1998.

Boyle JS: Field research: a collaborative model for practice and research. In Morse JM, editor: *Qualitative nursing research: a contemporary dialogue,* Newbury Park, Calif, 1991, Sage.

Burton CR: Living with stroke: a phenomenological study, *J Adv Nurs* 32(2): 301-309, 2000.

Caelli K: The changing face of phenomenological research: traditional and American phenomenology in nursing, *Qual Health Res* 10(3): 366-377, 2000.

Calvin A: Haemodialysis patients and end of life decisions: a theory of personal preservation, *J Adv Nurs* 46(5): 558-566, 2004.

Charmaz K: Grounded theory: objectivist and constructivist methods. In Denzin NK, Lincoln YS, editors: *Handbook of qualitative research,* ed 2, Thousand Oaks, Calif, 2000, Sage.

Chiu L: Lived experience of spirituality in Taiwanese women with breast cancer, *West J Nurs Res* 22(1): 29-53, 2000.

Christy TE: The methodology of historical research: a brief introduction, *Image J Nurs Sch* 24(3): 189-192, 1975.

Christy TE: The need for historical research in nursing, *Image: J Nurs Scholarship* 4: 227-228, 1981.

Cohen MZ, Kahn D, and Steeves R: *Hermeneutic phenomenological research: A practical guide for nurse researchers,* Thousand Oaks, Calif, 2000, Sage.

Colaizzi P: Psychological research as a phenomenologist views it. In Valle RS, King M, editors: *Existential phenomenological alternatives for psychology,* New York, 1978, Oxford University Press.

Crabtree BF, Miller WL: *Doing qualitative research,* Newbury Park, Calif, 1992, Sage.

Creswell JW: *Qualitative inquiry and research design: choosing among five traditions,* Thousand Oaks, Calif, 1998, Sage.

Dabbs ADV, Hoffman LA, Swigart V, Happ MB, Iacono AT, and Dauber JH: Using conceptual triangulation to develop an integrated model of the symptom experience of acute rejection after lung transplantation, *Adv Nurs Sci* 27(2): 138-149, 2004.

Denzin NK: The art and politics of interpretation. In Denzin NK and Lincoln YS, editors: *Collecting and interpreting qualitative materials,* Thousand Oaks, Calif, 1998, Sage.

Denzin NK, Lincoln YS: *The landscape of qualitative research,* Thousand Oaks, Calif, 1998, Sage.

Denzin NK, Lincoln YS: Introduction: the discipline and practice of qualitative research. In Denzin NK, Lincoln YS, editors: *Handbook of qualitative research,* ed 2, Thousand Oaks, Calif, 2000, Sage.

Fawcett J, Watson J, Neuman B, Hinton P, and Fitzpatrick JJ: On nursing theories and evidence, *J Nurs Scholarship* 33(2): 115-119, 2001.

Fontana JS: A methodology for critical science in nursing, *Adv Nurs Sci* 27(2): 93-101, 2004.

Giorgi A, Fischer CL, and Murray EL, editors: *Duquesne studies in phenomenological psychology,* Pittsburgh, 1975, Duquesne University Press.

Glaser BG, Strauss AL: *The discovery of grounded theory: strategies for qualitative research,* Chicago, 1967, Aldine.

Guba E, Lincoln Y: *Effective evaluation,* San Francisco, 1981, Jossey-Bass.

Holkup PA, Tripp-Reimer T, Salois EM, and Weinert C: Community-based participatory research: An approach to intervention research with a Native American community, *Adv Nurs Sci* 27(3): 162-175, 2004.

Hunter AJ, Chandler GE: Adolescent resilience, *Image J Nurs Sch* 31(3): 243-247, 1999.

Keeling AW: Blurring the boundaries between medicine and nursing: coronary care nursing, circa the 1960s, *Nurs Hist Rev* 12: 139-164, 2004.

Kleinman A: Local worlds of suffering: an interpersonal focus for ethnographies of illness experience, *Qual Health Res* 2(2): 127-134, 1992.

Kushner KE, Morrow R: Grounded theory, feminist theory, critical theory: toward theoretical triangulation. *Adv Nurs Sci* 26(1): 30-43, 2003.

Liehr P, Marcus MT: Qualitative approaches to research. In LoBiondo-Wood G, Haber J: *Nursing research: methods, critical appraisal, and utilization,* ed 5, 2002, St Louis, Mosby.

Liehr P et al.: Psychometric testing of the adolescent version of the Cook-Medley Hostility Scale, *Iss Compr Pediatr Nurs* 23(2): 103-116, 2000.

Lusk B: Historical methodology for nursing research, *Image J Nurs Sch* 29(4): 355-359, 1997.

Marcus MT, Walker T, Swint JM, Smith BP, Brown C, Busen N, Edwards T, Liehr P, Taylor WC, and von Sternberg K: Community-based participatory research to prevent substance abuse and HIV/AIDS in African American adolescents, *J Interprofess Pract* 2004 (in press).

Mead M: *Coming of age in Samoa,* New York, 1949, New American Library, Mentor Books.

Meadows LM, Dodendorf DM: Data management and interpretation using computers to assist. In Crabtree B, Miller WL, editors: *Doing qualitative research,* ed 2, Thousand Oaks, Calif, 1999, Sage.

Melnyk BM, Fineout-Overholt E: *Evidence-based practice in nursing and healthcare,* Philadelphia, 2005, Lippincott Williams & Wilkins.

Morse JM: The contracted relationship: ensuring protection of anonymity and confidentiality, *Qual Health Res* 8(3): 301-303, 1998.

O'Brien B, Evans M, and White-McDonald E: Isolation from "being alive": coping with severe nausea and vomiting of pregnancy, *Nurs Res* 51(5): 302-308, 2002.

Orne RM et al.: Living on the edge: a phenomenological study of medically uninsured working Americans, *Res Nurs Health* 23(3): 204-212, 2000.

Parse RR, Coyne AB, and Smith MJ: *Nursing research: qualitative and quantitative methods,* Bowie Md, 1985, Brady.

Pasco ACY, Morse JM, and Olson JK: Cross-cultural relationships between nurses and Filipino Canadian patients, *J Nurs Scholarship* 36(3): 239-246, 2004.

Philips JM, Cohen MZ, and Tarzian AJ: African American women's experiences with breast cancer screening, *J Nurs Scholarship* 33(2): 135-140, 2001.

Richardson L: Writing: a method of inquiry. In Denzin NK, Lincoln YS, editors: *Handbook of qualitative research,* ed 2, Thousand Oaks, Calif, 2000, Sage.

Sandelowski M: Using qualitative research, *Qual Health Res* 14(10): 1366-1386, 2004.

Sandelowski M, Barroso J: Creating metasummaries of qualitative findings, *Nurs Res* 52: 226-233, 2003.

Schreiber R, Stern PN, and Wilson C: Being strong: How black West-Canadian women manage depression and its stigma, *J Nurs Scholarship* 32(1): 39-45, 2000.

Smith MJ, Liehr P: The theory of attentively embracing story. In Smith MJ, Liehr P, editors: *Middle range theory for nursing,* New York, 2003, Springer.

Spear HJ: A follow-up case study on teenage pregnancy: "Havin' a baby isn't a nightmare, but it's really hard, *Pediatr Nurs* 30(2): 120-125, 2004.

Spiegelberg H: *The phenomenological movement,* vols I and II, The Hague, 1976, Martinus Nijhoff.

Spradley JP: *The ethnographic interview,* New York, 1979, Holt, Rinehart, and Winston.

Stake RE: *The art of case study research,* Thousand Oaks, Calif, 1995, Sage.

Stake RE: Case studies. In Denzin NK, Lincoln YS, editors: *Handbook of qualitative research,* ed 2, Thousand Oaks, Calif, 2000, Sage.

Strauss AL: *Qualitative analysis for social scientists,* New York, 1987, Cambridge University Press.

Strauss A, Corbin J: *Basics of qualitative research: grounded theory procedures and techniques,* Newbury Park, Calif, 1990, Sage.

Strauss A, Corbin J: Grounded theory methodology. In Denzin NK, Lincoln YS, editors: *Handbook of qualitative research,* Thousand Oaks, Calif, 1994, Sage.

Strauss A, Corbin J, editors: *Grounded theory in practice,* Thousand Oaks, Calif, 1997, Sage.

Stringer ET: *Action research,* ed 2, Thousand Oaks, Calif, 1999, Sage.

Swanson KM: Research-based practice with women who have had miscarriages, *Image J Nurs Sch* 31(4): 339-345, 1999.

Tarzian AJ: Caring for dying patients who have air hunger, *J Nurs Scholarship* 32(2): 137-143, 2000.

Tedlock B: Ethnography and ethnographic representation. In Denzin NK, Lincoln YS, editors: *Handbook of qualitative research,* ed 2, Thousand Oaks, Calif, 2000, Sage.

van Kaam A: *Existential foundations in psychology,* New York, 1969, Doubleday.

van Manen M: *Researching lived experience: Human science for an action sensitive pedagogy,* Albany, NY, 1990, State University of New York.

Vidick AJ, Lyman SM: Qualitative methods: their history in sociology and anthropology. In Denzin NK, Lincoln YS, editors: *The landscape of qualitative research: theories and issues,* Thousand Oaks, Calif, 1998, Sage.

Waltz CF, Strickland O, and Lenz E: Measurement in nursing research, ed 3, Philadelphia, 1991, F.A. Davis.

FOR FURTHER STUDY

Go to your Companion CD for review activities for this chapter.

evolve Go to Evolve at http://evolve.elsevier.com/LoBiondo/ for WebLinks, Content Updates, and additional research articles, for practice in reviewing and critiquing.

8

HELEN J. STREUBERT SPEZIALE

Evaluating Qualitative Research

KEY TERMS

auditability
credibility
fittingness

saturation
theoretical sampling
transferability

trustworthiness

LEARNING OUTCOMES

After reading this chapter, the student should be able to do the following:
- Identify the influence of stylistic considerations on the presentation of a qualitative research report.
- Identify the criteria for critiquing a qualitative research report.
- Evaluate the strengths and weaknesses of a qualitative research report.
- Describe the applicability of the findings of a qualitative research report.
- Construct a critique of a qualitative research report.

STUDY RESOURCES

Go to your Companion CD for review activities for this chapter.

evolve Go to Evolve at http://evolve.elsevier.com/LoBiondo/ for Weblinks, Content Updates, and additional research articles for practice in reviewing and critiquing.

Nursing knowledge is accelerating at an unprecedented rate. The contributions nursing scientists are making to health care are evident in nursing, medical, health care, and business journals. Nurse researchers are partnering at an ever-increasing rate with other health professionals to develop, implement, and evaluate a variety of evidence-based interventions to improve client outcomes. The methods used to develop evidence-based practice include quantitative, qualitative, and mixed research approaches. In addition to the increase in number of research studies and publications is an increasingly successful number of funded research studies. The willingness of private and public entities to invest in nursing research attests to its quality and potential for affecting health care outcomes of individuals, families, groups, and communities. Although quantitative, qualitative, and mixed research methods are all important to the ongoing development of a sound evidence-based practice, this chapter will focus on qualitative research.

Qualitative and quantitative research methods come from strong traditions in the physical and social sciences. Both types of research are different in their purpose, approach, analysis, and conclusions. Therefore the use of each requires an understanding of the traditions upon which the methods are based. The historical development of the methods identified as qualitative or quantitative can be discovered in this and other texts. This chapter aims to demonstrate a set of criteria that can be used to determine the quality of a qualitative research report. To achieve this, a published research report, as well as critiquing criteria, will be presented. The criteria then will be used to demonstrate the process of critiquing a qualitative research report.

STYLISTIC CONSIDERATIONS

Qualitative research differs from quantitative research in some very fundamental ways. Qualitative researchers represent a basic level of inquiry that seeks to discover and understand concepts, phenomena, or cultures. Creswell (2003) states that, "qualitative research is exploratory and researchers use it to explore a topic when the variables and theory base are unknown" (pp. 74-75). In a qualitative study you should not expect to find hypotheses; theoretical frameworks; dependent and independent variables; large, random samples; complex statistical procedures; scaled instruments; or definitive conclusions about how to use the findings. Because the intent of the research is to describe or explain phenomena or cultures, the report is generally written in a way that allows the researcher to convey the full meaning and richness of the phenomena or cultures being studied. Narrative—including subjective—comments are necessary to convey the depth and richness of the phenomena under study.

The goal of a qualitative research report is to describe in as much detail as possible the "insider's" or emic view of the phenomenon being studied. The **emic view** is the view of the person experiencing the phenomenon that reflects his/her culture, values, beliefs, and experiences. What the qualitative researcher hopes to produce in the report is an understanding of what it is like to experience a particular phenomenon or be part of a specific culture. One of the most effective ways to help the reader understand the emic view is to use quotes reflecting the phenomenon as experienced. For this reason the qualitative research report has a more conversational tone than a quantitative report. In addition, data are frequently reported using concepts or phrases that are called themes (see Chapter 7). A theme is a label. Themes represent a way of describing large quantities of data in a condensed format. To clearly demonstrate the application of a theme and how it helps the reader understand the emic view, the following is offered from a report published by Fair (2003). Fair's purpose is to offer "explanations of rheumatoid arthritis (RA) from young women's perceptions of the illness experience and providers understanding of the disease" (p. 339). The following quote is used by Fair to demonstrate the theme *"It changed me."*

> It is really difficult having RA. It totally changed my life. . . . Before, I was really physical. I rode my bike everywhere. . . . I was a performance artist. . . . And then, getting sick put the brakes on everything. . . . I didn't have the energy to go to rehearsal anymore. And I was cranky and wanted to be invisible. I did therapy for like years just so I could be visible again (p. 341).

The richness of the narrative provided in a qualitative research study cannot be shared in its entirety in a journal publication. Page limitations imposed by journals frequently limit research reports to 15 pages. Despite this limitation, it is the qualitative researcher's role to illustrate the richness of the data and to convey to the audience the relationship between the themes identified and the quotes shared. This will be essential in order to document the rigor of the research, which is called **trustworthiness** in a qualitative research study. It is important to point out that it is challenging to convey the depth and richness of the findings of a qualitative study in a published research report with stringent page limitations. A perusal of the nursing and health care literature will demonstrate a commitment by qualitative researchers and journal editors to publish qualitative research findings.

There are some journals that by virtue of their readership are committed to publication of more lengthy reports. *Qualitative Health Research* is an example of a journal that provides the opportunity for longer research reports. Guidelines for publication of research reports are generally listed in each nursing journal or are available from the journal editor. It is important to note that criteria for publication of research reports are not based on a specific type of research method (i.e., quantitative or qualitative). The primary goal of journal editors is to provide their readers with high-quality, informative, timely, and interesting articles. To meet this goal, regardless of the type of research report, editors prefer to publish manuscripts that have scientific merit, present new knowledge, and engage their readership. The challenge for the qualitative researcher is to meet these editorial requirements within the page limit imposed by the journal of interest.

Nursing journals do not generally offer their reviewers specific guidelines for evaluating qualitative and quantitative research reports. The editors make every attempt to see that reviewers are knowledgeable in the method and subject matter of the study. This determination is often made, however, based on the reviewer's self-identified area of interest. It is important to know that research reports are often evaluated based on the ideas or philosophic viewpoints held by the reviewer. The reviewer may have strong feelings about particular types of qualitative or quantitative research methods. Therefore it is important to clearly state the qualitative approach used and, if appropriate, its philosophical base. Fundamentally, principles for evaluating research are the same. Reviewers are concerned with the plausibility and trustworthiness of the researcher's account of the research and its potential and/or actual relevance to current or future theory and practice (Horsburgh, 2003, p. 308). Box 8-1 provides general guidelines for reviewing qualitative research. Box 8-2 provides guidelines for evaluating grounded theory. For information on

specific guidelines for evaluation of phenomenology, ethnography, grounded theory, and historical and action research, see Speziale and Carpenter (2003). If you are interested in additional information on the specifics of qualitative research design, please see Chapters 6 and 7.

APPLICATION OF QUALITATIVE RESEARCH FINDINGS IN PRACTICE

The purpose of qualitative research is to describe, understand, or explain phenomena or cultures. Phenomena are those things that are perceived by our senses. For example, pain or losing a loved one are considered phenomena. Unlike quantitative research, prediction and control of phenomena are not the aim of the qualitative inquiry. Therefore qualitative results are applied differently than more traditional quantitative research findings. Barbour and Barbour (2003) state "rather than seeking to import and impose templates and methods devised for another purpose, qualitative researchers and reviewers should look . . . for inspiration from their own modes of working and collaborating and seek to incorporate these, forging new and creative solutions to perennial problems, rather than hoping that these will simply disappear in the face of application of pre-existing sets of procedures" (p. 185). Further, Barbour and Barbour (2003) and Schepner-Hughes (1992) offer that qualitative research can provide the opportunity to give voice to those who have been disenfranchised and have no history. Therefore the application of qualitative findings will necessarily be context-bound (Russell and Gregory, 2003). This means that if a qualitative researcher studies the pain experience of individuals undergoing bone marrow biopsy, the application of these findings is confined to individuals who are similar to those in the study.

 EVIDENCE-BASED PRACTICE TIP

Nurses using qualitative research findings should ask whether the evidence provided in the study enhances their understanding of particular patient care situations.

BOX 8-1   CRITIQUING CRITERIA: QUALITATIVE RESEARCH

STATEMENT OF THE PHENOMENON OF INTEREST

1. What is the phenomenon of interest and is it clearly stated for the reader?
2. What is the justification for using a qualitative method?
3. What are the philosophic underpinnings of the research method?

PURPOSE

1. What is the purpose of the study?
2. What is the projected significance of the work to nursing?

METHOD

1. Is the method used to collect data compatible with the purpose of the research?
2. Is the method adequate to address the phenomenon of interest?
3. If a particular approach is used to guide the inquiry, does the researcher complete the study according to the processes described?

SAMPLING

1. What type of sampling is used? Is it appropriate given the particular method?
2. Are the informants who were chosen appropriate to inform the research?

DATA COLLECTION

1. Is data collection focused on human experience?
2. Does the researcher describe data-collection strategies (i.e., interview, observation, field notes)?
3. Is protection of human participants addressed?
4. Is saturation of the data described?
5. What are the procedures for collecting data?

DATA ANALYSIS

1. What strategies are used to analyze data?
2. Has the researcher remained true to the data?
3. Does the reader follow the steps described for data analysis?
4. Does the researcher address the credibility, auditability, and fittingness of the data?

Credibility

a. Do the participants recognize the experience as their own?
b. Has adequate time been allowed to fully understand the phenomenon?

Auditability

a. Can the reader follow the researcher's thinking?
b. Does the researcher document the research process?

Fittingness

a. Are the findings applicable outside of the study situation?
b. Are the results meaningful to individuals not involved in the research?
c. Is the strategy used for analysis compatible with the purpose of the study?

FINDINGS

1. Are the findings presented within a context?
2. Is the reader able to apprehend the essence of the experience from the report of the findings?
3. Are the researcher's conceptualizations true to the data?
4. Does the researcher place the report in the context of what is already known about the phenomenon? Was the existing literature on the topic related to the findings?

CONCLUSIONS, IMPLICATIONS, AND RECOMMENDATIONS

1. Do the conclusions, implications, and recommendations give the reader a context in which to use the findings?
2. How do the conclusions reflect the study findings?
3. What are the recommendations for future study? Do they reflect the findings?
4. How has the researcher made explicit the significance of the study to nursing theory, research, or practice?

Qualitative research findings can be used to create solutions to practical problems (Glesne, 1999). Qualitative research also has the ability to contribute to the evidenced-based practice literature (Gibson and Martin, 2003; Cesario, Morin, and Santa-Donato, 2002). For instance, in the development of a grounded theory representing some phenomenon, the theory may provide a profound description of the process a particular group may go through to arrive at a certain point. In the article on the following pages, Keating-Lefler and Wilson (2004) demonstrate this when they describe the process that single, unpartnered, Medicaid-eligible first-time mothers go through as they move through the first 3 postpartum months. The findings of this study can provide important insights that inform the practice of nurses working with similar patient populations. It is important to view research findings within context, whether quantitative or qualitative. For instance, a quantitative study of pain in children with chronic disease (see Appendix B) should not be viewed as having direct application to adults suffering with this same disease. The findings must be used within context, or additional studies must be conducted to validate the applicability of the findings across situations and patient populations. This is true in qualitative research, as well. Nurses who wish to use the findings of qualitative research in their practice must validate them, through thorough examination and synthesis of the literature on the topic, through their own observations, or through interaction with groups similar to the study participants, to determine whether the findings accurately reflect the experience.

Morse, Penrod, and Hupcey (2000) offer "qualitative outcome analysis (QOA) [as a] systematic means to confirm the applicability of clinical strategies developed from a single qualitative project, to extend the repertoire of clinical interventions, and evaluate clinical outcomes" (p. 125). Using this process, the researcher employs the findings of a qualitative study to develop interventions and then to test those selected. Qualitative outcome analysis allows the researcher/clinician to implement interventions based on the client's expressed experience of a particular clinical phenomenon. Morse, Penrod, and Hupcey state, "QOA may be considered a form of participant action research" (p. 129). Application of knowledge discovered during qualitative data collection adds to our understanding of clinical phenomena by using interventions that are based on the client's experience. QOA is considered a form of evaluation research and as such has the potential to add to

evidence-based practice literature either at Level V or at Level VI depending on how the study is designed.

Another use of qualitative research findings is to initiate examination of important concepts in nursing practice, education, or administration. Caring as a concept has been studied using qualitative approaches. Caring is considered a significant concept in nursing. Therefore studying its multiple dimensions is important. Wilkin and Slevin (2004) explored the meaning of caring for intensive care nurses. The researchers posit that although caring has been studied extensively, little research has been conducted in the highly technological area of critical care. The study adds to the existing body of knowledge on caring and extends the current state of the science by examining a specific area of nursing practice and the experience of caring by critical care nurses. This type of study is at Level V or VI, which includes either systematic reviews or single studies that are descriptive or qualitative in their design (see Chapter 2).

EVIDENCE-BASED PRACTICE TIP

Qualitative research studies can be used to guide practice when they are applied within context. The question the nurse should ask is the following: "Does this study provide me with a direction for caring for a particular patient group?"

Finally, qualitative research can be used to discover evidence about phenomena of interest that can lead to instrument development. When qualitative methods are used to direct the development of structured measurement instruments, it is usually part of a larger empirical research project . Instrument development from qualitative research studies is useful to practicing nurses because it is grounded in the reality of human experience with a particular phenomenon and informs item development.

CRITIQUE *of a Qualitative Research Study*

The study *The Experience of Becoming a Mother for Single, Unpartnered, Medicaid-Eligible, First-Time Mothers* by Rebecca Keating-Lefler and Margaret E. Wilson, published in *Journal of Nursing Scholarship* (2004), is critiqued. The article is presented in its entirety and followed by the critique on p. 184.

THE EXPERIENCE OF BECOMING A MOTHER FOR SINGLE, UNPARTNERED, MEDICAID-ELIGIBLE, FIRST-TIME MOTHERS

Rebecca Keating-Lefler, Margaret E. Wilson

Purpose: To understand the experience of becoming a mother for single, unpartnered, Medicaid-eligible, first-time mothers in the United States and to discover the basic social psychological problem and process experienced by the mothers during the first 3 months postpartum.

Design: Grounded theory.

Methods: Semi-structured interviews were conducted and audiotaped with 20 single, unpartnered, Medicaid-eligible, first-time mothers at 1, 2, and 3 months postpartum. Data analysis was completed using the constant comparative method of data analysis.

Findings: The women used the basic social psychological process of "reformulating life" to manage their "grieving of multiple losses." "Reformulating life" included "believing in future possibilities," "submerging self in the mother role," "daring to dream life's options," "development of a new self-definition, identity, and future," and "risking a new life course: attempting new roles." Social support and personal resilience facilitated the basic social psychological process of "reformulating life."

Conclusions: Single, unpartnered, Medicaid-eligible, first-time mothers in this study managed their "grieving multiple losses" by "reformulating life." The uniqueness of this substantive theory is the relationship between pregnancy, loss, and grief.

Journal of Nursing Scholarship, 2004; 36:1, 23-29.
© 2004 Sigma Theta Tall International

[*Key words: Medicaid-eligible mothers, loss, grief*]

Significant sociocultural, socioeconomic, and sociopolitical changes have taken place during the last 2 decades in the United States (US) that greatly affect single, Medicaid-eligible mothers. The proportion of births to unmarried women in 2002 was 34.4% (Martin et al., 2003), which is an 86% increase since the early 1980s. Social scholars have predicted that if the rate of births to single women continues at the same pace it will increase to one-half of all births in 2005 (Ludtke, 1997). Single, poor women and their children are the largest group of Americans at the lowest portion of the economic structure (Sidel, 1996).

Recent changes in welfare policy have further decreased the number of people entitled to benefits, including Medicaid, since the 1996 reform act. One in 10 families now are below the poverty line, and the great divide between the wealthy and the poor is increasing (Quindlen, 2002). Single, poor women and their families end to be marginalized in the social, political, and health care systems (Hildebrandt, 2002), and their interests are inadequately represented (Banerjee, 2002).

Understanding the needs and concerns of low-income, single mothers and the effect poverty has on their health and well-being and that of their children is of vital importance to their futures. It is the first step toward developing interventions and policies to address their physical, emotional, and environmental health disparities. "The personal experience of every woman has worth and should be understood in all its complexity and richness. Understanding women's experience in the social and political context of their lives in necessary" (Thompson, 1992). The purposes of this grounded theory study were (a) to understand the experience of becoming a mother for single, unpartnered, Medicaid-eligible, first-time mothers during the first 3 months postpartum; and (b) to discover the basic social psychological problems

Rebecca Keating-Lefler, PhD. Gamma Pi, Assistant Professor, **Margaret E. Wilson,** PhD, *Gamma Pi*, Associate Professor, both at the University of Nebraska Medical Center, Omaha, NE Correspondence to Dr. Keating-Lefler, 8518 North 48 Circle, Omaha, NE 68152. E-mail: rkeating@unmc.edu
Accepted for publication July 30, 2003.

these women encountered being a mother, and the processes they use to manage the problems. This understanding should lead to a substantive theory about their experience.

BACKGROUND

Many factors contribute to the fall into poverty for some single mothers. Many women are unable to maintain employment after childbirth. Women's earning capacity continues to be much less than that of men; many fathers do not pay child support; and changes in welfare regulations have resulted in diminished and limited public assistance for single mothers (Amato, 2000). Events of life such as divorce, death, illness, unemployment, unplanned pregnancy, and threatening and uncontrollable life events also can result in women's poverty (Ceballo & McLoyd, 2002).

Recent evidence links multiple adverse outcomes to single-mother status. Adverse outcomes may include a high incidence of depression, partner abuse, child abuse, substance abuse, low self-esteem, unemployment, financial distress, and high everyday stressors (Lutenbacher-Hall, 1998), Hildebrandt (2002) conducted interviews with 34 women who were enrolled in the new, work-based welfare program. Eighty-two percent of the women indicated that their health status suffered from "juggling" work and family responsibilities and from having insufficient finances. Ninety-two percent cited a lack of well-being after their forced work-based welfare and 50% indicated feelings of depression.

Single mothers, in the context of poverty and inadequate resources, juggle employment and the responsibility for maintaining their family's health and well-being (Hildebrandt, 2002). Their families often go without adequate food, shelter, health care services and other basic necessities of life (Lens, 2002). Populations whose health status continually suffers are those with the highest poverty rates (Avison, 1997). In the United States those people are single women and their children (Amato, 2000).

Brown and Moran (1997) interviewed 300 married mothers and 101 single mothers and found that single mothers were twice as likely to live in a state of financial hardship and to experience depressive symptoms. Davies, Avison, and McAlpine (1997) interviewed 518 single mothers and 502 married mothers and found that single mothers reported much higher lifetime rates of depression. Avison (1997) said that research on the mental health of single mothers has resulted in two important conclusions. First, single mothers do experience higher levels of psychological distress because of their exposure to high stress and physical and emotional and financial challenges. And, second, a direct association exists between single motherhood and poverty. Changes in society, attitudes toward single mothers, recent restrictions on welfare assistance, and the context in which each single poor mother lives affect her ability to function in the role of mother and to provide a healthy, nurturing environment for herself and her children.

METHODS

Grounded theory methodology was used to further the understanding of the experience of becoming a mother for single, unpartnered, Medicaid-eligible, first-time mothers and to generate a substantive theory to explain the basic social psychological problem and process encountered by the women during their first 3 months postpartum.

Setting and Sample

Permission from the institutional review board of a university in the U.S. midwest was obtained to conduct the study. Consultation with an expert on grounded theory methods was ongoing. Purposive sampling was used to identify eligible participants. Participants, recruited from a large obstetrical and gynecological clinic, were over 19 years of age and English speaking. All were Medicaid-eligible, first-time mothers, in their 9th month of pregnancy when they were invited to participate. Eighteen of the women were unpartnered. Further theoretical sampling through interviews with two single, first-time, Medicaid-eligible mothers with partners provided relevant data that were useful in the generation and saturation of categories and also in describing the challenges of unpartnered women's experiences.

Data Collection

Interviews were conducted in the homes of the participants at 1, 2, and 3 months postpartum and each interview lasted from 1 to 1½ hours. Interviews were audiotaped and transcribed verbatim with names and other identifying features removed from the transcripts. Saturation of the codes and categories was achieved with 20 participants. The beginning interview request used to prompt descriptions from the participants was: "Please tell me what the experience of becoming a mother has been like for you and how has it affected your life." More specific questions were asked to produce detailed responses.

Data Analysis

The constant comparative method of data analysis (Glaser, 1978; Polit & Tatano-Beck, 2004) was used in this grounded theory study. All research activities, beginning with data collection and continuing through the process of analysis, were done simultaneously. The primary purpose of the constant comparative method of data analysis was the discovery of the basic social psychological problem (core variable) and process, and the properties related to it (Glaser, 1978; Polit & Tatano-Beck, 2004).

The process of coding started with the development of level I codes. Exact words of the participants often become the level I codes (Glaser, 1978; Polit & Tatano-Beck, 2004). Level II codes, or categories, are the outcome of combining level I codes that mesh with one another (Glaser, 1978; Polit & Tatano-Beck, 2004). Level III codes provide the linkage or the relationships between the codes and categories and are the theoretical constructs identified in the experience and knowledge of the researcher.

Trustworthiness of Data

Credibility, the criterion against which the truth-value of a study is judged (Guba & Lincoln, 1981; Polit & Tatano-Beck, 2004), was enhanced by spending a minimum of 1 hour with each participant during the interviews. Spending adequate time with participants allowed understanding the context of their lives. Informant checking also assisted in establishing credibility by returning outcomes of the analysis to participants for confirmation of findings.

Auditability is a more fitting criterion than reliability in qualitative research (Guba & Lincoln, 1981; Polit & Tatano-Beck, 2004). Auditability began with careful attention to development of an audit trail at the beginning of the research process and included the recording and organization of all data including tapes, transcripts, field notes, memos, codes, categories, and other documentation. The generated data in the audit trail are essential to the ultimate establishment of trustworthiness. Confirmability was also established by the development of the audit trail.

Participants

The ages of the 20 participants ranged from 19 to 35, with an average age of 23. Fifteen of the participants were Caucasian (75%) and five were African American (25%). Three participants had not completed high school, and 17 had high school diplomas. Five had attended some college or professional school, and one had a college degree. Despite multiple attempts, locating all participants for all interview times was not possible. Nine participants completed only one interview at 1 month postpartum. Two women completed two interviews at 1 and 2 months postpartum. Nine women participated in all three interviews for a total of 40 completed interviews.

FINDINGS

The analysis and interpretation of participant's descriptions of their experience of becoming a mother resulted in the basic social psychological problem (core variable) titled "Grieving multiple losses." The described losses began to occur for participants at the moment they discovered they were pregnant. Each woman struggled with her decision to keep the child. The structure of the losses the participants experienced is described through the following categories.

Multiple Losses

The loss of relationships included the loss of their family of origin, which for some meant the loss of any contact with their parents and family because of complete rejection. "I knew I wasn't going to have the support of my family. My dad wouldn't even talk to me. He didn't even acknowledge that I existed."

Another traumatic relationship loss was the loss of the boyfriend. Some participants had complete loss of contact. Others occasionally had contact resulting in negative interactions. Most of the women described feelings of resentment and anger for their boyfriends' choices.

"There is no excuse for his irresponsibility. I used to think it was because his dad died or it was because he was kicked our of the house or something like that. But it's not because of any of that. It's because he chooses not to grow up and look outside of himself."

The dream for a shared future with the father of the baby was lost. Having a baby became a lonely, frightening, unpredictable, isolated journey. Some of the participants felt completely abandoned.

"When I was pregnant I used to lay here at night and wish that somebody would get excited about my tummy growing or would rub it. I did crave that and I'm sure other single people would like to have someone to talk to when they're feeling down. It was the most disheartening experience of my whole life."

Participants described the loss of relationships with friends. They no longer has shared interests with friends and were unable to make many new acquaintances because they were quite isolated. "Once you have a kid I think nobody thinks you want to go out with them and they never come to see you. They disappear."

One important consequence of the loss of relationships was the loss of support. Some of the mothers lost all support while others occasionally found support from various people. Fear of harmful and negative responses from the ex-boyfriend made some of the women choose not to ask for his support. The women also felt a lack of support in infant caregiving. "Everything in your life changes, from going to the grocery store to your personal hygiene, cleaning your house, everything. When you're by yourself, there's no help: Period. That pretty much sums it up. And she depends to tally, totally on you."

A powerful relationship loss described by the women was the loss of their relationship with themselves. The women described a loss of a sense of self, who they were, and who they would become. They struggled with that loss and the slow and difficult process of redefining and giving meaning to self, their experience, and their life. "This is just not what I had pictured for myself, where I had pictured myself being. It was so contrary to what I'd been working for the whole rest of my life." "I don't know if I know anymore what I want for myself, for the future. I used to have everything completely planned out. Now I don't know where I'm going or who I'll be."

The women described a loss of their dreams. The dream of a future with the father of the baby was a crushing loss. Other losses included their hopes and dreams for jobs, future professions, and financial security. Their desires to attend college were put on hold indefinitely with a pessimistic outlook for future possibilities of achieving an education. Dreams were fractured. The reconstruction of life dreams was hindered by new demands and challenges.

Each participant experienced the loss of her job when the baby was born. All of the mothers worried about when they would be able to work again and what type of job they would be able to find. Losing the ability to work for a period of time drained the financial resources. The uncertainty about future employment caused an overpowering fear and insecurity about many areas of life. The most basic human needs of safety and security were difficult to meet.

The women described the extreme difficulties they faced when attempting to discover their eligibility for welfare assistance and Medicaid, applying for the assistance, and maintaining benefits because of numerous "road blocks" encountered from the welfare system. This struggle compounded their loss of financial stability and loss of security and remained a challenging and unsettling problem throughout the 3 months.

Many of the women lost their homes and their means of transportation. The difficulty in locating participants over time might have been because of their inability to keep and maintain a secure home. Many of the women did not own a car, which forced them to rely on others for transportation. Those who did own a car verbalized the inability to drive because gas was unaffordable.

All of the women discussed their loss of physical and emotional well-being. They described feeling constant fatigue, headaches, nausea, loss of appetite, sadness, fear, anxiety, and depression.

Reformulating Life

The basic social psychological problem of "Grieving multiple losses" led participants to the basic social psychological process of "Reformulating life" (see Figure).

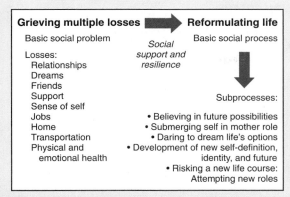

Figure. The substantive theory and major theoretical constructs.

Two factors that facilitated the process were social support and individual resilience. Support has been identified in the literature for decades as buffering and assisting people during the grief response (Cohen, Hettler, & Park, 1997). The perception of the presence of social support assisted participants to face challenges and it also stimulated resilience. The ability to experience stress and to deal with it effectively has been described as resilience behavior. Resilience allows personal growth in the face of difficult challenges (Holahan, Moos, & Bonin, 1997).

During the 3 months all participants were trying to rediscover and maintain a sense of equilibrium and balance in life that they had felt before the pregnancy and birth of the baby. All of the women were trying to give meaning to and redefine the new reality of life and existence in the world as an unmarried mother. Over the 3 months, all participants were incorporating their new life reality into their everyday existence. Each mother worked through the process of "reformulating life" at her own personal pace and achieved success at differing times during the 3-month period. The meaning of each of the losses to the women, the amount of available support, and the participant's resilience determined the temporality of the process.

The process of "reformulating life" included five subprocesses: (a) believing in future possibilities; (b) submerging self in the mother role; (c) daring to dream life's options; (d) the development of a new self-definition, identity, and future; and, (e) risking a new life course: attempting new roles.

The first subprocess was "believing in future possibilities." Numerous issues and concerns troubled the women as they wrestled with decisions about what would be best for their lives and the lives of their babies. Not one of the participants believed that she was in a place of security and comfort and could easily take on the responsibility of providing for another person. Each woman was at a personal life stage when she was still wondering who she would become. All were trying to give meaning to life and to find their places in the personal, educational, professional, social, and economic world. Now that they were becoming mothers they were trying to give meaning to that experience as well. Self-examination, courage, and belief in future possibilities were necessary to make the decision that they would keep the baby and become a mother. "I'm not seeing him (the boyfriend). And I won't be any time soon. I've got something else to take care of. I've got other things to worry about right now. Just her and myself and our future."

The second subprocess, "submerging self in the mother role," evolved after the birth. Each participant was able to recall her experiences since the discovery of the pregnancy, examine the multiple consequences of the pregnancy, give meaning to her situation, and begin reformulating life by focusing first on caring for her baby. "Well, considering everything, I think I am doing pretty well. It's hard some days. When I'm, exhausted and I need to get a break and I just want to go to sleep. Then it gets really hard. I didn't think it would be this hard."

By being submerged in the role of mother, each participant actively became involved in the care of the infant and in incorporating the role of mother into her self-definition. Viewing the self as a mother is a process of synthesis into one's self-definition that develops over time. Eventually feeling comfort with caregiving and understanding the needs and the personality of the infant lead to further development of self-esteem in the mother (Sawyer, 1999). The evolving belief in self allowed the participants to move into subprocess three.

The third subprocess, "daring to dream life's options," began after the women were able to see themselves as mother, function as mother, and approve of themselves as mother. That progress allowed the women to begin to consider their own personal life options and reevaluate themselves and their life courses. Believing in the possibility of future relationships and remembering previous goals stimulated hope. The cognitive processing of what life was like before the baby, what their dreams and desires were for their futures, and what possible means of achieving those goals were assisted the women in reworking their life options. "Now I'm figuring out the nursing classes for next semester. I'm pretty excited and it feels like I'm going in the right direction at least. I'm moving on."

The fourth subprocess, "the development of a new self-definition, identity, and future" was becoming evident when the women began believing in their abilities, themselves as women and mothers, and their future possibilities. These beliefs allowed the emergence of their new self-definition and identity. Realizing their own self-worth and thinking about themselves and their own personal needs were necessary steps in the further development of their new identity and their future possibilities. "The stuff I'm doing now is completely everything. I think the best job I'm doing is mothering my child." This process was slow because of the cumulative challenges that were the consequences of the multiple losses. All participants were still attending to this sub-process at 3 months postpartum and likely it was still evolving at 1 year.

The final subprocess, "risking a new life course and attempting new roles," began when each woman was ready to consider finding a new job, returning to school, and thinking about adding roles to her life. The achievement of a level of confidence in the ability to function competently in the maternal role and also to incorporate other roles successfully occurred at different rates for the participants. "The hardest part was keeping everything together at the very beginning. When I wasn't feeling well. Now that I'm well I feel like I'm back!"

Thinking through and verbalizing thoughts about how they could achieve other roles was a step toward further self-development. The participants' resilience and problem solving ability gave them hope for the future and that of the new baby, and allowed them to "risk a new life course."

DISCUSSION

The experience of becoming a mother for participants in this study involved multiple losses that were the consequence of unplanned pregnancy; birth; being a single, unpartnered, low-income mother; and having minimal social support. The losses affected the women's mental, physical, and environmental health. The losses challenged the women's ability to maintain their home, safety, and security. The lack of support and financial resources isolated the women and threatened their ability to function as mothers.

Loss has been incorporated into a few theories on motherhood but not in the life-encompassing ways the participants in this study described. Rogan, Schmied, Barclay, Everitt, and Wyllie (1997) conducted focus groups with 55 first-time married mothers and asked them what becoming a mother was like. They reported that women experienced a profound reconstruction of their self-identity. One identified category, titled "loss," indicared a loss of time the women had to spend with their spouse, the loss of their previous lifestyle, and the loss of their past self and life. These findings are similar to those of Rubin (1984), who described the loss of former self in her "maternal tasks." Participants in both studies were married women with adequate supports.

A link between loss and the onset of depression in mothers has been reported. Lewis and Nicolson (1998) reported the findings of two qualitative studies with women prenatally and during the postpartum period. Their purpose was to learn from the women what their transition to motherhood was like, what their understanding of prenatal and postpartum depression was, and if they believed they experienced either. They reported that the women experienced a loss of autonomy, identity, independence, power, and freedom. However, the respondents believed their reactions to the losses were pathologic because they were "supposed" to feel that being a mother was a happy event. Only in retrospect did they identify feeling depressed by the losses.

The authors said the majority of women who suffer from postpartum depression do not believe they are ill. The women believe they are exhausted, overworked, and irritable. Therefore, depression in mothers might be better explained as a response to the multiple tasks and the expectations of motherhood. Motherhood itself might be that which is depressing (Lewis & Nicolson, 1998). Thinking in these terms necessitates change in describing and understanding postpartum depression in general, based on the subjective experiences of mothers.

Jack (1991) interviewed women about their personal experiences of depression and found that the women's feelings of "loss of self," which they identified as depression, were caused by their need to subordinate their own needs and fulfill expectations as the caregivers for others. Cairney, Boyle, Offord, and Racine (2003) examined the effect of stress and social support on the relationship between being a single mother and depression. They found that single mothers were more likely to have suffered from depression over a 12-month period and to report higher levels of stress and lower levels of perceived social support than were partnered mothers. Multivariate analyses showed that stress and social support, together, accounted for almost 40% of the relationship between being a single mother and experiencing depression. Single mothers have a prevalence rate of depressive episodes three times higher than any other group of people. Women who are single, socially isolated, poor, and live in unsafe environments are more likely to experience depression during the 1st year postpartum than are women who have support systems and are more affluent (Targosz et al., 2003). Children from single-mother families are at increased risk for multiple adverse physical and emotional health outcomes. Single-mother status increases the child's risk for psychosocial morbidity, social difficulties, and academic problems. When low-income status and the presence of depression in the mother are added to the scenario, the ability of the women to provide optimal, supportive, and appropriate parenting to their children becomes more challenged (Lipman, Boyle, Dooley, & Offord, 2002).

Studies focused on women's health during and after pregnancy are increasing, yet few show single, low-income women's self-described health and illness experiences (Im & Meleis, 2001). What is clearly missing is a focus on gender issues that are embedded in the daily lives of women, which incorporate social, historical, and cultural contexts that affect all aspects of women's life experiences and perspectives.

The complexity of the issues of poverty and single motherhood present a unique challenge. Experiencing multiple losses during the process of becoming a mother puts women at risk for physical and emotional health problems, including the onset of depression. How and when nurses screen mothers during the postpartum period should be evaluated. Women might benefit from assessment of their subjective experiences of motherhood periodically throughout the 1st year postpartum. Ongoing evaluation might decrease the chances that depression goes undetected, and women and their children would be monitored for indicators of potential risk factors for poor outcomes. Discovering the individual, subjective experiences of women who identify themselves as feeling depressed is important, in relation to their individual parenting experience. Discovery of their subjective experience is necessary to identify their critical needs and to specify appropriate interventions.

Maternal child nurses should become knowledgeable about available resources for families and about welfare and Medicaid guidelines. Nurses' participation in the development of health policies to address the care that is available for single, low-income women and their children would benefit families. The mental and physical health of single mothers affects their children's health, growth, development, and home environment. Health policy to allow the extension of nurse visit follow up through the 1st year postpartum could have positive effects on parenting and on child and maternal health outcome. Olds, Henderson, Kitzman, and Cole (1995), in their extensive longitudinal studies with low-income mothers and their children, found that nurse home visitation programs during the first 2 years of the child's life had enduring effects on the child's health and well-being, on the safety of the home environment, and on the quality of the parental caregiving. Home visitation programs have received increased attention as a means of assisting low-income families and also in preventing child abuse and neglect (Olds, 2003).

Continual monitoring of maternal parenting outcomes, welfare and health care system utilization and improvement of social support for low-income families is important. Such interventions could facilitate the transition to parenthood and move single, low-income mothers and their families closer to a state of health and social well-being. Society could benefit from new approaches to the needs of single, low-income families. The largely economic response induced by recent welfare reform has not pulled single, low-income women out of poverty, nor has it improved their standard of living.

CONCLUSIONS

This grounded theory study was conducted to understand the personal experiences of becoming a mother in the context of these participants' lives. The uniqueness of this substantive theory is its inclusion of the relationship between pregnancy, motherhood, multiple losses, and grief as described by the participants. Pregnancy has been thought of as a developmental stage that results in great feelings of happiness and fulfillment. That description may be far from the reality of the experience for single, poor women without partners who comprise over 1/3 of American women having children today. Their experience of motherhood may be problematic, traumatic, and may include some very difficult, negative and challenging issues.

This basic social psychological problem and process shows the intensity of the vulnerability of single, low-income women and their children. Multiple issues must be addressed to improve the physical, emotional, social, and financial states of single, low-income mothers and their families. These single women and their families had minimal levels of social support, tended to live in isolation, and needed intervention and assistance.

One limitation of this study, and a concern with all research involving vulnerable populations, is that the retention of participants was a challenge. Encouraging participants to provide two or three contact persons for follow-up in case they cannot be located would be helpful in future studies.

In the next phase of this program of study, interviews will be conducted with single, low-income mothers, welfare employees, and healthcare providers who work with single mothers to determine multiple perspectives about the effectiveness of the health and social systems in assisting families during pregnancy and after birth. Findings will facilitate development of an intervention program to provide ongoing assessment, information, support, and guidance for single, low-income women and their families.

REFERENCES

Amato P (2000): Diversity within single-parent families. In D.H. Demo, K.R. Allen, and M.A. Fine (Eds.), *Handbook of family diversity: Family structure and family diversity* (pp. 149-172). New York: Oxford University Press.

Avison WR (1997): Single motherhood and mental health: Implications for primary prevention. *Canadian Medical Association Journal*, 156(5): 661-663.

Banerjee MM (2002): Voicing realities and recommending reform in Personal Responsibility and Work Opportunity Reconciliation Act. *Social Work*, 47(3): 315-328.

Brown GW, and Moran PM (1997): Single mothers, poverty and depression. *Psychological Medicine*, 27: 21-33.

Cairney J, Boyle M, Offord DR, and Racine Y (2003): Stress, social support and depression in single and married mothers. *Social Psychiatry and Psychiatric Epidemiology*, 38(8): 442-449.

Ceballo R, and McLoyd V (2002): Social support and parenting in poor dangerous neighborhoods. *Child Development*, 73(4): 1310-1321.

Cohen LH, Hettler TR, and Park CL (1997): *Social support, personality, and life stress adjustment.* In G.R. Pierce, B. Lahey, I.G. Sarason, and B.R. Sarason (Eds.), Sourcebook of social support and personality. New York: Plenium.

Davies L, Avison WR, and McAlpine DD (1997): Significant life experiences and depression among single and married mothers. *Journal of Marriage and the Family*, 59: 294-308.

Glaser B (1978): *Theoretical sensitivity.* Mill Valley, CA: Sociology Press.

Guba EG, and Lincoln Y, (1981): *Effective evaluation.* San Francisco: Jossey-Bass.

Hildebrandt E (2002): The health effects of work-based welfare. *Journal of Nursing Scholarship*, 34: 363-368.

Holahan CJ, Moos RH, and Bonin L (1997): Social support, coping, and psychological adjustment: A resources model. In GR Pierce, B. Lahey, L.G. Sarason, and BR Sarason (Eds.), Sourcebook of social support and personality. New York: Plenium.

Im EO, and Meleis AI (2001): An international Imperative for gender-sensitive theories in women's health. *Journal of Nursing Scholarship*, 33: 309-314.

Jack DC (1991): *Silencing the self.* Cambridge, MA: Harvard University Press.

Lens V (2002): Temporary assistance for needy families: What went wrong and what to do next. *Social Work*, 47(3): 279-292.

Lewis SE, and Nicolson P (1998): Talking about early motherhood: Recognizing loss and reconstructing depression. *Journal of Reproductive and Infant Psychology*, 16(2/3). 177-198.

Ludtke M (1997): *On our own. Unmarried motherhood in America*. New York: Random House.

Lutenbacher M, and Hall LA (1998): The effects of maternal psychosocial factors on parenting attitudes of low-income, single mothers with young children. *Nursing Research*, 47(1): 25-34.

Martin JA, Hamilton BE, Sutton PD, Ventura SJ, Menacker F, and Munson ML (2003): Births: Final data for 2002. U.S. Department of Health and Human Services National Vital Statistics Reports, 52(10): 1-5.

Nicholson P (2001): *Postnatal depression: Facing the paradox of loss, happiness and motherhood*. Philadelphia: Wilkins, Jack, & Sons.

Pearce D (2000): Rights and wrongs of welfare reform: A feminist approach. *Affilia*, 15: 133-152.

Polit DF, and Tatano-Beck C (2004): *Nursing research: Principles and methods*. Philadelphia: Lippincott, Williams & Wilkins.

Quindlen A (2002): Staring across a great divide. Newsweek, 140(1): 64.

Rogan F, Shnied V, Barclay L, Everitt L, and Wyllie A (1977). Becoming a mother: Developing a new theory of early motherhood, *Journal of Advanced Nursing*, 25, 877-885.

Rubin R (1984): *Maternal identity and the maternal experience*. New York: Springer.

Sawyer LM (1999): Engaged mothering: The transition to motherhood for a group of African American women. *Journal of Transcultural Nursing*, 10: 14-21.

Sidel R (1996): The enemy within: A commentary on the demonization of difference. American Orthopsychiatric Association, 66: 490-495.

Targosz S, Bebbington P, Lewis G, Brugha T, Jenldns R, Farrell M, et al. (2003): Lone mothers, social exclusion and depression. *Psychological Medicine*, 33(4): 715-722.

Thompson L (1992): Feminist methodology for family studies. *Journal of Marriage and the Family*, 54: 3-18.

INTRODUCTION TO THE CRITIQUE

The research report *The Experience of Becoming a Mother for Single, Unpartnered, Medicaid-Eligible, First-Time Mothers* (Keating-Lefler and Wilson, 2004) is critically examined for its rigor as a grounded theory study, its contribution to nursing, and its usefulness in practice. The criteria identified in Box 8-2 are used to guide the critique. These criteria are specific for grounded theory research.

Statement of the Phenomenon of Interest

Keating-Lefler and Wilson (2004) clearly state the phenomenon of interest. The researchers report that they are interested in understanding the experience of becoming a mother for single, unpartnered, Medicaid-eligible, first-time mothers during the first 3 months postpartum.

A clear case is made for the number of single, poor women having children and the way that they are marginalized by social, political, and health care systems. The researchers further demonstrate the importance of the research in the context of improving health care to this group and also giving voice to a population that is often anonymous.

Keating-Lefler and Wilson (2004) inform their readers that the reason for using grounded theory is because of their interest in discovering the basic social psychological problems encountered by the participants and how these problems are managed. According to Carpenter (2003), "basic social psychologic processes (BSPs) illustrate the social processes that emerge from data analysis" (p. 111) in grounded theory research. Therefore it is appropriate to use this approach. The work of Keating-Lefler and Wilson is also important because recently more nurse theorists and researchers are requesting the development of middle ranged theories as a more clinically applicable level of theory development (Alligood and Tomey, 2002; McKenna, 1997; Young, Taylor, and McLaughlin-Renpenning, 2001). Keating-Lefler and Wilson's findings have the potential to add to the literature in the area of mothering as well as the middle range theory base.

BOX 8-2 CRITIQUING CRITERIA: GROUNDED THEORY

STATEMENT OF THE PHENOMENON OF INTEREST

1. What is the phenomenon of interest and is it clearly stated for the reader?
2. What is the justification for using a grounded theory method?

PURPOSE

1. What is the explicit purpose for conducting the research?
2. What is the projected significance of the work to nursing?

METHOD

1. Is the method used to collect data compatible with the purpose of the research?
2. Is the method adequate to address the research topic?
3. What approach is used to guide the inquiry? Does the researcher complete the study according to the processes described?

SAMPLING

1. What type of sampling procedure is used? Is it appropriate for the method?
2. What major categories emerged?
3. What were some of the events, incidents, or actions that pointed to some of these major categories?
4. What were the categories that led to theoretical sampling?
5. After the theoretical sampling was done, how representative did the categories prove to be?

DATA GENERATION

1. What were the data-collection strategies? Were they appropriate for a grounded theory study?

2. How did theoretical formulations guide data collection?
3. How were human subjects protected?

DATA ANALYSIS

1. What strategies were used to analyze the data?
2. How does the researcher address the credibility, auditability, and fittingness of the data?
3. Does the researcher clearly describe how and why the core category was selected?

EMPIRICAL GROUNDING OF THE STUDY FINDINGS

1. Are concepts grounded in the data?
2. How are the concepts systematically related?
3. Are conceptual linkages described and are the categories well developed? Do they have conceptual density?
4. Are the theoretical findings significant? If yes, to what extent?
5. Was data collection comprehensive and analytical? Were interpretations conceptual and broad?
6. Is there sufficient variation to allow for applicability in a variety of contexts related to the phenomenon investigated?
7. How does the researcher relate the study findings to existing literature?

CONCLUSIONS, IMPLICATIONS, AND RECOMMENDATIONS

1. How do the conclusions, implications, and recommendations give readers a context in which to use the findings?
2. Do the conclusions reflect the study findings?
3. What are the recommendations for future research? Are they appropriate?
4. Is the significance of the study to nursing practice made explicit?

From Streubert HJ: Evaluating the qualitative research report. In LoBiondo-Wood G, Haber J, editors: *Nursing research: methods, critical appraisal, and utilization,* ed 4, pp 445-465, St Louis, 1998, Mosby; Strauss A, Corbin J: *Basics of qualitative research: grounded theory procedures and techniques,* Newbury Park, Calif, 1990, Sage. Adapted with permission.

Purpose

The researchers offer two purposes for their research: (1) "to understand the experience of becoming a mother for single, unpartnered, Medicaid-eligible, first-time mothers during their first three months postpartum; and (2) to discover the basic social psychological problems these women encountered being a mother, and the processes they used to manage the problem" (p. 23). These are appropriate purposes for grounded theory. The understanding of the experience will lead to the development of theory. Generally, it is not necessary to state that you are interested in understanding a phenomenon when it will lead to theory development. It is *only* through understanding of the experience that you will be capable of developing a substantive grounded theory of the phenomenon.

Although the significance of the study to nursing is not explicitly stated, there are many statements that imply the significance of the work. Some of these include the relationship between poverty and maternal-child health, the importance of understanding how losses experienced by these mothers affect their health care decisions, the value of being knowledgeable about available resources, and the need for understanding the advocacy role of nurses for this population.

METHOD

The method identified for this study is grounded theory. The authors offer that their intention is to develop a substantive theory to explain the social psychological problem and the processes used by the women during the first 3 months postpartum to overcome the problem. This is appropriate and yields the expected result. What is lacking from the declaration of method is mention of the tradition upon which the study is based. The references in the data analysis section are primarily to Glaser. The leading grounded theorists identified in most of the grounded theory literature are Glaser and also Strauss and Corbin. The work of Glaser (1978, 1992, 1998, 2001) has been described as inductive as opposed to the work of Strauss and Corbin (1990, 1998), which has been described as inductive-deductive (Maijala, Paavilainen, and Astedt-Kurki, 2003).

For the reader to know whether the research approach was executed fully and properly, it is necessary to return to the original work of Glaser (1978), because little is offered in the text of the manuscript regarding the specifics of the method. The authors also refer to Polit and Beck (2004) as the reference for their data analysis.

However, these authors are not grounded theorists. They are authors of a nursing research text. The references for methodology should be primary sources.

The authors state in the *Setting and Sample* section of the paper that consultation with an expert in grounded theory was ongoing. This is important because it informs the reader that the researchers recognize that they are not experts in the methodology so they have enlisted the help of someone who is. For the novice reader, a primary source on grounded theory is necessary to fully understand the research process.

Sampling

Keating-Lefler and Wilson report that purposive sampling was used. This is an appropriate sampling procedure for a grounded theory study (see Chapter 12). Purposive or purposeful sampling provides the qualitative researcher with the opportunity to recruit participants who are knowledgeable about the phenomenon under study. Participants in the study are recruited for the purpose of providing rich descriptions based on their personal experiences. In this case, Keating-Lefler and Wilson recruited single, Medicaid-eligible, unpartnered, first-time mothers. They state that saturation was achieved at the completion of 20 interviews. Saturation is a term used in qualitative research to signify the repeating nature of information and the end of data collection (see Chapters 6 and 12).

The researchers also state that theoretical sampling was used following the initial purposive sampling. **Theoretical sampling** is used primarily in grounded theory. Individuals are interviewed in an effort to further develop specific aspects of the emerging theory. This too is a traditional method of sampling for grounded theory. Keating-Lefler and Wilson do state that theoretical sampling "provided relevant data that were useful in the generation and saturation of categories and also in describing the challenges unpartnered women experience" (p. 24). The authors did not discuss how representative the categories proved to be after using this sampling procedure. For the reader to fully appreciate the use of theoretical sampling, it is important to explain what led to theoretical sampling and how it impacted theory development. The limited explanation of the use of theoretical sampling may be a result of the page limit imposed by the journal, which was described earlier.

Data Generation

Keating-Lefler and Wilson report that before data collection, permission to conduct the study was obtained from the institutional review board of a midwestern university. The interview process was initiated with a simple question: "Please tell me what the experience of becoming a mother has been like for you and how has it affected your life?" (Keating-Lefler and Wilson, 2004, p. 24). This question was followed up with more specific questions in order to obtain a full description of the participant's experiences. Interviews lasted between 1 and 1.5 hours. The interviews were audiotaped and transcribed. The questions and means of recording the interviews were appropriate.

Interviews were planned for the participants at 1-month, 2-month, and 3-month intervals. The researchers discovered that this was not possible. Of the 20 women, 9 completed all the interviews, 9 completed only the 1-month interview, and 2 completed interviews in months 1 and 2 but not month 3. Despite the dropout rate, the researchers report that saturation was achieved with 20 participants. One of the ways to assure credibility of the findings is to have a period of prolonged engagement with the subject matter. Given that the researchers met with the participants several times for a respectable length of time, it is logical to conclude that adequate engagement occurred without completion of the planned 60 interviews. Also, they report that saturation occurred at 20 participants, further attesting to the adequacy of contact.

The researchers do not report how their theoretical formulations guided ongoing data collection.

Data Analysis

Data generation and analysis are iterative processes in grounded theory. Data collection is followed by data analysis, which is followed by more data collection. The analysis leads the researcher to ask other questions of the data in order to build a strong theory. Keating-Lefler and Wilson report that they used the constant comparative method. True to this strategy, the researchers report that data collection and analysis were completed simultaneously. They further describe how theoretical coding was used to guide theory development. The researchers narrate the development of their ideas by describing the concepts that support their conceptual categories. This is further substantiated through the use of the participants' quotes.

Generally speaking, the measure of rigor in qualitative research is its **credibility, auditability, and fittingness/transferability.** In some sources, confirmability is offered as the fourth criterion for trustworthiness. These terms are defined in Chapter 7. In this study, the researchers report that credibility was obtained by the amount of time spent with the informants and by doing informant checks. Informant checks are also called member checks. Member checking is a process of returning to the informants and asking them whether the data reported represent their experience of the phenomenon under study.

Auditability (also called the audit trail) is the second check for rigor. The question to ask is as follows: Did the researcher present enough information for me to see how the raw data lead to the interpretation? Fittingness or transferability of the data is based on asking the following question: Is there enough detail here for me to evaluate the relevance and importance of these data for my own practice or for use in research or theory development? Keating-Lefler and Wilson share with readers how they developed their audit trail. It is still a criterion that is judged based on the reader's ability to follow the logical development of ideas.

Keating-Lefler and Wilson further state that confirmability was established by the development of the audit trail. Yonge and Stewin (1988) state that confirmability is a criterion of neutrality. If the study has credibility, auditability, and fittingness, it is has confirmability. Lincoln and Guba (1985) use the term confirmability in a manner similar to that of Keating-Lefler and Wilson; that is, they use the term confirmability as a process criterion documented through the audit trail.

Finally, when judging the quality of data analysis, the reader must ask the following: Has the researcher shared enough with me so that I can judge why the core variable or BSP was selected? The core category or BSP in this study is "grieving multiple losses." This variable accounts for the variation in patterns of behavior. In this article, the authors provide readers with a rich contextual narrative. In addition to sharing the core variable and the subprocesses, Keating-Lefler and Wilson use the concept of basic social psychological problems that lead to the basic social psychological process to help the reader understand the substantive theory. A novice reader will be challenged by the terminology used to describe the development of the grounded theory without the assistance of a knowledgeable qualitative researcher or a resource text on the method. Despite the use of unfamiliar terms to describe data analysis, the researchers do an excellent job of building their case for the substantive theory using informant comments and description of how data were synthesized.

Empirical Groundings of the Study: Findings

In this section of the critique, the reader must ask whether the concepts are grounded in the data. Does the researcher use the informant's words to guide the development of concepts? In each section of the research report, the authors offer some comment from the informant that helps the reader understand the choice of theoretical constructs. For example, in the paragraph that describes the third subprocess, daring to dream life's options, Keating-Lefler and Wilson use the following quote to illustrate the label selected: "Now I'm figuring out the nursing classes for next semester. I'm pretty excited and feel like I'm going in the right direction at least. I'm moving on" (p. 27).

The other critique questions ask the reader about the relationship between concepts. In this case, the reader can clearly gauge the relationship between concepts by reading the text of the article and viewing the figure that illustrates the theory. One limitation in the theory is the researcher's focus on the two theoretical conceptualizations: grieving multiple losses (basic social psychological problem) and reformulating life (basic social psychological process). There is reference to the fact that moving from grieving losses to reformulating life requires social support and resilience. These concepts are limitedly discussed in the article.

The conceptual terms used to describe the types of losses experienced are not necessarily unexpected: relationships, dreams, friends, support, sense of self, jobs, home, transportation, and physical and mental health. The subprocesses identified under reformulating life are more complex and include the following: believing in future possibilities; submerging self in the mother role; daring to dream life's options; development of new self-definition, identity, and future; and risking a new life course: attempting new roles. Given that the work presented is based on a phenomenon not previously studied, the theory is an initial attempt to describe a very complex process. The relationships between and among subprocess are clear. However, concepts will need to be further developed to fully realize the applicability of the theory in practice. This is not a flaw in the study but rather part of the developmental processes required of midrange theories (see Chapter 5). The study can still be viewed as a Level V or VI study. The figure used to illustrate the theory does not provide the reader with a clear understanding of the process.

It is difficult to judge the significance of the theory based on the presentation. The data offered relative to the developmental changes in the women in this study are critically important work. Further development and utilization of the theory will be needed for it to be judged adequate in describing the process of becoming a mother for this group of women with extremely complex life situations. The findings of this study are important to practice because as a Level V or VI research study, it informs practice in an area that was formally unknown or limitedly known.

 EVIDENCE-BASED PRACTICE TIP

Qualitative studies are helpful in answering research questions about a concept or phenomenon that is not well understood or adequately covered in the literature

Conclusions, Implications, and Recommendations

The implications for this study are included in the *Discussion* section of the report. They relate to understanding the experience of being a single, Medicaid-eligible, first-time mother. The researchers provide recommendations on how the findings can be helpful in caring for this population. As such, the study findings provide evidence to nurses on how what was discovered can be useful. This is very important given the necessity of providing evidence-based care.

The conclusions and recommendations are noted in the section labeled *Conclusions*. In this section, the researchers tell the reader why the newly developed theory is unique. Primarily they state that the relationships between pregnancy, motherhood, multiple losses, and grief have not been linked in the way they are in this study and, as such, provide understanding of this vulnerable patient population.

Discussion of how to use the theory is lacking. The researchers fulfill their first purpose of the study but leave the reader wanting to know more about how the theory will be useful. To fully realize the quality of the evidence presented, researchers should focus on offering clear direction to the reader on how the findings can be applied in practice. Also disappointing is the fact that the researchers do not describe how they plan to validate the theory. Rather, they offer their plans for future study, which are focused on interviewing a variety of individuals including single, low-income mothers, and health care providers who care for these mothers "to determine multiple perspectives about the effectiveness of the health and social systems in assisting families during pregnancy and after birth" (p. 28). Keating-Lefler and Wilson indicate that they will use the data from this and the planned study to develop interventions to support low-income women. When implemented, the findings of the proposed research can lead to Level II, III, or IV evidence. Although this is an important research direction, the reader is left without a clear understanding of why grounded theory was used if the plan was not to further refine and test the theory. Given the conclusions, the researchers would achieve the same outcome by using phenomenology as the method since the purpose of phenomenology is to understand human experience.

The findings of the study are valuable. The future direction for research based on the study is appropriate. However, the conclusions of the study leave the reader without a clear understanding of the purpose of developing a substantive theory if there is no plan to use the theory or further develop it.

 EVIDENCE-BASED PRACTICE TIP

Qualitative research may generate basic knowledge, hypotheses, and theories to be used in the design of other types of qualitative or quantitative studies. On the other hand, it is not necessarily a preliminary step to some other type of research. It is a complete and valuable end product in itself.

Critical Thinking Challenges

- Discuss the similarities and differences between the stylistic considerations of reporting a qualitative study as opposed to a quantitative study in a professional journal.
- Are critiques of qualitative studies by consumers of research, either in the role of student or practicing nurse, valid? Which type of qualitative study is the most difficult for consumers of research to critique? Discuss what assumptions you made to make this determination.
- Discuss how one would go about incorporating qualitative research in evidence-based practice? Give an example.

REFERENCES

Alligood MR, Tomey AM: *Nursing theory: utilization & application,* ed 2, St Louis, 2002, Mosby.

Barbour RS, Barbour M: Evaluating and synthesizing qualitative research: the need to develop a distinctive approach, *J Eval Clin Pract* 9(2): 179-186, 2003.

Carpenter DR: Grounded theory as method. In Speziale HJS, Carpenter DR: *Qualitative research in nursing: advancing the humanistic imperative,* ed 3, pp 107-122, Philadelphia, 2003, Lippincott.

Cesario S, Morin K, and Santa-Donato A: Evaluating the level of evidence of qualitative research, *J Obstet Gynecol Neonat Nurs* 31(6): 708-714, 2002.

Creswell JW: *Research design: qualitative, quantitative, and mixed methods approaches,* ed 2, Thousand Oaks, Calif, 2003, Sage.

Fair BS: Contrasts in patients' and providers' explanations of rheumatoid arthritis, *J Nurs Scholarship* 35(4): 339-344, 2003.

Gibson BE, Martin DK: Qualitative research and evidence-based physiotherapy practice, *Physiotherapy* 89(6): 350-358, 2003.

Glaser BG: *Theoretical sensitivity: advances in methodology of grounded theory,* Mill Valley, Calif, 1978, Sociology Press.

Glaser BG: *Basics of grounded theory analysis. Emergence vs. forcing,* Mill Valley, Calif, 1992, Sociology Press.

Glaser BG: *Doing grounded theory: issues and discussions,* ed 2, Mill Valley, Calif, 1998, Sociology Press.

Glaser BG: *The grounded theory perspective: conceptualizing contrasted with description,* Mill Valley, Calif, 2001, Sociology Press.

Glesne C: *Becoming qualitative researchers: an introduction,* ed 2, New York, 1999, Longman.

Horsburgh D: Evaluation of qualitative research, *J Clin Nurs* 12: 307-312, 2003.

Keating-Lefler R, Wilson ME: The experience of becoming a mother for single, unpartnered, Medicaid-eligible, first-time mothers, *J Nurs Scholarship* 36(1): 23-29, 2004.

Lincoln YS, Guba E: *Naturalistic inquiry,* Beverly Hills, Calif, 1985, Sage.

Maijala H, Paavilainen E, and Astedt-Kurki P: The use of grounded theory to study interaction, *Nurs Res* 11(2): 40-58, 2003.

McKenna H: *Nursing theories and models,* London, 1997, Routledge.

Morse JM, Penrod J, and Hupcey JE: Qualitative outcome analysis: evaluating nursing interventions for complex clinical phenomena, *J Nurs Scholarship* 32(2): 125-130, 2000.

Polit DF, Beck CT: *Nursing research: principles and methods,* ed. 7, Philadelphia, 2004, Williams & Wilkins.

Russell CK, Gregory DM: Evaluation of qualitative research studies, *Evidence-Based Nurs* 6(2): 36-40, 2003.

Schepner-Hughes N: *Death without weeping: the violence of everyday life in Brazil,* Berkeley, Calif, 1992, University of California Press.

Speziale HJS, Carpenter DR: *Qualitative research in nursing: advancing the humanistic imperative,* ed 3, Philadelphia, 2003, Lippincott.

Strauss A, Corbin J: *Basics of qualitative research. Grounded theory procedures and techniques,* Newbury Park, Calif, 1990, Sage.

Strauss A, Corbin J: *Basics of qualitative research. Techniques and procedures for developing grounded theory*, Thousand Oaks, Calif, 1998, Sage.

Streubert HJ: Evaluating the qualitative research report. In LoBiondo-Wood G, Haber J, editors: *Nursing research: methods, critical appraisal and utilization,* ed 4, pp 445-465, St Louis, 1998, Mosby.

Wilkin K, Slevin E: The meaning of caring to nurses: an investigation into the nature of caring work in an intensive care unit, *J Clin Nurs* 13(1): 50-59, 2004.

Yonge O, Stewin L: Reliability and validity: misnomers for qualitative research, *Can J Nurs* 20(2): 61-67, 1988.

Young A, Taylor SG, and McLaughlin-Renpenning K: *Connections: nursing research, theory and practice,* St Louis, 2001, Mosby.

FOR FURTHER STUDY

Go to your Companion CD for review activities for this chapter.

evolve Go to Evolve at http://evolve.elsevier.com/LoBiondo/ for WebLinks, Content Updates, and additional research articles, for practice in reviewing and critiquing.

PART III

PROCESSES RELATED TO QUANTITATIVE RESEARCH

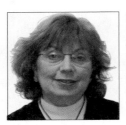

Lauren Aaronson, PhD, RN, FAAN
Professor
School of Nursing and Department
of Health Management in the
School of Nursing
University of Kansas
Kansas City, Kansas

In 1995 I was honored with the Distinguished Contribution to Research Award from the Midwest Nursing Research Society. This required a public lecture about my career to over 700 of my closest friends and colleagues. Knowing these talks can be very boring to those not into one's own area of research, I decided to try something different. Although I am known most for my expertise in quantitative methods, this challenge clearly called for a qualitative approach—and so I reviewed my professional history from first deciding to study nursing and through all my subsequent experiences. In the tradition of grounded theory, four themes emerged: 'Confronting Lies,' 'Blind Faith,' 'Self-Observation,' and 'A Little Bit of Luck.' I titled that talk, "Girls Don't Need Trigonometry and Other Lies." As I reflect on those themes today, I must acknowledge that they still hold true.

We all come to where we are via many different paths. Some are blessed to know exactly what they want to do from early on and set about making that happen. Others have a compelling experience that sets the course of their life's work. Still others wander through life responding to challenges encountered and changing paths as new options occur. There is no correct path; just whatever is right for each of us. I clearly fall into the third group.

When I was in my undergraduate nursing program and was asked what area of nursing I wanted to go into, I always responded: "Not sure, but not psych and not peds." Then I took my psychiatric nursing rotation and fell in love with the area ('Self-Observation'). It was

looking like a good thing that I was on that path where you could keep changing direction!

In the late '60's and early '70's I enjoyed an exciting career in all areas of psychiatric nursing: inpatient, outpatient, day care, and, with the advent of deinstitutionalization, consultation with the chronically mentally ill. It was a vibrant time in this clinical area in Los Angeles, and I still cherish my experiences working in community mental health ('A Little Bit of Luck'). Along the way I realized my job really called for a master's degree, and so I enrolled in the Community Mental Health Clinical Nurse Specialist program at UCLA.

While in that program I was introduced to research and chose to do a master's thesis rather than a research project. Once again, I fell in love—this time with research. For my master's thesis, "Sexism and Clinical Judgment" (my feminism was awakened by then), I created vignettes of situations in which I varied the sex, sex-role behavior, and psychopathology, and asked male and female psychiatric clinicians from nursing, medicine, social work, and psychology to rate how likely the described person was in need of professional help for an emotional problem. The entire research process opened a whole new world to me.

Although I was very passionate about my clinical work at that time, I knew then that I had to go on for my doctorate because RESEARCH was where I could combine all my loves: science, people, math (in the form of statistics), and, much to my surprise, teaching (something I dabbled in while in my master's program).

Along this new path I discovered all that sociology had to offer, especially the top-rated quantitative methods program at the University of Washington ('A Little Bit of Luck'). I was accepted into that program and was privileged to study under some of the greats in sociology and research methods, Hubert M. Blalock, Jr., Herbert Costner, Richard Emerson, and Karen Cook, to name just some. I also took advantage of a new doctoral opportunity program in health services research open to doctoral students from all different fields and was additionally fortunate to study with Stephen Shortell.

By this time I had developed my interest in studying health behavior, combining my clinical interest in human behavior and decision-making with my new knowledge of health services and medical sociology. One day, Professor Shortell handed me some papers and said: "You should apply for this." I was clueless about what it really was, but I could see it was a way to help support my dissertation research on health behavior decision-making among pregnant women. Using my 'Blind Faith' approach, I took his advice unquestioningly and prepared my first real federal research grant application. I was fortunate to get funded ('A Little Bit of Luck'), and thus launched my grant writing and research career.

I experienced a bit of déjà vu during my first year as an assistant professor at the University of Michigan. I was speaking with a former mentor from the School of Nursing at the University of Washington, Dr. Helen Nakagawa (now Kogan Budzynski), about my plans to submit a new grant proposal the following summer to the Division of Nursing (this was before the National Institute of Nursing Research was established). She simply said: "If you can you should submit it now for the February 1st deadline." Despite a very full plate with new teaching assignments, I once again employed my 'Blind Faith' approach and worked night and day to get that proposal out the door for follow-up work on the health outcomes of the participants in my dissertation research and their babies. And once again I was fortunate to get funded ('A Little Bit of Luck').

I continued my research on the health behaviors and health outcomes of pregnant women and extended my focus on healthy behaviors to a randomized control dietary intervention for hypercholesterolemia, which was privately funded. In 1989 I was challenged with yet another wonderful opportunity. I was offered the position of Associate Dean for Research at the University of Kansas School of Nursing, under the new dean at the time, Dr. Eleanor Sullivan, who was planning to launch a major effort to enhance and increase the research activities at that school. My

growing interest in helping others develop their research programs and in providing methodological expertise and support made this an exciting option ('Self-Observation'), and I enjoyed 11 years in that position, taking a nascent program into mainstream research activity with over $2 million in extramural funding annually.

Along the way, I led an effort by our faculty to get one of only two Exploratory Research Centers on Symptom Management funded in 1992 by the National Institute of Nursing Research (NINR). We focused on biobehavioral studies of fatigue management because fatigue was a symptom around which we could bring together several faculty members with different interests.

In 2000 I realized it was time for a change ('Self-Observation') and requested to step down from the associate dean role and assume responsibilities of a full-time faculty member. This afforded me the opportunity to work more closely with colleagues on specific research projects. Since then, I have been fortunate to work with Dr. Geri Neuberger on a large randomized clinical trial of an exercise intervention for persons with rheumatoid arthritis (funded by the NINR) that explored the impact of exercise on their symptoms of fatigue, pain, and depression, as well as their behavior adopting the exercise intervention. More recently I have been working with Dr. Karen Wambach on another NINR-funded randomized clinical trial of an intervention to promote the initiation and longer duration of breastfeeding by disadvantaged adolescent mothers, bringing me full circle back to my earlier work with a pregnant and early postpartum population. And, as I write this story, we are waiting to hear about the review and funding decision on a proposal submitted to the National Institutes of Health (NIH) with Dr. Katherine Grobe for a randomized controlled trial of an exercise intervention for manual wheelchair users.

In December 2003 I was again confronted with another exciting opportunity: Dr. Patricia Grady, director of the NINR, invited me to come to the NINR on an Interagency Personnel Act Agreement, where the NINR would contract for my time from my university and I get to work at the NIH in Bethesda, Maryland. I am functioning as a senior advisor to Dr. Grady with responsibilities for involving NINR and the extramural nursing science community in the new NIH efforts called "The NIH Roadmap for Research" and on another trans-NIH project, "The Public Trust Initiative," which Dr. Grady cochairs. You can read about the NIH Roadmap on the website: http://nihroadmap.nih.gov/; information about the Public Trust Initiative can be found on the website: http://publictrust.nih.gov/.

There are many paths to take with a nursing background and within the nursing profession. Research provides the scientific foundation for our practice and offers a wealth of opportunity for those who choose that path. Sometimes I marvel at all the rich experiences I have had and look forward to those experiences yet to come. The themes of my career have withstood the test of time. I encourage all to 'Confront Lies,' because with a little hard work you can do whatever you set out to do. Also, engage in 'Self-Observation' and go where your heart leads you; nursing and nursing research offer so many wonderful options. I wish you all 'A Little Bit of Luck,' and urge you to judiciously employ some 'Blind Faith' in the direction and advice of your trusted teachers and mentors. If so, you too will have a rewarding career with a sense of accomplishment and contribution.

GERI LOBIONDO-WOOD

Introduction to Quantitative Research

KEY TERMS

constancy
control
control group
dependent variable
experimental group
external validity
extraneous or mediating variable
history

homogeneity
independent variable
instrumentation
internal validity
intervening variable
intervention fidelity
maturation
measurement effects

mortality
pilot study
randomization
reactivity
selection
selection bias

LEARNING OUTCOMES

After reading this chapter, the student should be able to do the following:
- Define research design.
- Identify the purpose of research design.
- Define control as it affects research design.
- Compare and contrast the elements that affect control.
- Begin to evaluate what degree of control should be exercised in research design.
- Define internal validity.
- Identify the threats to internal validity.
- Define external validity.
- Identify the conditions that affect external validity.
- Identify the links between study design and evidence-based practice.
- Evaluate research design using critiquing questions.

STUDY RESOURCES

Go to your Companion CD for review activities for this chapter.

evolve Go to Evolve at http://evolve.elsevier.com/LoBiondo/ for Weblinks, Content Updates, and additional research articles for practice in reviewing and critiquing.

The word *design* implies the organization of elements into a masterful work of art. In the world of art and fashion, design conjures up images of processes and techniques that are used to express a total concept. When an individual creates, process and form are employed. The form, process, and degree of adherence to structure depend on the aims of the creator. The same can be said of the research process. The research process does not need to be a sterile procedure, but one where the researcher develops a masterful work within the limits of a research question and the related theoretical basis. The framework that the researcher creates is the design. When reading a study, the research consumer should be able to recognize that the research question, purpose, literature review, theoretical framework, and hypothesis all interrelate with, complement, and assist in the operationalization of the design (Figure 9-1). The degree to which there is a fit between these design elements strengthens the study and also the consumer's confidence in the evidence provided by the findings and their potential applicability to practice.

Nursing is concerned with a variety of structures that require varying degrees of process and form, such as the provision of quality, cost-effective patient care, responses of patients to disease, and factors that affect caregivers. When patient care is administered, the nursing process is used. Previous chapters stress the importance of theory and subject matter knowledge. How a researcher structures, implements, or designs a study affects the results of a research project.

For the consumer to understand the implications and the use of research, the central issues in the design of a research project should be understood. This chapter provides an overview of the meaning, purpose, and issues related to quantitative research design, and Chapters 10 and 11 present specific types of quantitative designs.

PURPOSE OF RESEARCH DESIGN

The purpose of the research design is to provide the plan for answering research questions. The design in quantitative research then becomes the vehicle for hypothesis testing or answering research questions. The design involves a plan, as well as structure and strategy. These three design concepts guide a researcher in writing the hypotheses or research questions, conducting the project, and analyzing and evaluating the data. The overall purpose of the research design is twofold: to aid in the solution of research questions and to maintain control. All research attempts to answer questions. The design coupled with the methods and analysis is the mechanism for finding solutions to research questions. *Control* is defined as the measures that the researcher uses to hold the conditions of the study uniform and avoid possible impingement of bias on the **dependent variable** or outcome.

A research example that demonstrates how the design can aid in the solution of a research question and maintain control is the study by Koniak-Griffin et al. (2003; see Appendix A). The aims of the study were to evaluate the 2-year postbirth infant health and maternal outcomes in Latina and African-American adolescents who partici-

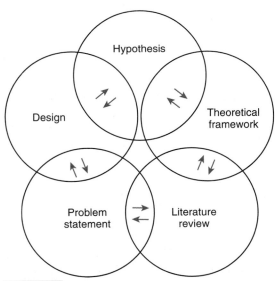

Figure 9-1. Interrelationships of design, research question, literature review, theoretical framework, and hypothesis.

pated in an early intervention program (EIP) of home visitation by public health nurses as compared to adolescents who received the traditional public health nursing care. The researchers randomly assigned subjects who fit the study's inclusion criteria to either the EIP or the traditional care group. The two interventions were clearly defined and developed for the study. By establishing the specific sample criteria and subject eligibility (inclusion criteria) and by clearly describing, designing, and distinguishing the experimental intervention from traditional care, the researchers were able to maintain control over the study's conditions. A variety of considerations, including the type of design chosen, affect the accomplishment of the study. These considerations include objectivity in the conceptualization of the research question, accuracy, feasibility, control of the experiment, internal validity, and external validity. There are statistical principles behind the many forms of control, but it is more important that the research consumer have a clear conceptual understanding.

The type of design used in a study also affects its application to practice. The next two chapters present a number of experimental, quasiexperimental, and nonexperimental designs. As you will recall from Chapter 2, the type of design used in a study is linked to the level of evidence and, in turn, how a study's findings contribute to evidence-based practice. As you critically appraise the design, you must also take into account other aspects of a study's design. These aspects are reviewed in this chapter. How they are applied depends on the type of design (see Chapters 10 and 11).

OBJECTIVITY IN THE RESEARCH QUESTION CONCEPTUALIZATION

Objectivity in the conceptualization of the research question is derived from a review of the literature and development of a theoretical framework (see Figure 9-1). Using the literature, the researcher assesses the depth and breadth of available knowledge on the question. The litera-

ture review and theoretical framework should demonstrate to the reader that the researcher reviewed the literature with a critical and objective eye (see Chapters 4 and 5), because this affects the type of design chosen. For example, a question about the relationship of the length of a breast-feeding teaching program may suggest either a correlational or an experimental design (see Chapters 10 and 11), whereas a question regarding the physical changes in a woman's body during pregnancy and the maternal perception of the unborn child may suggest a survey or correlation study (see Chapter 11). Therefore the literature review should reflect the following:

- When the question was studied
- What aspects of the question were studied
- Where it was investigated and with what populations
- By whom it was investigated
- The gaps or inconsistencies in the literature

 HELPFUL HINT

A review that incorporates the aspects presented here allows the consumer to judge the objectivity of the research question and therefore whether the design chosen matches the question.

ACCURACY

Accuracy in determining the appropriate design is also accomplished through the theoretical framework and review of the literature (see Chapters 4 and 5). Accuracy means that all aspects of a study systematically and logically follow from the research question. The beginning researcher is wise to answer a question involving a few variables that will not require the use of sophisticated designs. The simplicity of a research project does not render it useless or of a lesser value for practice. Although the project is simple, the researcher should not forego accuracy. The consumer should feel that the researcher chose a design that was consistent with the research question and offered the maximum amount of control. The issues of control are discussed later in this chapter. Also, many clinical questions have not yet been researched. Therefore a preliminary or pilot study would be a wise approach. The key is the accuracy, validity, and objectivity used by the researcher in attempting to answer the question. Accordingly, when reading research one should read various types of studies and assess how and if the criteria for each step of the research process were followed. Research consumers will find that many nursing journals publish not only sophisticated clinical research projects but also smaller clinical studies that can be applied to practice.

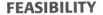 Carfoot, Williamson, and Dickson (2004) conducted an example of a preliminary **pilot study** that investigated a clinical problem. The researchers wanted to test the effect of a breast-feeding intervention that included skin-to-skin contact in healthy new mothers. This pilot study was done to test the feasibility of the intervention that would be used in a larger follow-up study, to assist with sample size estimation for the larger follow-up study, and to help the researchers decide what would be an adequate number of research assistants to employee in order to ensure success in a larger clinical study. The idea for the study grew from clinical observations and the literature suggesting that skin-to-skin contact during breast-feeding has little effect on length of breast-feeding initiation or duration. The researchers from their practice felt differently and also felt that past research was limited due to the type of designs used and the sample size. To remedy the issue the researchers decided first to conduct a pilot study to assess if their ideas and intervention were useful. The researchers learned a great deal from this pilot study. The pilot study helped to identify several areas of the intervention that needed to be amended, enabled the researchers to test an instrument that they wished to use in the follow-up study, and also helped to determine the sample size for future studies. Pilot studies such as this one are invaluable for maintaining accuracy and provide important information for future inquiry that is feasible and well grounded.

FEASIBILITY

When critiquing the research design one also needs to be aware of the pragmatic consideration of feasibility. Sometimes the reality of feasibility does not truly sink in until one does research. It is important to consider feasibility when reviewing a study, including availability of the subjects, timing of the research, time required for the subjects to participate, costs, and analysis of the data (Table 9-1). As indicated above, a major objective of the Carfoot, Williamson, and Dickson (2004) pilot study was to test the feasibility of implementing the skin-to-skin intervention. Before conducting a large experimental study, such as a randomized clinical trial, it is helpful to first conduct a pilot study with a small number of subjects to determine the feasibility of subject recruitment, the intervention, the data-collection protocol, the likelihood that subjects will complete the study, the reliability and validity of new measurement tools, and the costs of the study. These pragmatic considerations are not presented as a step in the research process as are the theoretical framework or methods, but they do affect every step of the process and, as such, should be considered when assessing a study. The student researcher may or may not have monies or accessible services. When critiquing a study, note the credentials of the author and whether the investigation was part of a student project or part of a fully funded grant project. If the project was a student project, the standards of critiquing are applied more liberally than for a doctorally prepared, experienced researcher or clinician. Finally, the pragmatic issues raised affect the scope and breadth of an investigation and the strength of evidence generated, and therefore its generalizability.

CONTROL

A researcher attempts to use a design to maximize the degree of control over the tested variables. **Control** involves holding the conditions of the study constant and establishing specific sam-

TABLE 9-1 **Pragmatic Considerations in Determining the Feasibility of a Research Question**

Factor	Pragmatic Consideration
Time	The research question must be one that can be studied within a realistic period of time. All researchers have deadlines for completion of a project. The scope of the research question must be circumscribed enough to provide ample time for the completion of the entire project. Research studies generally take longer to complete than anticipated.
Subject availability	The researcher must determine whether a sufficient number of eligible subjects will be available and willing to participate in the study. If one has a captive audience (e.g., students in a classroom), it may be relatively easy to enlist their cooperation. When a study involves the subjects' independent time and effort, they may be unwilling to participate when there is no apparent reward for doing so. Other potential subjects may have fears about harm or confidentiality and be suspicious of the research process in general. Subjects with unusual characteristics are often difficult to locate. People are generally fairly cooperative about participating, but a researcher should consider enlisting a larger subject pool than actually needed to prepare for subject unavailability. At times, when reading a research report the researcher may note how the inclusion criteria were liberalized or the number of subjects was altered, probably as a result of some unforeseen pragmatic consideration.
Facility and equipment availability	All research projects require some kind of equipment. The equipment may be questionnaires, telephones, stationery, stamps, technical equipment, or some other apparatus. Most research projects require the availability of some kind of facility. The facility may be a hospital site for data collection or a laboratory space or computer center for data analysis.
Money	Many research projects require some expenditure of money. Before embarking on a study the researcher probably itemized the expenses and projected the total cost of the project. This provides a clear picture of the budgetary needs for items like books, stationery, postage, printing, technical equipment, telephone and computer charges, and salaries. These expenses can range from about $200 for a small-scale student project to hundreds of thousands of dollars for a large-scale federally funded project.
Researcher experience	The selection of the research problem should be based on the nurse's experience and interest. It is much easier to develop a research study related to a topic that is either theoretically or experientially familiar. Selecting a research question that is of interest to the researcher is essential for maintaining enthusiasm when the project has its inevitable ups and downs.
Ethics	Research questions that place unethical demands on subjects may not be feasible for study. Researchers must take ethical considerations seriously. The consideration of ethics may affect the choice of the design and methodology.

pling criteria as described by Van Cleve, et al. (2004) (see Appendix B):

- The same instruments were used with all subjects and the instruments had established reliability and validity (Chapter 15).
- The data-collection methods were standardized for each subject.
- The research associates who assisted with data collection were trained and assessed for standardization of procedures (interrater reliability; see Chapter 15).
- Children were invited to participate if they were between the ages of 7 and 14 years, had been diagnosed with acute lymphocytic leukemia within the past month, and were English or Spanish speaking.
- Children were excluded if they did not have another chronic illness associated with pain,

a fulminating disease, a known cognitive disability, or inability to cope with the burden of research tasks as determined by the primary nurse.

The Koniak-Griffin et al. (2003) study also reflects constancy of data collection in the sections that describe both the early intervention program (EIP) group and the traditional public health nursing care (TPHNC) group. The description of the groups and how they differed from each other was clearly presented. An efficient design can maximize results, decrease errors, and control preexisting conditions that may affect outcomes. To accomplish these tasks, the research design and methods should demonstrate the researcher's efforts at control. These studies illustrate how the investigators planned the design to apply controls. Control is important in all designs. When various research designs are critiqued, the issue of control is always raised but with varying levels of flexibility. The issues discussed here will become clearer as you review the various types of designs discussed in later chapters (see Chapters 10 and 11). Control is accomplished by ruling out extraneous or mediating variables that compete with the independent variables as an explanation for a study's outcome. An **intervening, extraneous, or mediating variable** is one that interferes with the operations of the variables being studied (e.g., age and gender as in the Van Cleeve, et. al., 2004 study of chronically ill youth). Means of controlling extraneous variables include the following:

- Use of a homogeneous sample
- Use of consistent data-collection procedures
- Manipulation of the independent variable
- Randomization

The following example illustrates and defines these concepts:

An investigator might be interested in how a new stop-smoking program (independent variable) affects smoking behavior (dependent variable). The independent variable is assumed to affect the outcome or dependent variable. An investigator needs to be relatively sure that the

decrease in smoking is truly related to the stop-smoking program rather than to some other variable, such as motivation. The design of the research study alone does not inherently provide control. However, an appropriately designed study with the necessary controls can increase an investigator's ability to answer a research question. These examples illustrate how appropriate control strengthens a research study and offers you as a reader: (1) more confidence in the evidence provided by the findings, (2) a perspective about the degree to which the findings are generalizeable, and (3) an assessment of readiness for use in practice.

 EVIDENCE-BASED PRACTICE TIP

As you read studies it is important to assess if the study includes a tested intervention and whether the report contains a clear description of the intervention and how it was controlled. If the details are not clear, it should make you think that the intervention may have been administered differently among the subjects, therefore affecting the interpretation of the results.

Homogeneous Sampling

In the stop-smoking study, extraneous variables may affect the dependent variable. The characteristics of a study's subjects are common extraneous variables. Age, gender, length of time smoked, amount smoked, and even smoking rules may affect the outcome in the stop-smoking example. These variables may therefore affect the outcome, even though they are extraneous or outside of the study's design. As a control for these and other similar problems, the researcher's subjects should demonstrate **homogeneity** or similarity with respect to the extraneous variables relevant to the particular study (see Chapter 12). Extraneous variables are not fixed but must be reviewed and decided on, based on the study's purpose and theoretical base. By using a sample of homogeneous subjects, the researcher has used a straightforward step of control.

For example, in the study described earlier by Koniak-Griffin et al. (2003), the researchers ensured homogeneity of the sample based on age and demographics. This control step limits the generalizability or application of the outcomes to other populations when analyzing and discussing the outcomes (see Chapter 18). Results can then be generalized only to a similar population of individuals. You may say that this is limiting. This is not necessarily so because no treatment or program may be applicable to all populations, and the consumer of research findings must take the differences in populations into consideration.

 HELPFUL H I N T

When reviewing studies remember that it is better to have a "clean" study that can be used to make generalizations about a specific population than a "messy" one that can generalize little or nothing.

If the researcher feels that one of the extraneous variables is important, it may be included in the design. In the smoking example, if individuals are working in an area where smoking is not allowed and this is considered to be important, the researcher could build it into the design and set up a control for it. This can be done by comparing two different work areas: one where smoking is allowed and one where it is not. The important idea to keep in mind is that before the data are collected, the researcher should have identified, planned for, or controlled the important extraneous variables.

Constancy in Data Collection

Another basic, yet critical, component of control is constancy in data-collection procedures. **Constancy** refers to the notion that the data-collection procedures should reflect to the consumer a cookbook-like recipe of how the researcher controlled the conditions of the study. This means that environmental conditions, timing of data collection, data-collection instruments, and data-collection procedures used to gain the data are the same for each subject (see Chapters 12 and 14). Constancy in data collection is also referred to as **intervention fidelity** (Santacroce et al, 2004). An example of a well-controlled study was done by Defloor and DeSchuijmer (2000). The objective of this study was to assess the effect of the type of operating table mattress and surgical position on interface pressures in healthy adults. The investigators solicited healthy volunteers and tested five types of mattresses and four different positions in which patients are often placed during extensive surgery (i.e., >2 hours in length). To control conditions, the investigators randomized the order of mattresses and the positions for every subject, and each measurement was performed after 1 minute of immobilization. The system used to measure pressure was standardized prior to every measurement and with every manipulation of the measuring mat, and the interface measurements were done twice for each subject to test the reliability of the measurement. A review of this study shows that data were collected from each subject in the same manner and under the same conditions. This type of control aided the investigators' ability to draw conclusions, have discussions, and cite the need for further research in this area. For the consumer it demonstrates a clear, consistent, and specific means of data collection. When psychosocial interventions are implemented, researchers will often describe the training of interventionists and/or data collectors that took place to ensure constancy. They might also indicate that an intervention manual was used to script a standardized approach to intervention or data collection. For example, in a pilot study that preceded a full randomized clinical trial, Hoskins and colleagues (2001) tested the differential effectiveness of a phase-specific educational video versus telephone counseling in promoting physical, emotional, and social adjustment of women with breast cancer and their partners. Nurse interventionists were trained using a standardized intervention training manual; tape recordings were used for supervision to ensure adherence of all nurse interventionists to the video and telephone counseling protocols.

Manipulation of Independent Variable

A third means of control is manipulation of the **independent variable.** This refers to the administration of a program, treatment, or intervention to only one group within the study and not to the other subjects in the study. The first group is known as the **experimental group,** and the other group is known as the **control group.** In a control group the variables under study are held at a constant or comparison level. For example, suppose a researcher wants to study ways to improve maternal and infant outcomes postbirth for Latina and African-American adolescents and their infants, as in the Koniak-Griffin et al. (2003, Appendix A) study. The research team using past literature and research developed an experimental intervention that they believed would improve outcomes. The research team randomly assigned subjects to the *experimental group* (the group who received EIP) and to the *control group* (the group who received traditional public health nursing care). Experimental and quasiexperimental designs use manipulation. These designs are used to test whether a treatment or intervention impacts patient outcomes. Nonexperimental designs do not manipulate the independent variable. This does not decrease the usefulness of a nonexperimental design, but the use of a control group in an experimental or quasiexperimental design is related to the level of the research question, the theoretical framework. For example, Van Cleve et al. (2004, Appendix B) used a nonexperimental study to examine the pain experience, management strategies, and outcomes during the first year after diagnosis of leukemia. This study did not manipulate the pain experience (that would be unethical) but studied how children responded to both the treatment experience and pain over the first year of treatment.

 HELPFUL HINT

Be aware that the lack of manipulation of the independent variable does not mean a weaker study. The level of the question, the amount of theoretical work, and the research that has preceded the project all affect the researcher's choice of the design. If the question is amenable to a design that manipulates the independent variable, it increases the power of a researcher to draw conclusions; that is, if all of the considerations of control are equally addressed.

Randomization

Researchers may also choose other forms of control, such as randomization. **Randomization** is used when the required number of subjects from the population is obtained in such a manner that each subject in a population has an equal chance of being selected. Randomization eliminates bias, aids in the attainment of a representative sample, and can be used in various designs (see Chapters 10 and 12). The study by Ratner et al. (2004) wanted to examine the effectiveness of an intervention to help smokers who were elective surgery patients abstain from smoking, maintain abstinence postoperatively, and achieve long-term smoking cessation. After obtaining consent to participate in the study from the patients preoperatively, the researchers randomly assigned each patient to either routine care (control group) or the smoking cessation intervention (experimental group). Koniak-Griffin et al. (2003) also used randomization in their study (Appendix A).

Randomization can also be done with paper-and-pencil types of instruments. By randomly ordering items on the instruments, the investigator can assess if there is a difference in responses that can be related to the order of the items. This may be especially important in longitudinal studies where bias from giving the same instrument to the same subjects on a number of occasions can be a problem (see Chapter 11).

QUANTITATIVE CONTROL AND FLEXIBILITY

The same level of control cannot be exercised in all types of designs. At times, when a researcher wants to explore an area in which little or no literature on the concept exists, the researcher will probably use an exploratory design or a qualitative study (see Chapters 6 through 8). In this type of study the researcher is interested in describing or categorizing a phenomenon in a group of individuals. Beginning in 1986, Swanson began developing the theory of caring, first in her work with women who had experienced a miscarriage. Over the years Swanson has used both qualitative and different quantitative designs to develop the middle range theory of caring (see Kristen Swanson Research Vignette on p. 128). Swanson's beginning qualitative exploratory research with the subsequent testing of interventions with quantitative designs and the subsequent publications of these works is an excellent example of moving theory along a research continuum that ranged from a qualitative to a quantitative program of research to readiness for application of evidence to practice. In critiquing Swanson's various studies the issues of control would be viewed differently based on the design of each study.

If it is determined from a review of a study that the researcher intended to conduct a correlation study, or a study that looks at the relationship between or among the variables, then the issue of control takes on a different importance (see Chapter 11). Control must be exercised as strictly as possible. At this intermediate level of design, it should be clear to the reviewer that the researcher considered the extraneous variables that may affect the outcomes.

All aspects of control are strictly applied to studies that use an experimental design (see Chapter 10). The reviewer should be able to locate in the research report how the researcher met the following criteria (i.e., the conditions of the research were constant throughout the study, assignment of subjects was random, and experimental and control groups were used). The

Koniak-Griffin et al. (2003) study, which was previously discussed, is an example in which the aspects of control were addressed. Because of the control exercised in the study, the reviewer can see that all issues related to control were considered and the extraneous variables were addressed.

 EVIDENCE-BASED PRACTICE TIP

Remember that establishing evidence for practice is determined by assessing the validity of each step of the study, assessing if the evidence assists in planning patient care, and assessing if patients respond to the evidence-based care.

INTERNAL AND EXTERNAL VALIDITY

When reading research, one must feel that the results of a study are valid, based on precision, and faithful to what the researcher wanted to measure. For a study to form the basis of further research, practice, and theory development, it must be credible and dependable. There are two important criteria for evaluating the credibility and dependability of the results: internal validity and external validity. Threats to validity are listed in Box 9-1, and discussion follows.

Internal Validity

Internal validity asks whether the independent variable really made the difference or the change in the dependent variable. To establish internal validity the researcher rules out other factors or threats as rival explanations of the relationship between the variables. There are a number of threats to internal validity, and these are considered by researchers in planning a study and by consumers before implementing the results in practice (Campbell and Stanley, 1966). Research consumers should note that the threats to internal validity are most clearly applicable to experimental designs, but attention to factors that can

9-1 THREATS TO VALIDITY

INTERNAL VALIDITY
History
Maturation
Testing
Instrumentation
Mortality
Selection bias

EXTERNAL VALIDITY
Selection effects
Reactive effects
Measurement effects

compromise outcomes should be considered to some degree in all quantitative designs. If these threats are not considered, they could negate the results of the research. How these threats may affect specific designs are addressed in Chapters 10 and 11. Threats to internal validity include history, maturation, testing, instrumentation, mortality, and selection bias. Table 9-2 provides examples of the threats to internal validity.

History

In addition to the independent variable, another specific event that may have an effect on the dependent variable may occur either inside or outside the experimental setting; this is referred to as **history.** For example, in a study of the effects of a breast-feeding teaching program on the length of time of breast-feeding, an event such as government-sponsored advertisements on the importance of breast-feeding featured on television and in newspapers may be a threat of history.

Another example may be that of an investigator testing the effects of a testicular self-examination teaching program on the incidence of testicular self-examination. Concurrently, a famous movie star or news correspondent is diagnosed as having testicular cancer. The occurrence of this diagnosis in a public figure engenders a great deal of media and press attention. In the course of the media attention, medical experts are interviewed widely and the importance of testicular self-examination is supported. If the researcher finds that testicular self-examination behavior is improved, the researcher may not be able to conclude that the change in behavior is the result of the teaching program because it may be the result of the diagnosis given to the known figure and the resultant media coverage. An example of history from a published study can be found in the Bull, Hansen, and Gross (2000) study (see Table 9-2).

Maturation

Maturation refers to the developmental, biological, or psychological processes that operate within an individual as a function of time and are external to the events of the investigation. For example, suppose one wishes to evaluate the effect of a specific teaching method on baccalaureate students' achievements on a skills test. The investigator would record the students' abilities before and after the teaching method. Between the pretest and posttest, the students have grown older and wiser. The growth or change is unrelated to the investigation and may explain the differences between the two testing periods rather than the experimental treatment.

Maturation could also occur in a study focused on investigating the relationship between two methods of teaching about children's knowledge of self-care measures. Posttests of student learning must be conducted in a relatively short time period after the teaching sessions are completed. A relatively short interval allows the investigator to conclude that the results were the result of the design of the study and not maturation in a population of children who are learning new skills rapidly. It is important to remember that maturation is more than change due to an age-related developmental process but could be related to physical changes as well (see Table 9-2).

Testing

Taking the same test repeatedly could influence subjects' responses the next time a measure is

TABLE **9-2 Examples of Internal Validity Threats**

Threat	Example
History	Bull, Hansen, and Gross (2000) tested a teaching intervention in one hospital and compared outcomes to those of another hospital in which usual care was given. During the final months of data collection, the control hospital implemented a congestive heart failure critical pathway; as a result, data from the control hospital (cohort four) were not included in the analysis.
Maturation	In the Koniak-Griffin et al. study (2003) the lack of change in some of the variables and changes in other variables may have been due to the general maturation changes experienced by new mothers. In a study of wound healing, Wikblad and Anderson (1995) controlled for the possibility of maturation in a study of wound healing processes. Normal wound healing could have been a threat to the findings, but the researchers developed a careful data-collection plan to control for the threat of maturation.
Testing	A researcher measured acute pain with a repeated measure's design during a lengthy procedure. The researcher would have to consider the results in light of the possible bias of repeating the pain measurements over a short period of time. The measurements may have primed the patients' responses, and the practice of reporting pain repeatedly on the same instrument during a procedure may have influenced the results.
Instrumentation	Inoue and associates (2004) studied biochemical hypoglycemia in female nurses during shift work in Japan. The nurses determined their own blood glucose levels 12 times, at 4 points during 3 shifts. The researchers noted that the study depended on self-testing and self-reporting of blood glucose levels, and thus it was difficult to document the validity of the data. Even though the study was well developed and subjects were ensured confidentiality, the researchers still were concerned with this threat to the study's validity. Holditch-Davis et al (2003) examined the development of eight infant behaviors in preterm infants. Data collectors were trained and assessed for interrater reliability, thus avoiding the threat of instrumentation.
Mortality	Miles and associates (2003) studied the efficacy of an HIV self-care symptom intervention for emotional distress and perceptions of health among low-income African-American mothers with HIV. There were 3 interventions over a 6-month period. During the course of the study, of the 50 subjects in the control group, 37 were available at time 2 and 29 at time 3. Of the 59 subjects in the experimental group, 37 were available at time 2 and 30 at time 3. The investigators noted that they, like other researchers, had difficulty with attrition in studies of high-risk, low-income populations, such as drug-dependent Afrcian-American women and home care for individuals with HIV. The investigators noted the loss and the potential reasons for the loss. Though they lost subjects, they still had adequate numbers to analyze the data and arrive at useful conclusions.
Selection bias	Koniak-Griffin et al. (2003, Appendix A) controlled for selection bias by establishing selection criteria and by having an experimental and a control group. In the Davison et al. study (2003, Appendix D), while the investigators tried to control for bias the urologists only referred patients to the study who they thought would be interested in accessing information and willing to participate.

completed. For example, the effect of taking a pretest on the subject's posttest score is known as testing. The effect of taking a pretest may sensitize an individual and improve the score of the posttest. Individuals generally score higher when they take a test a second time, regardless of the treatment. The differences between posttest and pretest scores may not be a result of the independent variable but rather of the experience gained through the testing. For example, in a pilot study investigating the effect of a video and telephone counseling intervention for women with breast cancer and their partners mentioned earlier (Hoskins et al., 2001), pretests and posttests assessing the increase in health-relevant information were administered before and after the video intervention. It was difficult to determine conclusively if the significant increase in knowledge was due to the video or the effect of taking the test more than once. Table 9-2 provides another example.

Instrumentation

Instrumentation threats are changes in the measurement of the variables or observational techniques that may account for changes in the obtained measurement. For example, a researcher may wish to study various types of thermometers (e.g., tympanic, digital, electronic, chemical indicator, plastic strip, and mercury) to compare the accuracy of using the mercury thermometer to other temperature-taking methods. To prevent instrumentation threat, a researcher must check the calibration of the thermometers according to the manufacturer's specifications before and after data collection.

Another example that fits into this area is related to techniques of observation or data collection. If a researcher has several raters collecting observational data, all must be trained in a similar manner so that they collect data using a standardized approach, thereby ensuring treatment fidelity. Lack of treatment fidelity weakens the strength of the findings.

If data collectors are not similarly trained, or even if they are similarly trained but unable to conduct the study as planned, a lack of consistency may occur in their ratings, and therefore a threat to internal validity will occur. For an example, see Table 9-2. At times, even though the researcher takes steps to prevent problems of instrumentation, this threat may still occur. When a critiquer finds such a threat, it must be evaluated within the total context of the study.

Mortality

Mortality is the loss of study subjects from the first data-collection point (pretest) to the second data-collection point (posttest). If the subjects who remain in the study are not similar to those who dropped out, the results could be affected. The loss of subjects may be from the sample as a whole, or in a study that has both an experimental and a control group, there may be differential loss of subjects. Differential loss of subjects means that more of the subjects in one group dropped out than the other group. In a study of the ways a media campaign affects the incidence of breast-feeding, if most dropouts were non-breast-feeding women, the perception given could be that exposure to the media campaign increased the number of breast-feeding women, whereas it was the effect of experimental mortality that led to the observed results. See Table 9-2 for an example of a study in which mortality may have influenced the results.

Selection Bias

If the precautions are not used to gain a representative sample, **selection bias** could result from the way the subjects were chosen. Selection effects are a problem in studies in which the individuals themselves decide whether to participate in a study. Suppose an investigator wishes to assess if a new stop-smoking program contributes to smoking cessation. If the new program is offered to all, chances are only individuals who are more motivated to learn about how to stop smoking will take part in the program. Assessment of the effectiveness of the program is problematic, because the investigator cannot be sure if the new program encouraged smoking-cessation behaviors or if only highly motivated individuals joined the program. To avoid selection bias, the researcher could randomly assign subjects to either the new teaching method group or a control group that receives a different type of instruction. Table 9-2 provides another example of selection bias.

 HELPFUL H I N T

The list of internal validity threats is not exhaustive. More than one threat can be found in a study, depending on the type of study design. Finding a threat to internal validity in a study does not invalidate the results and is usually acknowledged by the investigator in the "Results" or "Discussion" section of the study.

 EVIDENCE-BASED PRACTICE TIP

Avoiding threats to internal validity when conducting clinical research can be quite difficult at times. Yet this reality does not render studies that have threats useless. Take them into consideration and weigh the total evidence of a study for not only its statistical meaningfulness but also its clinical meaningfulness.

External Validity

External validity deals with possible problems of generalizability of the investigation's findings to additional populations and to other environmental conditions. External validity questions under what conditions and with what types of subjects the same results can be expected to occur. The goal of the researcher is to select a design that maximizes both internal and external validity. This is not always possible; if this is the case, the researcher must establish a minimum requirement of meeting the criteria of external validity.

The factors that may affect external validity are related to selection of subjects, study conditions, and type of observations. These factors are termed effects of selection, reactive effects, and effects of testing. The reader will notice the similarity in the names of the factors of selection and testing to those of the threats to internal validity. When considering factors as internal threats, the reader assesses them as they relate to the *independent* and *dependent* variables within the study, and when assessing them as external threats, the reader considers them in terms of the *generalizability* or use outside of the study to other populations and settings. The Critical Thinking Decision Path for threats to validity displays the way threats to internal and external validity can interact with each other. It is important to remember that this path is not exhaustive of the type of threats and their interaction. Problems of internal validity are generally easier to control. Generalizability issues are more difficult to deal with because it means that the researcher is assuming that other populations are similar to the one being tested. External validity factors include effect of selection, reactivity effects, and effect of testing.

CRITICAL THINKING DECISION PATH | Potential Threats to a Study's Validity

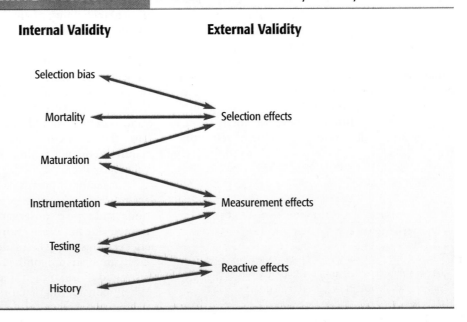

 EVIDENCE-BASED PRACTICE TIP

Generalizability depends on who actually participates in a study. Not everyone who is approached actually participates, and not everyone who agrees to participate completes a study. As you review studies, think about how well this group reflects the population of interest.

Selection Effects

Selection refers to the generalizability of the results to other populations. An example of the effects of selection occurs when the researcher cannot attain the ideal sample population. At times, numbers of available subjects may be low or not accessible to the researcher; the researcher may then need to choose a nonprobability method of sampling over a probability method (see Chapter 12). Therefore the type of sampling

method used and how subjects are assigned to research conditions affect the generalizability to other groups or the external validity.

Examples of selection effects are depicted when researchers note any of the following:

- "Without a control group, investigators can not conclude with certainty that the benefits reported were actually the result of the information counseling session" (Davison et al., 2004; Appendix D).
- "The use of a small convenience sample of primarily White, English speaking, well-educated mothers of pre-schoolers, most of whom were connected with community services, limits the generalizability of findings to those of similar characteristics" (Sgarbossa and Ford-Gilboe, 2004).
- "The sample size was small and the findings descriptive in nature" (LoBiondo-Wood et al., 2004).

These remarks caution the reader but also point out the usefulness of the findings for practice and future research aimed at building the data in these areas.

Reactive Effects

Reactivity is defined as the subjects' responses to being studied. Subjects may respond to the investigator not because of the study procedures but merely as an independent response to being studied. This is also known as the Hawthorne effect, which is named after Western Electric Corporation's Hawthorne plant, where a study of working conditions was conducted. The researchers developed several different working conditions (i.e., turning up the lights, piping in music loudly or softly, and changing work hours). They found that no matter what was done, the workers' productivity increased. They concluded that production increased as a result of the workers' realization that they were being studied rather than because of the experimental conditions. For example, in a study by Ratner et al. (2004) that tested an intervention to help smokers abstain from smoking before and after surgery, smokers were randomized to a counseling intervention and nicotine replacement program, and the control group received usual hospital care. At the end of the study the researchers found that the control had a relatively high abstinence rate. They concluded that because the control group was aware of their group assignment, they tried to demonstrate that they could do as well as the treatment group, even though they did not receive the intervention.

Measurement Effects

Administration of a pretest in a study affects the generalizability of the findings to other populations and is known as **measurement effects.** Just as pretesting affects the posttest results within a study, pretesting affects the posttest results and generalizability outside the study. For example, suppose a researcher wants to conduct a study with the aim of changing attitudes toward AIDS. To accomplish this, an education program on the risk factors for AIDS is incorporated. To test whether the education program changes attitudes toward AIDS, tests are given before and after the teaching intervention. The pretest on attitudes allows the subjects to examine their attitudes regarding AIDS. The subjects' responses on follow-up testing may differ from those of individuals who were given the education program and did not see the pretest. Therefore when a study is conducted and a pretest is given, it may prime the subjects and affect their ability to generalize to other situations.

> **HELPFUL** H I N T
>
> When reviewing a study, be aware of the internal and external threats to validity. These threats do not make a study useless—but actually more useful—to you. Recognition of the threats allows researchers to build on data and consumers to think through what part of the study can be applied to practice. Specific threats to validity depend on the type of design and generalizations the researcher hopes to make.

There are other threats to external validity that depend on the type of design and methods of sampling used by the researcher, but these are beyond the scope of this text. Campbell and Stanley (1966) offer detailed coverage of the issues related to internal and external validity.

Critiquing the design of a study requires one to first have knowledge of the overall implications that the choice of a particular design may have for the study as a whole (see Critiquing Criteria box below). Researchers want to consider the level of evidence provided by the design and how the study can be used to improve or change practice. Minimizing threats to internal and external validity enhances the strength of evidence for any quantitative design. The concept of the research design is an all-inclusive one that parallels the concept of the theoretical framework. The research design is similar to the theoretical framework in that it deals with a piece of the research study that affects the whole. For one to knowledgeably critique the design in light of the entire study, it is important to understand the factors that influence the choice and the implications of the design. In this chapter, the meaning, purpose, and important factors of design choice, as well as the vocabulary that accompanies these factors, have been introduced.

Several criteria for evaluating the design can be drawn from this chapter. One should remember that the criteria are applied differently with various designs. Different application does not mean that the consumer will find a haphazard approach to design. It means that each design has particular criteria that allow the consumer to classify the design by type (e.g., experimental or nonexperimental). These criteria must be met and addressed in conducting an experiment. The particulars of specific designs are addressed in Chapters 10 and 11. The following discussion primarily pertains to the overall evaluation of a quantitative research design.

The research design should reflect that an objective review of the literature and the establishment of a theoretical framework guided the choice of the design. There is no explicit statement regarding this in a research study. A consumer can evaluate this by critiquing the theoretical framework (see Chapter 5) and literature review (see Chapter 4). Is the question new and not extensively researched? Has a great deal been done on the question, or is it a new or different way of looking at an old question? Depending on the level of the question, the investigators make certain choices. For example, in their study assessing the pressure-reducing effects of five operating-table mattresses, Defloor and DeSchuijmer (2000) decided to have nonsurgical volunteers test the mattresses rather than patients undergoing surgery. This choice allowed the researchers to look for differences in a controlled, comparative manner.

CRITIQUING CRITERIA   *Quantitative Research*

1. Is the type of design employed appropriate?
2. Does the researcher use the various concepts of control that are consistent with the type of design chosen?
3. Does the design used seem to reflect the issues of economy?
4. Does the design used seem to flow from the proposed research question, theoretical framework, literature review, and hypothesis?
5. What are the threats to internal validity?
6. What are the controls for the threats to internal validity?
7. What are the threats to external validity?
8. What are the controls for the threats to external validity?
9. Is the design appropriately linked to the levels of evidence hierarchy?

The consumer should be alert for the means investigators use to maintain control (e.g., homogeneity in the sample, consistent data-collection procedures, how or if the independent variable was manipulated, and whether randomization was used). As you can see in Chapter 10, all of these criteria must be met for an experimental design. As you begin to understand the types of designs (i.e., experimental, quasiexperimental, and nonexperimental designs such as survey and relationship designs), you will find that control is applied in varying degrees, or—as in the case of a survey study—the independent variable is not manipulated at all (see Chapter 11). The level of control and its applications presented in Chapters 10 and 11 provide the remaining knowledge to fully critique the aspects of a study's design.

Once it has been established whether the necessary control or uniformity of conditions has been maintained, the consumer must determine whether the study is believable or valid. The consumer should ask whether the findings are the result of the variables tested—and thus internally valid—or whether there could be another explanation. To assess this aspect, the threats to internal validity should be reviewed. If the investigator's study was systematic, well grounded in theory, and followed the criteria for each of the processes, the consumer will probably conclude that the study is internally valid.

In addition, the consumer must know whether a study has external validity or generalizability to other populations or environmental conditions. External validity can be claimed only after internal validity has been established. If the credibility of a study (internal validity) has not been established, a study cannot be generalized (external validity) to other populations. Determination of external validity goes hand-in-hand with the sampling frame (see Chapter 12). If the study is not representative of any one group or phenomena of interest, external validity may be limited or not present at all. The consumer will find that establishment of internal and external validity requires not only knowledge of the threats to internal and external validity but also knowledge of the phenomena being studied. Knowledge of the phenomena being studied allows critical judgments to be made about the linkage of theories and variables for testing. The consumer should find that the design follows from the theoretical framework, literature review, research question, and hypotheses. The consumer should feel, on the basis of clinical knowledge and knowledge of the research process, that the investigators are not comparing apples to oranges.

Critical Thinking Challenges

- Would you support or refute the following statement: "All research attempts to solve problems"?
- As a consumer of research, you recognize that control is an important concept in the issue of research design. You are critiquing an assigned experimental study as part of your "open book" midterm exam. From what is written, you cannot determine how the researchers kept the conditions of the study constant. How does this affect the study's use in an evidence-based practice model?
- Box 9-1 lists six major threats to the internal validity of an experimental study. Prioritize them and defend the one that you have made the essential, or number one, threat to address in a study.
- You will be critiquing the research design of an assigned study for the first time as a consumer of research. How does the research design influence the findings of evidence in the study?
- How do threats to external validity contribute to the strength and quality of evidence provided by the findings of a research study?

KEY POINTS

- The purpose of the design is to provide the format of a masterful and creative piece of research.
- There are many types of designs. No matter which type of design the researcher uses, the purpose always remains the same.
- The research consumer should be able to locate within the study a sense of the question that the researcher wished to answer. The question should be proposed with a plan or scheme for the accomplishment of the investigation. Depending on the question, the consumer should be able to recognize the steps taken by the investigator to ensure control.
- The choice of the specific design depends on the nature of the question. Specification of the nature of the research question requires that the design reflects the investigator's attempts to maintain objectivity, accuracy, pragmatic considerations, and, most important, control.
- Control affects not only the outcome of a study but also its future use. The design should also reflect how the investigator attempted to control threats to both internal and external validity.

- Internal validity must be established before external validity can be established. Both are considered within the sampling structure.
- No matter which design the researcher chooses, it should be evident to the reader that the choice was based on a thorough examination of the research question within a theoretical framework.
- The design, research question, literature review, theoretical framework, and hypothesis should all interrelate to demonstrate a woven pattern.
- The choice of the design is affected by pragmatic issues. At times, two different designs may be equally valid for the same question.
- The choice of design affects the study's level of evidence.

REFERENCES

Bull MJ, Hansen HE, and Gross CR: A professional-patient partnership model of discharge planning with elders hospitalized with heart failure, *App Nurs Res* 13(1): 19-28, 2000.

Campbell D, Stanley J: *Experimental and quasi-experimental designs for research,* Chicago, 1966, Rand-McNally.

Carfoot S, Williamson PR, and Dickson R: The value of a pilot study in breast-feeding research, *Midwifery* 20(2): 188-193, 2004.

Defloor T, DeSchuijmer DS: Preventing pressure ulcers: an evaluation of four operating-table mattresses, *Appl Nurs Res* 13: 134-141, 2000.

Holditch-Davis D, Brandon DH, and Schwartz T: Development of behaviours in preterm infants: relation to sleeping and waking, *Nurs Res* 52(5): 3007-317, 2003.A

Hoskins CN, Haber J, Budin WC, Cartwright-Alcarase F, Kowalski MO, Panke J, and Maislin G: Breast cancer: education, counseling and adjustment. A pilot study, *Psychol Rep* 89: 677-704, 2001.

Inoue K, Kakehashi Y, Oomori S, and Koizumi A: Endemic hypoglycemia among female nurses, *Res Nurs Health* 27: 87-96, 2004.

LoBiondo-Wood G, Williams L, and McGhee C: Liver transplantation in children: maternal and family stress, coping and adaptation, *J Specialists Pediatr Nurs* 9: 59-66, 2004.

Miles MS, Holditch-Davis D, Eron J, Black BP, Pederson C, and Harris DA: An HIV self-care symptom management intervention for African American mothers, *Nursing* 52: 350-360, 2003.

Ratner PA, Johnson JL, Richardson CG, Bottorff JL, Moffat B, Mackay M, Foonoff D, Kingsbury K, Miller C, and Budz B: Efficacy of a smoking cessation intervention for elective surgical patients, *Res Nurs Health* 27: 148-161, 2004.

Santacroce SJ, Maccarelli LM, and Grey M: Intervention fidelity, *Nurs Res* 53(1): 63-66, 2004.

Sgarbossa RN, Ford-Gilboe M: Mother's friendship quality, parental support, quality of life, and family health led by adolescent mothers with preschool children, *J Family Nurs* 10: 212-232, 2004.

Wikblad K, Anderson B: Comparison of three wound dressings in patients undergoing heart surgery, *Nurs Res* 44: 312-316, 1995.

FOR FURTHER STUDY

🔘 Go to your Companion CD for review activities for this chapter.

evolve Go to Evolve at http://evolve.elsevier.com/LoBiondo/ for WebLinks, Content Updates, and additional research articles, for practice in reviewing and critiquing.

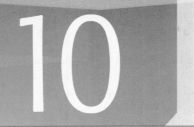

10

ROBIN WHITTEMORE

MARGARET GREY

Experimental and Quasiexperimental Designs

KEY TERMS

a priori
after-only design
after-only nonequivalent control
   group design
antecedent variable
control
dependent variable
design

evaluation research
experiment
experimental design
independent variable
intervening variable
manipulation
mortality
nonequivalent control group design

one group (pretest-posttest) design
quasiexperimental design
randomization
Solomon four-group design
testing
time series design
true or classic experiment

LEARNING OUTCOMES

After reading this chapter, the student should be able to do the following:

- List the criteria necessary for inferring cause-and-effect relationships.
- Distinguish the differences between experimental and quasiexperimental designs.
- Define internal validity problems associated with experimental and quasiexperimental designs.
- Describe the use of experimental and quasiexperimental designs for evaluation research.
- Critically evaluate the findings of selected studies that test cause-and-effect relationships.
- Apply levels of evidence to experimental and quasiexperimental designs.

STUDY RESOURCES

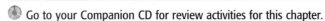

Go to your Companion CD for review activities for this chapter.

evolve Go to Evolve at http://evolve.elsevier.com/LoBiondo/ for Weblinks, Content Updates, and additional research articles for practice in reviewing and critiquing.

RESEARCH PROCESS

One of the fundamental purposes of scientific research in any profession is to determine cause-and-effect relationships. In nursing, for example, we are concerned with developing effective approaches to maintaining and restoring wellness. Testing such nursing interventions to determine how well they actually work—that is, evaluating the outcomes in terms of efficacy and cost-effectiveness—is accomplished by using **experimental** and **quasiexperimental designs.** These designs differ from nonexperimental designs in one important way: the researcher actively seeks to bring about the desired effect and does not passively observe behaviors or actions. In other words, the researcher is interested in making something happen, not merely observing customary patient care. Experimental and quasiexperimental studies are also important to consider in relation to evidence-based practice because they provide Level II and Level III evidence. It is the findings of such studies that provide the validation of a clinical practice intervention and the rationale for changing specific aspects of practice (see Chapters 19 and 20).

Experimental designs are particularly suitable for testing cause-and-effect relationships because they help eliminate potential alternative explanations (threats to validity) for the findings. To infer causality requires that the following three criteria be met:

- The causal variable and effect variable must be associated with each other.
- The cause must precede the effect.
- The relationship must not be explainable by another variable.

When you critique studies that use experimental and quasiexperimental designs, the primary focus is on the validity of the conclusion that the experimental treatment, or **independent variable,** caused the desired effect on the outcome, or **dependent variable.** The validity of the conclusion depends on just how well the researcher has controlled the other variables that

may explain the relationship studied. Thus the focus of this chapter is to differentiate between experimental and quasiexperimental designs and to explain how the various types of experimental and quasiexperimental designs control extraneous variables.

It should be made clear, however, that most research in nursing is not experimental. Considerable preliminary research is required to test the complex cause-and-effect relationships of nursing interventions (Whittemore and Grey, 2002). For example, an experimental design requires that all of the relevant variables have been defined so that they can be manipulated and studied. In most problem areas in nursing, this requirement has not been met. Therefore nonexperimental designs used in identifying variables and determining their relationship to each other often need to be done before experimental studies are performed.

The purpose of this chapter is to acquaint you with the issues involved in interpreting studies that use **experimental design** and **quasiexperimental design.** These designs are listed in Box 10-1. The Critical Thinking Decision Path in the illustration below shows an algorithm that influences a researcher's choice of experimental or quasiexperimental design.

BOX 10-1   SUMMARY OF EXPERIMENTAL AND QUASIEXPERIMENTAL RESEARCH DESIGNS

EXPERIMENTAL DESIGNS

1. True experiment (pretest-posttest control group) design
2. Solomon four-group design
3. After-only design

QUASIEXPERIMENTAL DESIGNS

1. Nonequivalent control group design
2. After-only nonequivalent control group design
3. One group (pretest-posttest) design
4. Time series design

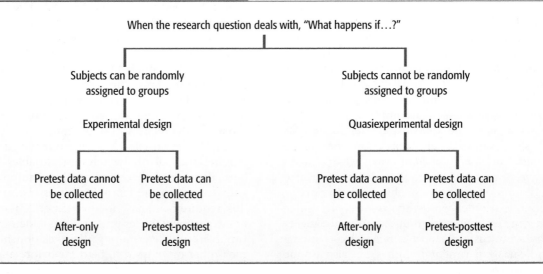

CRITICAL THINKING DECISION PATH   Experimental and Quasiexperimental Design

When the research question deals with, "What happens if...?"

Subjects can be randomly assigned to groups

Experimental design

Pretest data cannot be collected → After-only design

Pretest data can be collected → Pretest-posttest design

Subjects cannot be randomly assigned to groups

Quasiexperimental design

Pretest data cannot be collected → After-only design

Pretest data can be collected → Pretest-posttest design

TRUE EXPERIMENTAL DESIGN

An **experiment** is a scientific investigation that makes observations and collects data according to explicit criteria. A **true experimental design** has three identifying properties—**randomization, control,** and **manipulation**. These properties allow for other explanations of the phenomenon to be ruled out and thereby provide the strength of the design for testing cause-and-effect relationships.

A research study using an experimental design is commonly called a *randomized clinical trial* (RCT). An RCT or experimental design is considered to be the best research design, "the gold standard", for providing information about cause-and-effect relationships. An individual RCT generates Level II evidence in the hierarchy of evidence because of the minimal bias introduced by this design (see Chapter 9). The higher a design on the evidence hierarchy, the more likely the results are to offer an unbiased estimate of the effect of an intervention and the more confident you are that the intervention will be effective and produce the same results over and over again (see Chapters 2, 4, 9, and 20).

Randomization

Randomization, or random assignment to a group, involves the distribution of subjects to either the experimental or the control group on a purely random basis. That is, each subject has an equal and known probability of being assigned to any group. Random assignment may be done individually or by groups (Coleman et al., 2003; Grey et al., 2000). Random assignment to experimental or control groups allows for the elimination of any systematic bias in the groups with respect to attributes that may affect the dependent variable being studied. The procedure for randomization assumes that any important intervening variables will be equally distributed between the groups and, as discussed in Chapter 9, minimizes variance and decreases selection bias. Randomization helps to attribute any group differences that emerge in the study to the treatment or experimental condition. Note that random assignment to groups is different from random sampling discussed in Chapter 12.

Control

Control means the introduction of one or more constants into the experimental situation. Control is acquired by manipulating the causal or independent variable, by randomly assigning subjects to a group, by very carefully preparing experimental protocols, and by using comparison groups. In experimental research the comparison group is the control group, or the group that receives the usual treatment, rather than the innovative experimental one.

Manipulation

As discussed previously, experimental designs are characterized by the researcher "doing something" to at least some of the involved subjects. This "something," or the independent variable, is manipulated by giving it (the experimental treatment) to some participants in the study and not to others or by giving different amounts of it to different groups. The independent variable might be a treatment, a teaching plan, or a medication that must be clearly defined. It is the effect of this **manipulation** that is measured to determine the result of the experimental treatment on the dependent variable.

The concepts of randomization, control, and manipulation and their application to experimental design are sometimes confusing. To see the way randomization, control, and manipulation allow researchers to have confidence in the causal inferences they make about findings by allowing them to rule out other potential explanations, the use of these properties is illustrated in one report.

Koniak-Griffin and associates (2003) (see Appendix A) used a randomized controlled experiment to study if an early intervention program of home visitation by public health nurses would improve postbirth infant and maternal outcomes. Latina and African-American adolescent mothers were randomly assigned to one of two groups: the experimental group, who received the early intervention program (EIP) and intensive home visitation by public health nurses from pregnancy through 1-year postbirth; or a control group, who received traditional public health nursing care (TPHNC). The use of random assignment means that all the patients who met the study criteria had an equal and known chance of being assigned to the control or the experimental group. The use of random assignment to groups helps ensure that the two study groups are comparable on preexisting factors that might affect the outcome of interest, such as age, educational level, and marital status. It is important to note that the researchers checked statistically whether the procedure of random assignment did produce groups that were similar with regard to important factors.

Both groups received public health nursing care; however, the treatment group received a more structured and time-intensive program of care developed to improve maternal self-care behaviors and caretaking, to improve infant health outcomes, to prevent repeat pregnancy, and to improve maternal social competence. Thus in this study, the early intervention program was the manipulated treatment or the independent variable. Dependent variables consisted of infant (infant hospitalization, infant emergency room visits, and immunizations) and maternal (substance use, repeat pregnancies, continuation in education, social competence, interaction with infants, and environment of the home) outcomes.

The experimental criteria of control were exhibited in this study by having a control group to provide a comparison against which the experimental group could be evaluated. In addition, the early intervention program was thoroughly described, which assists the reader in understanding the nature of the experimental treatment, and was consistently delivered, which helps to ensure that all members of the experimental group received similar treatment.

In addition, the use of the experimental design allowed the researchers to rule out many of the potential threats to internal validity of the findings, such as selection, history, and maturation (see Chapter 9). By clearly and carefully controlling the experimental intervention by the use of standard protocols and recordings, the investigators were able to make the assertion that the intervention was effective in improving infant outcomes and selected aspects of maternal health and life-course. The Level II evidence provided by the findings of this RCT helps public health nurses make EIP versus TPHNC program resource allocation decisions with more certainty.

The strength of the true experimental design, in this case the RCT, lies in its ability to help the researcher control the effects of any extraneous variables that might constitute threats to internal validity. Such extraneous variables can be either antecedent or intervening. The **antecedent variable** occurs before the study but may affect the dependent variable and confuse the results. Factors such as age, socioeconomic status, and educational level might be important antecedent variables in nursing research because they may affect dependent variables such as recovery and ability to manage health or illness needs. In the study by Koniak-Griffin and associates (2003), antecedent variables that might affect the dependent variables included ethnicity, age, educational level, and marital status. Random assignment to groups helps ensure that groups will be similar with regard to these variables so that differences in the dependent variable may be attributed to the experimental treatment. It should be noted, however, that the researcher should check and report how the groups actually compared on such variables. Koniak-Griffin and associates (2003) clearly stated in their article that these variables at study entry were similar between both the experimental and control groups. An **intervening variable** extraneous or mediating occurs during the course of the study and is not part of the study, but it affects the dependent variable and could affect the study outcomes. An example of an intervening variable that might affect the outcomes of this study

(Koniak-Griffin et al., 2003) is a change in health care status in any of the participants, such as a newly diagnosed medical condition or mental illness. Certainly, if care provided to patients changed in any major way while the study was being implemented, the study also would be affected.

Types of Experimental Designs

There are many different experimental designs (Campbell and Stanley, 1966). Each is based on the classic design called the true experiment diagrammed in Figure 10-1, *A*. Above the description diagram, symbolic notations are routinely used. **R** represents random assignment (for both the experimental and the control group). **O** signifies observation via data collection on the dependent variable. O_1 signifies pretest data collection whereas O_2 represents posttest data collection. **X** represents the group exposure to the intervention. Therefore in this figure, you will note that subjects were assigned randomly (**R**) to the experimental or the control group. The experimental treatment (**X**) was given only to those in the experimental group, and the pretests (O_1) and posttests (O_2) are those measurements of the dependent variables that were made before and after the experimental treatment was performed. All true experimental designs have subjects randomly assigned to groups, have an experimental treatment introduced to some of the subjects, and have the effects of the treatment observed. Designs vary primarily in the number of observations that are made.

⚗️ **EVIDENCE-BASED PRACTICE TIP**

In health care research, the term randomized clinical trial (RCT) is often used to refer to a true experimental design. These designs are being utilized more frequently in nursing research, which is critical to evidence-based practice initiatives.

A. True or classic experiment

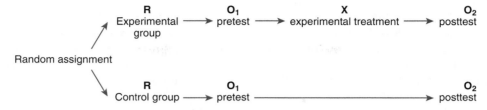

B. Solomon four-group design

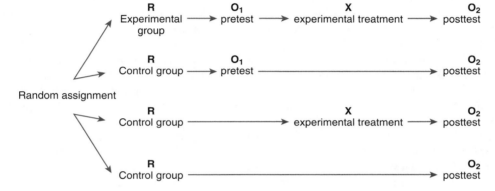

C. After-only experimental design

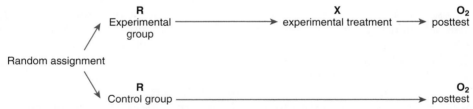

Figure 10-1. Comparison of experimental designs. **A,** True or classic experiment. **B,** Solomon four-group design. **C,** After-only experimental design.

As shown in Figure 10-1, *A,* in a **true or classic experiment**, subjects are randomly assigned to the two groups, experimental and control, so that antecedent variables are controlled. Then pretest measures or observations are made so that the researcher has a baseline for determining the effect of the independent variable. The researcher then introduces the experimental variable to one of the groups and measures the dependent

variable again to see whether it has changed. The control group gets no experimental treatment but also is measured later for comparison with the experimental group. The degree of difference between the two groups at the end of the study indicates the confidence the researcher has that a causal link exists between the independent and dependent variables. Because random assignment and the control inherent in this design minimize the effects of many threats to internal validity, it is a strong design for testing cause-and-effect relationships. However, the design is not perfect. Some threats cannot be controlled in true experimental studies (see Chapter 9). People tend to drop out of studies that require their participation over an extended period of time. The influence over the outcome of an experiment from people dropping out or dying is commonly known as the **mortality** effect. If there is a difference in the number or type of people who drop out of the experimental group from that of the control group, a mortality effect might explain the findings. When reading such a work, it is important to examine the sample and the results carefully to see if dropouts or deaths occurred. **Testing** also can be a problem in these studies, because the researcher is usually giving the same measurement twice and subjects tend to score better the second time just by learning the test. Researchers can get around this problem in one of two ways: they might use different forms of the same test for the two measurements, or they might use a more complex experimental design called the Solomon four-group design.

The **Solomon four-group design,** shown in Figure 10-1, *B*, has two groups that are identical to those used in the classic experimental design, plus two additional groups: an experimental after-group and a control after-group. As the diagram shows, all four groups have randomly assigned (**R**) subjects as in all experimental studies. However, the addition of these last two groups helps rule out testing threats to internal validity that the before and after groups may experience. Suppose a researcher is interested in the effects of some counseling on chronically ill patients' self-esteem, but just measurement of self-esteem (O_1) may influence how the subjects report themselves. For example, the items on the questionnaire might make the subjects think more about how they view themselves so that the next time they fill out the questionnaire (O_2), their self-esteem might appear to have improved. In reality, however, their self-esteem may be the same as it was before; it just looks different

because they took the test before. The use of this design with the two groups that do not receive the pretest allows for evaluating the effect of the pretest on the posttest in the first two groups. Although this design helps evaluate the effects of testing, the threat of mortality remains a problem as with the classic experimental design. Swanson (1999) used a Solomon four-group design to test the effects of caring-based counseling, measurement, and time on the integration of loss (from miscarriage) and women's emotional well-being in the first year after miscarrying. She studied four groups: two treatment groups and two control groups.

A less frequently used experimental design is the **after-only design,** shown in Figure 10-1, *C.* This design, which is sometimes called the posttest-only control group design, is composed of two randomly assigned groups (**R**), but unlike the true experimental design, neither group is pretested or measured. Again, the independent variable is introduced to the experimental group (**X**) and not to the control group. The process of randomly assigning the subjects to groups is assumed to be sufficient to ensure a lack of bias so that the researcher can still determine whether the treatment (**X**) created significant differences between the two groups (**O**). This design is particularly useful when testing effects are expected to be a major problem, when outcomes cannot be measured beforehand (i.e., postoperative pain management), and when the number of available subjects is too limited to use a Solomon four-group design. When this design is used, it is important that researchers carefully examine the two groups to ensure that the groups were equivalent at baseline, so that they could be assured that random assignment has yielded equivalent groups.

EVIDENCE-BASED PRACTICE TIP

RCTs, as true experimental designs, minimize bias and are considered the most appropriate research design to answer questions about the effectiveness of an intervention.

Field and Laboratory Experiments

Experiments also can be classified by setting. Field experiments and laboratory experiments share the properties of control, randomization, and manipulation, and they use the same design characteristics, but they are conducted in different environments. Laboratory experiments take place in an artificial setting created specifically for the purpose of research. In the laboratory, the researcher has almost total control over the features of the environment, such as temperature, humidity, noise level, and subject conditions. On the other hand, field experiments are exactly what the name implies—experiments that take place in some real, preexisting social setting such as a hospital or clinic where the phenomenon of interest usually occurs. Because most experiments in the nursing literature are field experiments and control is such an important element in the conduct of experiments, it should be obvious that studies conducted in the field are subject to treatment contamination by factors specific to the setting that the researcher cannot control. However, studies conducted in the laboratory are by nature "artificial," because the setting is created for the purpose of research. Thus laboratory experiments, although stronger with respect to internal validity questions than field work studies, suffer more from problems with external validity. For example, a subject's behavior in the laboratory may be quite different from the person's behavior in the real world—a dichotomy that presents problems in generalizing findings from the laboratory to the real world. When research reports are read, therefore, it is important to consider the setting of the experiment and what impact it might have on the findings of the study.

Consider the study comparing a wound treatment gel to a placebo gel for the management of pressure sores (Hirshberg et al., 2001). This study could have been done in a laboratory using animals, which would have allowed complete control over the external environment of the study, a variable that might be important in studying wound healing. However, there is no guarantee that the results found in a study in a laboratory would be applicable to patients in hospital settings, so the study would lose some external validity.

 HELPFUL H I N T

Look for evidence of preestablished inclusion and exclusion criteria for the study participants.

Advantages and Disadvantages of the Experimental Design

As previously discussed, experimental designs are the most powerful design for testing cause-and-effect relationships. This is because of the design's ability to control the experimental situation. Therefore the design offers better corroboration of a true treatment effect. Such studies are important because one of nursing's major research priorities is documenting outcomes to provide a basis for changing or supporting current nursing practice (see Chapter 1). In the study by Koniak-Griffin and associates (2003), the authors were able to conclude from their findings that the early intervention program for pregnant Latina and African-American adolescents is useful in improving infant health outcomes and select maternal health and lifestyle outcomes. Their study helps support using an early intervention program with other racial or ethnic groups and in other geographical settings. Similarly, in a review of seven randomized clinical trials, Brooten and associates (2002) were able to conclude that an advanced practice nurse intervention consistently improved patient outcomes and reduced health care costs with women with high-risk pregnancies and elders with acute and chronic illnesses. These studies and others like them allow nurses to anticipate in a scientific manner the outcomes of their actions and provide the basis for effective evidence-based practice.

Still, experimental designs are not the ones most commonly used in nursing research for several reasons. First, experimentation assumes that all of the relevant variables involved in a phenomenon have been identified. For many areas of nursing research, this simply is not the case, and descriptive studies need to be completed before experimental interventions can be applied. Second, these designs have some significant disadvantages.

One problem with an experimental design is that many variables important in predicting outcomes of nursing care are not amenable to experimental manipulation. It is well-known that health status varies with age and socioeconomic status. No matter how careful a researcher is, no one can assign subjects randomly by age or a certain level of income. In addition, some variables may be technically manipulable, but their nature may preclude actually doing so. For example, the ethics of a researcher who tried to randomly assign groups for the study of the effects of cigarette smoking and asked the experimental group to smoke two packs of cigarettes a day would be seriously questioned. It is also potentially true that such a study would not work because nonsmokers randomly assigned to the smoking group would be unlikely to comply with the research task.

Another problem with experimental designs is that they may be difficult or impractical to perform in field settings. It may be quite difficult to randomly assign patients from a hospital unit to different groups when nurses might talk to each other about the different treatments. Experimental procedures also may be disruptive to the usual routine of the setting. If several nurses are involved in administering the experimental program, it may be impossible to ensure that the program is administered in the same way to each subject.

Because of these problems in carrying out true experiments, researchers frequently turn to another type of research design to evaluate cause-and-effect relationships. Such designs, because they look like experiments but lack some of the control of the true experimental design, are called quasiexperiments.

QUASIEXPERIMENTAL DESIGNS

Quasiexperimental designs are also intended to test cause-and-effect relationships; however, in a quasiexperimental design, full experimental control is not possible. Quasiexperiments are research designs in which the researcher initiates an experimental treatment but some characteristic of a true experiment is lacking. Random assignment to the treatment or control groups may not have been undertaken, or there may not be a control group at all. These characteristics of a true experiment may not be possible because of the nature of the independent variable or the nature of the available subjects.

Without all of the characteristics associated with a true experiment, internal validity may be compromised, and the ability to determine that the treatment caused the changes observed in outcomes is weakened. Therefore the basic problem with the quasiexperimental approach is a weakened confidence in making causal assertions. Because of the lack of some controls in the research situation, quasiexperimental designs are subject to contamination by many, if not all, of the threats to internal validity discussed in Chapter 9. As a result, Level III evidence is provided by studies that use quasiexperimental designs. Because full experimental control is not possible, confidence is weakened that the findings generated were the result of the intervention itself rather than the result of other extraneous variables.

 HELPFUL H I N T

Remember that researchers often make trade-offs and sometimes use a quasiexperimental design instead of an experimental design because it may be pragmatically impossible to randomly assign subjects to groups. Not using the "purest" design does not decrease the value of the study even though it may decrease the strength of the findings.

Types of Quasiexperimental Designs

There are many different quasiexperimental designs. Only the ones most commonly used in nursing research are discussed in this book. Again, the symbols and notations introduced earlier in the chapter are used. Refer back to the true experimental design shown in Figure 10-1, *A*, and compare it with the **nonequivalent control group design** shown in Figure 10-2, *A*. Note that this design looks exactly like the true experiment except that subjects are not randomly assigned to groups. Suppose a researcher is interested in the effects of a new diabetes edu-

cation program on the physical and psychosocial outcomes of patients newly diagnosed with diabetes. If conditions were right, the researcher might be able to randomly assign subjects to either the group receiving the new program or the group receiving the usual program, but for any number of reasons, that design might not be possible. For example, nurses on the unit where patients are admitted might be so excited about the new program that they cannot help but include the new information for all patients. So the researcher has two choices—to abandon the experiment or to conduct a quasiexperiment. To

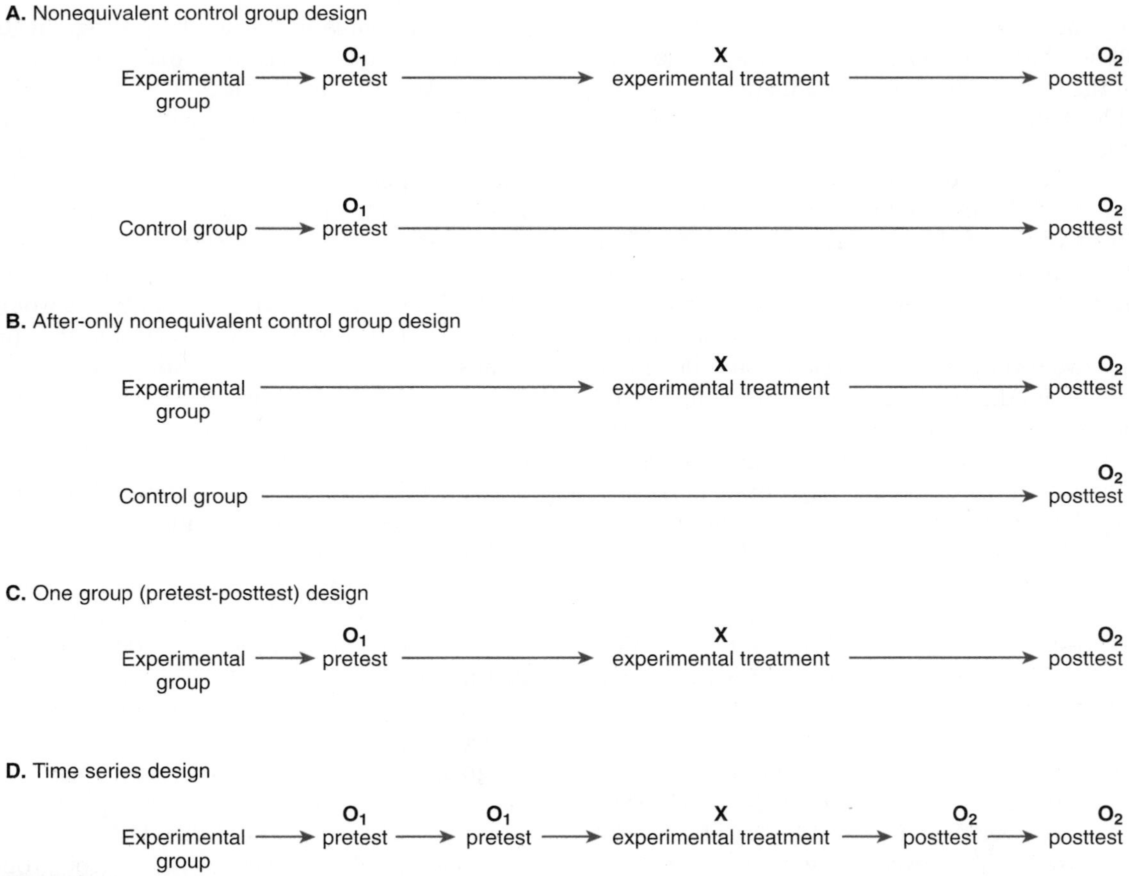

A. Nonequivalent control group design

$$
\begin{array}{cccc}
 & O_1 & X & O_2 \\
\text{Experimental} \longrightarrow \text{pretest} \longrightarrow \text{experimental treatment} \longrightarrow \text{posttest} \\
\text{group} & & &
\end{array}
$$

$$
\begin{array}{ccc}
 & O_1 & O_2 \\
\text{Control group} \longrightarrow \text{pretest} \longrightarrow \text{posttest}
\end{array}
$$

B. After-only nonequivalent control group design

$$
\begin{array}{ccc}
 & X & O_2 \\
\text{Experimental} \longrightarrow \text{experimental treatment} \longrightarrow \text{posttest} \\
\text{group} & &
\end{array}
$$

$$
\begin{array}{c}
O_2 \\
\text{Control group} \longrightarrow \text{posttest}
\end{array}
$$

C. One group (pretest-posttest) design

$$
\begin{array}{cccc}
 & O_1 & X & O_2 \\
\text{Experimental} \longrightarrow \text{pretest} \longrightarrow \text{experimental treatment} \longrightarrow \text{posttest} \\
\text{group} & & &
\end{array}
$$

D. Time series design

$$
\begin{array}{cccccc}
 & O_1 & O_1 & X & O_2 & O_2 \\
\text{Experimental} \longrightarrow \text{pretest} \longrightarrow \text{pretest} \longrightarrow \text{experimental treatment} \longrightarrow \text{posttest} \longrightarrow \text{posttest} \\
\text{group} & & & & &
\end{array}
$$

Figure 10-2. Comparison of quasiexperimental designs. **A,** Nonequivalent control group design. **B,** After-only nonequivalent control group design. **C,** One group (pretest-posttest) design. **D,** Time series design.

conduct a quasiexperiment the researcher might find a similar unit that has not been introduced to the new program and study the newly diagnosed patients with diabetes who are admitted to that unit as a comparison group. The study would then involve this type of design.

The nonequivalent control group design is commonly used in nursing research studies conducted in field settings. The basic problem with this design is the weakened confidence the researcher can have in assuming that the experimental and comparison groups are similar at the beginning of the study. Threats to internal validity, such as selection, maturation, testing, and mortality, are possible with this design. However, the design is relatively strong because the gathering of the data at the time of pretest allows the researcher to compare the equivalence of the two groups on important antecedent variables before the independent variable is introduced. In the previous example, the motivation of the patients to learn about their medical condition might be important in determining the effect of the diabetes education program. The researcher could include in the measures taken at the outset of the study some measure of motivation to learn. Then differences between the two groups on this variable could be tested, and if significant differences existed, they could be controlled statistically in the analysis. Nonetheless, the strength of the causal assertions that can be made on the basis of such designs depends on the ability of the researcher to identify and measure or control possible threats to internal validity.

Now suppose that the researcher did not think to measure the subjects before the introduction of the new treatment (or the researcher was hired after the new program began) but later decided that it would be useful to have data demonstrating the effect of the program. Perhaps, for example, a third party asks for such data to determine whether they should pay the extra cost of the new teaching program. Sometimes, the outcomes simply cannot be measured before the intervention, as with prenatal interventions that are expected to impact birth outcomes. The study

that could be conducted would look like the **after-only nonequivalent control group design,** shown in Figure 10-2, *B.*

This design is similar to the after-only experimental design, but randomization is not used to assign subjects to groups. This design makes the assumption that the two groups are equivalent and comparable before the introduction of the independent variable (**X**). Thus the soundness of the design and the confidence that we can put in the findings depend on the soundness of this assumption of preintervention comparability. Often it is difficult to support the assertion that the two nonrandomly assigned groups are comparable at the outset of the study because there is no way of assessing its validity.

In the example of the teaching program for patients with newly diagnosed diabetes, measuring the subjects' motivation after the teaching program would not tell us whether their motivations differed before they received the program, and it is possible that the teaching program would motivate individuals to learn more about their health problem. Therefore the researcher's conclusion that the teaching program improved physical status and psychosocial outcome would be subject to the alternative conclusion that the results were an effect of preexisting motivations (selection effect) in combination with greater learning in those so motivated (selection-maturation interaction). Nonetheless, this design is frequently used in nursing research because opportunities for data collection are often limited and because it is particularly useful when testing effects may be problematic. Consider again the example of the experiment conducted by Koniak-Griffin and associates (2003). Suppose that they had not randomly assigned the participants to the early intervention program, but rather took all patients before a certain point and assigned them to the control group and then assigned all new patients to the experimental treatment. The study would then be an example of an after-only nonequivalent control group design. If the authors had chosen to conduct the study with this design and had found the same results, they would have been less confident of the results because selection effects may have been more problematic.

A study by Hall and colleagues (2004) used an after-only quasiexperimental design to test the preliminary efficacy of an adult learning theory-based training curriculum with adult peritoneal dialysis outpatients. New patients starting peritoneal dialysis were trained using the experimental curriculum or a conventional training program. Because patients were new to peritoneal dialysis, there were no preintervention data available for comparison (i.e., infection rate), so a quasiexperimental after-only design was used. The two groups were compared on outcomes after the program completion, and the patients who participated in the theory-based training curriculum had fewer exit site infections, better fluid balance, and better adherence to treatment than those in the conventional program. Thus the researchers were able to demonstrate the preliminary efficacy of this new program in improving patient outcomes in peritoneal dialysis.

Another quasiexperimental design is a **one-group (pretest-posttest) design** (Figure 10-2, *C*), which is used by researchers when only one group is available for study. Data are collected before and after an experimental treatment on one group of subjects. In this type of design, there is no control group and no randomization, which are important characteristics that enhance the internal validity of the study. Therefore it becomes important that the evidence generated by the findings of this type of quasiexperimental design is interpreted with careful consideration of the design limitations.

Davison and colleagues (2003) (see Appendix D) conducted a one-group (pretest-posttest) design to determine the benefits of providing individualized information, based on a computerized assessment, to men newly diagnosed with prostate cancer and their spouses. While improvements in psychological status and treatment decision making were reported, the likelihood of alternative explanations is high with this type of design (i.e., any individualized attention provided to subjects in this situation may be ben-

eficial, or it is possible that psychological distress would have improved over time without any intervention). However, this study allowed the researchers to evaluate the feasibility and potential benefits of using a computerized program to help focus and individualize counseling sessions. The researchers clearly identify the limitations of the study design and report that a subsequent study is being undertaken using an experimental design to test this potentially effective intervention.

Another approach used by researchers when only one group is available is to study that group over a longer period of time. This quasiexperimental design is called a **time series design,** and it is illustrated in Figure 10-2, *D*. Time series designs are useful for determining trends. Data are collected multiple times before the introduction of the treatment to establish a baseline point of reference on outcomes. The experimental treatment is introduced, and data are collected multiple times afterward to determine a change from baseline. The broad range and number of data-collection points helps to rule out alternative explanations, such as history effects. However, a testing threat to validity is present due to multiple data-collection points, and without a control group, the threats of selection and maturation cannot be ruled out (see Chapter 9).

> **HELPFUL** HINT
>
> One of the reasons replication is so important in nursing research is that so many problems cannot be subjected to experimental methods. Therefore the consistency of findings across many populations helps support a cause-and-effect relationship even when an experiment cannot be conducted.

Advantages and Disadvantages of Quasiexperimental Designs

Given the problems inherent in interpreting the results of studies using quasiexperimental designs, you may be wondering why anyone would use them. Quasiexperimental designs are used frequently because they are practical, feasible, and generalizable. These designs are more adaptable to the real-world practice setting than the controlled experimental designs. In addition, for some hypotheses, these designs may be the only way to evaluate the effect of the independent variable of interest.

The weaknesses of the quasiexperimental approach involve mainly the inability to make clear cause-and-effect statements. However, if the researcher can rule out any plausible alternative explanations for the findings, such studies can lead to increased knowledge about causal relationships. Researchers have several options for ruling out these alternative explanations. They may control extraneous variables (alternative events that could explain the findings) **a priori** (before initiating the intervention) by design. There are also methods to control extraneous variables statistically. In some cases, common sense knowledge of the problem and the population can suggest that a particular explanation is not plausible. Nonetheless, it is important to replicate such studies to support the causal assertions developed through the use of quasiexperimental designs.

The literature on cigarette smoking is an excellent example of how findings from many studies, experimental and quasiexperimental, can be linked to establish a causal relationship. A large number of well-controlled experiments with laboratory animals randomly assigned to smoking and nonsmoking conditions have documented that lung disease will develop in smoking animals. Although such evidence is suggestive of a link between smoking and lung disease in humans, it is not directly transferable because animals and humans are different. However, we cannot randomly assign humans to smoking and nonsmoking groups for ethical and other reasons. So researchers interested in this problem have to use quasiexperimental data to test their hypotheses about smoking and lung disease. Several different quasiexperimental designs have been used to study this problem, and all had similar results—a causal relationship

does exist between cigarette smoking and lung disease. Note that the combination of results from both experimental and quasiexperimental studies led to the conclusion that smoking causes cancer because the studies together meet the causal criteria of relationship, timing, and lack of an alternative explanation. Nonetheless, the tobacco industry has taken the stand that because the studies on humans are not true experiments, there may be another explanation for the relationships that have been found. For example, they suggest that the tendency to smoke is linked to the tendency for lung disease to develop and smoking is merely an unimportant intervening variable. The reader needs to study the evidence from multiple studies to determine whether the cause-and-effect relationship postulated is believable.

 EVIDENCE-BASED PRACTICE TIP

Experimental designs are considered Level II and quasiexperimental designs are considered Level III. Quasiexperimental designs are lower on the hierarchy of evidence due to lack of some research control, which limits the ability to make confident cause-and-effect statements that influence clinical decision making.

EVALUATION RESEARCH AND EXPERIMENTATION

As the science of nursing expands and the cost of health care rises, nurses and other health professionals have become increasingly concerned with the ability to document the costs and the benefits of nursing care (see Chapter 1). This is a complex process, but at its heart is the ability to evaluate or measure the outcomes of nursing care. Such studies usually are associated with quality assurance, quality improvement, and evaluation. Studies of evaluation or quality assurance do exactly what the name implies—such studies are concerned with the determination of the quality of nursing and health care and with assurance that the public is receiving high-quality care.

Quality assurance and quality improvement in nursing are a present and important topic for nursing care. Experimentation techniques are just beginning to be applied to the study of the delivery of nursing care. Many early quality assurance studies documented whether nursing care met predetermined standards. More recently, the goal of quality improvement studies is to evaluate the effectiveness of nursing interventions and to provide direction for further improvement in the achievement of quality clinical outcomes and cost effectiveness.

Evaluation research is the use of scientific research methods and procedures to evaluate a program, treatment, practice, or policy; it uses analytical means to document the worth of an activity. Such research is not a different design. Evaluation research uses both experimental and quasiexperimental designs (as well as nonexperimental designs) for the purpose of determining the effect or outcomes of a program (see Chapter 19). Bigman (1961) listed the following purposes and uses of evaluation research:

1. To test whether and how well the project's objectives are met
2. To determine the reasons for specific successes and failures
3. To direct the course of experiment with techniques for increasing effectiveness
4. To uncover principles underlying a successful program
5. To base further research on the reasons for the relative success of alternative techniques
6. To redefine the means to be used for attaining objectives and to redefine subgoals, in light of research findings

Evaluation studies may be formative and/or summative. Formative evaluation refers to assessment of a program as it is being implemented; usually the focus is on evaluation of the process of a program rather than the outcomes. Summative evaluation refers to the assessment of the outcomes of a program that is conducted after completion of the initial program.

Majumdar and colleagues (2004) used a summative evaluation with an experimental design to evaluate the effectiveness of a cultural sensitivity training program (delivered to health care providers) on the knowledge and attitudes of health care providers and on the satisfaction and health outcomes of patients from different minority groups whose providers received the training. In contrast, Marshall and colleagues (2001) used formative evaluation to describe the process of care associated with implementing venous leg ulcer guidelines in primary health care. Knowledge related to summative (outcomes) and formative (process) evaluation of programs is important in translating research into clinical practice.

The use of experimental and quasiexperimental designs in quality improvement and evaluation studies allows for the determination of not only whether care is adequate but also which method of care is best under certain conditions. Furthermore, such studies can be used to determine whether a particular type of nursing care is cost effective, that is, not only that the health benefits of the care are reached but also that the care is achieved at a cost less than or equal to the projected expenditure. Duren-Winfield and colleagues (2000) describe the background of an ongoing cost-effectiveness analysis of an exercise program for patients with chronic respiratory disease. In an era of health care reform and cost containment for health expenditures, it has become increasingly important to evaluate the relative costs and benefits of new programs of care. Therefore nursing costs and cost savings will be important outcomes to evaluate in future studies.

 HELPFUL H I N T

Think of quality assurance and quality improvement projects as research-related activities that enhance the ability of nurses to generate cost and quality outcome data. These outcome data contribute to documenting the way nursing practice makes a difference.

Experimental and Quasiexperimental Designs

As discussed earlier in the chapter, various designs for research studies differ in the amount of control the researcher has over the antecedent and intervening variables that may impact the results of the study. True experimental designs, which provide Level II evidence, offer the most possibility for control, and preexperimental designs (Levels IV, V, or VI) offer the least. Quasiexperimental designs, which provide Level III evidence, fall somewhere in between. Research designs must balance the needs for internal validity and external validity to produce useful results. In addition, judicious use of design requires that the chosen design be appropriate to the problem, free of bias, and capable of answering the research question.

Questions that the reader should pose when reading studies that test cause-and-effect relationships are listed in the following Critiquing Criteria box. All of these questions should help

CRITIQUING CRITERIA *Experimental and Quasiexperimental Designs*

1. What design is used in the study?
2. Is the design experimental or quasiexperimental?
3. Is the problem one of a cause-and-effect relationship?
4. Is the method used appropriate to the problem?
5. Is the design suited to the setting of the study?

Experimental Designs

1. What experimental design is used in the study, and is it appropriate?
2. How are randomization, control, and manipulation applied?
3. Are there any reasons to believe that there are alternative explanations for the findings?
4. Are all threats to validity, including mortality, addressed in the report?
5. Whether the experiment was conducted in the laboratory or a clinical setting, are the findings generalizable to the larger population of interest?

Quasiexperimental Designs

1. What quasiexperimental design is used in the study, and is it appropriate?
2. What are the most common threats to the validity of the findings of this design?
3. What are the plausible alternative explanations, and have they been addressed?
4. Are the author's explanations of threats to validity acceptable?
5. What does the author say about the limitations of the study?
6. Are there other limitations related to the design that are not mentioned?

Evaluation Research

1. Does the study identify a specific problem, practice, policy, or treatment that it will evaluate?
2. Are the outcomes to be evaluated identified?
3. Is the problem analyzed and described?
4. Is the program to be analyzed described and standardized?
5. Is measurement of the degree of change (outcome) that occurs identified?
6. Is there a determination of whether the observed outcome is related to the activity or to some other cause(s)?

the reader judge whether it can be confidently believed that a causal relationship exists.

For studies in which either experimental or quasiexperimental designs are used, first try to determine the type of design that was used. Often a statement describing the design of the study appears in the abstract and in the methods section of the paper. If such a statement is not present, the reader should examine the paper for evidence of the following three characteristics: control, randomization, and manipulation. If all are discussed, the design is probably experimental. On the other hand, if the study involves the administration of an experimental treatment but does not involve the random assignment of subjects to groups, the design is quasiexperimental. Next, try to identify which of the various designs within these two types of designs was used. Determining the answer to these questions gives you a head start, because each design has its inherent threats to validity and this step makes it a bit easier to critically evaluate the study. The next question to ask is whether the researcher required a solution to a cause-and-effect problem. If so, the study is suited to these designs. Finally, think about the conduct of the study in the setting. Is it realistic to think that the study could be conducted in a clinical setting without some contamination?

The most important question to ask yourself as you read experimental studies is the following: "What else could have happened to explain the findings?" Thus it is important that the author provide adequate accounts of how the procedures for randomization, control, and manipulation were carried out. The paper should include a description of the procedures for random assignment to such a degree that the reader could determine just how likely it was for any one subject to be assigned to a particular group. The description of the independent variable also should be detailed. The inclusion of this information helps the reader decide if it is possible that the treatment given to some subjects in the experimental group might be different from

what was given to others in the same group. In addition, threats to validity, such as testing and mortality, should be addressed. Otherwise there is the potential for the findings of the study to be in error and less believable to the reader.

 HELPFUL HINT

Remember that mortality is a problem in most experimental studies because data are usually collected more than once. The researcher should demonstrate that the groups are equivalent when they enter the study and that subjects who do not complete the study are not different from subjects who complete the study.

This question of potential alternative explanations or threats to internal validity for the findings is even more important when critically evaluating a quasiexperimental study because quasiexperimental designs cannot possibly control many plausible alternative explanations. A well-written report of a quasiexperimental study systematically reviews potential threats to the validity of the findings. Then the reader's work is to decide if the author's explanations make sense.

When critiquing evaluation research, the reader should look for a careful description of the program, policy, procedure, or treatment being evaluated. In addition, the reader may need to determine the design used to evaluate the program and assess the appropriateness of the design for the evaluation. Once the design has been determined, the reader assesses threats to validity for the appropriate design in determining the appropriateness of the author's conclusions related to the outcomes. As with all research, studies using these designs need to be generalizable to a larger population of people than those actually studied. Thus it is important to decide whether the experimental protocol eliminated some potential subjects and whether this affected not only internal validity but also external validity.

Critical Thinking Challenges

- Discuss the barriers to nurse researchers meeting the three criteria of a true experimental design.
- How is it possible to have a research design that includes an experimental treatment intervention and a control group, yet is not considered a true experimental study? How does this affect the usefulness of the findings in an evidence-based practice?
- Argue your case for supporting or not supporting the following claim, include examples with your rationale: "A study that does not use true experimental design does not decrease the value of the study even though it may decrease the utility of the findings in practice."
- Respond to the following question. Why are experimental studies considered the best evidence for an evidence-based practice model? Justify your answer.

KEY POINTS

- Experimental designs or randomized clinical trials provide the strongest evidence (Level II) in terms of whether an intervention or treatment impacts patient outcomes.
- Two types of design commonly used in nursing research to test hypotheses about cause-and-effect relationships are experimental and quasi-experimental designs. Both are useful for the development of nursing knowledge because they test the effects of nursing actions and lead to the development of prescriptive theory.
- True experiments are characterized by the ability of the researcher to control extraneous variation, to manipulate the independent variable, and to randomly assign subjects to research groups.
- Experiments conducted either in clinical settings or in the laboratory provide the best evidence in support of a causal relationship because the following three criteria can be met: (1) the independent and dependent variables are related to each other; (2) the independent variable chronologically precedes the dependent variable; and (3) the relationship cannot be explained by the presence of a third variable.
- Researchers frequently turn to quasiexperimental designs to test cause-and-effect relationships because experimental designs often are impractical or unethical.
- Quasiexperiments may lack either the randomization or the comparison group characteristics

of true experiments, or both of these factors. Their usefulness in studying causal relationships depends on the ability of the researcher to rule out plausible threats to the validity of the findings, such as history, selection, maturation, and testing effects.

- The level of evidence (Level III) provided by quasiexperimental designs weakens confidence that the findings were the result of the intervention rather than extraneous variables.
- The overall purpose of critiquing such studies is to assess the validity of the findings and to determine whether these findings are worth incorporating into the nurse's personal practice.

REFERENCES

Bigman SK: Evaluating the effectiveness of religious programs, *Rev Relig Res* 2: 99-110, 1961.

Brooten D et al.: Lessons learned from testing the quality cost model of advanced practice nursing (APN) transitional care, *J Nurs Scholarship* 34: 369-375, 2002.

Campbell D, Stanley J: *Experimental and quasiexperimental designs for research,* Chicago, 1966, Rand-McNally.

Coleman EA et al.: The Delta Project: increasing breast cancer screening among rural minority and older women by targeting rural healthcare providers, *Oncol Nurs Forum* 30: 669-677, 2003.

Davison BJ et al.: Provision of individualized information to men and their partners to facilitate treatment decision making in prostate cancer, *Oncol Nurs Forum* 30(1): 107-114, 2003.

Duren-Winfield V et al.: Cost-effectiveness analysis methods for the REACT study, *West J Nurs Res* 22: 460-474, 2000.

Grey M et al.: Coping skills training for youth with diabetes mellitus has long-lasting effects on metabolic control and quality of life, *J Pediatr* 137: 107-113, 2000.

Hall G et al.: New directions in peritoneal dialysis patient training, *Nephrol Nurs J* 31: 159-163, 2004.

Hirshberg J et al.: TGF-s3 in the treatment of pressure ulcers: a preliminary report, *Adv Skin Wound Care* 14: 91-95, 2001.

Koniak-Griffin et al.: Nurse visitation for adolescent mothers, *Nurs Res* 52(2): 127-136, 2003.

Majumdar B et al.: Effects of cultural sensitivity training on health care provider attitudes and patient outcomes, *J Nurs Scholarship* 36: 161-166, 2004.

Marshall JL et al.: The implementation of venous leg ulcer guidelines: process analysis of the intervention used in a multi-centre, pragmatic, randomized, controlled trial, *J Clin Nurs* 10: 758-766, 2001.

Swanson K: Effects of caring, measurement, and time on miscarriage impact and women's well-being, *Nurs Res* 48: 288-298, 1999.

Whittemore R, Grey M: The systematic development of nursing interventions, *J Nurs Scholarship* 34: 115-120, 2002.

FOR FURTHER STUDY

Go to your Companion CD for review activities for this chapter.

evolve Go to Evolve at http://evolve.elsevier.com/LoBiondo/ for WebLinks, Content Updates, and additional research articles, for practice in reviewing and critiquing.

11

GERI LOBIONDO-WOOD

JUDITH HABER

Nonexperimental Designs

KEY TERMS

cohort
correlational study
cross-sectional studies
developmental studies
ex post facto studies

longitudinal studies
meta-analysis
methodological research
nonexperimental research designs
prospective studies

psychometrics
relationship/difference studies
retrospective studies
secondary analysis
survey studies

LEARNING OUTCOMES

After reading this chapter, the student should be able to do the following:

- Describe the overall purpose of nonexperimental designs.
- Describe the characteristics of survey, relationship, and difference designs.
- Define the differences between survey, relationship, and difference designs.
- List the advantages and disadvantages of surveys and each type of relationship and difference designs.
- Identify methodological, secondary analysis, and meta-analysis types of research.
- Identify the purposes of methodological, secondary analysis, and meta-analysis types of research.
- Discuss relational inferences versus causal inferences as they relate to nonexperimental designs.
- Identify the criteria used to critique nonexperimental research designs.
- Apply the critiquing criteria to the evaluation of nonexperimental research designs as they appear in research reports.
- Apply levels of evidence to nonexperimental designs.

STUDY RESOURCES

Go to your Companion CD for review activities for this chapter.

evolve Go to Evolve at http://evolve.elsevier.com/LoBiondo/ for Weblinks, Content Updates, and additional research articles for practice in reviewing and critiquing.

Many phenomena of interest and relevant to nursing do not lend themselves to an experimental design. For example, nurses studying pain may be interested in the amount of pain, variations in the amount of pain, and patient responses to postoperative pain. The investigator would not design an experimental study that would potentially intensify a patient's pain just to study the pain experience. Instead, the researcher would examine the factors that contribute to the variability in a patient's postoperative pain experience using a nonexperimental design. Nonexperimental designs are used in studies in which the researcher wishes to construct a picture of a phenomenon; explore events, people, or situations as they naturally occur; or test relationships and differences among variables. Nonexperimental designs may construct a picture of a phenomenon at one point or over a period of time.

In experimental research the independent variable is manipulated; in nonexperimental research it is not. In nonexperimental research the independent variables have naturally occurred, so to speak, and the investigator cannot directly control them by manipulation. In contrast, in an experimental design the researcher actively manipulates one or more variables, and in a nonexperimental design the researcher explores relationships or differences among the variables. Nonexperimental research requires a clear, concise research problem or hypothesis that is based on a theoretical framework. Even though the researcher does not actively manipulate the variables, the concepts of control (see Chapter 9) should be considered as much as possible. Nonexperimental research provides Level IV evidence. The strength of evidence provided by nonexperimental designs is not as strong as that for experimental designs because there is a different degree of control within the study; that is, the independent variable is not manipulated, subjects are not randomized, and there is no control group.

Researchers are not in agreement on how to classify nonexperimental studies. A continuum of quantitative research design is presented in Figure 11-1. Nonexperimental studies explore the relationships or the differences between variables. This chapter divides nonexperimental designs into survey studies and relationship/difference studies as illustrated in Box 11-1. These categories are somewhat flexible, and other sources may classify nonexperimental studies in a different way. Some studies fall exclusively within one of these categories, whereas other studies have characteristics of more than one category (see Table 11-1). As you read the research literature you will often find that researchers who are conducting a nonexperimental study use several design classifications. This chapter introduces the various types of nonexperimental designs and discusses their advantages and disadvantages, the use of nonexperimental research, the issues of causality, and the critiquing process as it relates to nonexperimental research. The Critical Thinking Decision Path shown below outlines the path to the choice of a nonexperimental design.

BOX 11-1   SUMMARY OF NONEXPERIMENTAL RESEARCH DESIGNS

I. SURVEY STUDIES

A. Descriptive
B. Exploratory
C. Comparative

II. RELATIONSHIP/DIFFERENCE STUDIES

A. Correlational studies
B. Developmental studies
   1. Cross-sectional
   2. Longitudinal and prospective
   3. Retrospective and ex post facto

Nonexperimental ⟶ Quasiexperimental ⟶ Experimental

Figure 11-1. Continuum of quantitative research design.

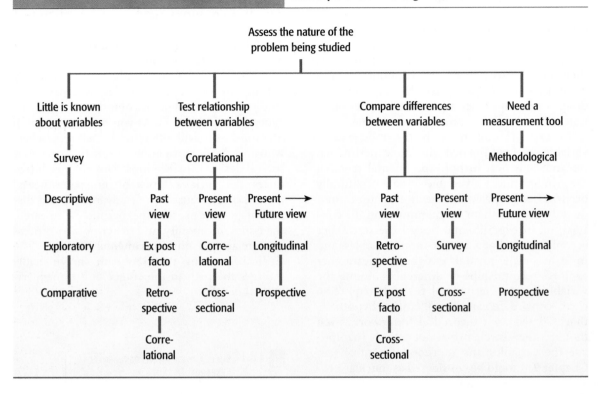

CRITICAL THINKING DECISION PATH | Nonexperimental Design Choice

 EVIDENCE-BASED PRACTICE TIP

When critically appraising nonexperimental studies, you need to be aware of possible sources of bias that can be introduced at any point in the study.

SURVEY STUDIES

The broadest category of nonexperimental designs is the survey study. **Survey studies** are further classified as descriptive, exploratory, or comparative. *Descriptive, exploratory,* or *comparative surveys* collect detailed descriptions of existing variables and use the data to justify and assess current conditions and practices or to

make plans for improving health care practices. The reader of research will find that the terms *exploratory, descriptive, comparative,* and *survey* are used either alone, interchangeably, or together to describe the design of a study (see Table 11-1). Investigators may use a descriptive or exploratory survey design to search for accurate information about the characteristics of particular subjects, groups, institutions, or situations or about the frequency of a phenomenon's occurrence, particularly when little is known about the phenomenon. The types of variables of interest can be classified as opinions, attitudes, or facts. Thimbault-Prevost, Jensen, and Hodgins (2000) conducted a survey study to explore the perceptions of nurses regarding do-not-resuscitate (DNR) decisions in the critical care setting. Studies such as this provide the basis for the development of educational programs that help health care professionals understand issues regarding DNR decisions.

Fact variables include attributes of individuals that are a function of their membership in society, such as gender, income level, political and religious affiliations, ethnicity, occupation, and educational level. Burns, Camaione, and Chatterton (2000) conducted a survey study that explored facts. The overall purpose of their study was to determine whether adult nurse practitioners (ANPs) met the objective of routinely counseling clients about physical activity. To accomplish this aim, the researchers conducted a national survey of 1000 ANPs. They asked the ANPs if they counseled people about physical activity, and if so, the ANPs were asked to describe the methods and guidelines they used to access and counsel clients about physical activity. The ANPs also were asked about the perceived barriers to physical activity counseling. The researchers noted that the significance of this study was to assess if nurse practitioners, who provide a significant amount of primary care, were meeting the national *Healthy People 2010* objective of promoting health. The results provide useful information about how nurses in advance roles are working toward improving health and preventing disease.

Surveys are comparative when they are used to determine differences between variables. Anderson, Higgins, and Rozmus (1999) conducted a comparative survey study that addressed an important dimension of health care—cost containment. They conducted a descriptive, comparative survey study to examine the length of stay in the intensive care unit (ICU) after coronary artery bypass graft (CABG) surgery relative to the number of hours postoperation, when ambulation occurred, and the overall postoperative length of hospital stay. This study assessed whether patients who ambulated earlier after surgery spent less time in the ICU. The study did find a significant difference between ICU length of stay and the time when ambulation began. This study, like the two previously discussed, does not manipulate variables but assesses data in order to provide data for future nursing intervention studies.

Data in survey research can be collected through a questionnaire or an interview (see Chapter 14). For example, Valente and Saunders (2004) wanted to explore nurses' knowledge and attitudes about suicide and to assess the barriers to suicide-risk management perceived by oncology nurses. They surveyed a random sample of 1200 nurses from the Oncology Nursing Society. Potential subjects were given a demographic inventory, the Suicide Opinion Questionnaire, a suicide attitude measure, and a vignette of a suicidal patient. Though there are standards of practice that identify the nurse's role in risk detection, intervention, and management, little is known about the barriers to fulfilling this role. This survey added to the body of literature that will aid in educating and supporting nurses in this role. Survey researchers study either small or large samples of subjects drawn from defined populations. The sample can be either broad or narrow and can be made up of people or institutions. For example, if a primary care rehabilitation unit based on a case management model were to be established in a hospital, a survey might be done on the prospective applicants' attitudes with regard to case management before the unit staff are selected. In a broader example, if a hospital were contemplating converting all patient care units to a case management model, a survey might be conducted to determine attitudes of a representative sample of nurses in the hospital toward case management. The data might provide the basis for projecting in-service needs of nursing regarding case management. The scope and depth of a survey are a function of the nature of the problem.

In surveys investigators attempt only to relate one variable to another, or assess differences between variables, but they do not attempt to determine causation. The two major advantages of surveys are that a great deal of information can be obtained from a large population in a fairly economical manner and that survey research information can be surprisingly accurate. If a sample is representative of the population (see Chapter 12), a relatively small number of subjects can provide an accurate picture of the population.

Survey studies have several disadvantages. First, the information obtained in a survey tends to be superficial. The breadth rather than the depth of the information is emphasized. Second, conducting a survey requires a great deal of expertise in various research areas. The survey investigator must know sampling techniques, questionnaire construction, interviewing, and data analysis to produce a reliable and valid study. Third, large-scale surveys can be time-consuming and costly, although the use of on-site personnel can reduce costs.

 HELPFUL HINT

Research consumers should recognize that a well-constructed survey can provide a wealth of data about a particular phenomenon of interest, even though causation is not being examined.

 EVIDENCE-BASED PRACTICE TIP

Evidence gained from a survey may be coupled with clinical expertise and applied to a similar population to develop an educational program to enhance knowledge and skills in a particular clinical area (e.g., a survey designed to measure the nursing staff's knowledge and attitudes about EBP where the data are used to develop an EBP staff development course).

RELATIONSHIP AND DIFFERENCE STUDIES

Investigators also endeavor to trace the relationships or differences between variables that can provide a deeper insight into a phenomenon. These studies can be classified as relationship or difference studies. The following types of **relationship/difference studies** are discussed: correlational studies and developmental studies.

Correlational Studies

In a **correlational study** an investigator examines the relationship between two or more variables. The researcher is not testing whether one variable causes another variable or how different one variable is from another variable. The researcher is testing whether the variables co-vary; that is, as one variable changes, does a related change occur in the other variable? The researcher using this design is interested in quantifying the strength of the relationship between the variables or in testing a hypothesis about a specific relationship. The positive or negative direction of the relationship is also a central concern (see Chapter 16 for an explanation of the correlation coefficient). For example, in their correlational study, Redeker, Ruggiero, and Hedges (2004) explored if there was a relationship between sleep patterns and physical functioning and emotional well-being 4 weeks and 8 weeks after cardiac surgery. The researchers noted that the previous research literature suggests that evidence of altered sleep patterns contributes to physical function, and emotional well-being. Yet researchers have not examined the separate contributions of sleep pattern alteration to physical function and emotional well-being in order to guide the future development of sleep-promoting interventions. In the theoretical framework and literature review, the researchers noted the importance of understanding sleep problem alterations, physical functioning, and well-being after cardiac surgery. Each step of this study was consistent with the aims of exploring a relationship among the variables.

It should be remembered that the researchers were not testing a cause-and-effect relationship. All that is known is that the researchers found a relationship and that one variable (sleep pattern alterations) varied in a consistent way with the variables of physical functioning and emotional well-being for the particular sample studied. When reviewing a correlational study, remember what relationship the researcher tested and notice whether the researcher implied a relationship that is consistent with the theoretical framework and hypotheses being tested. Correlational studies offer researchers and research consumers the following advantages:

- An increased flexibility when investigating complex relationships among variables
- An efficient and effective method of collecting a large amount of data about a problem
- A potential for evidence-based application in clinical settings
- A potential foundation for future, experimental research studies
- A framework for exploring the relationship between variables that cannot be inherently manipulated

The reader will find that the correlational design has a quality of realism and is particularly appealing because it suggests the potential for practical solutions to clinical problems. The following are disadvantages of correlational studies:

- The researcher is unable to manipulate the variables of interest.
- The researcher does not employ randomization in the sampling procedures because of dealing with preexisting groups, and therefore generalizability is decreased.
- The researcher is unable to determine a causal relationship between the variables because of the lack of manipulation, control, and randomization.
- The strength and quality of evidence is limited by the associative nature of the relationship between the variables.

A misuse of a correlational design would be if the researcher concluded that a causal relationship exists between the variables. In their study, Redeker and associates (2004) appropriately concluded that a relationship existed between the variables, not that patient's sleep patterns caused physical functioning and well-being changes.

The investigators also appropriately concluded that their findings extend those of previous research and suggest a focus for future intervention studies (e.g., Level II randomized clinical trial [RCT] or Level III quasiexperimental study) that promote sleep.

Correlational studies may be further labeled as *descriptive correlational or predictive correlational*. The study by Redeker et al. (2004) would be an example of descriptive correlational as the study's goal was to describe the relationship of variables over time. A study by Clark and associates (2004) that examined the influence of stroke survivor motor function, memory, and behavior changes and the family conflict surrounding stroke recovery on the mental and physical health of caregivers during the subacute recovery period is classified as a correlational, cross-sectional study. This study tested multiple variables to assess the relationship among the variables and the ability of the chosen variables to predict caregiver outcomes. The researchers concluded that several of the variables were able to predict (not cause) caregiver outcomes. This study would also be classified as predictive correlational.

Given the level of evidence provided by this study, the ability to generalize the findings has some limitations, but the authors do conclude with some very thoughtful recommendations for future studies in this area. This study is a well-presented example of a clinical study that uses a correlational design. The inability to draw causal statements should not lead the research consumer to conclude that a nonexperimental correlational study uses a weak design. In terms of evidence for practice, the researchers, based on the literature review and their findings, frame the utility of the results in light of previous research and therefore help to establish supportive evidence of the study's applicability to a specific patient population. A correlational design is a very useful design for clinical research studies because many of the phenomena of clinical interest are beyond the researcher's ability to manipulate, control, and randomize.

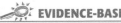 **EVIDENCE-BASED PRACTICE TIP**

Establishment of a strong relationship in predictive correlational studies often lends support for attempting to influence the independent variable in a future intervention study.

Developmental Studies

There are also classifications of nonexperimental designs that use a time perspective. Investigators who use **developmental studies** are concerned not only with the existing status and the relationship and differences among phenomena at one point in time but also with changes that result from elapsed time. The following three types of developmental study designs are discussed: cross-sectional, longitudinal or prospective, and retrospective or ex post facto. Remember that in the literature, however, studies may be designated by more than one design name. This practice is accepted because many studies have elements of several nonexperimental designs. Table 11-1 provides examples of studies classified with more than one design label.

Cross-Sectional Studies

Cross-sectional studies examine data at one point in time, that is, data collected on only one occasion with the same subjects rather than with the same subjects at several time points. For example, Nyamathi and associates (2000) studied the type of social support reported by homeless women and examined the characteristics of homeless women with different types of support. The data were collected from 1302 sheltered homeless women. Each woman (subject) met with an investigator on one occasion when the questionnaires were administered. The goal was to explore what types of support were associated with psychosocial profiles, health behaviors, and use of medical care.

Another cross-sectional study approach is to simultaneously collect data on the study's

TABLE 11-1 **Examples of Studies with More than One Design Label**

Design Type	Study's Purpose
Descriptive with repeated measures	To evaluate the impact of intervention dosage on client outcomes in different case management models within substance abuse (Huber et al., 2003)
Descriptive, correlational	To examine relationships among mothers' resilience, family health-promoting activity, and mothers' health-promoting lifestyle practices in families with preschool children (Monteith and Ford-Gilboe, 2002)
Correlational, cross-sectional	To examine the influence of stroke survivors' motor function, memory, and behavior changes as well as family conflict surrounding stroke recovery on the mental and physical health of caregivers during the subacute recovery period (Clark et al., 2004)
Descriptive, longitudinal	To examine the pain experience management strategies and outcomes during the first year after diagnosis of acute leukemia (Van Cleve et al., 2004)
Correlational, predictive	To determine whether pain, depression, and fatigue are significant factors in the return of older adults to functional status after having major abdominal surgery, and examination of self-perception of recovery in the first 3 months following discharge from the hospital (Zalon, 2004)
Prospective, comparative, longitudinal	To prospectively describe patient outcomes and caregiving experiences after early discharge following elective abdominal aortic aneurysm repair using a standard or endovascular grafting system procedure (Jones et al., 2002)

variables from different subject groups. An example of a cross-sectional study with different groups is one conducted by Stastny et al. (2004). This study assessed newborn placement practices of the mother and nursery staff and their inter-relationship in the hospital setting. Clinically this is an important study because past research has shown that the most modifiable infant care sudden infant death syndrome (SIDS) risk factor appears to be prone sleeping position. Thus understanding what is taught and how the infor-mation is given and used is important. The cohorts were nurses from different hospitals nurseries in Orange County, California. Nurses and mothers of newborns from the hospitals completed the study's questionnaire on one occasion, and then responses were compared between the different groups of mothers and nurses.

Cross-sectional studies can explore relation-ships and correlations, or differences and com-parisons, or both. For instance, the study by Nyamathi and associates (2000) about homeless women and social support posed research ques-tions that allowed them to explore both differ-ences and relationships among and between variables.

 EVIDENCE-BASED PRACTICE TIP

Replication of significant findings in nonexperimental studies, using similar and/or different populations, increases your confidence in the conclusions offered by the researcher and the strength of evidence generated by consistent findings from more than one study.

Longitudinal/Prospective Studies

In contrast to the cross-sectional design, **longi-tudinal** or **prospective studies** collect data from the same group at different points in time. Prospective or longitudinal studies also explore differences and relationships. Longitudinal studies also are referred to as a *repeated measures*

or *cohort* studies (see Chapter 20). For instance, the investigator conducting a study with diabetic children could elect to use a longitudinal design. In that case the investigator could collect yearly data or follow the same children over a number of years to compare changes in the variables at different ages. By collecting data from each subject at yearly intervals, a longitudinal per-spective of the diabetic process is accomplished. As another example of a longitudinal study, LoBiondo-Wood, Williams, and McGhee (2004) collected data on 2 occasions at least 5 years apart (pretransplatation and at least 5 years after the child's transplantation) from a sample of 15 mothers whose children had received a liver transplant. The purpose of the study was to examine the relationship of family stress, sever-ity of the stressors, uncertainty, coping, and family adaptation over the 5-year period from pretransplantation to posttransplanatation.

Van Cleve and associates (2004, Appendix B) conducted a descriptive longitudinal study whose purpose was to examine the pain experi-ence, management strategies, and outcomes during the first year after the diagnosis of acute leukemia in children. Data were collected on a total of seven occasions over a period of 1 year to look for differences that may have existed among the subjects at each time period.

Cross-sectional and longitudinal designs have many advantages and disadvantages. When assessing the appropriateness of a cross-sectional study versus a longitudinal study, the research consumer should first assess the nature of the research question: What is the researcher's goal in light of the theoretical framework and the strength of evidence that will be provided by the findings? For example, in the study of a family's adaptation to transplantation, the researchers are exploring a developmental process; therefore a longitudinal design seems more appropriate. Longitudinal research allows clinicians to assess the incidence of a problem over time and poten-tial reasons for changes in the variables of study. However, the disadvantages inherent in a longi-tudinal design also must be considered. Data collection may be of long duration and costs therefore high because of the time it takes for the subjects to progress to each data-collection point. In the family adaptation to liver transplantation study, it took the researchers approximately 6 years to collect the data for the total sample. Internal validity threats such as testing and mortality also are ever-present and unavoidable in a longitudinal study. Subject loss to follow-up and attrition, whether due to drop out or death, may lead to unintended sample bias that affects external validity and generalizability of the findings.

These realities make a longitudinal design costly in terms of time, effort, and money. There is also a chance of confounding variables that could affect the interpretation of the results. Subjects in such a study may respond in a socially desirable way that they believe is congruent with the investigator's expectations (see Hawthorne Effect in Chapters 9 and 10). However, despite the pragmatic constraints imposed by a longitudinal study, the researcher should proceed with this design if the theoretical framework supports a longitudinal developmental perspective.

One advantage of a longitudinal study is that each subject is followed separately and thereby serves as his or her own control; other advantages are increased depth of responses can be obtained and early trends in the data can be analyzed. The researcher can assess changes in the variables of interest over time, and both relationships and differences can be explored between variables.

Cross-sectional studies, when compared to longitudinal studies, are less time-consuming, less expensive, and thus more manageable for the researcher. Because large amounts of data can be collected at one point, the results are more readily available. In addition, the confounding variable of maturation, resulting from the elapsed time, is not present. However, the investigator's ability to establish an in-depth developmental assessment of the interrelationships of the phenomena being studied is lessened. Thus the researcher is unable to determine whether the change that occurred is related to the change that

was predicted because the same subjects were not followed over a period of time. In other words, the subjects are unable to serve as their own controls (see Chapter 9). In summary, longitudinal studies begin in the present and end in the future, and cross-sectional studies look at a broader perspective of a cross section of the population at a specific point in time.

 EVIDENCE-BASED PRACTICE TIP

The quality of evidence provided by a longitudinal cohort study is stronger than that from other nonexperimental designs because the researcher can determine the incidence of a problem and its possible causes.

Retrospective/Ex Post Facto Studies

Retrospective studies are essentially the same as **ex post facto studies.** Epidemiologists primarily use the term *retrospective,* whereas social scientists prefer the term *ex post facto* (see Chapter 20). In either case, the dependent variable already has been affected by the independent variable, and the investigator attempts to link present events to events that have occurred in the past. When scientists wish to explain causality or the factors that determine the occurrence of events or conditions, they prefer to employ an experimental design. However, they cannot always manipulate the independent variable, X, or use random assignments. In cases in which experimental designs that test the effect of an intervention or condition cannot be employed, ex post facto studies may be used. Ex post facto literally means "from after the fact." Ex post facto or retrospective studies also are known as *case control, causal-comparative* studies or *comparative* studies. As we discuss this design further, you will see that many elements of ex post facto research are similar to quasiexperimental designs because they explore differences between variables (Campbell and Stanley, 1963).

In retrospective/ex post facto studies, a researcher hypothesizes, for instance, that X

(cigarette smoking) is related to and a determinant of *Y* (lung cancer), but *X*, the presumed cause, is not manipulated and subjects are not randomly assigned to groups. Rather, a group of subjects who have experienced *X* (cigarette smoking) in a normal situation is located and a control group of subjects who have not experienced *X* is chosen. The behavior, performance, or condition (lung tissue) of the two groups is compared to determine whether the exposure to *X* had the effect predicted by the hypothesis. Table 11-2 illustrates this example. Examination of Table 11-2 reveals that although cigarette smoking appears to be a determinant of lung cancer, the researcher is still not able to conclude a causal relationship exists between the variables because the independent variable has not been manipulated and subjects were not randomly assigned to groups.

Kearney and associates (2004) conducted a retrospective study in which they explored the role of substance abuse (smoking, alcohol, and drug use) and weight gain of 15 pounds during pregnancy as potential mediators of the relation between recent partner abuse and infant birth weight and to explore the role of demographic factors as moderators for the impact of abuse on infant birth weight. Data on the variables were abstracted from the medical records of 1969 women who had been screened for domestic abuse during pregnancy. From the data gathered, recent physical or psychological abuse had a small but significant effect on birth weight and single marital status was the strongest demographic predictor of decreased infant weight.

A study by Bezanson and associates (2004) is another example of a retrospective study. The researchers noted that Medicare recipients, especially those 80 years and older, are increasingly undergoing coronary artery bypass graft (CABG) surgery. Consistent with this, they noted that there is an association between older age and the need for prolonged mechanical ventilation (MV), yet it is unclear what other physical characteristics may contribute to prolonged ventilation in this population. The purpose of this investigation consistent with the study's research question was to develop and validate a model for prolonged mechanical intervention using selected presurgical patient characteristics. The researchers reviewed 548 charts of Medicare recipients 65 years of age and older undergoing CABG surgery. They collected demographic data as well as data related to history of heart disease and other chronic conditions, preoperative status, and history of prior vascular or CABG surgery. The researchers presented conclusions and developed an exploratory model that provides nurses with a preliminary indication of factors that place Medicare recipients at risk for late extubation. The researchers also correctly stipulated that the model requires further development and testing.

The advantages of the retrospective/ex post facto design are similar to those in the correlational design. The additional benefit of the ex post facto design is that it offers a higher level of control than a correlational study, thereby increasing the confidence the research consumer would have in the evidence provided by the

TABLE **11-2 Paradigm for the Ex Post Facto Design**

Groups (Not Randomly Assigned)	Independent Variable (Not Manipulated by Investigator)	Dependent Variable
Exposed group: Cigarette smokers	X Cigarette smoking	Y_e Lung cancer
Control group: Nonsmokers		Y_c No lung cancer

findings. For example, in the cigarette smoking study, a group of nonsmokers' lung tissue samples are compared with samples of smokers' lung tissue. This comparison enables the researcher to establish the existence of a differential effect of cigarette smoking on lung tissue. However, the researcher remains unable to draw a causal linkage between the two variables, and this inability is the major disadvantage of the retrospective/ex post facto design.

Another disadvantage of retrospective research is the problem of an alternative hypothesis being the reason for the documented relationship. If the researcher obtains data from two existing groups of subjects, such as one that has been exposed to X and one that has not, and the data support the hypothesis that X is related to Y, the researcher cannot be sure whether X or some extraneous variable is the real cause of the occurrence of Y. As such, the impact or effect of the relationship cannot be estimated accurately. Finding naturally occurring groups of subjects who are similar in all respects except for their exposure to the variable of interest is very difficult. There is always the possibility that the groups differ in some other way, such as exposure to other lung irritants, such as asbestos, that can affect the findings of the study and produce spurious results. Consequently, the reader of such a study needs to cautiously evaluate the conclusions drawn by the investigator.

 HELPFUL H I N T

When reading research reports, the reader will note that at times researchers classify a study's design with more than one design type label. This is correct because research studies often reflect aspects of more than one design label.

Longitudinal/prospective (**cohort**) studies are less common than retrospective studies. This may be explained by the fact that it can take a long time for the phenomenon of interest to become evident in a prospective study. For example, if researchers were studying pregnant women who regularly consume alcohol, it would take 9 months for the effect of low birth weight in the subjects' infants to become evident and much longer to collect the data from the total sample size needed. The problems inherent in a prospective study are therefore similar to those of a longitudinal study. However, longitudinal/prospective studies are considered to be stronger than retrospective studies because of the degree of control that can be imposed on extraneous variables that might confound the data.

 HELPFUL H I N T

Remember that nonexperimental designs can test relationships, differences, comparisons, or predictions, depending on the purpose of the study.

PREDICTION AND CAUSALITY IN NONEXPERIMENTAL RESEARCH

A concern of researchers and research consumers are the issues of prediction and causality. Researchers are interested in explaining cause-and-effect relationships, that is, estimating the effect of one phenomenon on another. Historically, researchers have said that only experimental research can support the concept of causality. For example, nurses are interested in discovering what causes anxiety in many settings. If we can uncover the causes, we could perhaps develop interventions that would prevent or decrease the anxiety. Causality makes it necessary to order events chronologically; that is, if we find in a randomly assigned experiment that event 1 (stress) occurs before event 2 (anxiety) and that those in the stressed group were anxious while those in the unstressed group were not, we can say that the hypothesis of stress causing anxiety is supported by these empirical observations. If these results were found in a nonexperimental study where some subjects underwent the stress of surgery and were anxious and others did not have surgery and were not anxious, we would say that there is an association or relationship between stress (surgery) and anxiety. But on the basis of the results of a nonexperimental study, we could say that the stress of surgery caused the anxiety.

Many variables (e.g., anxiety) that nurse researchers wish to study cannot be manipulated, nor would it be wise or ethical to try to manipulate them. Yet there is a need to have studies that can assert a predictive or causal sequence; in light of this need, many nurse researchers are using several analytical techniques that can explain the relationships among variables to establish predictive or causal links. These techniques are called *causal modeling, model testing,* and *associated causal analysis techniques* (Kaplan, 2000). The reader of research also will find the terms *path analysis, LISREL, analysis of covariance structures, structural equation modeling (SEM), and hierarchical linear modeling (HLM)* used to describe the statistical techniques (see Chapter 16) used in these studies. Lyons and associates (2004) used HLM in their study to determine whether pessimism and optimism can be used as early warning signs for negative changes in caregiver depressive symptoms and physical health over a 10-year period. To test if pessimism and depression were predictive, the researchers asked the subjects to respond to questionnaires that corresponded to the variables in the study at the beginning of the study (year 0) and after 2 years and 10 years. The study results showed that caregiver pessimism early in the caregiver role was found to be a warning sign for poor current and future caregiver health. High baseline pessimism signaled high levels of baseline depression symptoms and poor health as well as a decline in health over the 10 years of the study. The results of this long-term study aid both future research and the design and testing of nursing interventions.

Researchers at times want to make a forecast or prediction about how patients will respond to an intervention or a disease process or how successful individuals will be in a particular setting

or field of specialty. In this case, a model may be tested to assess which independent variables can best explain the dependent variable(s). For example, Poss (2000) wanted to analyze the relationship between variables (susceptibility, severity, barriers, benefits, cues to action, normative beliefs, subjective norm, attitude, and intention) from the Health Belief Model and the Theory of Reasoned Action and participation by Mexican migrant workers in a tuberculosis (TB) screening program. The researcher recruited subjects who had participated in a tuberculosis education program and interviewed them to assess which of the independent variables predicted their intention and behavior to participate in the TB screening program.

In another example, Stuifbergen, Seraphine, and Roberts (2000) tested an explanatory model of variables influencing health promotion and quality of life in persons living with multiple sclerosis (MS). The variables of the model were developed from previous systematic study and further tested in this study. The researchers explained the development of the model and the premise of the study. The explanation provided by the researchers allows the reader of the study to clearly understand the purpose and aim of the research and the test of the model using SEM. Although the research does not test a cause-and-effect relationship between the chosen independent predictor variables and the dependent criterion variable, it does demonstrate a theoretically meaningful model of how variables work together in a group in a particular situation.

As nurse researchers develop their programs of research in a specific area, more studies that test models are available. The statistics used in model-testing studies are advanced, but the beginning reader should be able to read the article and understand the purpose of the study and if the model generated was logical and developed with a solid basis from the literature and past research. This section cites several studies that conducted sound tests of theoretical models. A full description of the techniques and principles of causal modeling is beyond the scope of this text; if you want to read about these advanced techniques, a book such as that by Kaplan (2000) is appropriate to consult.

 HELPFUL H I N T

Nonexperimental clinical research studies have progressed to the point where prediction models are used to explore or test relationships between independent and dependent variables.

 EVIDENCE-BASED PRACTICE TIP

Research studies that use nonexperimental designs that provide Level IV evidence often precede and provide the foundation for building a program of research that leads to experimental designs that test the effectiveness of nursing interventions.

ADDITIONAL TYPES OF QUANTITATIVE STUDIES

Other types of quantitative studies complement the science of research. These additional types of designs provide a means of viewing and interpreting phenomena that gives further breadth and knowledge to nursing science and practice. The additional types are methodological, meta-analysis, and secondary analysis.

Methodological Research

 Methodological research is the development and evaluation of data-collection instruments, scales, or techniques. As you will find in succeeding chapters (see Chapters 14 and 15), methodology greatly influences research and the evidence produced.

The most significant and critically important aspect of methodological research addressed in measurement development is called **psychometrics.** Psychometrics deals with the theory and development of measurement instruments (such as questionnaires) or measurement techniques (such as observational techniques) through the research process. Psychometrics thus deals with the measurement of a concept, such as anxiety, quality of life, or caregiver burden, with reliable and valid tools (see Chapter 15 for a discussion of reliability and validity). Psychometrics is a critical issue for nurse researchers. Nurse researchers have used the principles of psychometrics to develop and test measurement instruments that focus on nursing phenomena. Nurse researchers also use instruments developed by other disciplines such as psychology and sociology. Sound measurement tools are critical to the reliability and validity of a study. Although a study's purpose, problems, and procedures may be clear and the data analysis correct and consistent, if the measurement tool that was used by the researcher has inherent psychometric problems, the findings are rendered questionable or limited.

The main problem for nurse researchers is locating appropriate measurement tools. Many of the phenomena of interest to nursing practice and research are intangible, such as interpersonal conflict, resilience, quality of life, coping, and symptom management. The intangible nature of various phenomena, yet the recognition of the need to measure them, places methodological research in an important position. Methodological research differs from other designs of research. First, it does not include all of the research process steps as discussed in Chapter 2. Second, to implement its techniques the researcher must have a sound knowledge of psychometrics or must consult with a researcher knowledgeable in psychometric techniques. The methodological researcher is not interested in the relationship of the independent variable and dependent variable or in the effect of an independent variable on a dependent variable. The methodological researcher is interested in identifying an intangible construct (concept) and making it tangible with a paper-and-pencil instrument or observation protocol.

A methodological study basically includes the following steps:

- Defining the construct/concept or behavior to be measured
- Formulating the tool's items
- Developing instructions for users and respondents
- Testing the tool's reliability and validity

These steps require a sound, specific, and exhaustive literature review to identify the theories underlying the construct. The literature review provides the basis of item formulation. Once the items have been developed, the researcher assesses the tool's reliability and validity (see Chapter 15).Various aspects of these procedures may differ according to the tool's use, purpose, and stage of development.

As an example of methodological research, Barnason and associates (2002) first identified the concept of self-efficacy; they defined this concept as the degree of confidence of post-coronary artery bypass graft (CABG) patients to successfully perform specific activities. They were specifically interested in how this behavior manifested itself in CABG patients. The researchers defined the concept conceptually and operationally and followed up by testing the instrument for reliability and validity (see Chapter 15). Common considerations that researchers incorporate into methodological research are outlined in Table 11-3. Many more examples of methodological research can be found in nursing research literature and many nursing journals. Psychometric or methodological studies are found primarily in journals that report research. The *Journal of Nursing Measurement* is devoted to the publication of information on instruments, tools, and approaches for

TABLE 11-3 **Common Considerations in the Development of Measurement Tools**

Consideration	Example
The well-constructed scale, test, interview schedule, or other form of index should consist of an objective, standardized measure of samples of a behavior that has been clearly defined. Observations should be made on a small but carefully chosen sampling of the behavior of interest, thus permitting us to feel confident that the samples are representative.	In their study of the development of a self-efficacy instrument for CABG patients, Barnason et al. (2002) developed 20 items that evolved to the current 15-item version in 3 phases of testing. The scale also was based on a thorough review of the self-efficacy theoretical framework and the research literature.
The tool should be standardized; that is, it should be a set of uniform items and response possibilities that are uniformly administered and scored.	In the study by Barnason et al. (2002), the items are rated based on a patient's perception of confidence (self-efficacy) in his/her ability to perform the stated behavior of each item; each item is scored using a Likert scale ranging from 1 to 4 points. The total score is obtained by summation of the ratings for each response. A higher score indicates the strength of efficacy expectations for CABG surgery recovery.
The items of a measurement tool should be unambiguous; they should be clear-cut, concise, exact statements with only one idea per item. Negative stems or items with negatively phrased response possibilities result in a double negative and ambiguity in meaning and scoring.	In constructing a tool to measure job satisfaction, a nurse scientist writes the following: "I never feel that I don't have time to provide good nursing care." The response format consists of "Agree," "Undecided," and "Disagree." It is very likely that a response of "Disagree" will not reflect the respondent's true intent because of the confusion that is created by the double negatives.

Continued

TABLE **11-3 Common Considerations in the Development of Measurement Tools—cont'd**

Consideration	Example
The type of items used in any one test or scale should be restricted to a limited number of variations. Subjects who are expected to shift from one kind of item to another may fail to provide a true response as a result of the distraction of making such a change.	Mixing true-or-false items with questions that require a yes-or-no response and items that provide a response format of five possible answers is conducive to a high level of measurement error.
Items should not provide irrelevant clues. Unless carefully constructed, an item may furnish an indication of the expected response or answer. Furthermore, the correct answer or expected response to one item should not be given by another item.	An item that provides a clue to the expected answer may contain value words that convey cultural expectations, such as: "A good wife enjoys caring for her home and family."
The items of a measurement tool should not be made difficult by requiring unnecessarily complex or exact operations. Furthermore, the difficulty of an item should be appropriate to the level of the subjects being assessed. Limiting each item to one concept or idea helps accomplish this objective.	A test constructed to evaluate learning in an introductory course in research methods may contain an item that is inappropriate for the designated group, such as: "A nonlinear transformation of data to linear data is a useful procedure before testing a hypothesis of curvilinearity."
The diagnostic, predictive, or measurement value of a tool depends on the degree to which it serves as an indicator of a relatively broad and significant area of behavior, known as the universe of content for the behavior. As already emphasized, a behavior must be clearly defined before it can be measured. The definition is developed from the universe of content, that is, the information and research findings that are available for the behavior of interest. The items should reflect that definition. To what extent the test items appear to accomplish this objective is an indication of the validity of the instrument.	Two nurse researchers, A and B, are studying the construct of quality of life. Each has defined this construct in a different way. Consequently, the measurement tool that each nurse devises will include different questions. The questions on each tool will reflect the universe of content for quality of life as defined by each researcher.
The instrument also should adequately cover the defined behavior. The primary consideration is whether the number and nature of items in the sample are adequate. If there are too few items, the accuracy or reliability of the measure must be questioned. In general, there should be a minimum of 10 items for each independent aspect of the behavior of interest.	Very few people would be satisfied with an assessment of such traits as intelligence if the scales were limited to three items.
The measure must prove its worth empirically through tests of reliability and validity.	A researcher should demonstrate to the reader that the scale is accurate and measures what it purports to measure (see Chapter 15).

measurement of variables. The specific procedures of methodological research are beyond the scope of this book, but the reader is urged to look closely at the tools used in studies.

Meta-Analysis

Meta-analysis is not a design per se, but a research method based on a strict scientific approach that takes the results of many studies in a specific area, synthesizes their findings, and statistically summarizes the data to obtain a precise estimate of the effect (impact) of the results of the studies included in the systematic review (Whittemore, 2005). Each study is a unit of analysis. The goal is to bring together all the studies concerning a particular clinical question and, using rigorous inclusion and exclusion criteria, analyze those studies that are similar, analyze results in order to quantify the effectiveness of the intervention under study. This method is more powerful because it is a rigorous process of evidence summarization rather than an effect estimate derived from single studies alone. Johnston (2005) notes that the meta-analysis of a number of randomized clinical trials (RCTs) gives due weight to the sample size of the studies included and provides an estimate of treatment effect; that is, it asks whether the intervention really makes a difference. Meta-analysis is a type of systematic review that provides the most powerful and useful evidence available to guide practice, that is, Level I evidence (see Chapters 2, 4, 19, and 20).

When the research consumer critically appraises a meta-analysis, some of the questions to consider are the following:

- Does the meta-analysis address a focused research question?
- Are there specific inclusion and exclusion criteria for judging the studies?
- Was there any publication bias?
- Are the studies included homogeneous?
  similar design
  similar interventions
  similar outcome measures

Think about the meta-analysis method as one that progressively sifts and sorts data until the highest quality of evidence is used to arrive at the conclusions. First the researcher combines the results of all the studies that focus on a specific question. The studies considered of lowest quality are then excluded and the data are reanalyzed. This process is repeated sequentially, excluding studies until only the studies of highest quality available are included in the analysis. An alteration in the overall results as an outcome of this sifting and sorting process suggests how sensitive the conclusions are to the quality of studies included (Johnston, 2005; Stevens, 2001).

Such considerations determine whether or not it is reasonable to combine the studies for analysis. The consumer of research should note that a researcher who conducts a meta-analysis does not conduct the original analysis of data in the area but rather takes the data from already published studies and synthesizes the information by following a set of controlled and systematic steps. Meta-analysis can be used to synthesize both nonexperimental and experimental research studies.

Finally, evidence-based practice requires that you, the research consumer, determine, based on the strength and quality of the evidence provided by the meta-analysis coupled with your clinical expertise and patient values, whether or not you would consider a change in practice. For example, a meta-analysis by Edwards, Hailey, and Maxwell (2004) addressed the clinical question, "Do psychological interventions (education, individual cognitive behavioral or psychotherapeutic programs, or group support) improve survival and psychological outcomes in women with metastatic breast cancer?" The results of the meta-analysis are reported as follows:

A search was conducted of published and unpublished RCTs in any language that assessed the effectiveness of psychological or psychosocial interventions in women with breast cancer. Data sources included the following: Cochrane

Breast Cancer Group Trials Register, Cochrane Central Register of Controlled Trials, Medline, CINAHL, PsychINFO, and SIGLE; references of relevant studies and reviews; hand searches of relevant journals; and known authors in the field. Two reviewers assessed the quality of individual RCTs using the Jadad scale and another method score that was more relevant for trials of psychological interventions.

The main results of the meta-analysis indicate that five studies ($n = 636$) met the selection criteria; two studies assessed cognitive behavioral group interventions and three assessed supportive-expressive group therapy. Meta-analysis using a fixed effects model showed that group psychological interventions did not differ from usual care for survival at 1, 5, or 10 years. Cognitive behavioral therapy did not differ from usual care for anxiety (1 trial), self-esteem (1 trial), or mood state (1 trial) at 6 months. Supportive-expressive group therapy improved scores on the Courtauld Emotional Control scale at 8 months (1 trial) and reduced reported pain assessed using a 10-point visual analogue scale (meta-analysis of 2 trials; weighted mean difference 0.75 reduction, 95%, CI 0.63 to 0.86) compared with usual care. The groups did not differ in mood states at 10 to 12 months (2 trials) or quality of life at 1 year (1 trial). The authors concluded that existing evidence does not support a survival benefit for women with metastatic breast cancer who received group psychological interventions compared to those who received usual care. Evidence on the effects on various aspects of psychological functioning is mixed.

A commentary by Haber (2004) notes that because of the diverse nature of the RCTs and participants, the authors used a rigorous approach to data analysis that considered the heterogeneity and scarcity of data in the field as potential factors that could affect the meta-analysis. Potential modifiers, such as family history of breast cancer, age, time of diagnosis of metastasis, variation in length of follow-up, and failure to follow-up, were also considered.

Although the evidence suggests some short-term psychosocial benefits, these benefits were not maintained in the longer term. Haber concludes the commentary by commenting on the disappointing results considering the conceptually logical and anecdotal evidence of the benefits of such psychosocial interventions. Considering the human and financial resource commitment of breast cancer services to psychosocial interventions, the lack of evidence supporting the efficacy of this approach justifies evaluation of traditional programming and resource allocation for this patient population.

Systematic reviews that use multiple RCTs to combine study results offer stronger evidence, Level I, in estimating the magnitude of an effect for an intervention (see Chapter 2, Table 2-3). The strength of evidence provided by systematic reviews has become the "heart and soul" of evidence-based practice (Stevens, 2001).

 EVIDENCE-BASED PRACTICE TIP

EBP methods such as meta-analysis increase a nurse's ability to manage the ever-increasing volume of information produced in order to develop the best practices that are evidence-based.

Secondary Analysis

Secondary analysis also is not a design but rather a form of research in which the researcher takes previously collected and analyzed data from *one* study and reanalyzes the data for a *secondary* purpose. The original study may be either an experimental or a nonexperimental design. For example, Gift and associates (2003) conducted a secondary analysis of a longitudinal study. The original study collected data from a National Institutes of Health (NIH) sponsored longitudinal panel study of patients with newly diagnosed cancer (Given & Given, 1993-1998). The purpose of the original study was to examine lung cancer patients' symptoms, functional status, and depression and family caregivers' reactions over time. The research team generated a number of research question from the original data to explore symptom clusters over time, assess the severity of the symptoms over time, and explore if physiological factors related to lung cancer predict symptom clusters and if the severity of the cluster symptoms was predictive of death. Though the data have limited generalizability to a larger group of cancer patients, the data coupled with the original data form a base for beginning to answer important clinical issues related to symptom management in this population.

 HELPFUL HINT

As you read the literature, you will find labels such as outcomes' research, needs' assessments, evaluation research, and quality assurance. These studies are not designs per se. These studies use either experimental or nonexperimental designs. Studies with these labels are designed to test the effectiveness of health care techniques, programs, or interventions. When reading such a research study, the reader should assess which design was used and if the principles of the design, sampling strategy, and analysis are consistent with the study's purpose.

CRITIQUING GUIDE   *Nonexperimental Designs*

Criteria for critiquing nonexperimental designs are presented in the accompanying Critiquing Criteria box. When critiquing nonexperimental research designs, the consumer should keep in mind that such designs offer the researcher the least amount of control. As such, the level of evidence provided by nonexperimental designs is not as strong as evidence generated by experimental designs where manipulation, randomization, and control are used. The first step in critiquing nonexperimental research is to determine which type of design was used in the study. Often a statement describing the design of the study appears in the abstract and in the methods section of the report. If such a statement is not present, the reader should closely examine the paper for evidence of which type of design was employed. The reader should be able to discern

that either a survey or a relationship design was used, as well as the specific subtype. For example, the reader would expect an investigation of self-concept development in children from birth to 5 years of age to be a relationship study using a longitudinal design.

Next, the reader should evaluate the theoretical framework and underpinnings of the study to determine if a nonexperimental design was the most appropriate approach to the problem. For example, many of the studies on pain discussed throughout this text are suggestive of a nonmanipulative relationship between pain and any of the independent variables under consideration. As such, these studies suggest a nonexperimental correlational, longitudinal, or cross-sectional design. Investigators will use one of these designs to examine the relationship between the variables in naturally occurring groups. Sometimes the reader may think that it would have been more appropriate if the investigators had used an experimental or quasiexperimental design. However, the reader must recognize that pragmatic or ethical considerations also may have guided the researchers in their choice of design (see Chapters 9 and 13).

Then the evaluator should assess whether the problem is at a level of experimental manipulation. Many times researchers merely wish to examine if relationships exist between variables. Therefore when one critiques such studies, the purpose of the study should be determined. If the purpose of the study does not include describing a cause-and-effect relationship, the researcher should not be criticized for not looking for one. However, the evaluator should be wary of a nonexperimental study in which the researcher suggests a cause-and-effect relationship in the findings.

Finally, the factor or factors that actually influence changes in the dependent variable can be ambiguous in nonexperimental designs. As with all complex phenomena, multiple factors can contribute to variability in the subjects' responses. When an experimental design is not used for controlling some of these extraneous variables that can influence results, the researcher must strive to provide as much control of them as possible within the context of a nonexperi-

mental design. For example, when it has not been possible to randomly assign subjects to treatment groups as an approach to controlling an independent variable, the researcher may use a strategy of matching subjects for identified variables. For example, in a study of infant birth weight, pregnant women could be matched on variables such as weight, height, smoking habits, drug use, and other factors that might influence birth weight. The independent variable of interest, such as the type of prenatal care, would then be the major difference in the groups. The reader would then feel more confident that the only real difference between the two groups was the differential effect of the independent variable because the other factors in the two groups were theoretically the same. However, the consumer should remember also that there might be other influential variables that were not matched, such as income, education, and diet. Threats to internal and external validity represent a major influence on the interpretation of a nonexperimental study because they impose limitations on the generalizability of the results and their applicability to practice.

If the consumer is critiquing one of the additional types of research discussed, it is important first to identify the type of research used. Once the type of research is identified, its specific purpose and format need to be understood. The format and methods of secondary analysis, methodological research, and meta-analysis vary; knowing how they vary allows a consumer to assess whether the process was applied appropriately. Some of the basic principles of these methods were presented in this chapter. The specific criteria for evaluating these designs are beyond the scope of this text, but the references provided will assist in this process. Even though the format and methods vary, it is important to remember that all research has a central goal: to answer questions scientifically and provide the strongest, most consistent evidence possible.

Critical Thinking Challenges

- Discuss which type of nonexperimental design might help validate the defining characteristics of a particular nursing diagnosis you use in practice. Do you think it is possible to use nurses and patients/clients as the subjects in this type of study?
- The midterm assignment for your research course is to critique an assigned quantitative study. To proceed, you must first decide what the study's overall type is. You think it is an ex post facto nonexperimental design; the others think it is an experimental design because it has several explicit hypotheses. How would you convince them that you are correct?
- You are completing your senior practicum on a surgical step-down unit. The nurses completed an evidence-based practice protocol for patient-controlled analgesics (PCAs). Some of the nurses want to implement it immediately, while others want to implement it with only some of the patients. You think that it should be implemented as a research study. Discuss what type of research design would be useful and whether either of the methods chosen by the nurses to implement the protocol should be considered in the research study.
- You are part of a journal club at your hospital. Your group has been looking at a phenomenon specific to your patient population and noticed that there are 20 correlational studies on the topic. Your group decides to do a meta-analysis of the data. What steps need to be considered in doing the meta-analysis? What level of evidence would you expect to obtain with this method? Explain your answer.

KEY POINTS

- Nonexperimental research designs are used in studies that construct a picture or make an account of events as they naturally occur. The major difference between nonexperimental and experimental research is that in nonexperimental designs the independent variable is not actively manipulated by the investigator.

- Nonexperimental designs can be classified as either survey studies or relationship/difference studies.
- Survey studies and relationship/difference studies are both descriptive and exploratory in nature.
- Survey research collects detailed descriptions of existing phenomena and uses the data either to

justify current conditions and practices or to make more intelligent plans for improving them.

- Relationship studies endeavor to explore the relationships between variables that provide deeper insight into the phenomena of interest.
- Correlational studies examine relationships.
- Developmental studies are further broken down into categories of cross-sectional, longitudinal, prospective, retrospective, and ex post facto studies.
- Methodological research, secondary analysis, and meta-analysis are examples of other means of adding to the body of nursing research. Both the researcher and the reader must consider the advantages and disadvantages of each design.
- Nonexperimental research designs do not enable the investigator to establish cause-and-effect relationships between the variables. Consumers must be wary of nonexperimental studies that make causal claims about the findings unless a causal modeling technique is used.
- Nonexperimental designs also offer the researcher the least amount of control. Threats to validity represent a major influence on the interpretation of a nonexperimental study because they impose limitations on the generalizability of the results and as such should be fully assessed by the critical reader.
- The critiquing process is directed toward evaluating the appropriateness of the selected nonexperimental design in relation to factors such as the research problem, theoretical framework, hypothesis, methodology, and data analysis and interpretation.
- Though nonexperimental designs do not provide the highest level of evidence (Level I), they do provide a wealth of data that become useful pieces for formulating both Level I and Level II studies that are aimed at developing and testing nursing interventions.

REFERENCES

Anderson B, Higgins L, and Rozmus C: Critical pathways: application to selected patient outcomes following coronary bypass graft, *Appl Nurs Res* 12(4): 168-174, 1999.

Barnason S, Zimmerman L, Atwood J, Nieveen J, and Schmaderer M: Development of a self-efficacy instrument for coronary artery bypass graft patients, *J Nurs Meas* 10: 123-133, 2002.

Bezanson JL, Weaver M, Kinney MR, Waldrum M, and Weintraub WS: Presurgical risk factors for late extubation in Medicare recipients after cardiac surgery, *Nur Res* 53: 46-52, 2004.

Burns KJ, Camaione DN, and Chatterton CT: Prescription of physical activity by adult nurse practitioners: a national survey, *Nurs Outlook* 48(1): 28-33, 2000.

Campbell DT, Stanley JC: *Experimental and quasi-experimental designs for research,* Chicago, 1963, Rand-McNally.

Clark PC, Dunbar SB, Shields CG, Viswanathan B, Aycock DM, and Wolf SL: Influence of stroke survivor characteristics and family conflict surrounding recovery on caregivers' mental and physical health, *Nurs Res* 53: 406-413, 2004.

Edwards AG, Hailey S, and Maxwell M: Psychological interventions for women with metastatic breast cancer, *Cochrane Database Systematic Rev* 2004(2): CD004253, 2004.

Given BA, Given CW: Family home care: A community-based model [1993-1998]. Funded by the U.S. Department of Health and Human Services, National Center for Nursing Research and AHCPR (grant # RO1 NR/CAO1915).

Gift AG, Stommel M, Jablonski A, and Gien W: A cluster of symptoms over time in patients with lung cancer, *Nurs Res* 52: 393-400, 2003.

Haber J: Commentary: Psychological interventions for women with metastatic breast cancer, *Evidence-Based Nurs* 7(4): 111, 2004.

Huber DL, Vaughan-Sarrazin M, Vaughn T, and Hall JA: Evaluating the impact of case management dosage, *Nurs Res* 52: 276-288, 2003.

Johnston L: Critically appraising quantitative evidence. In Melnyk BM, Fineout-Overholt E, editors: *Evidence-based practice in nursing and healthcare,* Philadelphia, 2005, Lippincott Williams & Wilkins.

Jones MA, Hoffman LA, Makaroun MS, Zullo TG, and Chelluri L: Early discharge following abdominal aortic aneurysm repair: impact on patients and caregivers, *Res Nurs Health* 25: 345-356, 2002.

Kaplan D: *Structure equation modeling: foundations and extensions,* Thousand Oaks, Calif, 2000, Sage.

Kearney MH, Munron BH, Kelly U, and Hawkins JW: Health behaviors as mediators for the effect of partner abuse on infant birth weight, *Nur Res* 53: 36-45, 2004.

LoBiondo-Wood G, Williams L, and McGhee C: Liver transplantation in children: maternal and family stress, coping and adaptation, *J Specialists Ped Nurs* 9: 59-66, 2004.

Lyons KS, Stewart BJ, Archbold PG, Carter JH, and Perrin NA: Pessimism and optimism as early warning signs for compromised health for caregivers of patients with Parkinson's Disease, *Nurs Res* 53: 354-362, 2004.

Nyamathi A et al.: Type of social support among homeless women: its impact on psychological resources, health and health behaviors, and use of health services, *Nurs Res* 49(6): 318-326, 2000.

Poss JE: Factors associated with participation by Mexican migrant farmworkers in a tuberculosis screening program, *Nurs Res* 49(1): 20-28, 2000.

Redeker NS, Ruggiero JS, and Hedges C: Sleep is related to physical function and emotional well-being after cardiac surgery, *Nurs Res* 53: 154-162, 2004.

Stastny PF, Ichinose TY, Thayer SD, Olson RJ, and Keens TG: Infant sleeping position by nursery staff and mothers in newborn hospital nurseries, *Nurs Res* 53: 122-129, 2004.

Stevens KR: Systematic reviews: the heart of evidence-based practice, *AACN Clin Issues: Adv Pract Acute Clin Care* 12: 529-538, 2001.

Stuifbergen AK, Seraphine A, and Roberts G: An explanatory model of health promotion and quality of life in chronic disabling conditions, *Nurs Res* 49(3): 122-129, 2000.

Thimbault-Prevost J, Jensen LA, and Hodgins M: Critical care nurses' perceptions of DNR status, *J Nurs Scholarship* 32(3): 259-266, 2000.

Valente S, Saunders JM: Barriers to suicide risk management in clinical practice: a national survey of oncology nurses, *Issues Mental Health Nurs* 25: 629-648, 2004.

Van Cleve L, Bossert E, Beecroft P, Adlard K, Alvarez O, and Savedra MC: The pain experience of children with leukemia during the first year after diagnosis, *Nurs Res* 53: 1-10, 2004.

Whittemore R: Combing evidence in nursing research, *Nurs Res* 54: 56-62, 2005.

Zalon ML: Correlates of recovery among older adults after major addominal surgery, *Nurs Res* 53: 99-106, 2004.

FOR FURTHER STUDY

🌐 Go to your Companion CD for review activities for this chapter.

evolve Go to Evolve at http://evolve.elsevier.com/LoBiondo/ for WebLinks, Content Updates, and additional research articles, for practice in reviewing and critiquing.

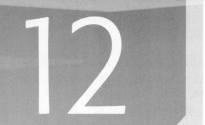

Sampling

KEY TERMS

accessible population
convenience sampling
data saturation
delimitations
element
eligibility criteria
matching
multistage (cluster) sampling
network (snowball effect) sampling

nonprobability sampling
pilot study
population
probability sampling
purposive sampling
quota sampling
random selection
representative sample
sample

sampling
sampling frame
sampling interval
sampling unit
simple random sampling
snowball effect
stratified random sampling
systematic sampling
target population

LEARNING OUTCOMES

After reading this chapter, the student should be able to do the following:

- Identify the purpose of sampling.
- Define population, sample, and sampling.
- Compare and contrast a population and a sample.
- Discuss the eligibility criteria for sample selection.
- Define nonprobability and probability sampling.
- Identify the types of nonprobability and probability sampling strategies.
- Compare the advantages and disadvantages of specific nonprobability and probability sampling strategies.
- Discuss the contribution of nonprobability and probability sampling strategies to strength of evidence provided by study findings.
- Discuss the factors that influence determination of sample size.
- Discuss the procedure for drawing a sample.
- Identify the criteria for critiquing a sampling plan.
- Use the critiquing criteria to evaluate the "Sample" section of a research report.

STUDY RESOURCES

Go to your Companion CD for review activities for this chapter.

evolve Go to Evolve at http://evolve.elsevier.com/LoBiondo/ for Weblinks, Content Updates, and additional research articles for practice in reviewing and critiquing.

ampling is the process of selecting representative units of a population for study in a research investigation. Although sampling is a complex process, it is a familiar one. In our daily lives, we gather knowledge, make decisions, and formulate predictions based on sampling procedures. For example, nursing students may make generalizations about the overall quality of nursing professors as a result of their exposure to a sample of nursing professors during their undergraduate programs. Patients may make generalizations about a hospital's food or quality of nursing care during a 1-week hospital stay. It is apparent that limited exposure to a limited portion of these phenomena forms the basis of our conclusions, and so much of our knowledge and decisions are based on our experience with samples.

Scientists also derive knowledge from samples. Many problems in scientific research cannot be solved without employing sampling procedures. For example, when testing the effectiveness of a medication for patients with asthma, the drug is administered to a sample of the population for whom the drug is potentially appropriate. The scientist must come to some conclusions without administering the drug to every known patient with asthma or every laboratory animal in the world. But because human lives are at stake, the scientist cannot afford to arrive casually at conclusions that are based on the first dozen patients available for study. The consequences of arriving at erroneous conclusions or making generalizations from a small nonrepresentative sample are much more severe in scientific investigations than in everyday life. Consequently, research methodologists have expended considerable effort to develop sampling theories and procedures that produce accurate and meaningful information. Essentially, researchers sample representative segments of the population because it is rarely feasible or necessary to sample the entire population of interest to obtain relevant information.

This chapter will familiarize the research consumer with the basic concepts of sampling as they primarily pertain to the principles of quantitative research design, nonprobability and probability sampling, sample size, and the related critiquing process. Sampling issues that relate to qualitative research designs are mainly discussed in Chapter 7.

SAMPLING CONCEPTS

Population

A **population** is a well-defined set that has certain specified properties. A population can be composed of people, animals, objects, or events. For example, if a researcher is studying undergraduate nursing students, the type of educational preparation of the population must be specified. In this instance, the population consists of undergraduate students enrolled in a baccalaureate nursing program. Examples of other possible populations might be all of the female patients admitted to a certain hospital for lumpectomies for treatment of breast cancer during the year 2005, all of the children with diabetes in the state of New York, or all of the men and women with a diagnosis of bipolar disorder in the United States. These examples illustrate that a population may be broadly defined and potentially involve millions of people or narrowly specified to include only several hundred people.

The reader of a research report should consider whether the researcher has identified the population descriptors that form the basis for the inclusion (eligibility) or exclusion (delimitations) criteria that are used to select the sample from the array of all possible units—whether people, objects, or events. These four terms—inclusion or eligibility criteria and exclusion criteria or delimitations—are used synonymously when considering subject attributes that would lead a researcher to specify inclusion or exclusion criteria. Consider the population previously defined as undergraduate nursing students enrolled in a baccalaureate program. Would this population include both part-time and full-time students? Would it include students who had previously earned a bachelor's degree in another major such as English? What about foreign students? Would freshmen through seniors qualify? Insofar as it is possible, the researcher must demonstrate that the exact criteria used to decide whether an individual would be classified as a member of a given population have been specifically delineated. The population descriptors that provide the basis for inclusion (eligibility) criteria should be evident in the sample; that is, the characteristics of the population and the sample should be congruent. The degree of congruence is evaluated to assess the representativeness of the sample. For example, if a population is defined as full-time, American-born, senior nursing students enrolled in a baccalaureate nursing program, the sample would be expected to reflect these characteristics.

Think about the concept of inclusion or eligibility criteria applied to a research study where the subjects are patients. For example, participants in a study investigating the pain experience of children with leukemia during the first year after diagnosis (Van Cleve et al., 2004) (see Appendix B) had to meet the following inclusion (eligibility) criteria:

1. Age—between 4 and 17 years
2. Diagnosis—acute lymphocytic leukemia within 1 month of diagnosis
3. Health status—no other existing chronic illnesses associated with pain, a fulminating disease, a known cognitive disability
4. Status—ability to cope with the burden of research tasks as determined by the primary nurse
5. Language—English or Spanish speaking

Inclusion or eligibility criteria may also be viewed as exclusion criteria or delimitations, those characteristics that restrict the population to a homogeneous group of subjects. Examples of exclusion criteria or delimitations include the following: gender, age, marital status, socioeconomic status, religion, ethnicity, level of education, age of children, health status, and diagnosis. In a study investigating factors associated with levels of knowledge about heart failure and related treatment in a diverse group of patients (Artinian et al., 2002), the researchers established the following exclusion criteria:

- History of documented dementia or mental illness
- Self-reported substance abuse
- On hemodyalysis
- In terminal stages of cancer

These exclusion criteria or delimitations were selected because of their potential effect on the accurate assessment of knowledge about the health problem under consideration: heart failure. Let us consider the effect of a co-occurring health problem such as dementia on the subject's ability to master information about their heart failure. If level of knowledge was assessed in patients who had a primary or secondary diagnosis of heart failure, and who also had dementia, the accuracy of that assessment would be confounded by their degree of cognitive impairment (e.g., knowledge acquisition, retention, and application). Heterogeneity of this sample group would decrease the strength of the evidence and inhibit the researchers' ability to interpret the findings meaningfully and make generalizations. It is much wiser to study only one homogeneous group or include specific groups as distinct subsets of the sample and study the groups comparatively, as was the case in the study by Artinian and colleagues (2002).

For example, in a study investigating the effectiveness of advanced practice nursing (APN) support by telephone on cardiac surgery patients during the first 5 weeks following hospital discharge, the sample consisted of 186 individuals who had been admitted to a large teaching hospital and had undergone coronary artery bypass graft (CABG) surgery (Trammer and Parry, 2004). The sample subjects were randomly assigned to two groups that were studied comparatively. Group I ($n = 94$), the intervention group, consisted of postdischarge CABG patients who received weekly APN-initiated follow-up telephone calls for 5 weeks that were individually tailored in response to the patient's symptoms, concerns, and recovery. Group II ($n = 92$), the control group, consisted of postdischarge CABG patients who received the usual care provided to patients undergoing CABG surgery at that hospital. The subjects recruited to the study met the following inclusion criteria that maximized the likelihood of having a homogeneous sample:

- Had undergone their first elective or emergent cardiac surgery
- Had no unexpected cardiac complications that necessitated an unexpected stay in the ICU
- Were oriented to time, place, and person
- Had no history of acute or chronic psychiatric problems as assessed through medical records and by discussion with the health care team
- Were able to read, write, and speak English
- Were capable of responding over the telephone

Remember that inclusion and exclusion criteria are not established in a casual or meaningless way but are established to control for extraneous variability or bias that would limit the strength of evidence contributed by the sampling plan in relation to the experimental design of the study. Each inclusion or exclusion criterion should have a rationale, presumably related to a potential contaminating effect on the dependent variable. The careful establishment of sample inclusion or exclusion criteria will increase the precision of the study and strength of evidence, thereby contributing to the accuracy and generalizability of the findings (see Chapter 9).

The population criteria establish the **target population,** that is, the entire set of cases about which the researcher would like to make generalizations. A target population might include all undergraduate nursing students enrolled in generic baccalaureate programs in the United States. Because of time, money, and personnel, however, it is often not feasible to pursue a research study using a target population. An **accessible population,** one that meets the population criteria and that is available, is used instead. For example, an accessible population might include all full-time generic baccalaureate students attending school in Indiana. Pragmatic factors must also be considered when identifying a potential population of interest.

It is important to know that a population is not restricted to human subjects. It may consist of hospital records; blood, urine, or other specimens taken from patients at a clinic; historical documents; or laboratory animals. For example, a population might consist of all the blood test specimens collected from patients in the Crestview Hospital hypertension clinic or all of the patient charts on file who had been screened during pregnancy for intimate partner abuse. It is apparent that a population can be defined in a variety of ways. The important point to remember is that the basic unit of the population must be clearly defined because the generalizability of the findings will be a function of the population criteria.

HELPFUL HINT

Often, researchers do not clearly identify the population under study, or the population is not clarified until the "Discussion" section when the effort is made to discuss the group (population) to which the study findings can be generalized.

EVIDENCE-BASED PRACTICE TIP

Consider whether the choice of participants was biased, thereby influencing the strength of evidence provided by the outcomes of the study.

Samples and Sampling

Sampling is a process of selecting a portion or subset of the designated population to represent the entire population. A **sample** is a set of elements that make up the population; an **element** is the most basic unit about which information is collected. The most common element in nursing research is individuals, but other elements (e.g., places or objects) can form the basis of a sample or population. For example, a researcher was planning a study that compared the effectiveness of different nursing interventions on reducing falls in the elderly in long term care facilities (LTCs). Four LTCs, each using a different treatment protocol, were identified as the sampling units rather than the nurses themselves or the treatment alone.

The purpose of sampling is to increase the efficiency of a research study. The novice reviewer of research reports must realize that it would not be feasible to examine every element or unit in the population. When sampling is done properly, the researcher can draw inferences and make generalizations about the population without examining each unit in the population. Sampling procedures that entail the formulation of specific criteria for selection ensure that the characteristics of the phenomena of interest will be, or are likely to be, present in all of the units being studied. The researcher's efforts to ensure that the sample is representative of the target population strengthens the evidence generated by the sample composition, which puts the researcher in a stronger position to draw conclusions that are generalizable to the population and applicable to practice (see Chapter 9).

After having reviewed a number of research studies, you will recognize that samples and sampling procedures vary in terms of merit. The foremost criterion in evaluating a sample is its representativeness. A **representative sample** is one whose key characteristics closely approximate those of the population. If 70% of the population in a study of child-rearing practices consisted of women and 40% were full-time employees, a representative sample should reflect these characteristics in the same proportions.

It must be understood that there is no way to guarantee that a sample is representative without obtaining a database about the entire population. Because it is difficult and inefficient to assess a population, the researcher must employ sampling strategies that minimize or control for sample bias. If an appropriate sampling strategy is used, it almost always is possible to obtain a reasonably accurate understanding of the phenomena under investigation by obtaining data from a sample.

 EVIDENCE-BASED PRACTICE TIP

Determining whether the sample is representative of the population being studied will influence the research consumer's interpretation of the evidence provided by the findings and decision making about their relevance to his or her patient population and practice setting.

TYPES OF SAMPLES

Sampling strategies are generally grouped into two categories: nonprobability sampling and probability sampling. In **nonprobability sampling,** elements are chosen by nonrandom methods. The drawback of this strategy is that there is no way of estimating each element's probability of being included in the samples. Essentially, there is no way of ensuring that every element has a chance for inclusion in the nonprobability sample. **Probability sampling** uses some form of random selection when the sample units are chosen. This type of sample enables the researcher to estimate the probability that each element of the population will be included in the sample. Probability sampling is the more rigorous type of sampling strategy and is more likely to result in a representative sample. The remainder of this section is devoted to a discussion of different types of nonprobability and probability sampling strategies. A summary of sampling strategies appears in Table 12-1. You may wish to refer to this table as the various nonprobability and probability strategies are discussed in the following sections.

 HELPFUL HINT

Research articles are not always explicit about the type of sampling strategy that was used. If the sampling strategy is not specified, assume that a convenience sample was used for a quantitative study and a purposive sample was used for a qualitative study.

TABLE 12-1 **Summary of Sampling Strategies**

Sampling Strategy	Ease of Drawing Sample	Risk of Bias	Representativeness of Sample
NONPROBABILITY			
Convenience	Very easy	Greater than any other sampling strategy	Because samples tend to be self-selecting, representativeness is questionable
Quota	Relatively easy	Contains unknown source of bias that affects external validity	Builds in some representativeness by using knowledge about population of interest
Purposive	Relatively easy	Bias increases with greater heterogeneity of population; conscious bias is also a danger	Very limited ability to generalize because sample is handpicked
PROBABILITY			
Simple random	Laborious	Low	Maximized; probability of nonrepresentativeness decreases with increased sample size
Stratified random	Time-consuming	Low	Enhanced
Cluster	Less time-consuming than simple or stratified	Subject to more sampling errors than simple or stratified	Less representative than simple or stratified
Systematic	More convenient and efficient than simple, stratified, or cluster sampling	Bias in the form of nonrandomness can be inadvertently introduced	Less representative if bias occurs as result of coincidental nonrandomness

Nonprobability Sampling

Due to lack of randomization, the nonprobability sampling strategy is less generalizable than the probability sampling strategy, and it tends to produce less representative samples. Such samples are more feasible for the researcher to obtain, however, and many samples—not only in nursing research but also in other disciplines—are nonprobability samples. When a nonprobability sample is carefully chosen to reflect the target population, through the careful use of inclusion and exclusion criteria, the research consumer can have more confidence in the representativeness of the sample and the external validity of the findings. The three major types of nonprobability sampling are the following:

convenience, quota, and purposive sampling strategies.

Convenience Sampling

Convenience sampling is the use of the most readily accessible persons or objects as subjects in a study. The subjects may include volunteers, the first 100 patients admitted to hospital X with a particular diagnosis, all of the people enrolled in program Y during the month of September, or all of the students enrolled in course Z at a particular university during 2005. The subjects are convenient and accessible to the researcher and are thus called a convenience sample. For example, a researcher studying health promotion and cardiovascular health in adult monozygotic twins used a convenience sample of 77 monozygotic twins ranging in age from 20 to 60 years who had attended a special conference, met the eligibility criteria, and volunteered to participate in the study (Wynd, Murrock, and Zeller, 2004). Another researcher, studying the effect of a nursing intervention that sought to determine if providing individualized information to men who are newly diagnosed with prostate cancer and their partners would lower their levels of psychological distress and enable them to become more active participants in treatment decision making, used a sample of 80 couples referred to the Prostate Centre at Hospital X in British Columbia and who met the eligibility criteria (Davison et al., 2003) (see Appendix D). The advantage of a convenience sample is that it is easier for the researcher to obtain subjects. The researcher may have to be concerned only with obtaining a sufficient number of subjects who meet the same criteria.

The major disadvantage of a convenience sample is that the risk of bias is greater than in any other type of sample (see Table 12-1). Because convenience samples use voluntary participation, this fact increases the probability of researchers recruiting those people who feel strongly about the issue being studied, which may favor certain outcomes (Sousa, Zauszniewski, and Musil, 2004). In this case, the following questions must be raised: What motivated some of the people to participate and others not to participate (self-selection)? What kind of data would have been obtained if nonparticipants had also responded? How representative are the people who did participate in relation to the population? What kind of confidence can you have in the evidence provided by the findings? For example, a researcher may stop people on a street corner to ask their opinion on some issue, place advertisements in the newspaper, or place signs in local churches, community centers, or supermarkets indicating that volunteers are needed for a particular study. A study examining prevention or treatment of osteoporosis in postmenopausal women who had completed treatment (except for Tamoxifen) for breast cancer, and for whom hormone replacement therapy was contraindicated, recruited subjects from breast cancer support groups, physician referrals, and local television and radio announcements (Waltman et al., 2003). In order to assess the degree to which a convenience sample approximates a random sample, a researcher can compare the convenience sample data to known population data in terms of percentages. In this manner the researcher checks for the representativeness of the convenience sample and the extent to which bias is or is not evident (Cochran, 1977; Sousa, Zauszniewski, and Musil, 2004).

Because acquiring research subjects is a problem that confronts many nurse researchers, innovative recruitment strategies may be used. For example, a researcher may even offer to pay the participants for their time. A unique method of accessing and recruiting subjects is the use of online computer networks (e.g., disease-specific chat rooms and bulletin boards). In the evidence hierarchy located in Table 2-3, nonprobability sampling is most commonly associated with quantitative nonexperimental or qualitative studies that contribute Level IV through Level VI evidence.

The evaluator of a research report should recognize that the convenience sample strategy, although the most common, is the weakest form of sampling strategy with regard to strength of evidence and generalizability. The use of this strategy should be avoided whenever possible. When a convenience sample is used, caution should be exercised in analyzing and interpreting the data. When critiquing a research study that has employed this sampling strategy, the reviewer should be justifiably skeptical about the external validity of the findings and applicability of the findings (see Chapter 9).

Quota Sampling

Quota sampling refers to a form of nonprobability sampling in which knowledge about the population of interest is used to build some representativeness into the sample (see Table 12-1). A quota sample identifies the strata of the population and proportionally represents the strata in the sample. For example, the data in Table 12-2 reveal that 20% of the 5000 nurses in city X are diploma graduates, 40% are associate degree students, and 40% are baccalaureate graduates. Each stratum of the population should be proportionately represented in the sample. In this case the researcher used a proportional quota sampling strategy and decided to sample 10% of a population of 5000 (i.e., 500 nurses). Based on the proportion of each stratum in the population, 100 diploma graduates, 200 associate degree graduates, and 200 baccalaureate graduates were the quotas established for the 3 strata. The researcher recruited subjects who met the eligibility criteria of the study until the quota for each stratum was filled. In other words, once the researcher obtained the necessary 100 diploma graduates, 200 associate degree graduates, and 200 baccalaureate graduates, the sample was complete in light of the research design, as well as other pragmatic matters, such as economy.

The researcher systematically ensures that proportional segments of the population are included in the sample. The quota sample is not randomly selected (i.e., once the proportional strata have been identified, the researcher obtains subjects until the quota for each stratum has been filled) but does increase the representativeness of the sample. This sampling strategy addresses the problem of overrepresentation or underrepresentation of certain segments of a population in a sample.

The characteristics chosen to form the strata are selected according to a researcher's judgment based on knowledge of the population and the literature review. The criterion for selection should be a variable that reflects important differences in the dependent variables under investigation. Age, gender, religion, ethnicity, medical diagnosis, socioeconomic status, level of completed education, and occupational rank are among the variables that are likely to be important stratifying variables in nursing research investigations. For example, McConnell and colleagues (2003) sought to describe patterns of change in physical functioning on a quarterly basis over 1 year among long-term nursing home residents stratified into seven groups according to their level of cognitive impairment on admission.

The critiquer of a research study seeks to determine whether the sample strata appropriately reflect the population under consideration and whether the stratifying variables are homogeneous enough to ensure a meaningful comparison of differences among strata. Even when the preceding factors have been addressed by the researcher, the evaluator must remember that as a nonprobability sample, the quota strategy contains an unknown source of bias that affects external validity.

The problem is that those who choose to participate may not be typical of the population with regard to the variables being measured. There is no way to assess the biases that may be operating. In cases where the phenomena under investigation are relatively homogeneous within the population, the risk of bias may be minimal.

TABLE 12-2 **Numbers and Percentages of Students in Strata of a Quota Sample of 5000 Graduates of Nursing Programs in City X**

	Diploma Graduates	**Associate Degree Graduates**	**Baccalaureate Graduates**
Population	1000 (20%)	2000 (40%)	2000 (40%)
Strata	100	200	200

In heterogeneous populations, however, the risk of bias is great.

Purposive Sampling

Purposive sampling is an increasingly common strategy in which the researcher's knowledge of the population and its elements is used to hand-pick the cases to be included in the sample. The researcher usually selects subjects who are considered to be typical of the population. For example, in a qualitative research study by Burns (2004) examining the problems and coping strategies of blacks on hemodialysis, a purposive sample of 102 black patients who were over the age of 18 and had a confirmed diagnosis of end-stage renal disease (ESRD) requiring hemodialysis was recruited at a community hemodialysis center. These participants were used because they were typical (homogeneous) of the population under consideration, which enhances the representativeness of this nonprobability sampling strategy used to describe a specific, and often underrepresented, minority population.

A purposive sample is used also when a highly unusual group is being studied, such as a population with a rare genetic disease (e.g., progeria). In this case, the researcher would describe the sample characteristics precisely to ensure that the reader will have an accurate picture of the subjects in the sample. This type of sample can also be used to study the differential effect of risk factors in a specific population longitudinally. For example, same-sex monozygotic (MZ) twin pairs who met the eligibility criteria were recruited into a study examining relationships among cardiovascular health indicators and health promoting behaviors in adult MZ twins. The researchers examined the differential effect of variables potentially influencing cardiovascular health through a health assessment survey that included questions about smoking status, alcohol and caffeine consumption, history of diabetes, and demographic variables such as the degree to which the MZ twins grew up in similar environments. The findings showed that both genetic and behavioral factors contributed to cardiovascular risk and cardiovascular health in participants.

In another situation, the researcher may wish to interview individuals who reflect different ends of the range of a particular characteristic. For example, Van Cleve and colleagues (2004) explored children's pain experience, management strategies, and outcomes during the first year after a diagnosis of acute lymphocytic leukemia; 95 children between the ages of 4 and 17 years who met the eligibility criteria constituted the sample.

Today, computer networks (e.g., online services) can be of great value in helping researchers access and recruit subjects for purposive samples. One researcher investigating the relationship between job stress, job performance, and social support among hospital nurses recruited a convenience sample of staff nurses who were accessible over the Internet. The researcher subscribed to a variety of listservs to compile a list of nurses' names and their e-mail addresses. A total of 3050 e-mail addresses were collected. From this list of possible participants, nurses who currently were working as hospital staff nurses, who had worked as staff nurses for at least 6 months in the last 3 years, and who were eligible to participate in the study, 2509 agreed to enroll in the study (AbuAlRub, 2004). Online support group bulletin boards that facilitate recruitment of subjects for purposive samples exist for people with cancer, rheumatoid arthritis, systemic lupus erythematosus, HIV/AIDS, bipolar disorder, Lyme disease, and many others.

The researcher who uses a purposive sample assumes that errors of judgment in overrepresenting or underrepresenting elements of the population in the sample will tend to balance out. There is no objective method, however, for determining the validity of this assumption. The evaluator must be aware of the fact that the more heterogeneous the population, the greater the chance of bias being introduced in the selection of a purposive sample. As indicated in Table

12-1, conscious bias in the selection of subjects remains a constant danger. Therefore the findings from a study using a purposive sample should be regarded with caution. As with any nonprobability sample, the ability to generalize from the evidence provided by the findings is very limited. The following are several instances when a purposive sample may be appropriate:

- The effective pretesting of newly developed instruments with a purposive sample of divergent types of people
- The validation of a scale or test with a known-group technique
- The collection of exploratory data in relation to an unusual or highly specific population, particularly when the total target population remains an unknown to the researcher
- The collection of descriptive data (e.g., as in qualitative studies) that seek to describe the lived experience of a particular phenomenon (e.g., postpartum depression; caring, hope, or surviving childhood sexual abuse)
- The focus of the study population relates to a specific diagnosis (e.g., type I diabetes, multiple sclerosis) or condition (e.g., legal blindness, terminal illness) or demographic characteristic (e.g., same-sex twin pairs)

Even when the use of a purposive sample is appropriate, the researcher, as well as the critiquer, should be cognizant of the limitations of this sampling strategy.

Probability Sampling

The primary characteristic of probability sampling is the random selection of elements from the population. **Random selection** occurs when each element of the population has an equal and

independent chance of being included in the sample. In the hierarchy of evidence, probability sampling, which is most closely associated with experimental and quasiexperimental designs, represents the strongest type of sampling strategy. The research consumer has greater confidence that the sample is representative rather than biased and more closely reflects the characteristics of the population of interest. Four commonly used probability sampling strategies are simple random sampling, stratified random sampling, cluster sampling, and systematic sampling.

Random selection of sample subjects should not be confused with random assignment of subjects. The latter, as discussed in Chapter 10, refers to the assignment of subjects to either an experimental or a control group on a purely random basis.

Simple Random Sampling

Simple random sampling is a laborious and carefully controlled process. Because more complex probability designs incorporate the principles of simple random sampling in their procedures, the principles of this strategy are presented.

The researcher defines the population (a set), lists all of the units of the population (a **sampling frame**), and selects a sample of units (a subset) from which the sample will be chosen. For example, if American hospitals specializing in the treatment of cancer were the sampling unit, a list of all such hospitals would be the sampling frame. If certified adult nurse practitioners (NPs) constituted the accessible population, a list of those nurses would be the sampling frame.

Once a list of the population elements has been developed, the best method of selecting a sample is to employ a table of random numbers containing columns of digits, such as the one appearing in Figure 12-1. Such tables can be generated by computer programs. After assigning consecutive numbers to units of the population, the researcher starts at any point on the table of random numbers and reads consecutive

1000 random integers between 0 and 99																				
40	23	0	29	10	94	17	58	12	85	13	25	80	84	72	74	54	63	55	31
32	98	49	23	74	97	51	42	21	87	48	64	54	38	84	68	14	17	35	48
84	34	84	14	53	65	67	37	2	45	84	21	71	34	10	80	72	27	11	13
86	37	24	89	23	4	44	40	72	81	44	69	25	44	34	34	34	75	50	50
50	58	85	8	22	24	73	20	63	35	60	87	91	92	96	80	19	22	87	24
1	87	43	82	9	31	40	88	33	28	82	73	18	6	48	64	59	45	34	3
21	19	42	76	84	67	29	68	8	66	93	89	96	28	12	14	38	47	52	65
32	66	33	21	81	97	39	76	67	27	97	22	76	89	41	11	91	29	6	66
16	82	42	75	35	42	92	90	77	24	21	8	36	16	5	54	89	51	57	85
74	32	63	65	93	96	18	36	82	72	39	69	37	97	51	17	36	71	38	30
50	94	4	66	17	37	10	53	8	29	67	74	88	38	11	59	60	91	56	17
71	47	81	18	53	98	7	87	29	37	22	93	13	6	95	7	95	71	14	6
71	93	48	16	33	19	46	21	60	44	52	91	52	58	10	9	41	31	35	18
20	94	13	99	45	6	53	54	1	25	79	28	1	48	36	26	68	37	59	7
75	22	69	56	62	40	64	45	40	99	94	14	98	84	22	38	24	87	43	71
16	87	41	0	88	83	11	37	71	78	22	39	43	37	75	84	84	11	55	58
92	90	80	2	30	37	85	55	56	50	3	71	24	13	62	74	82	44	90	32
96	89	31	32	37	45	70	67	80	55	58	9	55	60	61	55	86	44	27	77
38	29	36	94	65	39	56	29	29	65	88	13	71	38	71	8	81	66	31	44
20	6	61	66	90	13	70	60	92	53	87	49	34	42	14	47	75	33	26	9
63	44	94	21	14	13	41	80	39	72	29	3	25	89	44	88	13	49	18	58
13	32	93	90	31	75	86	95	18	51	61	59	84	95	67	54	40	30	29	63
26	35	48	81	19	24	36	36	76	16	46	5	93	41	97	46	79	54	95	49
89	74	96	95	94	69	31	60	16	69	76	42	28	71	69	34	46	55	20	42
50	39	28	64	20	68	60	33	92	82	61	70	5	68	95	88	12	85	18	94
55	86	5	96	87	69	75	93	54	79	0	57	45	8	86	59	25	21	9	29
75	35	1	2	86	62	70	83	85	13	97	37	13	73	16	38	36	23	54	11
74	50	1	77	87	92	68	87	57	36	17	47	0	97	78	72	72	45	54	51
34	24	35	13	26	42	22	75	47	2	34	87	15	50	65	27	5	72	28	68
73	33	42	65	91	24	44	84	71	55	70	1	27	30	8	61	65	61	18	92
7	55	12	6	61	17	23	95	91	58	60	30	35	61	34	27	75	44	35	64
10	94	18	4	3	19	21	37	28	55	76	25	10	29	80	64	8	81	20	32
20	48	92	87	95	58	57	73	42	1	12	81	94	85	63	97	24	19	93	51
81	10	92	49	70	15	76	4	36	92	62	99	78	32	86	74	43	22	98	46
66	67	82	94	67	75	16	88	84	98	0	52	37	0	43	9	0	51	2	62
64	92	36	11	3	52	44	65	45	67	97	86	92	2	50	5	93	66	73	40
36	29	98	46	88	23	28	44	8	71	69	43	53	16	87	21	56	23	37	24
15	11	82	30	59	94	23	30	40	25	87	26	24	30	44	53	33	65	72	55
89	57	49	79	83	88	42	45	41	93	38	24	15	80	97	18	61	12	13	42
23	36	65	9	64	26	93	37	26	44	42	17	45	68	27	77	74	56	49	34
9	93	90	61	45	40	75	85	64	66	36	89	72	43	99	90	92	10	10	85
53	94	30	31	62	92	82	30	94	56	40	4	50	53	9	74	87	2	36	36
18	69	77	38	89	78	30	68	71	92	22	93	91	74	52	1	97	69	71	42
50	20	76	36	6	20	75	56	36	5	14	70	9	78	23	33	91	33	25	72
30	46	1	10	16	72	69	26	94	39	80	36	36	68	92	74	22	74	41	42
59	47	7	92	77	55	2	12	5	24	0	30	25	62	83	36	92	96	36	75
93	22	3	20	82	44	16	69	98	72	30	57	77	15	90	29	32	38	3	48
9	55	27	41	40	94	77	14	54	10	25	75	1	74	72	15	69	80	33	58
70	8	3	5	46	89	28	86	40	6	25	40	81	26	63	97	87	48	26	41
19	6	89	31	80	60	13	89	17	69	38	93	58	55	54	69	74	33	8	55

Figure 12-1. A table of random numbers.

numbers in any direction (i.e., horizontally, vertically, or diagonally). When a number is read that corresponds with the written unit on a card, that unit is chosen for the sample. The investigator continues to read until a sample of the desired size is drawn. The advantages of simple random sampling are as follows:

- The sample selection is not subject to the conscious biases of the researcher.
- The representativeness of the sample in relation to the population characteristics is maximized.
- The differences in the characteristics of the sample and the population are purely a function of chance.
- The probability of choosing a nonrepresentative sample decreases as the size of the sample increases.

Simple random sampling was used in a study examining exercise behavior and functional outcomes in men and women 5 to 6 years following coronary artery bypass graft (CABG) surgery. All individuals who were 21 years of age and older and who were scheduled for CABG surgery at a large Midwestern hospital were enumerated and randomly selected for recruitment to the Post CABG Biobehavioral study. In an effort to achieve a sample broadly representative of the population undergoing CABG surgery at this site, patients were included in the study regardless of age or medical condition at the time of surgery (Treat-Jacobson and Lindquist, 2004).

Consumers must remember that despite the use of a carefully controlled sampling procedure that minimizes error, there is no guarantee that the sample will be representative. Factors such as sample heterogeneity and subject dropout may jeopardize the representativeness of the sample despite the most stringent random sampling procedure. In a study examining family perspectives about the final month of life for Oregon decedents dying in hospitals, nursing homes, and private homes, all death certificates for all Oregon deaths occurring in the 14 months between November 1996 and December 1997 were systematically randomly sampled, excluding decedents under age 18 years and deaths attributable to sucicide, homicide, or accident, or those undergoing medical examiner review. Out of a sampling frame of $n = 24,074$, the systematic random sample yielded 1458 death certificates. A potential factor jeopardizing representativeness of this sample is due to the fact that although the name of a family contact is listed on each death certificate, Oregon death certificates do not list an address or telephone number for family contacts. As a result, case finding for family contacts was unsuccessful for 44% of the sample (Tolle et al., 2000).

The major disadvantage of simple random sampling is that it is a time-consuming and inefficient method of obtaining a random sample. (Consider the task of listing all of the baccalaureate nursing students in the United States.) With random sampling, it may also be impossible to obtain an accurate or complete listing of every element in the population. Imagine trying to obtain a list of all completed suicides in New York City for the year 2005. It often is the case that although suicide may have been the cause of death, another cause (e.g., cardiac failure) appears on the death certificate. It would be difficult to estimate how many elements of the target population would be eliminated from consideration. The issue of bias would definitely enter the picture despite the researcher's best efforts. Thus the evaluator of a research paper must exercise caution in generalizing from reported findings, even when random sampling is the stated strategy, if the target population has been difficult or impossible to list completely.

Stratified Random Sampling

Stratified random sampling requires that the population be divided into strata or subgroups. The subgroups or subsets that the population is divided into are homogeneous. An appropriate number of elements from each subset are randomly selected on the basis of their proportion in the population. The goal of this strategy is to achieve a greater degree of representativeness.

Stratified random sampling is similar to the proportional stratified quota sampling strategy discussed earlier in the chapter. The major difference is that stratified random sampling uses a random selection procedure for obtaining sample subjects. Figure 12-2 illustrates the use of stratified random sampling.

The population is stratified according to any number of attributes, such as age, gender, ethnicity, religion, socioeconomic status, or level of education completed. The variables selected to make up the strata should be adaptable to homogeneous subsets with regard to the attributes being studied. The following criteria can be used in the selection of a stratified sample:

- Is there a critical variable or attribute that provides a logical basis for stratifying the sample?
- Does the population list contain sufficient information about the attributes that will be used to divide the sample into subsets?
- Is it appropriate for each subset to be equal in size, or is it more appropriate for each subset

to be proportionally stratified based on the proportion of each subset in the population?
- If proportional sampling is being used, is there a sufficient number of subjects in each subset for basing meaningful comparisons?
- Once the subset comparison has been determined, are random procedures used for selection of the sample?

As illustrated in Table 12-1, several advantages to a stratified sampling strategy are the following: (1) the representativeness of the sample is enhanced; (2) the researcher has a valid basis for making comparisons among subsets if information on the critical variables has been available; and (3) the researcher is able to oversample a disproportionately small stratum to adjust for their underrepresentation, statistically weigh the data accordingly, and continue to make legitimate comparisons.

The obstacles encountered by a researcher using this strategy include the following: (1) the difficulty of obtaining a population list containing complete critical variable information; (2)

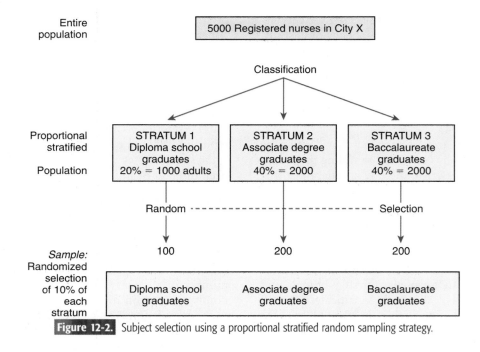

Figure 12-2. Subject selection using a proportional stratified random sampling strategy.

the time-consuming effort of obtaining multiple enumerated lists; (3) the challenge of enrolling proportional strata; and (4) the time and money involved in carrying out a large-scale study using a stratified sampling strategy. The critiquer must question the appropriateness of this sampling strategy to the problem under investigation. For example, Bath and colleagues (2000) conducted a mail survey to determine the extent to which hospitals complied with a national advisory committee recommendation about having hepatitis B screening policies and rubella immunization programs for pregnant women during an early prenatal visit. Using as a sampling frame a 1990 list of 5580 medical surgical hospitals from the American Hospital Association, the population was stratified by number of beds ($n = 500$) and affiliation with a medical school (yes/no). The sample size for each stratum was calculated to detect a 10% difference in proportions among strata with 95% confidence and 80% power. Of the 986 hospitals with labor and delivery programs in the sample, 858 (87%) responded. This study is a good example of how researchers can mathematically attempt to represent all strata proportionately in the study sample. In another example, researchers sought to determine the differential effect of early versus late extubation from mechanical ventilation (MV) in Medicare recipients after cardiac surgery (Bezanson et al., 2004). A total of 272 participants were randomly selected to comprise an estimation sample; an additional 272 participants comprised an independent validation sample. Participants were stratified into two study groups:

- Group 1 (early extubation)—equal to or less than 5 hours ($N = 205$)
- Group 2 (late extubation)—more than 5 hours ($N = 343$)

Multistage Sampling (Cluster Sampling)

Multistage (cluster) sampling involves a successive random sampling of units (clusters) that progress from large to small and meet sample eligibility criteria. The first-stage **sampling unit** consists of large units or clusters. The second-stage sampling unit consists of smaller units or clusters. Third-stage sampling units are even smaller. For example, if a sample of nurse practitioners (NPs) is desired, the first sampling unit would be a random sample of hospitals, obtained from an American Hospital Association list, that meet the eligibility criteria (e.g., size, type). The second-stage sampling unit would consist of a list of pediatric nurse practitioners (PNPs) practicing at each hospital selected in the first stage (i.e., the list obtained from the vice president for nursing at each hospital). The criteria for inclusion in the list of PNPs were as follows: (1) certified PNP with at least 2 years experience as an PNP; (2) at least 75% of the PNP's time spent in providing direct patient care in pediatric primary care practices; and (3) full-time employment at the hospital. The second-stage sampling strategy called for random selection of two PNPs from each hospital who met the previously mentioned eligibility criteria.

When multistage sampling is used in relation to large national surveys, states are used as the first-stage sampling unit, followed by successively smaller units such as counties, cities, districts, and blocks as the second-stage sampling unit, and finally households as the third-stage sampling unit.

Sampling units or clusters can be selected by simple random or stratified random sampling methods. Suppose that the hospitals, described in the example above, were grouped into 4 strata according to size (i.e., number of beds), as follows: (1) 200 to 299; (2) 300 to 399; (3) 400 to 499; and (4) 500 or more. Stratum 1 comprised 25% of the population; stratum 2 comprised 30% of the population; stratum 3 comprised 20% of the population; and stratum 4 comprised 25% of the population. This means that either a simple random or a proportional, stratified sampling strategy is used to randomly select hospitals that would proportionately represent the population of hospitals in the American Hospital Association list.

The main advantage of cluster sampling, as illustrated in Table 12-1, is that it is considerably more economical in terms of time and money than other types of probability sampling, particularly when the population is large and geographically dispersed or a sampling frame of the elements is not available. There are two major disadvantages, as follows: (1) more sampling errors tend to occur than with simple random or stratified random sampling; and (2) the appropriate handling of the statistical data from cluster samples is very complex.

The critiquer of a research report will need to consider whether the use of cluster sampling is justified in light of the research design, as well as other pragmatic matters, such as economy. For example, in a study investigating nurses attitudes and practice related to hospice care, a cross-sectional design was used to survey nurses employed in one of six Connecticut hospitals from 1998 to 1999. Selection of eligible nurses involved a two-stage sampling strategy. First, 6 hospitals were randomly selected from all Connecticut community hospitals with more than 200 licensed medical and surgical beds. Second, 30 nurses were randomly selected from each hospital according to specified eligibility criteria. Eligible nurses were staff nurses who were employed full-time (at least 30 hours per week) at the hospital for at least 6 months before the study, and who were assigned to medical, cardiology, pulmonology, or oncology units. Nurses who declined to participate were replaced by other randomly selected eligible nurses until 30 nurses per hospital mailed in completed questionnaires. The resulting response rate was 82% (180 of 219 completed). Nonresponders did not differ significantly from responders by hospital affiliation, type of patient care unit, or gender (Cramer et al., 2003). The fact that nonresponders did not differ from participants completing the study provides evidence suggesting that enrollee versus non-enrollee bias did not significantly influence the survey outcomes.

Systematic Sampling

Systematic sampling refers to a sampling strategy that involves the selection of every "kth" case drawn from a population list at fixed intervals, such as every tenth member listed in the directory of the American Psychiatric Nurses Association. Systematic sampling might be used to sample every "kth" person to enter a hospital lobby or be hospitalized with a diagnosis of congestive heart failure in 2005. When systematic sampling is used, the population must be narrowly defined in order to be considered as a probability sample, for example, all those people entering or leaving a hospital lobby. If senior citizens were sampled systematically upon entering a hospital lobby, the resulting sample would not be called a probability sample, because not every senior citizen would have a chance of being selected. As such, systematic sampling can sometimes represent a nonprobability sampling strategy.

Systematic sampling strategies can be designed, however, to fulfill the requirements of a probability sample. First, the listing of the population (sampling frame) must be random in relation to the variable of interest. For example, subjects were being selected from every tenth hospital room for a study on patient satisfaction with nursing care. Every tenth room happens to be a private room in the hospital where the study is being conducted. It is possible that the responses of patients in private rooms with regard to patient satisfaction might be different from those of patients in semiprivate rooms. Because of the nonrandom arrangement of the rooms, bias may have been introduced.

Second, the first element or member of the sample must be selected randomly. In this case, the researcher—who has a population list or sampling frame—first divides the population (N) by the size of the desired sample (n) to obtain the sampling interval width (k). The **sampling interval** is the standard distance between the elements chosen for the sample. For example, to select a sample of 50 family nurse practitioners from a population of 500 family nurse practitioners, the sampling interval would be as follows:

$$k = \frac{500}{50} = 10$$

Essentially, every tenth case on the family nurse practitioner list would be sampled. Once the sampling interval has been determined, the researcher uses a table of random numbers (see Figure 12-1) to obtain a starting point for the selection of the 50 subjects. If the population size is 500 and a sample size of 50 is desired, a number between 1 and 500 is randomly selected as the starting point. In this instance, if the first number is 51, the family nurse practitioners corresponding to numbers 51, 61, 71, and so forth would be included in the sample of 50. Another procedure recommended in many texts is to randomly select the first element from within the first sampling interval. If the sampling interval is 5, a number between 1 and 5 is selected as the random starting point. For example, the number 3 is randomly chosen. Keeping in mind the sampling interval of 5, the next elements selected would correspond to the numbers 8, 13, 18, and so on, until the sample was obtained. Although this procedure is technically correct, choosing a random starting point from across the total population of elements is more attractive because every element has a chance to be chosen for the sample during the first selection step.

Systematic sampling and simple random sampling are essentially the same type of procedure. The advantage of systematic sampling is that the results are obtained in a more convenient and efficient manner (see Table 12-1). The disadvantage of systematic sampling is that bias in the form of nonrandomness can inadvertently be introduced to the procedure. This problem may occur if the population list is arranged so that a certain type of element is listed at intervals that coincide with the sampling interval. As an example, if every tenth nursing student on a population list of all types of nursing students in New Mexico was a baccalaureate student and the sampling interval was 10, baccalaureate students would be overrepresented in the sample. Cyclical fluctuations are also a factor. For example, if a list of nursing students using the college library each day to do computer literature searches is kept, a biased sample will probably be obtained if every seventh day is chosen as the sampling interval because fewer and perhaps different nursing students probably use the library on Sundays than on weekdays. Therefore caution must be exercised about departures from randomness as they affect the representativeness of the sample and, as a result, affect the external validity of the study.

The critiquer will want to note whether a satisfactory random selection procedure was carried out. If randomization was not used, the systematic sampling may have become a nonprobability quota sample. It is important to be cognizant of this issue because the implications related to interpretation and generalizability are drastically altered if the evaluator is dealing with a nonprobability sample. For example, in their study Cho et al. (2003) sought to determine the effects of nurse staffing on adverse events including morbidity, mortality, and medical costs. The study used two existing databases: California Hospital Financial Data and 1997 data for the state of California released by the Agency for Healthcare Research and Quality (AHRQ). The selection of hospitals and patients strived to create a sample that included homogeneous hospital and patient groups while representing the majority of the target population. Hospitals were stratified by ownership, hospital size, teaching affiliation, and location; nurse staffing was stratified by type of care unit (e.g., medical-surgical acute care, medical-surgical intensive care, and coronary care). Patient characteristics were stratified by Diagnositc Related Group (DRG) and selected demographic variables. Because randomization was not used at any phase of this multilevel sampling procedure, the evaluator would consider this to be a nonprobability stratified sample with the external validity limitations of that sampling strategy (see Chapter 9).

In contrast, in a study investigating the effect of comprehensive, multidisciplinary maternity care (Genesis program) on maternity outcomes in a matched sample of pregnant women of low socioeconomic class, a systematic sampling procedure was used (Lowry and Beikirch, 1998). Data on Genesis clients were retrieved by a retrospective chart review in which the sample was randomly selected from 1200 charts of the women who presented for prenatal care during the first fully operational year of the Genesis program and who delivered between July 1, 1991 and July 1, 1992. Every sixth chart was reviewed for a total of 200 Genesis records and a similar number of matched subject charts for subjects who had received care from county public health units and one of the local migrant clinics. Because random selection was used in this example of systematic sampling, the critiquer could have more confidence in the generalizability of the findings to a similar target population.

 EVIDENCE-BASED PRACTICE TIP

The sampling strategy, whether probability or nonprobability, must be appropriate to the design and evaluated in relation to the level of evidence provided by the design.

Special Sampling Strategies

Several special sampling strategies are used in nonprobability sampling. **Matching** is a special strategy used to construct an equivalent comparison sample group by filling it with subjects who are similar to each subject in another sample group in relation to preestablished variables such as age, gender, level of education, medical diagnosis, or socioeconomic status. Theoretically, any variable other than the independent variable that could affect the dependent variable should be matched. In reality, the more variables matched, the more difficult it is to obtain an adequate sample size. For example, in a study examining the effect of an ankle strengthening and walking exercise program on improving fall-related outcomes in the elderly, Schoenfelder and Rubenstein (2004) recruited participants from 10 private, urban nursing homes in eastern Iowa.

Participants were matched in pairs by Risk Assessment for Falls Scale II scores and then randomly assigned within each pair to the intervention or control group.

Networking sampling, sometimes referred to as snowballing, is a strategy used for locating samples that are difficult or impossible to locate in other ways. This sampling strategy takes advantage of social networks and the fact that friends tend to have characteristics in common. When a few subjects with the necessary eligibility criteria are found, the researcher asks for their assistance in getting in touch with others with similar criteria. For example, Ugarriza (2002) used networking and snowballing to obtain participants for a study gathering information from postpartum depressed mothers on their perceptions of their condition and to compare those responses with the biomedical view of postpartum depression. Thirteen new mothers were recruited for the study from the practices of nurse midwives and other health providers such as childbirth educators who maintained contact with the new mothers after delivery. The 13 mothers assisted in snowball sampling by referring 17 other postpartum depressed mothers to the study. In another study examining the stress process in everyday life for African-American adults, Brown (2004) recruited participants at churches, cultural events, community organizations, beauty salons, and barber shops, via the internet and newspaper ads, as well as word-of-mouth referrals by interview participants—all of which capture the essence of the **network (snowball effect) sampling** strategy that resulted in a sample of 211 middle-class African-Americans ranging in age from 25 to 79. Today, online computer networks, as described in the section on purposive sampling and in this last example, can be used to assist researchers in acquiring otherwise difficult to locate subjects, thereby taking advantage of the networking or snowball effect. The Critical Thinking Decision Path illustrates the relationship between the type of sampling strategy and the appropriate generalizability.

CRITICAL THINKING DECISION PATH   Assessing the Relationship between the Type of Sampling Strategy and the Appropriate Generalizability

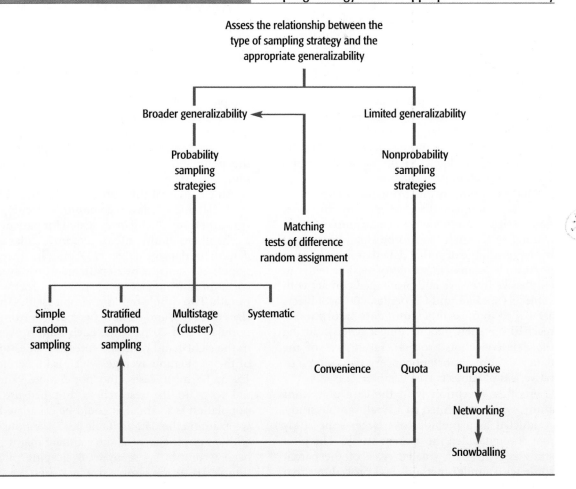

 HELPFUL H I N T

Look for a brief discussion of a study's sampling strategy in the "Methods" section of a research article. Sometimes there is a separate subsection with the heading "Sample," "Subjects," or "Study Participants." A statistical description of the characteristics of the actual sample often does not appear until the "Results" section of a research article.

SAMPLE SIZE

There is no single rule that can be applied to the determination of a sample's size. When arriving at an estimate of sample size, many factors, such as the following, must be considered:

- The type of design used
- The type of sampling procedure used
- The type of formula used for estimating optimum sample size

- The degree of precision required
- The heterogeneity of the attributes under investigation
- The relative frequency that the phenomenon of interest occurs in the population (i.e., a common vs. a rare health problem)
- The projected cost of using a particular sampling strategy

The sample size should be determined before the study is conducted. A general rule of thumb is always to use the largest sample possible. The larger the sample, the more representative of the population it is likely to be; smaller samples produce less accurate results.

One exception to this principle occurs when using certain qualitative designs. In this case, sample size is not predetermined. Sample sizes in qualitative research tend to be small because of the large volume of verbal data that must be analyzed and because this type of design tends to emphasize intensive and prolonged contact with subjects (Speziale and Carpenter, 2003). Subjects are added to the sample until **data saturation** is reached (i.e., new data no longer emerge during the data-collection process). Fittingness of the data is a more important concern than representativeness of subjects (see Chapter 7).

Another exception is in the case of a **pilot study,** which is defined as a small sample study, conducted as a prelude to a larger-scale study that is often called the "parent study." The pilot study is typically a smaller scale of the parent study with similar methods and procedures that yield preliminary data that determine the feasibility of conducting a larger-scale study and establish that sufficient scientific evidence exists to justify subsequent, more extensive research (Jaireth, Hogerney, and Parsons, 2000). For example, Hoskins and associates (2001) conducted a pilot study, "Breast Cancer: Education, Counseling and Adjustment," using a small sample ($n = 12$) to determine the feasibility of and to analyze preliminary data about the differential effect of a standardized phase-specific educational and telephone counseling intervention

for women with breast cancer and their partners prior to conducting the parent study, a randomized clinical trial that would have a sample size of $n = 280$.

The principle of "larger is better" holds true for both probability and nonprobability samples. Results based on small samples (under 10) tend to be unstable—the values fluctuate from one sample to the next. Small samples tend to increase the probability of obtaining a markedly nonrepresentative sample. As the sample size increases, the mean more closely approximates the population values, thus introducing fewer sampling errors.

An example of this concept is illustrated by a study in which the average monthly sleeping pill consumption is being investigated for patients on a rehabilitation unit after a cerebrovascular accident. The data in Table 12-3 indicate that the population consists of 20 patients whose average consumption of sleeping pills is 15.15 per month. Two simple random samples with sample sizes of 2, 4, 6, and 10 have been drawn from the population of 20 patients. Each sample average in the right-hand column represents an estimate of the population average, which is known to be 15.15. In most cases, the population value is unknown to the researchers, but because the population is so small, it could be calculated. As we examine the data in Table 12-3, we note that with a sample size of 2, the estimate might have been wrong by as many as 8 sleeping pills in sample 1B. As the sample size increases, the averages get closer to the population value, and the differences in the estimates between samples A and B also get smaller. Large samples permit the principles of randomization to work effectively (i.e., to counterbalance atypical values in the long run).

It is possible to estimate the sample size with the use of a statistical procedure known as power analysis (Cohen, 1977). It is beyond the scope of this chapter to describe this complex procedure in great detail, but a simple example will illustrate its use. Koniak-Griffin and colleagues

TABLE 12-3 **Comparison of Population and Sample Values and Averages in Study of Sleeping Pill Consumption**

Number in Group	Group	Number of Sleeping Pills Consumed (Values Expressed Monthly)	Average
20	Population	1, 3, 4, 5, 6, 7, 9, 11, 13, 15, 16, 17, 19, 21, 22, 23, 25, 27, 29, 30	15.15
2	Sample 1A	6, 9	7.5
2	Sample 1B	21, 25	23.0
4	Sample 2A	1, 7, 15, 25	12.0
4	Sample 2B	5, 13, 23, 29	17.5
6	Sample 3A	3, 4, 11, 15, 21, 25	13.3
6	Sample 3B	5, 7, 11, 19, 27, 30	16.5
10	Sample 4A	3, 4, 7, 9, 11, 13, 17, 21, 23, 30	13.8
10	Sample 4B	1, 4, 6, 11, 15, 17, 19, 23, 25, 27	14.8

(2003) wanted to determine the effect of an early intervention program (EIP) versus traditional public health nursing care (TPHNC) on 2-year postbirth infant health and maternal outcomes in a population of Latina and African-American adolescent mothers (Appendix A). Adolescent mothers who met the eligibility criteria were randomly assigned to an experimental group or a control group. How many patients should be used in the study? When using power analysis, the researcher must estimate how large of a difference will be observed between the groups (i.e., the difference in selected infant health outcomes, including number of hospitalizations, emergency department visits, and immunizations, and in maternal outcomes of social competence, education, and employment status after the experimental EIP program was implemented). If a small difference is expected, the sample must be large (in this case, 184 patients in each group) to ensure that the differences, the effect, will actually be revealed in a statistical analysis. If a medium-size difference is expected, the total sample size would be 144, that is, 72 in each group. When expected differences are large, it does not take a very large sample to ensure that differences will be revealed through statistical analysis. Power analysis is an advanced statistical technique that is commonly used by researchers and is a requirement for external funding. When

it is not used, research consumers will have less confidence provided by the findings because the research study may be based on a sample that is too small. A researcher may commit a type II error of accepting a null hypothesis when it should have been rejected if the sample is too small (see Chapter 17). No matter how high a research design is located on the hierarchy of evidence (e.g., Level II—experimental design consisting of a randomized clinical trial), the findings of a study, and the generalizability, are weakened when power analysis is not calculated to ensure an adequate sample size to determine the effect of the intervention.

Despite the principles related to determining sample size that have been identified, the consumer should be aware that large samples do not ensure representativeness or accuracy. A large sample cannot compensate for a faulty research design. The proportion of the population that is sampled does not provide a guarantee of accurate results. It is often possible to obtain accurate results from only a small fraction of a large population. For example, a 10% probability sample of a population containing 1500 elements will yield more precise results than a nonprobability 0.01% sample of a population with 100,000 elements.

The critiquer should evaluate the sample size in terms of the following: (1) how representative the sample is relative to the target population; (2) to whom the researcher wishes to generalize the results of the study. The goal of sampling is to have a sample as representative as possible with as little sampling error as possible. Unless representativeness is ensured, all the data in the world become inconsequential.

 HELPFUL H I N T

Remember to look for some rationale about the sample size and those strategies the researcher has used (e.g., matching, test of differences on demographic variables) to ascertain or build in sample representativeness.

 EVIDENCE-BASED PRACTICE TIP

Research designs and types of samples are often linked. The research consumer would expect to see experimental designs using probability sampling strategies; if a nonprobability purposive sampling strategy is used to recruit participants to such a study, the research consumer would expect random assignment to intervention and control groups to follow.

SAMPLING PROCEDURES

The criteria for drawing a sample vary according to the sampling strategy. Regardless of which strategy is used, it is important that the procedure be systematically organized. This organization will eliminate the bias that occurs when sample selection is carried out inconsistently. Bias in sample representativeness and generalizability of findings are important sampling issues that have generated national concern because the presence of these factors decreases confidence in the evidence provided by the findings and limits its applicability. Many of the landmark adult health studies (e.g., the Framingham heart study and the Baltimore longitudinal study on aging)

historically excluded women as subjects. Despite the all-male samples, the findings of these studies were generalized from males to all adults, in spite of the lack of female representation in the samples. Similarly, the use of largely Euro-American subjects in clinical trials limits the identification of variant responses to interventions or drugs in ethnic or racially distinct groups (Bailey et al., 2004; Ward, 2003). Findings based on Euro-American data cannot be generalized to African-Americans, Asians, Hispanics, or any other cultural group. Consequently, careful identification of the target population is a crucial step in the process. If a researcher wants to be able to draw conclusions about psychosocial stressors related to all patients with a first-time myocardial infarction, then both males and females must be included in the target population. When a researcher wants to be able to draw conclusions about the incidence of weight gain and diabetes in African-American psychiatric patients taking olanzapine (Zyprexa) compared to Euro-Americans, the target population must be diverse. Sometimes the target population has to be gender-specific, as when breast or prostate cancer or aspects of pregnancy or menopause are studied.

Several general steps, as illustrated in Figure 12-3, that will ensure a consistent approach by the researcher can be identified. Initially, the target population (i.e., the entire group of people or objects about whom the researcher wants to draw conclusions or make generalizations) must be identified. The target population may consist of all female patients with a first-time diagnosis of breast cancer, all children with asthma, all pregnant teenagers, or all doctoral students in the United States. Next, the accessible portion of the target population must be delineated. An accessible population might consist of all of the NPs in the state of California, all of the male patients with unstable angina admitted to hospital X during 2005, all of the pregnant teenagers in a specific prenatal clinic, or all of the children with acute lymphocytic leukemia under care at a specific children's hospital specializing in the

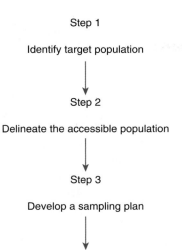

Step 1

Identify target population

Step 2

Delineate the accessible population

Step 3

Develop a sampling plan

Step 4

Obtain approval from Institutional Review Board

Figure 12-3. Summary of general sampling procedure.

treatment of cancer. Then a sampling plan or a protocol for actually selecting the sample from the accessible population is formulated. The researcher makes decisions about how subjects will be approached, what strategies will be used to recruit a diverse sample with minority representation, how the study will be explained, and who will select the sample—the researcher or a research assistant. Regardless of who implements the sampling plan, consistency in how it is done is paramount. The reader of a research study will want to find a description of the sample, as well as the sampling procedure, in the report. On the basis of the appropriateness of what has been reported, the critiquer can make judgments about the soundness of the sampling protocol,

which of course will affect the interpretations made about the evidence provided by the findings. Finally, once the accessible population and sampling plan have been established, permission is obtained from the institution's research board, which is commonly referred to as the Institutional Review Board. This permission provides free access to the desired population (see Chapter 13).

When an appropriate sample size, including power analysis for calculation of sample size, and sampling strategy have been used, the researcher can feel more confident that the sample is representative of the accessible population rather than biased; however, it is more difficult to feel confident that the accessible population is representative of the target population. Are NPs in California representative of all NPs in the United States? It is impossible to be sure about this. Researchers must exercise judgment when assessing typicality. Unfortunately there are no guidelines for making such judgments, and there is even less basis for the critiquer to make such evidence-based decisions. The best rule of thumb to use when evaluating the representativeness of a sample and its generalizability to the target population is to be realistic and conservative about making sweeping claims relative to the findings.

 HELPFUL H I N T

Remember to evaluate the appropriateness of the generalizations made about the study findings in light of the target population, the accessible population, the type of sampling strategy, and the sample size.

CRITIQUING GUIDE *Sampling*

The criteria for critiquing the sampling technique of a study are presented in the Critiquing Criteria box. The research consumer approaches the "Sample" section of a research report with a different perspective than the researcher. The consumer must raise two questions: (1) "If this study were to be replicated, would there be enough information presented about the nature of the population, the sample, the sampling strategy, and sample size of another investigator to carry out the study?" (2) "Are the previously mentioned factors about sampling appropriate in light of the particular research design, and if not, which sampling factors require modification, especially if the study is to be replicated?" The answers to those questions highlight the important link of the sample to the study findings and the strength of the evidence used to make clinical decisions about the applicability of the findings to clinical practice.

Sampling is considered to be one important aspect of the methodology of a research study. As such, data pertaining to the sample usually appear in the "Methodology" section of the research report. The sampling content presented should reflect the outcome of a series of decisions based on sampling criteria appropriate to the design of the study, as well as the options and limitations inherent in the context of the investigation. The following discussion will highlight several sampling criteria that the research consumer will want to consider when evaluating the merit of a sampling strategy as it relates to a specific research study.

Initially, the parameters or attributes of the study population should clearly specify to what population the findings may be generalized. In general, the target population of the study is not specifically identified by the researcher, but the nature of it is implied in the description of the accessible population and/or the sample. For example, if a researcher states that 100 subjects were randomly drawn from a population of women 14 years of age or older diagnosed with cervical intraepithelial neoplasia II or III and who were willing to postpone standard ablative

CRITIQUING CRITERIA *Sampling*

1. Have the sample characteristics been completely described?
2. Can the parameters of the study population be inferred from the description of the sample?
3. To what extent is the sample representative of the population as defined?
4. Are the criteria eligibility in the sample specifically identified?
5. Have sample delimitations been established?
6. Would it be possible to replicate the study population?
7. How was the sample selected? Is the method of sample selection appropriate?
8. What kind of bias, if any, is introduced by this method?
9. Is the sample size appropriate? How is it substantiated?
10. Are there indications that rights of subjects have been ensured?
11. Does the researcher identify the limitations in generalizability of the findings from the sample to the population? Are they appropriate?
12. Is the sampling strategy appropriate for the design of the study and level of evidence provided by the design?
13. Does the researcher indicate how replication of the study with other samples would provide increased support for the findings?

therapy and receive topical retinoic acid treatment at affiliated clinics within hospital system X during the year 2006, the critiquer can specifically evaluate the parameters of the population. Demographic characteristics of the sample (e.g., age, diagnosis, ethnicity, religion, level of education, socioeconomic status [SES], and marital status) should also be presented in either a tabled or a narrative summary because they provide further explication about the nature of the sample and enable the critiquer to evaluate the sampling procedure more accurately. For example, in their study titled "Nurse Visitation for Adolescent Mothers", Koniak-Griffin and colleagues (2003; see Appendix A) present detailed data summarizing demographic variables of importance. These data are reproduced as follows:

Participants had a mean age of 16.70 years (SD = 1.13) and were predominantly poor, unmarried, and from ethnic groups of color (Table 1). Of the young women who described themselves as Latina, 43 (the majority) were born in the United States (US), 17 in Mexico, and 3 in Central America. The average score on the Short Acculturation Scale, administered to Latinas who identified themselves as either "Spanish-speaking only" or "bilingual in Spanish and English" (n = 40), was 3.46 (SD = 0.81), representing a moderate degree of acculturation. At intake nearly half the adolescents were enrolled and attending school; however, more than 25% had dropped out. Histories of childhood physical abuse (n = 58, 57%) ranging from being slapped to being threatened with a weapon and of sexual abuse (n = 25, 25%) of varying degrees of severity (e.g., fondling to forced sexual intercourse) were reported. Twelve participants reported one or more suicide attempts within the previous year (see Appendix A).

This example illustrates how a detailed description of the sample both provides the critiquer with a frame of reference for the study population and sample and generates questions to be raised. For instance, the critiquer will note that the range of age from 14 to 19, with a mean age of 16.70, captures the age range of adolescent mothers, yet provides the homogeneity necessary to eliminate extraneous variability due to age. The evaluator who has this demographic sample information available is able to question a sampling strategy that does not also consider the differential effect of the mother's age on maternal and infant outcomes. It would seem logical that there might be a difference in the maternal and infant outcomes if the new mother is a teenager rather than a woman in her twenties or thirties.

It is also helpful if the researcher has presented a rationale for having elected to study one type of population vs. another. For example, given the fact that teen birth rates have declined sharply in recent years, by 22% from 1991 to 2000, why did the previously cited study focus on teen mothers between the ages of 14 and 19? To support their sample population choice, the authors report that Hispanic and African-American adolescents continue to have a much higher birth rate than non-Hispanic Caucasians. Adolescent mothers and their children may benefit from a home visitation program, as they often lack the resources needed to maintain health and reduce risk factors in their lives. Many of these women live in poverty, have low educational attainment, and lack social support. Moreover, their children have higher rates of morbidity and unintentional injuries, leading to more emergency room visits and hospitalizations during the first 3 years of life compared to children of adult mothers.

In a research study that uses a nonprobability sampling strategy, it is particularly important to fully describe the population and the sample in terms of who the study subjects are, the way they were chosen, and the reason they were chosen. If these criteria are adhered to, the degree of heterogeneity or homogeneity of the sample can be determined. The use of a homogeneous sample minimizes the amount of sampling error introduced, a problem particularly common in nonprobability sampling. When deciding about whether the findings of a study can be applied to patients in the nurse's practice, the degree to which the study participants are similar to the nurse's patients is important.

Next, the defined representativeness of the population should be examined. Probability sampling is clearly the ideal sampling procedure for ensuring the representativeness of a study population. Use of random selection procedures (e.g., simple random, stratified, cluster, or systematic sampling strategies) minimizes the occurrence of conscious and unconscious biases, which affect the researcher's ability to generalize about the findings from the sample to the population. The critiquer should be able to identify the type of probability strategy used and determine whether the researcher adhered to the criteria for a particular sampling plan. In experimental and quasiexperimental studies, the evaluator must also know whether or how the subjects were assigned to groups. If criteria for random assignment have not been followed, the reader has a valid basis for being cautious about the strength of evidence provided by the proposed conclusions of the study.

Although random selection is the ideal in establishing the representativeness of a study population, more often realistic barriers (e.g., institutional policy, inaccessibility of subjects, lack of time or money, and current state of knowledge in the field) necessitate the use of nonprobability sampling strategies. Many important research questions that are of interest to nursing do not lend themselves to levels of evidence provided by experimental designs and probability sampling. This is particularly true with qualitative research designs. A well-designed, carefully controlled study using a non-probability sampling strategy can yield accurate and meaningful evidence that makes a significant contribution to nursing's scientific body of knowledge. As the critiquer, you must ask a philosophical question: "If it is not possible or appropriate to conduct an experimental or quasiexperimental investigation that uses probability sampling, should the study be abandoned?" The answer usually suggests that it is better to carry out the investigation and be fully aware of the limitations of the methodology and evidence provided than to lose the knowledge that can be gained. The researcher is always able to move on to subsequent studies that reflect a stonger and more consistent level of evidence either by replicating the study or by using more stringent design and sampling strategies to refine the knowledge derived from a nonexperimental study.

The greatest difficulty in nonprobability sampling stems from the fact that not every element in the population has an equal chance of being represented in the sample. Therefore it is likely that some segment of the population will be systematically underrepresented. If the population is homogeneous on critical characteristics, such as age, gender, socioeconomic status, and diagnosis, systematic bias will not be very important. Few of the attributes that researchers are interested in, however, are sufficiently homogeneous to render sampling bias an irrelevant consideration.

Next, the sampling plan's suitability to the research design should be evaluated. Experimental and quasiexperimental designs use some form of random selection or random assignment of subjects to groups (see Chapter 10). The critiquer evaluates whether the researcher adhered to the principles of random selection and assignment. Lack of adherence to such principles compromises the representativeness of the sample and the external validity of the study. The following are questions the evaluator might pose relative to this issue:

- Has a random selection procedure (e.g., a table of random numbers) been identified?
- Has the appropriate random sampling plan been selected; that is, has a proportional stratified sampling plan been selected instead of a simple random sampling plan in a study where there is more than one distinct level that appears to be a critical variable for stratification (e.g., cognitive status, type of health care organization, functional status)?
- Has the particular random sampling plan been carried out appropriately; that is, if a

cluster sampling strategy was used, did the sampling units logically progress from the largest to the smallest?

Random sampling should not be looked on as a cure-all. Sometimes bias is inadvertently introduced even when the principle of random selection is used.

Nonexperimental designs often use nonprobability sampling strategies. In this instance, the question that can be raised by the critiquer is whether a nonexperimental design and a related nonprobability sampling plan were most appropriate for this study. It is sometimes true that if the researcher had used another type of design or sampling plan, he or she could have constructed a stronger study that would have provided a stronger level of evidence which allowed more generalizability and greater confidence to be placed in the findings. The critiquer, however, is rarely in a position to know what factors entered into the decision to plan one type of study vs. another.

When critiquing qualitative research designs, the evaluator applies criteria related to sampling strategies that are relevant for a particular type of qualitative study. In general, sampling strategies are purposive because the study of specific phenomena in their natural setting is emphasized; any subject belonging to a specified group is considered to represent that group. For example, when a qualitative study such as "Bone Marrow Transplantation: The Battle for Hope in the Face of Fear" (Cohen and Levy, 2000) is conducted, the specified group is people with cancer who are autologous bone marrow transplant survivors. The researcher's goal is to establish the meaning of their slices of life, that is, the typicality or atypicality of the observed events, behaviors, or responses in the lives of the bone marrow transplant survivors in order to better understand the effect of this treatment on their lives and how nursing can best meet their needs (see Chapters 6 and 7).

The evaluator should then determine whether the sample size is appropriate and its size is justifiable. It is common for the researcher to indicate in a research article how the sample size was determined. The method of arriving at the sample size and the rationale should be briefly mentioned. For example, in a study comparing the differential effectiveness of normal saline compared to heparinized saline for patency of intravenous locks in neonates, a researcher may state in a very detailed way:

Sample size was based on a 12-hour difference in the longevity of the IV lock. Power analysis for a Student's t-test determined an optimum sample size of 292 would provide a power of 0.80 with a two-tailed alpha less than 0.05 (Schultz, Drew, and Hewitt, 2002).

The importance of this example lies not in understanding every technical word cited, but in understanding that this type of statement or some abbreviated form of it meets the criteria stated at the beginning of the paragraph and should be evident in the research report.

Other considerations with respect to sample size, especially when the sample size appears to be small or inadequate and there is no stated rationale for the size, are as follows:

- How will the sample size affect the accuracy of the results?
- Is the sample size large enough to detect the effect of the intervention?
- Are any subsets or cells of the sample over-represented or underrepresented?
- Are any of the subsets so small as to limit meaningful comparisons?
- Has the researcher examined the effect of attrition or dropouts on the results?
- Has the researcher recognized and identified any limitations posed by the size of the sample?

Essentially, these criteria demand that the critiquer carefully scrutinize several important elements pertaining to sample size that have implications for the generalizability of the findings. Keep in mind that qualitative studies will not discuss predetermining sample size or method of arriving at sample size. Rather, sample size will tend to be small and a function of data saturation (see Chapter 7).

Finally, evidence that the rights of human subjects have been protected should appear in the "Sample" section of the research report. The critiquer will evaluate whether permission was obtained from an institutional review board that reviewed the study relative to the maintenance of ethical research standards (see Chapter 13). For example, the review board examines the research proposal to determine whether the introduction of an experimental procedure may be potentially harmful and therefore undesirable. The critiquer also examines the report for evidence of the subjects' informed consent, as well as protection of their confidentiality or anonymity. It is highly unusual for research studies not to demonstrate evidence of having met these criteria. Nevertheless, the careful critiquer will want to be certain that ethical standards that protect sample subjects have been maintained.

It is evident that there are many factors to consider when critiquing the "Sample" section of a research report. The type and appropriateness of the sampling strategy become crucial elements in the analysis and intepretation of data, in the conclusions derived from the findings, and in the generalizability of the findings from the sample to the population. As stated earlier in this chapter, the major purpose of sampling is to increase the efficiency of a research study by using a sample that is representative of the particular population so that every element need not be studied, and yet generalizing the findings from the sample to the population. The critiquer must justify that the sampling strategy used provided a valid basis for the findings and their generalizability in order to feel confident.

Critical Thinking Challenges

- A research classmate asks the instructor the following question: "Wouldn't it be better to study an entire population of patients with lung cancer instead of using a research sampling technique?" How would you answer this question? Explain how sampling will improve the strength and quality of the evidence provided by the findings? Include examples that will help the student see it from your point of view.
- A quasiexperimental study indicates that it used a convenience sample with random assignment. How is this possible? Would this be a nonprobability or probability sample? How does this type of sampling affect the evidence findings? Would this quasiexperimental study's findings be useful in evidence-based practice? Explain your answer.
- Your research class is having a debate on probability vs. nonprobability sampling in regard to desirability and feasibility. You are assigned to present the pros of nonprobability sampling in nursing research. What arguments would you use?
- Discuss the principle of "larger is better" and its relationship to "network" sampling and the sample size of qualitative studies. Include in your discussion the concept of "data saturation," as well as the use of computer technology.
- Your research classmate is arguing that a random sample is always better, even if it is small and represents only one site. Another student is arguing that a very large convenience sample representing multiple sites can be very significant. Which classmate would you defend and why? How would each scenario affect the strength and quality of the evidence provided by the findings?

KEY POINTS

- Sampling is a process that selects representative units of a population for study. Researchers sample representative segments of the population because it is rarely feasible or necessary to sample entire populations of interest to obtain accurate and meaningful information.
- Researchers establish eligibility criteria; these are descriptors of the population and provide the basis for selection of a sample. Eligibility criteria, which are also referred to as delimitations, include the following: age, gender, socioeconomic status, level of education, religion, and ethnicity.
- The researcher must identify the target population (i.e., the entire set of cases about which the researcher would like to make generalizations). Because of the pragmatic constraints, however, the researcher usually uses an accessible population (i.e., one that meets the population criteria and is available).
- A sample is a set of elements that makes up the population.
- A sampling unit is the element or set of elements used for selecting the sample. The foremost criterion in evaluating a sample is the representativeness or congruence of characteristics with the population.
- Sampling strategies consist of nonprobability and probability sampling.
- In nonprobability sampling, the elements are chosen by nonrandom methods. Types of nonprobability sampling include convenience, quota, and purposive sampling.
- Probability sampling is characterized by the random selection of elements from the population. In random selection, each element in the population has an equal and independent chance of being included in the sample. Types of probability sampling include simple random, stratified random, cluster, and systematic sampling.
- Sample size is a function of the type of sampling procedure being used, the degree of precision required, the type of sample estimation formula being used, the heterogeneity of the study attributes, the relative frequency of occurrence of the phenomena under consideration, and cost.

- Criteria for drawing a sample vary according to the sampling strategy. Systematic organization of the sampling procedure minimizes bias. The target population is identified, the accessible portion of the target population is delineated, permission to conduct the research study is obtained, and a sampling plan is formulated.
- The critiquer of a research report evaluates the sampling plan for its appropriateness in relation to the particular research design and level of evidence generated by the design.
- Completeness of the sampling plan is examined in light of potential replicability of the study. The critiquer evaluates whether the sampling strategy is the strongest plan for the particular study under consideration.
- An appropriate systematic sampling plan will maximize the efficiency of a research study. It will increase the strength, accuracy, and meaningfulness of the evidence provided by the findings and enhance the generalizability of the findings from the sample to the population.

REFERENCES

AbuAlRub RF: Job stress, job performance, and social support among hospital nurses, *J Nurs Scholarship* 36(1): 73-78, 2004.

Artinian NT, Magnan M, Christian W, and Lange MP: What do patients know about their heart failure?, *Appl Nurs Res* 15(4): 200-208, 2002.

Bailey JM, Bieniasz ME, Kmak D, Brenner DE, and Ruffin MT: Recruitment and retention of economically underserved women to a cervical cancer prevention trial, *Appl Nurs Res* 17(1): 55-60, 2004.

Bath SK, Singleton JA, Strikas RA, Stevenson JM, McDonald LL, and Williams WW: Performance of US hospitals on recommended screening and immunization practices for pregnant and postpartum women, *Am J Infect Control* 28(5): 327-332, 2000.

Bezanson JL, Weaver M, Kinney MR, Waldrum M, and Weintrau WS: Presurgical risk factors for late extubation in Medicare recipients after cardiac surgery, *Nurs Res* 53(1): 46-52, 2004.

Brown DJ: Everyday life for Black American adults: stress, emotions, and blood pressure, *West J Nurs Res* 26(5): 499-514, 2004.

Burns D: Physical and psychosocial adaptation of blacks on hemodialysis, *Appl Nurs Res* 17(2): 118-124, 2004.

Cho SH, Ketefian S, Barkauskas VH, and Smith DG: The effects of nurse staffing on adverse events, morbidity, mortality, and medical costs, *Nurs Res* 52(2): 71-79, 2003.

Cochran WG: *Sampling technique,* ed 3, New York, 1977, Wiley.

Cohen J: *Stastistical power analysis for the behavioral sciences,* New York, 1977, Academic Press.

Cohen MZ, Levy CD: Bone marrow transplantation: the battle for hope in the face of fear, *Oncol Nurs Forum* 27(3): 473-480, 2000.

Cramer LD, McCorkle R, Cherlin E, Johnson-Hurzler R, and Bradley EH: Nurses' attitudes and practice related to hospice care, *J Nurs Scholarship* 35(3): 249-255, 2003.

Davison BJ, Goldenberg SL, Gleave ME, and Degner LF: Provision of individualized information to men and their partners to facilitate treatment decision making in prostate cancer, *Oncol Forum* 30(1): 107-114, 2003.

Hoskins CN et al.: Breast cancer: education, counseling and adjustment: a pilot study, *Psychol Rep* 89: 677-704, 2001.

Jaireth N, Hogerney M, and Parsons C: The role of the pilot study: a case illustration from cardiac nursing research, *Appl Nurs Res* 13(2): 92-96, 2000.

Koniak-Griffin D, Verzemnieks IL, Anderson NLR, Brecht ML, Lesser J, Kim S, and Turner-Pluta C: Nurse visitation for adolescent mothers: two-year infant and maternal outcomes, *Nurs Res* 52(2): 127-136, 2003.

Lowry LW, Beikirch P: Effect of comprehensive care on pregnancy outcomes, *Appl Nurs Res* 11(2): 55-61, 1998.

McConnell ES, Branch LG, Sloane RJ, and Pieper CF: Natural history of change in physical function among long-stay nursing home residents, *Nurs Res* 52(2): 119-126, 2003.

Schoenfelder DP, Rubenstein LM: An exercise program to improve fall-related outcomes in elderly nursing home residents, *Appl Nurs Res* 17(1): 21-31, 2004.

Schultz AA, Drew D, and Hewitt H: Comparison of normal saline and heparinized saline for patency of IV locks in neonates, *Appl Nurs Res* 15(1): 28-34, 2002.

Sousa VD, Zauszniewski JA, and Musil CM: How to determine whether a convenience sample represents the population, *Appl Nurs Res* 17(2): 130-133, 2004.

Speziale S, Carpenter DR: *Qualitative research in nursing,* ed 2, Philadelphia, 2003, Lippincott.

Tolle SW et al.: Family reports of barriers to optimal care of the dying, *Nurs Res* 49(6): 310-317, 2000.

Trammer JE, Parry MJE: Enhancing postoperative recovery of cardiac surgery patients: a randomized clinical trial of an advanced practice nursing intervention, *West J Nurs Res* 26(5): 515-532, 2004.

Treat-Jacobson D, Lindquist RA: Functional recovery and exercise behavior in men and women 5 to 6 years following coronary artery bypass graft (CABG) surgery, *West J Nurs Res* 26(5): 479-498, 2004.

Ugarriza DN: Postpartum depressed women's explanation of depression, *J Nurs Scholarship* 34(3): 227-233, 2002.

Van Cleve L, Bossert E, Beecroft P, Allard K, Alvarez O, and Savedra MC: The pain experience of children with leukemia during the first year after diagnosis, *Nurs Res* 53(1): 1-10, 2004.

Waltman NL, Twiss JJ, Ott CD, Gross GJ, Lindsey AM, Moore TE, and Berg K: Testing an intervention for preventing osteoporosis in postmentopausal breast cancer survivors, *J Nurs Scholarship* 35(4): 333-338, 2003.

Ward LS: Race as a variable in cross-cultural research, *Nurs Outlook* 51(3): 120-125, 2003.

Wynd CA, Murrock CJ, and Zeller RA: Health promotion and cardiovascular health in adult monozygotic twins, *J Nurs Scholarship* 36(2): 140-145, 2004.

FOR FURTHER STUDY

Go to your Companion CD for review activities for this chapter.

evolve Go to Evolve at http://evolve.elsevier.com/LoBiondo/ for WebLinks, Content Updates, and additional research articles, for practice in reviewing and critiquing.

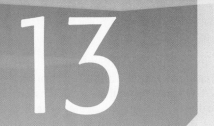

JUDITH HABER

Legal and Ethical Issues

KEY TERMS

animal rights
anonymity
assent
beneficence
benefits

confidentiality
consent
ethics
informed consent
institutional review boards (IRBs)

justice
product testing
respect for persons
risk/benefit ratio
risks

LEARNING OUTCOMES

After reading this chapter, the student should be able to do the following:

- Describe the historical background that led to the development of ethical guidelines for the use of human subjects in research.
- Identify the essential elements of an informed consent form.
- Evaluate the adequacy of an informed consent form.
- Describe the institutional review board's role in the research review process.
- Identify populations of subjects who require special legal and ethical research considerations.
- Appreciate the nurse researcher's obligations to conduct and report research in an ethical manner.
- Describe the nurse's role as patient advocate in research situations.
- Discuss the nurse's role in ensuring that FDA guidelines for testing of medical devices are followed.
- Discuss animal rights in research situations.
- Critique the ethical aspects of a research study.

STUDY RESOURCES

Go to your Companion CD for review activities for this chapter.

evolve Go to Evolve at http://evolve.elsevier.com/LoBiondo/ for Weblinks, Content Updates, and additional research articles for practice in reviewing and critiquing.

"In the 'court of imagination,' where Americans often play out their racial politics, a ceremony, starring a southern white President of the United States offering an apology and asking for forgiveness from a 94- year-old African-American man, seemed like a fitting close worthy in its tableaux quality of a William Faulkner or Toni Morrison novel. The reason for this drama was the federal government's May 16th formal ceremony of repentance tendered to the aging and ailing survivors of the infamous Tuskegee Syphilis Study. The study is a morality play for many among the African-American public and the scientific research community, serving as our most horrific example of a racist 'scandalous story' . . . when government doctors played God and science went mad. At the formal White House gathering, when President William J. Clinton apologized on behalf of the American government to the eight remaining survivors of the study, their families, and heirs seemingly a sordid chapter in American research history was closed 25 years after the study itself was forced to end. As the room filled with members of the Black Congressional Caucus, cabinet members, civil rights leaders, members of the Legacy Committee, the Centers for Disease Control (CDC), and five of the survivors, the sense of a dramatic restitution was upon us" (Reverby, 2000).

Nurses are in an ideal position to promote patients' awareness of the role played by research in the advancement of science and improvement in patient care. Embedded in our professional Code of Ethics (ANA, 2001) is the charge to protect patients from harm; the codes not only are the rules and regulations regarding the involvement of human research subjects to ensure that research is conducted legally and ethically, but also address the conduct of the people who are supposed to be governed by the rules. Researchers themselves and caregivers providing care to patients, who also happen to be research subjects, must be fully committed to the tenets of informed consent and patients' rights. The principle "the ends justify the means" must never be tolerated. Researchers and caregivers of research subjects must take every precaution to protect people being studied from physical or mental harm or discomfort. It is not always clear what constitutes harm or discomfort.

The focus of this chapter is the legal and ethical considerations that must be addressed before, during, and after the conduct of research. Informed consent, institutional review boards,

and research involving vulnerable populations—the elderly, pregnant women, children, prisoners, persons with AIDS, and animals—are discussed. The nurse's role as patient advocate, whether functioning as researcher, caregiver, or research consumer, is addressed.

ETHICAL AND LEGAL CONSIDERATIONS IN RESEARCH: A HISTORICAL PERSPECTIVE

Past Ethical Dilemmas In Research

Ethical and legal considerations with regard to research first received attention after World War II. When the reigning U.S. Secretary of State and Secretary of War learned that the trials for war criminals would focus on justifying the atrocities committed by Nazi physicians as "medical research," the American Medical Association was asked to appoint a group to develop a code of ethics for research that would serve as a standard for judging the medical atrocities committed by physicians on concentration camp prisoners.

The 10 rules included in what was called the Nuremberg Code appear in Box 13-1. Its definitions of the terms *voluntary, legal capacity, sufficient understanding,* and *enlightened decision* have been the subject of numerous court cases and presidential commissions involved in setting ethical standards in research (Creighton, 1977). The code that was developed requires informed consent in all cases but makes no provisions for any special treatment of children, the elderly, or the mentally incompetent. Several other international standards have followed, the most notable of which was the Declaration of Helsinki, which was adopted in 1964 by the World Medical Assembly and then later revised in 1975 (Levine, 1979).

In the United States, federal guidelines for the ethical conduct of research involving human subjects were not developed until the 1970s. Despite the supposed safeguards provided by the federal guidelines, some of the most atrocious, and hence memorable, examples of unethical research studies took place in the United States

13-1 ARTICLES OF THE NUREMBERG CODE

1. The voluntary consent of the human subject is absolutely essential.
2. The study should be such as to yield fruitful results for the good of society, unprocurable by other means of study, and not random and unnecessary in nature.
3. The experiment should be so designed and based on the results of animal experimentation and knowledge of the natural history of the disease or other problems under study that the anticipated results will justify the performance of the experiment.
4. The experiment should be conducted to avoid all unnecessary physical and mental suffering and injury.
5. No experiment should be conducted where there is a prior reason to believe that death or disabling injury will occur.
6. The degree of risk to be taken should never exceed that determined by the humanitarian importance of the problem to be solved by the experiment.
7. Proper preparations should be made and adequate facilities provided to protect the subject against . . . injury, disability, or death.
8. The experiment should be conducted only by scientifically qualified persons.
9. The human subject should be at liberty to bring the experiment to an end.
10. During the experiment, the scientist . . . if he or she has probable cause to believe that a continuation of the experiment is likely to result in injury, disability, or death to the experimental subject . . . will bring it to a close.

Modified from Katz J: *Experimentation with human beings,* New York, 1972, Russell Sage Foundation.

13-2 BASIC ETHICAL PRINCIPLES RELEVANT TO THE CONDUCT OF RESEARCH

RESPECT FOR PERSONS

People have the right to self-determination and to treatment as autonomous agents. Thus they have the freedom to participate or not participate in research. Persons with diminished autonomy are entitled to protection.

BENEFICENCE

Beneficence is an obligation to do no harm and maximize possible benefits. Persons are treated in an ethical manner, their decisions are respected, they are protected from harm, and efforts are made to secure their well-being.

JUSTICE

Human subjects should be treated fairly. An injustice occurs when a benefit to which a person is entitled is denied without good reason or when a burden is imposed unduly.

as recently as the 1990s. These examples are highlighted in Table 13-1. They are sad reminders of our own tarnished research heritage and illustrate the human consequences of not adhering to ethical research standards.

The conduct of harmful, illegal research made additional controls necessary. In 1973 the Department of Health, Education, and Welfare published the first set of proposed regulations on the protection of human subjects. The most important provision was a regulation mandating that an institutional review board (IRB) functioning in accordance with specifications of the department must review and approve all studies. The National Research Act, passed in 1974 (Public Law 93-348), created the National Commission for the Protection of Human Subjects of Biomedical and Behavioral Research. A major charge of the Commission was to identify the basic principles that should underlie the conduct of biomedical and behavioral research involving human subjects and to develop guidelines to ensure that research is conducted in accordance with those principles (Levine, 1986). Three ethical principles were identified as relevant to the conduct of research involving human

TABLE 13-1 **Highlights of Unethical Research Studies Conducted in the United States**

Research Study	Year(s)	Focus of Study	Ethical Principle Violated
Hyman vs. Jewish Chronic Disease Hospital case	1965	Doctors injected cancer-ridden aged and senile patients with their own cancer cells to study the rejection response.	Informed consent was not obtained, and there was no indication that the study had been reviewed and approved by an ethics committee. The two physicians claimed that they did not wish to evoke emotional reactions or refusals to participate by informing the subjects of the nature of the study (Hershey and Miller, 1976).
Ivory Coast, Africa, AIDS/AZT case	1994	In clinical trials supported by the U.S. government and conducted in the Ivory Coast, Dominican Republic, and Thailand, some pregnant women infected with the HIV virus were given placebo pills rather than AZT, a drug known to prevent mothers from passing on the virus to their babies. Babies born to these mothers were in danger of contracting a fatal disease unnecessarily.	Subjects who consented to participate and who were randomized to the control group were denied access to a medication regimen with a known benefit. This violates the subjects' right to fair treatment and protection (French, 1997; Wheeler, 1997).
Midgeville, Georgia, case	1969	Investigational drugs were used on mentally disabled children without first obtaining the opinion of a psychiatrist.	There was no review of the study protocol or institutional approval of the program before implementation. (Levine, 1986).
Tuskegee, Alabama, Syphilis Study	1932-1973	For 40 years the United States Public Health Service conducted a study using two groups of poor black male sharecroppers. One group consisted of those who had untreated syphilis; the other group was judged to be free of the disease. Treatment was withheld from the group having syphilis even after penicillin became generally available and accepted as effective treatment in the 1950s. Steps were taken to prevent the subjects from obtaining it. The researcher wanted to study the untreated disease.	Many of the subjects who consented to participate in the study were not informed about the purpose and procedures of the research. Others were unaware that they were subjects. The degree of risk outweighed the potential benefit. Withholding of known effective treatment violates the subjects' right to fair treatment and protection from harm (Levine, 1986).
San Antonio Contraceptive Study	1969	In a study examining the side effects of oral contraceptives, 76 impoverished Mexican-American women were randomly assigned to an experimental group receiving birth control pills or a control group receiving placebos. Subjects were	Principles of informed consent were violated; full disclosure of potential risk, harm, results, or side effects was not evident in the informed consent document. The potential risk outweighed the benefits of the study.

TABLE **13-1 Highlights of Unethical Research Studies Conducted in the United States—cont'd**

Research Study	Year(s)	Focus of Study	Ethical Principle Violated
		not informed about the placebo and attendant risk of pregnancy; 11 subjects became pregnant, 10 of whom were in the placebo control group.	The subjects' right to fair treatment and protection from harm was violated (Levine, 1986).
Willowbrook Hospital	1972	Mentally incompetent children ($n = 350$) were not admitted to Willowbrook Hospital, a residential treatment facility, unless parents consented to their children being subjects in a study examining the natural history of infectious hepatitis and the effect of gamma globulin. The children were deliberately infected with the hepatitis virus under various conditions; some received gamma globulin; others did not.	Principle of voluntary consent was violated. Parents were coerced to consent to their children's participation as research subjects. Subjects or their guardians have a right to self-determination; that is, they should be free of constraint, coercion, or undue influence of any kind. Many subjects feel pressured to participate in studies if they are in powerless, dependent positions (Rothman, 1982).
UCLA Schizophrenia Medication Study	1983 to present	In a study examining the effects of withdrawing psychotropic medications of 50 patients under treatment for schizophrenia, 23 subjects suffered severe relapses after their medication was stopped. The goal of the study was to determine if some schizophrenics might do better without medications that had deleterious side effects.	Although all subjects signed informed consent documents, they were not informed about how severe their relapses might be, or that they could suffer worsening symptoms with each recurrence. Principles of informed consent were violated; full disclosure of potential risk, harm, results, or side effects was not evident in the informed consent document. The potential risk outweighed the benefits of the study. The subjects' right to fair treatment and protection from harm was violated (Hilts, 1995).

subjects: the principles of **respect for persons, beneficence,** and **justice.** They are defined in Box 13-2. Included in a report issued in 1979, called the Belmont Report, these principles provided the basis for regulations affecting research sponsored by the federal government. The Belmont Report also served as a model for many of the ethical codes developed by scientific disciplines (National Commission, 1978).

In 1980 the Department of Health and Human Services (DHHS) developed a set of reg-ulations in response to the Commission's recommendations. These regulations were published in 1981 and have been revised several times with the latest revisions in 2004 (DHHS, 1983, 2005a). These regulations include the following:

- General requirements for informed consent
- Documentation of informed consent
- IRB review of research proposals
- Exempt and expedited review procedures for certain kinds of research
- Criteria for IRB approval of research

The 2001 regulations are part of the Code of Federal Regulations (CFR, 1983) Title 45 Part 46. These regulations are interpreted by the Office for Human Research Protection (OHRP), an agency that is part of the DHHS whose functions are outlined online at http://ohrp.osophs.dhhs. gov. CFR Title 21 Parts 50 and 56 and also CFR Title 45 Part 46 provide guidelines for the protection of human subjects in publicly and privately funded research to ensure privacy and confidentiality of information obtained from research. However, the potential of electronic access and transfer of an individual's health information has led to public concern about the possible abuse of individual health information in all health care contexts, including research. First enacted in 1996 and implemented with regulations on April 13, 2003, the Health Insurance Portability and Accountability Act (HIPPA) (Public Law 104-191) requires the health care profession to protect the privacy of patient information and create standards for electronic data exchange (Olson, 2003; DHHS, 2005b) (see www.hhs.gov/ocr/). These regulations will be discussed in detail in the sections on informed consent and institutional review later in this chapter.

In 1992 the National Institutes of Health (NIH) Office of Research Integrity was established to set standards for dealing with allegations of scientific misconduct (Office of Research Integrity, 2000). In 1993 Congress passed the NIH Revitalization Act, which, among other provisions, created a 12-member Commission on Research Integrity to propose new procedures for addressing scientific misconduct. A report, "Integrity and Misconduct in Research," issued by the Commission in 1995 proposed a new definition of scientific misconduct, additional protection for "whistle blowers," and a set of guidelines for handling allegations of scientific misconduct (Commission on Research Integrity, 1995; National Bioethics Advisory Commission, 1998; Ryan, 1996). In 1996 the ORI reviewed and revised the scientific misconduct policy to (1) make a uniform policy that could be used across

agencies of the federal government, (2) establish a policy that has the potential to affect the integrity of the research record, and (3) develop a protocol for handling allegations of research misconduct. Concurrently, President Clinton appointed members of the National Bioethics Advisory Commission, which provided guidance to federal agencies on the ethical conduct of current and future human biological and behavioral research related to such controversial issues as cloning, gene transfer, and stem cell research. The Commission concluded its 6-year charge to articulate a set of bioethical research issues in December 2001.

Current and Future Ethical Dilemmas in Research

On a national level, the ethical dilemmas in research for the twenty-first century concern biotechnology and the creation of an organizational culture that values and nurtures research ethics and the rights and equity of people who engage in research either as investigators or as subjects (Ulrich, Wallen, and Grady, 2002; Olsen, 2003).

In 1993 an executive order lifted the government's ban on fetal tissue research, which allowed the resumption of research into the testing of fetal tissue for use in the treatment of such diseases as Parkinson's, multiple sclerosis, cancer, and diabetes. However, in 2001 President George W. Bush supported a more restricted stem cell policy that heavily impacts research by making fewer federal research dollars available to fund stem cell research initiatives. More recently federal lawyers opined that support of stem cell research would not violate the federal ban on support of embryo research if researchers use stem cells that have already been isolated and derived from excess in vitro fertilization (IVF) blastocytes that would otherwise be destroyed, following appropriate informed consent and donation practices. Some states, particularly New Jersey and California via the Proposition 71 vote, are acting independently to ensure that all aspects of stem cell research, including state funding, are pursued in those states. The National Institutes of Health (NIH) has developed guidelines for stem cell research that include protection for couples whose in vitro embryos may be used in research (Andrews, 1999; Brainard, 2004).

In the past, women of childbearing potential were denied access to participation as subjects in drug or therapeutic studies because of the unknown potentially harmful effects of drugs and other therapies that were in various stages of testing on fetuses. Guidelines related to the inclusion of pregnant women as research subjects have been even more stringent. This policy has led to the exclusion of women from many important drug and research studies over the years. Currently researchers seeking funds from the NIH have to justify excluding women from such studies (Crane et al., 2004).

Similarly, inclusion of ethnic minorities in federally funded research studies also is a priority (Julion, Gross, and Barclay-McLaughlin, 2000; Mallory, Miles, Holditch-Davis, 2002; Ward, 2003). Although inclusion of racial minorities in clinical research funded by the NIH has been required since 1994, recent epidemiological evidence indicates that low-income minority women and men, particularly African-Americans, are underenrolled in research studies.

In 1993 the NIH issued guidelines requiring grantees to include enough women in clinical trials to determine whether and how experimental drugs affect them differently from men (McDonald, 1999). Also, in 1994 the Food and Drug Administration (FDA) allowed researchers to include AIDS-infected pregnant women, without the father's consent, in studies to determine whether the drug AZT would prevent transmission of the virus from mother to fetus (Wheeler, 1997).

Over the next decade many questions and controversies will arise in relation to the risks and benefits of the aforementioned areas of research and also as a result of ever-increasing technology in health care in areas that have not been defined as yet. Although these areas of research may seem far removed from nursing research and patient care, they will affect the type of patients nurses will care for and the type of clinical research nurses will conduct.

EVOLUTION OF ETHICS IN NURSING RESEARCH

The evolution of ethics in nursing research can be traced back to 1897 and the constitution of the Nurses' Associated Alumnae Organization. One of the first goals of this organization was to establish a code of ethics for the nursing profession. In 1900 Isabel Hampton Robb wrote *Nursing Ethics: For Hospital and Private Use.* In describing moral laws by which people must abide, she states:

> Etiquette, speaking broadly, means a form of behavior or manners expressly or tacitly required on particular occasions. It makes up the code of polite life and includes forms of ceremony to be observed, so that we invariably find in societies that a certain etiquette is required and observed either tacitly or by expressed agreement.

Clearly, Hampton Robb's comments reflect the norms of Victorian society. However, they also highlight a historical concern for ethical actions by nurses as health care providers (Robb, 1900).

In 1967 the American Nurses Association (ANA) charged its Committee on Research Studies with the task of developing guidelines for the nurse researcher in clinical research. In 1968 the Board of Directors approved the statement titled "The Nurse in Research: ANA Guidelines on Ethical Values." Not only were basic principles regarding the use of human subjects endorsed, but also the role of the nurse as investigator, as well as practitioner, was described.

The ANA established the Commission on Nursing Research in 1970. By doing so, it publicly affirmed nursing's obligation to support the advancement of scientific knowledge and reflected a commitment to support two sets of human rights: (1) the rights of qualified nurses to engage in research and have access to resources necessary for implementing scientific investigation; (2) the rights of all persons who are participants in research performed by investigators whose studies impinge on the patient care provided by nurses. The ANA emphasized human rights in terms of three domains: (1) right to freedom from intrinsic risk or injury, (2) right to privacy and dignity, and (3) right to anonymity.

The guidelines for human rights published by the ANA in 1985 reflect the nursing profession's code of ethics for research (ANA, 1985). Box 13-3 provides a summary of this document, one that helps ensure that research maintains ethical and scientific rigor. This document is relevant for all nurses; the nurse as a researcher or caregiver must assure patients that their human rights will be safeguarded. In fact, nurses, when interviewing for potential employment, should ask what is expected of them in terms of research

---

BOX 13-3   AMERICAN NURSES ASSOCIATION HUMAN RIGHTS GUIDELINES FOR NURSES IN CLINICAL AND OTHER RESEARCH

GUIDELINE 1: RIGHT TO SELF-DETERMINATION

Implementation

Where research participation is a condition of employment, nurses must be informed in writing of the nature of the activity involved in advance of employment. If nurses are not so informed, they must be given the opportunity of not participating in the research.

Potential of risk to others must be clarified in relation to the types of risk involved, the ways of recognizing when risk is present, and the ways in which to counteract potential and unnecessary danger.

GUIDELINE 2: RIGHT TO FREEDOM FROM RISK OR HARM

Implementation

Investigators must ensure freedom from risk or harm by estimating the potential physical or emotional risk and benefit involved. Vulnerable and captive subjects, such as students, patients, prisoners, the mentally incompetent, children, the elderly, and the poor, must be carefully monitored for sources of potential risk of injury so they can be protected.

GUIDELINE 3: SCOPE OF APPLICATION

Implementation

Guidelines for protection of human rights apply to all individuals, that is, subjects involved in research activities. The use of subjects with limited civil freedom usually can be justified only when there is benefit to them or others in similar circumstances.

GUIDELINE 4: RESPONSIBILITIES TO SUPPORT KNOWLEDGE DEVELOPMENT

Implementation

Nurses have an obligation to support the development of knowledge that expands the depth and breadth of the scientific knowledge or base of nursing practice.

GUIDELINE 5: INFORMED CONSENT

Implementation

The right to self-determination is protected when informed consent is obtained from the prospective subject or legal guardian.

GUIDELINE 6: PARTICIPATION ON INSTITUTIONAL REVIEW BOARDS

Implementation

As professionals accountable to the public who are the consumers of health care, nurses have an obligation to support the inclusion of nurses on institutional review boards (IRBs). Nurses also have an obligation to serve on IRBs to review ethical implications of proposed and ongoing research. All studies involving data collection from humans, animals, or records should be reviewed by a review board of health professionals and community representatives who ensure the protection of subjects' rights.

From American Nurses Association: *Guidelines for nurses in clinical and other research*, Kansas City, Mo, 1975, ANA.

responsibilities. For example, nurses might ask the following:

- Are nurses required to collect data or administer medications or treatments in double-blind clinical trials?
- Are written research protocols available as references?
- Has the IRB ruled on each protocol?
- Are nurses free to decline to participate without jeopardizing their position?
- What channels exist for addressing ethical concerns with regard to research being conducted?

Clearly, ignorance and naiveté together with ethical and legal guidelines for the conduct of research must never be an excuse for a nurse's failure to be familiar with and act on behalf of the patients whose human rights must, at all times, be safeguarded. Nurse researchers are often among the most responsible and conscientious investigators when it comes to respecting the rights of human subjects. All nurses should be aware that the tenets of the ANA's Code for Nurses (ANA, 2001) are integral with the ANA human rights' guidelines (ANA, 1985) mentioned earlier.

PROTECTION OF HUMAN RIGHTS

Human rights are the claims and demands that have been justified in the eyes of an individual or by a group of individuals. The term refers to the following five rights outlined in the ANA (in press) guidelines:

1. Right to self-determination
2. Right to privacy and dignity
3. Right to anonymity and confidentiality
4. Right to fair treatment
5. Right to protection from discomfort and harm

These rights apply to everyone involved in a research project, including research team members who may be involved in data collection, practicing nurses involved in the research setting, and subjects participating in the study. As consumers of research read a research article, they must realize any issues highlighted in Table 13-2 should have been addressed and resolved before a research study is approved for implementation.

 HELPFUL H I N T

Recognize that the right to personal privacy may be more difficult to protect when carrying out qualitative studies because of the small sample size and because the subjects' verbatim quotes are often used in the results/findings section of the research report to highlight the findings.

Procedures for Protecting Basic Human Rights

Informed Consent

Elements of informed consent illustrated by the ethical principles of respect and its related right to self-determination are outlined in Box 13-4 and Table 13-2. Nurses need to understand elements of informed consent so that they are knowledgeable participants in obtaining informed consents from patients and/or in critiquing this process as it is presented in research

BOX 13-4   ELEMENTS OF INFORMED CONSENT

1. Title of Protocol
2. Invitation to Participate
3. Basis for Subject Selection
4. Overall Purpose of Study
5. Explanation of Procedures
6. Description of Risks and Discomforts
7. Potential Benefits
8. Alternatives to Participation
9. Financial Obligations
10. Assurance of Confidentiality
11. In Case of Injury Compensation
12. HIPPA Disclosure
13. Subject Withdrawal
14. Offer to Answer Questions
15. Concluding Consent Statement
16. Identification of Investigators

From Code of Federal Regulations: Protection of human subjects, 45 CFR 46, *OPRR Reports*, Revised March 8, 1983.

TABLE **13-2 Protection of Human Rights**

Basic Human Right	Definition
Right to self-determination	Based on the ethical principle of respect for persons, people should be treated as autonomous agents who have the freedom to choose without external controls. An autonomous agent is one who is informed about a proposed study and is allowed to choose to participate or not to participate (Brink, 1992); subjects have the right to withdraw from a study without penalty. Subjects with diminished autonomy are entitled to protection. They are more vulnerable because of age, legal or mental incompetence, terminal illness, or confinement to an institution. Justification for use of vulnerable subjects must be provided.
Right to privacy and dignity	Based on the principle of respect, privacy is the freedom of a person to determine the time, extent, and circumstances under which private information is shared or withheld from others.
Right to anonymity and confidentiality	Based on the principle of respect, **anonymity** exists when the subject's identity cannot be linked, even by the researcher, with his or her individual responses (ANA, 1985). **Confidentiality** means that individual identities of subjects will not be linked to the information they provide and will not be publicly divulged.

Violation of Basic Human Right	Example
A subject's right to self-determination is violated through the use of coercion, covert data collection, and deception. • Coercion occurs when an overt threat of harm or excessive reward is presented to ensure compliance. • Covert data collection occurs when people become research subjects and are exposed to research treatments without knowing it. • Deception occurs when subjects are actually misinformed about the purpose of the research. • Potential for violation of the right to self-determination is greater for subjects with diminished autonomy; they have decreased ability to give informed consent and are vulnerable.	Subjects may feel that their care will be adversely affected if they refuse to participate in research. The Jewish Chronic Disease Hospital Study (see Table 13-1) is an example of a study in which patients and their doctors did not know that cancer cells were being injected. In the Milgrim (1963) Study, subjects were deceived when asked to administer electric shocks to another person; the person was really an actor who pretended to feel the shocks. Subjects administering the shocks were very stressed by participating in this study although they were not administering shocks at all. The Willowbrook Study (see Table 13-1) is an example of how coercion was used to obtain parental consent of vulnerable mentally retarded children who would not be admitted to the institution unless the children participated in a study in which they were deliberately injected with the hepatitis virus.
The Privacy Act of 1974 was instituted to protect subjects from such violations. These occur most frequently during data collection when invasive questions are asked that might result in loss of job, friendships, or dignity or might create embarrassment and mental distress. It also may occur when subjects are unaware that information is being shared with others.	Subjects may be asked personal questions such as the following: "Were you sexually abused as a child?" "Do you use drugs?" "What are your sexual preferences?" When questions are asked using hidden microphones or hidden tape recorders, the subjects' privacy is invaded because they have no knowledge that the data are being shared with others. Subjects also have a right to control access of others to their records.
Anonymity is violated when the subjects' responses can be linked with their identity.	Subjects are given a code number instead of using names for identification purposes. Subjects' names are never used when reporting findings.
Confidentiality is breached when a researcher, by accident or by direct action, allows an unauthorized person to gain access to study data that contain information about subject identity or responses that create a potentially harmful situation for subjects.	Breaches of confidentiality with regard to sexual preference, income, drug use, prejudice, or personality variables can be harmful to subjects. Data are analyzed as group data so that individuals cannot be identified by their responses.

Continued

TABLE 13-2 **Protection of Human Rights—cont'd**

Basic Human Right	Definition
Right to fair treatment	Based on the ethical principle of justice, people should be treated fairly and should receive what they are due or owed. Fair treatment is equitable selection of subjects and their treatment during the research study. This includes selection of subjects for reasons directly related to the problem studied vs. convenience, compromised position, or vulnerability. It also includes fair treatment of subjects during the study, including fair distribution of risks and benefits regardless of age, race, or socioeconomic status.
Right to protection from discomfort and harm	Based on the ethical principle of beneficence, people must take an active role in promoting good and preventing harm in the world around them, as well as in research studies. Discomfort and harm can be physical, psychological, social, or economic in nature. There are five categories of studies based on levels of harm and discomfort: 1. No anticipated effects 2. Temporary discomfort 3. Unusual level of temporary discomfort 4. Risk of permanent damage 5. Certainty of permanent damage

articles. Informed consent is documented by a consent form that is given to prospective subjects and must contain standard elements. It is critical to note that informed consent is not just giving a potential subject a consent form but is a process that must be completed with each subject.

Informed consent is the legal principle that, at least in theory, governs the patient's ability to accept or reject individual medical interventions designed to diagnose or treat an illness. It is also a doctrine that determines and regulates participation in research (Olson, 2003). The Code of Federal Regulations (FDA,1998a) defines the meaning of informed consent:

The knowing consent of an individual or his/her legally authorized representative, under circumstances that provide the prospective

Violation of Basic Human Right	Example
Injustices with regard to subject selection have occurred as a result of social, cultural, racial, and gender biases in society.	The Tuskegee Syphilis Study (1973), the Jewish Chronic Disease Study (1965), the San Antonio Contraceptive Study (1969), and the Willowbrook Study (1972) (see Table 13-1) all provide examples related to unfair subject selection.
Historically, research subjects often have been obtained from groups of people who were regarded as having less "social value," such as the poor, prisoners, slaves, the mentally incompetent, and the dying. Often subjects were treated carelessly, without consideration of physical or psychological harm.	Investigators should not be late for data-collection appointments, should terminate data collection on time, should not change agreed upon procedures or activities without consent, and should provide agreed upon benefits such as a copy of the study findings or a participation fee.
Subjects' right to be protected is violated when researchers know in advance that harm, death, or disabling injury will occur and thus the benefits do not outweigh the risk.	Temporary physical discomfort involving minimal risk includes fatigue or headache; emotional discomfort includes the expense involved in traveling to and from the data-collection site.
	Studies examining sensitive issues, such as rape, incest, or spouse abuse, might cause unusual levels of temporary discomfort by opening up current and/or past traumatic experiences. In these situations, researchers assess distress levels and provide debriefing sessions during which the subject may express feelings and ask questions. The researcher has the opportunity to make referrals for professional intervention. Studies having the potential to cause permanent damage are more likely to be medical rather than nursing in nature. A recent clinical trial of a new drug, a recombinant activated protein C (rAPC) (Zovan) for treatment of sepsis, was halted when interim findings from the Phase III clinical trials revealed a reduced mortality rate for the treatment group vs. the placebo group. Evaluation of the data led to termination of the trial to make available a known beneficial treatment to all patients.
	In some research, such as the Tuskegee Syphilis Study or the Nazi medical experiments, subjects experienced permanent damage or death.

subject or representative sufficient opportunity to consider whether or not to participate without undue inducement or any element of force, fraud, deceit, duress, or other forms of constraint or coercion.

No investigator may involve a human as a research subject before obtaining the legally effective informed consent of a subject or legally authorized representative. The study must be explained to all potential subjects, that is, the study's purpose; procedures; risks, discomforts, and benefits; and expected duration of participation (e.g., when the study's procedures will be implemented, how many times, and in what setting). Potential subjects must also be informed about any appropriate alternative procedures or treatments, if any, that might be advantageous to the subject. For example, in the Tuskegee Syphilis Study, the researchers should have disclosed that penicillin was an effective treatment for their disease. Any compensation for their participation must be delineated when there is more than minimal risk through disclosure about medical treatments and/or compensation that is available if injury occurs.

Prospective subjects must have time to decide whether to participate in a study. The researcher must not coerce the subject into participating. Nor may researchers collect data on subjects who have explicitly refused to participate in a study. An ethical violation of this principle is illustrated by the halting of eight experiments by the Food and Drug Administration (FDA) at the University of Pennsylvania's Institute for Human Gene Therapy 4 months after the death of an 18-year-old male, Jesse Gelsinger, who received experimental treatment as part of the Institute's research. The Institute could not document that all patients had been informed of the risks and benefits of the procedures. Furthermore, some patients who received the therapy should have been considered ineligible because their illnesses were more severe than allowed by the clinical protocols. Mr. Gelsinger had a non–life-threatening genetic disorder that permits toxic amounts of ammonia to build up in the liver. Nevertheless, he volunteered for an experimental treatment in which normal genes were implanted directly into his liver and he subsequently died of multiple organ failure. The Institute failed to report to the FDA that two patients in Mr. Gelsinger's trial had suffered severe side effects, including inflammation of the liver, as a result of their treatment; this should have triggered a halt to the trial (Brainard and Miller, 2000). Of course, subjects may discontinue participation or withdraw from a study at any time without penalty or loss of benefits.

The language of the consent form must be understandable. For example, the reading level should be no greater than eighth grade for adults, and the use of technical research language should be avoided. Federal guidelines also require that information given to subjects or their representatives must be in a language they can understand (DHHS, 2005b). According to the Code of Federal Regulations, subjects should in no way be asked to waive their rights or release the investigator from liability for negligence. The elements that need to be contained in an informed consent are listed in Box 13-4. It is important to note that many institutions, guided by HIPPA guidelines in developing their informed consent procedures, require additional elements.

 HELPFUL H I N T

Remember that research reports rarely provide readers with detailed information regarding the degree to which the researcher adhered to ethical principles, such as informed consent, because of space limitations in journals that make it impossible to describe all aspects of a study. Failure to mention procedures to safeguard subjects' rights does not necessarily mean that such precautions were not taken.

Investigators obtain **consent** through personal discussion with potential subjects. This process allows the person to obtain immediate answers to questions. However, consent forms, written in narrative or outline form, highlight elements that both inform and remind subjects of the nature of the study and their participation (Dubler and Post, 1998; Haggerty and Hawkins, 2000).

Assurance of anonymity and confidentiality (defined in Table 13-2) is usually conveyed in writing and describes the extent to which confidentiality of their records will be maintained. The right to privacy is also protected through protection of individually identifiable health information (IIHI). The DHHS developed guidelines to help researchers, health care organizations, health care providers, and academic institutions when they can use and disclose IIHI:

- The IIHI has to be deidentified under the HIPPA Privacy Rule.
- The data are part of a limited data set, and a data use agreement with the researcher is in place.
- The individual who is a potential research subject provides authorization for the researcher to use and disclose his or her protected health information (PHI).
- A waiver or alteration of the authorization requirement is obtained from the institutional review board (IRB).
- The consent form must be signed and dated by the subject. The presence of witnesses is not always necessary but does constitute evidence that the subject concerned actually signed the form. In cases in which the subject is a minor or is physically or mentally incapable of signing the consent, the legal guardian or representative must sign. The investigator also signs the form to indicate commitment to the agreement.

Generally the signed informed consent form is given to the subject. The researcher should keep a copy also. Some research, such as a retrospective chart audit, may not require informed consent—only institutional approval. In some cases when minimal risk is involved, the investigator may have to provide the subject only with an information sheet and verbal explanation. In other cases, such as a volunteer convenience sample, completion and return of research instruments provide evidence of consent. The IRB will help advise on exceptions to these guidelines, cases in which the IRB might grant waivers or amend its guidelines in other ways. The IRB makes the final determination regarding the most appropriate documentation format. Research consumers should note whether and what kind of evidence of informed consent has been provided in a research article.

HELPFUL HINT

Note that researchers often do not obtain written, informed consent when the major means of data collection is through self-administered questionnaires. The researcher usually assumes applied consent in such cases; that is, the return of the completed questionnaire reflects the respondent's voluntary consent to participate.

Institutional Review Board

Institutional review boards (IRBs) are boards that review research projects to assess that ethical standards are met in relation to the protection of the rights of human subjects. The National Research Act (1974) requires that such agencies as universities, hospitals, and other health care organizations (e.g., managed care companies) applying for a grant or contract for any project or program that involves the conduct of biomedical or behavioral research involving human subjects must submit with their application assurances that they have established an IRB, sometimes called a human subjects' committee, that reviews the research projects and protects the rights of the human subjects (FDA, 1998b). At agencies where no federal grants or contracts are awarded, there is usually a review mechanism similar to an IRB process, such as a research advisory committee. The National Research Act requires that the IRB have at least five members of various backgrounds to promote complete and adequate project review. The members must be qualified by virtue of their expertise and experience and reflect professional, gender, racial, and cultural diversity. Membership must include one member whose concerns are primarily nonscientific (lawyer, clergy, ethicist) and at least one member from outside the agency. Members of IRBs often have mandatory training in scientific integrity and prevention of scientific misconduct as do the principal investigator of a research study and his or her research team members. In an effort to protect research subjects, the HIPPA

Privacy Rule has made IRB requirements much more stringent for researchers to meet (Clinical Research Resources, 2004).

The IRB is responsible for protecting subjects from undue risk and loss of personal rights and dignity. For a research proposal to be eligible for consideration by an IRB, it must already have been approved by a departmental review group such as a nursing research committee that attests to the proposal's scientific merit and congruence with institutional policies, procedures, and mission. The IRB reviews the study's protocol to ensure that it meets the requirements of ethical research that appear in Box 13-5.

Most boards provide guidelines or instructions for researchers that include steps to be taken to receive IRB approval. For example, guidelines for writing a standard consent form or criteria for qualifying for an expedited rather than a full IRB review may be made available. The IRB has the authority to approve research, require modifications, or disapprove a research study. A researcher must receive IRB approval before beginning to conduct research. Institutional review boards have the authority to suspend or terminate approval of research that is not conducted in accordance with IRB requirements or that has been associated with unexpected serious harm to subjects (Pallikkathayll, Crighton, and Aaronson, 1998).

IRBs also have mechanisms for reviewing research in an expedited manner when the risk to research subjects is minimal (Code of Federal Regulations, 1983). An expedited review usually shortens the length of the review process. Keep in mind that although a researcher may determine that a project involves minimal risk, the IRB makes the final determination, and the research may not be undertaken until then. A full list of research categories eligible for expedited review is available from any IRB office. It includes the following:

- Collection of hair and nail clippings in a nondisfiguring manner
- Collection of excreta and external secretions including sweat

> **BOX 13-5** CODE OF FEDERAL REGULATIONS FOR IRB APPROVAL OF RESEARCH STUDIES
>
> To approve research, the IRB must determine that the following Code of Federal Regulations has been satisfied:
> 1. The risks to subjects are minimized.
> 2. The risks to subjects are reasonable in relation to anticipated benefits.
> 3. The selection of the subjects is equitable.
> 4. Informed consent, in one of several possible forms, must be and will be sought from each prospective subject or the subject's legally authorized representative.
> 5. The informed consent form must be properly documented.
> 6. Where appropriate, the research plan makes adequate provision for monitoring the data collected to ensure subject safety.
> 7. Where appropriate, there are adequate provisions to protect the privacy of subjects and the confidentiality of data.
> 8. Where some or all of the subjects are likely to be vulnerable to coercion or undue influence, such as persons with acute or severe physical or mental illness or persons who are economically or educationally disadvantaged, appropriate additional safeguards are included.

- Recording of data on subjects 18 years or older, using noninvasive procedures routinely employed in clinical practice
- Voice recordings
- Study of existing data, documents, records, pathological specimens, or diagnostic data

An expedited review does not automatically exempt the researcher from obtaining informed consent.

Under the HIPPA Privacy Rule (DHHS, 2003), IRBs can act on requests for a waiver or alteration of the authorization requirement for a research project. An altered authorization requirement occurs when an IRB approves a request that some, but not all, of the deidentification elements (e.g., name or address) be removed from the health information that is to be used in research. The researcher can also request a partial waiver of authorization, which allows the researcher to obtain personal health information (PHI) to contact and recruit potential subjects for a study.

The Federal Register is a publication that contains updated information about federal guidelines for research involving human subjects. Every researcher should consult an agency's research office to ensure that the application being prepared for IRB approval adheres to the most current requirements. Nurses who are critiquing published research should be conversant with current regulations to determine whether ethical standards have been met. The Critical Thinking Decision Path illustrates the ethical decision-making process an IRB might use in evaluating the risk/benefit ratio of a research study.

CRITICAL THINKING DECISION PATH   **Evaluating the Risk/Benefit Ratio of a Research Study**

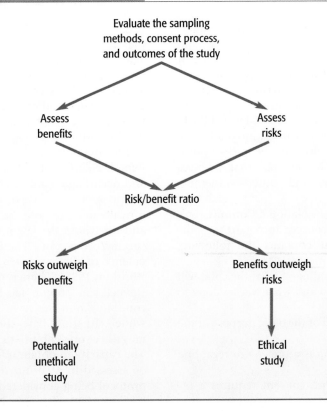

Protecting Basic Human Rights of Vulnerable Groups

Researchers are advised to consult their agency's IRB for the most recent federal and state rules and guidelines when considering research involving vulnerable groups who may have diminished autonomy such as the elderly, children, pregnant women, the unborn, those who are emotionally or physically disabled, prisoners, the deceased, students, and persons with AIDS (Baskin et al., 1998; Tigges, 2003; Haggerty and Hawkins, 2000; Dobratz, 2003; National Bioethics Advisory Commission, 1998). In addition, researchers should consult the IRB before planning research that potentially involves an oversubscribed research population, such as organ transplantation patients or AIDS patients, or "captive" and convenient populations, such as prisoners. It should be emphasized that use of special populations does not preclude undertaking research; extra precautions must be taken, however, to protect their rights (Levine, 1995). Davis (1981) reminds us that a society can be judged by the way it treats its most vulnerable people—a point worth remembering in research that involves children, the elderly, and other vulnerable groups.

Mitchell discussed the National Commission's concept of assent vs. consent in regard to pediatric research. **Assent** contains the following three fundamental elements:

1. A basic understanding of what the child will be expected to do and what will be done to the child
2. A comprehension of the basic purpose of the research
3. An ability to express a preference regarding participation

In contrast to assent, consent requires a relatively advanced level of cognitive ability. Informed consent reflects competency standards requiring abstract appreciation and reasoning regarding the information provided. The issue of assent vs. consent is an interesting one when one determines at what age children can make meaningful decisions about participating in research.

In terms of the work by Piaget regarding cognitive ability, children at age 6 and older can participate in giving assent. Children at age 14 and older, although not legally authorized to give sole consent unless they are emancipated minors, can make such decisions as capably as adults (Mitchell, 1984).

Federal regulations require parental permission whenever a child is involved in research unless otherwise specified, for example, in cases of child abuse or mature minors at minimal risk (Tigges, 2003). If the research involves more than minimal risk and does not offer direct benefit to the individual child, both parents must give permission. When individuals reach maturity, usually at 18 years of age in cases of research, they may render their own consent. They may do so at a younger age if they have been legally declared emancipated minors. Questions regarding this should be addressed by the IRB and/or research administration office and not left to the discretion of the researcher to answer.

The American Geriatrics Society Ethics Committee (1998), as an advocate for the vulnerable elderly who are of increasing dependence and declining cognitive ability, states that elders are precisely the class of persons who were historically and are potentially vulnerable to abuse and for whom the law must struggle to fashion specific protections. The issue of the legal competence of elders is often raised (Flaskerud and Winslow, 1998). There is no issue if the potential subject can supply legally effective informed consent. Competence is not a clear "black or white" situation. The complexity of the study may affect one's ability to consent to participate. The capacity to obtain informed consent should be assessed in each individual for each research protocol being considered (American Geriatrics Society, 1998). For example, an elderly person may be able to consent to participate in a simple observation study but not in a clinical drug trial.

The issue of the necessity of requiring the elderly to provide consent often arises. Dubler (1993) refers to research requirements for which some or all of the elements of informed consent may be waived:

1. The research involves no more than minimal risk to the subjects.
2. The waiver or alteration will not adversely affect the rights and welfare of the subjects.
3. The research could not feasibly be carried out without the waiver or alteration.
4. Whenever appropriate, the subjects will be provided with additional pertinent information after participation.

No vulnerable population may be singled out for study because it is simply convenient. For example, neither people with mental illness nor prisoners may be studied simply because they are an available and convenient group. Prisoners may be studied if the study pertains to them, that is, studies concerning the effects and processes of incarceration. Similarly, people with mental illness may participate in studies that focus on expanding knowledge about psychiatric disorders and treatments. Students also are often a convenient group. They must not be singled out as research subjects because of convenience; the research questions must have some bearing on their status as students.

Researchers and patient caregivers involved in research with vulnerable people are well advised to seek advice from appropriate IRBs, clinicians, lawyers, ethicists, and others. In all cases, the burden should be on the investigator to show the IRB that it is appropriate to involve vulnerable subjects in research.

💡 HELPFUL H I N T

Keep in mind that researchers rarely mention explicitly that the study participants were vulnerable subjects or that special precautions were taken to appropriately safeguard the human rights of this vulnerable group. Research consumers need to be attentive to the special needs of groups who may be unable to act as their own advocates or are unable to adequately assess the risk/benefit ratio of a research study.

SCIENTIFIC FRAUD AND MISCONDUCT

Fraud

Periodically articles reporting unethical actions of researchers appear in the professional and lay literature. Data may have been falsified or fabricated, or subjects may have been coerced to participate in a research study (Kevles, 1996; Office of Research Integrity Website, 2000; Tilden, 2000). In a climate of "publish or perish" in academic and scientific settings and declining research dollars, there is increasing pressure on academics and scientists to produce significant research findings. Job security and professional recognition are coveted, essential, and often predicated on being a productive scientist and prolific writer. These pressures have been known to overpower some people, who then take shortcuts, fabricate data, and falsify findings to advance their positions (Rankin and Esteves, 1997; Tilden, 2000).

The risks are many, including harming research subjects or basing clinical practice on false data. Nurses, as advocates of patient welfare and professional practice, should be aware that, albeit ideally rare, there are occasions when misconduct of the researcher is observed or suspected. In such cases, nurses must be advised to contact the appropriate group, such as the IRB, to ensure that this matter receives appropriate attention and review.

Misconduct

Of equal importance is the issue of basing practice on reports that appear in journals where subsequent research and reports on those subjects change the scientific basis for practice. Journals may print corrections or further research in follow-up reports that are buried, obscure, or underreported. A physician, Lawrence K. Altman (1988), stated, "Such shortcomings are critically important because the thousands of journals that cover a range of specialties are the central reservoir of scientific knowledge. They are the standard references for crediting discoveries and determining treatments." It is incumbent on nurses as patient advocates and research consumers to keep up-to-date on scientific reports related to nursing practice and adjust practice as directed by ever-evolving evidence-based research findings. In addition, it is the responsibility of the researcher to make sure that she or he keeps current with federal compliance regulations on prevention, detection, and inquiry into and adjudication of scientific misconduct. For example, the federal government is proposing to change the definition of misconduct, a change that will appear in the Federal Register when the change is approved by the Office of Research Integrity (ORI). How many researchers or research consumers regularly check the Federal Register or other government documents or websites to maintain their currency in legal and ethical research issues?

Unauthorized Research

At times, ad hoc or informal and unauthorized research does go on, including **product testing.** Although the testing may seem harmless, again it is not the purview of the investigator to make that determination. Nurses must carefully avoid being involved in unauthorized research for a number of reasons, including the following (Raybuck, 1997):

- These treatments or methods of care are usually not monitored as closely for untoward effects, hence exposing the client to unwarranted risk.
- Clients' rights to informed consent in clinical trials are not protected.
- The success or failure of these unrecorded trials contributes nothing to the organized scientific knowledge of the efficacy or complications of the treatment.
- The lack of independent quality supervision allows deviations from the adopted experimental program that may eliminate the program's effectiveness.

Sometimes the nurse plays the dual role of researcher and caregiver. In that situation, the nurse must question whether risks may be inherent in the research that do not exist in the care. Even when these risks are clearly identified—and they must be—the caregiver must be comfortable that the level of risk is acceptable and that the benefits outweigh the risks. Patients must feel comfortable in refusing to participate in the caregiver's research while continuing to require the nurse's care. It must be made clear to patients that they may refuse to participate or withdraw from the study at any time without consequence or compromise to their care or relationship to the institution. The nurse in this dual role must consider whether the research will incur additional expense for the patient, whether that is warranted, and whether the subject has been apprised of such expenses (Sailer, 1999).

PRODUCT TESTING

Nurses are often approached by manufacturers to test products on patients. They often assume the role of research coordinator in clinical drug or product trials (Raybuck, 1997). Nurses should be aware of the FDA guidelines and regulations for testing of medical devices before they initiate any form of clinical testing. Medical devices are classified under Section 513 in the Federal Food, Drug and Cosmetic Act according to the extent of control necessary to ensure safety and effectiveness of each device. Classes related to product testing are defined in Table 13-3.

It is important that nurses be aware of their own institution's policies for product testing. The class of the product will obviously make a difference to the institution's position. If a nurse suspects that, for example, a class II device is being tested in an ad hoc or unauthorized manner and without patient consent, this should be discussed with a supervisor or other appropriate authorities.

LEGAL AND ETHICAL ASPECTS OF ANIMAL EXPERIMENTATION

The federal laws that have been written to protect **animal rights** in research emanate from an

TABLE 13-3 **Classes Related to Product Testing**

Classes	Examples
CLASS I: GENERAL CONTROLS	
Included in class I are devices whose safety and effectiveness can be guaranteed reasonably by the general controls of the Good Manufacturing Practices Regulations. The regulations' part of the act ensures that manufacturers will follow specific guidelines for packaging, storing, and providing specific product instructions.	Ostomy supplies
CLASS II: PERFORMANCE STANDARDS	
General controls are insufficient in this case to ensure safety and efficacy of the product, and the manufacturer must provide this assurance in the form of information.	Cardiac pacemakers, sutures, surgical metallic mesh, and biopsy needles
CLASS III: PREMARKET APPROVAL	
This class includes devices whose safety and effectiveness are insufficiently ensured by general controls and for which performance standards are insufficient to ensure safety and effectiveness. These products are represented to be life sustaining or life supporting, are implanted into the body, or present a potential, unreasonable risk of illness or injury to the patient. Devices in this class are required to have approved applications for premarket approval. Extensive laboratory, animal, and human studies, which often require 2 to 3 years to complete, are required for class III devices.	Heart valves, bone cements, contact lenses, and implantable devices left in the body for 30 days or longer

interesting history of attitudes toward animals and the value people place on them. Animal activists (e.g., the Animal Liberation Front) and antivivisectionist societies began to gain considerable public attention in the 1970s. Of interest, however, is the fact that the oldest piece of legislation controlling animal experimentation goes back to 1876 in the United Kingdom. With the increase in the use of animals in research after World War II, a number of states passed legislation called "pound seizure laws" that allowed and even mandated the release of unclaimed animals from pounds to laboratories. The first pound seizure law was enacted in 1949; not until 1972 was the first law of that type repealed. In 1966 in the United States, the first Laboratory Animal Welfare Act was passed. The act did not deal with what we consider today to be some of the most salient issues related to animal experimentation (e.g., pain management), and amendments continued to be passed to address these concerns. The 1970 Animal Welfare Act provided for the establishment of an institutional Animal Care and Use Committee (ACUC), one member of which must be a veterinarian. The United States Department of Agriculture (USDA) oversees compliance with animal welfare acts and holds institutions' administrations accountable for such compliance.

In 1985 President Reagan signed PL 99-108, which contains the Improved Standards for the Laboratory Animals' Act. Provisions in the series of acts and amendments to acts pertaining to animal experimentation include, but are by no means limited to, the list that appears in Box 13-6 (PHS Policy on Humane Care, 1985).

This section serves only as an introduction to the concept of legal and ethical issues related to animal experimentation. Principles of protection of animal rights in research have evolved over time. Animals, unlike humans, cannot give informed consent, but other conditions related to their welfare must not be ignored. Nurses who encounter the use of animals in research should be alert to their rights.

BOX 13-6 BASIC PROVISIONS OF ACTS PERTAINING TO ANIMAL EXPERIMENTATION

1. The transportation, care, and use of animals should be in accordance with the Animal Welfare Act and other applicable federal laws, guidelines, and policies.
2. Procedures involving animals should be designed and performed with consideration of their relevance to human or animal health, the advancement of knowledge, or the good of society.
3. The animals selected for a procedure should be of an appropriate species and quality and the minimum number required to obtain valid results. Methods such as mathematical models, computer simulation, and in vitro biological systems should be considered.
4. Proper use of animals, including the avoidance or minimization of discomfort, distress, and pain when consistent with sound scientific practices, is imperative. Unless the contrary is established, investigators should consider that the procedures that cause pain or distress in human beings may cause pain or distress in other animals.
5. Procedures with animals that may cause more than temporary or slight pain or distress should be performed with appropriate sedation, analgesia, or anesthesia. Surgical or other painful procedures should not be performed on anesthetized animals paralyzed by chemical agents.
6. Animals that would otherwise suffer severe or chronic pain or distress that cannot be relieved should be painlessly killed at the end of the procedure or, if appropriate, during the procedure.
7. The living conditions of animals should be appropriate for their species and contribute to their health and comfort. Normally the housing, feeding, and care of all animals used for biomedical purposes must be directed by a veterinarian or other scientist trained and experienced in the proper care, handling, and use of the species being maintained or studied. In any case, veterinary care shall be provided as indicated.
8. Investigators and other personnel shall be appropriately qualified and experienced for conducting procedures on living animals. Adequate arrangements shall be made for their in-service training, including the proper and humane care and use of laboratory animals.
9. Where exceptions are required in relation to the provision of these principles, the decisions should not rest with the investigators directly concerned but should be made, with regard to principle 2, by an appropriate review group, such as an institutional animal research committee. Such exceptions should not be made solely for the purposes of teaching or demonstration.

CRITIQUING GUIDE *Legal and Ethical Aspects of a Research Study*

Research articles and reports often do not contain detailed information regarding the degree to which or all of the ways in which the investigator adhered to the legal and ethical principles presented in this chapter. Space considerations in articles preclude extensive documentation of all legal and ethical aspects of a research study. Lack of written evidence regarding the protection of human rights does not imply that appropriate steps were not taken.

The Critiquing Criteria box provides guidelines for evaluating the legal and ethical aspects of a research report. Although research consumers reading a research report will not see all areas explicitly addressed in the research article, they should be aware of them and should determine that the researcher has addressed them before gaining IRB approval to conduct the study. A nurse who is asked to serve as a member of an IRB will find the critiquing criteria useful in evaluating the legal and ethical aspects of the research proposal.

Information about the legal and ethical considerations of a study is usually presented in the methods section of a research report. The subsection on the sample or data-collection methods is the most likely place for this information. The author most often indicates in a few sentences that informed consent was obtained and that approval from an IRB or similar committee was granted. It is likely that a paper will not be accepted for publication without such a discussion. This also makes it almost impossible for unauthorized research to be published. Therefore when a research article provides evidence of having been approved by an external review committee, the reader can feel confident that the ethical issues raised by the study have been thoroughly reviewed and resolved.

To protect subject and institutional privacy, the locale of the study frequently is described in general terms in the sample subsection of the report. For example, the article might state that data were collected at a 1000-bed tertiary care center in the Southwest, without mentioning its name. Protection of subject privacy may be explicitly addressed by statements indicating that anonymity or confidentiality of data was maintained or that grouped data were used in the data analysis.

Determining whether participants were subjected to physical or emotional risk is often accomplished indirectly by evaluating the study's methods section. The reader evaluates the **risk/benefit ratio,** that is, the extent to which the benefits of the study are maximized and the risks are minimized such that subjects are protected from harm during the study (Dubler and Post, 1998; Pruchino and Hayden, 2000).

For example, the study by Melkus et al. (2004) compared the effect of a 6-week, cognitive-behavioral (CB), culturally competent diabetes mellitus (DM) intervention program for African-American women ($n = 25$) with Type 2 DM, led by advanced practice registered nurses trained in DM care and certified as DM educators on glycemic control, weight, body mass, and diabetes-related emotional distress. Results from this pilot study, using a one-group, pretest-postest, quasiexperimental design, demonstrate that women who participated in the CB intervention for 3 months had improved psychosocial and metabolic outcomes as measured by a significant decrease in diabetes-related distress, body mass index, and weight as well as decreased HbA1c levels to below 8%. The findings related to the outcomes of this low-cost intervention have implications for significant cost savings, at no risk and with potential significant benefit to both patients and health care institutions that treat community-residing minority women with Type 2 DM.

In another example, a study by LoBiondo-Wood and associates (2000) investigated the relationship between family stress, family coping, social support, perception of stress, and family adaptation in families of children undergoing liver transplants. The benefits to the participants were increased knowledge about the family stressors, strains, and resources needed by families during the long-term process of seeking a transplant for a chronically ill child. Risk was minimized because subjects were mothers of children being evaluated for a liver transplant; the children's usual regimen was not being altered in any way. LoBiondo-Wood and colleagues (2000) state that before interventions can be developed to assist such families during this crisis, clinicians need to understand how aspects of family life are affected. The evaluator could infer from a description of the method that the benefits were greater than the risks and subjects were protected from harm. The findings of the study highlighted the need to understand the impact of transplantation on the family as a whole. As health care providers move to cost containment and documentation of outcomes that affect the child's family and that family's ability to cope and care for a member with chronic health care needs, research needs to focus on what aspects of the child's care are compromised if the family's needs

are not addressed. The obligation to balance the risks and benefits of a study is the responsibility of the researcher. However, the research consumer reading a research report also should be confident that subjects have been protected from harm.

When considering the special needs of vulnerable subjects, research consumers should be sensitive to whether the special needs of groups, unable to act on their own behalf, have been addressed. For instance, has the right of self-determination been addressed by the informed consent protocol identified in the research report? For example, in a study by Koenes and Karshmer (2000) comparing whether the incidence of depression was greater among blind adolescents than a sighted comparison group, the study was approved by the institutional committee for review of research involving human subjects, as well as the school administrators and parents or guardians who had to provide written consent for subject participation. Actual student participation was entirely voluntary; they were invited to participate in a study designed to "explore stress and its impact on adolescence." All students were individually recruited, and 22 adolescents who had been legally blind since birth and 29 sighted adolescents participated in the study.

When qualitative studies are reported, verbatim quotes from informants often are incorporated into the findings section of the article. In such cases, the reader will evaluate how effectively the author protected the informant's identity, either by using a fictitious name or by withholding information such as age, gender, occupation, or other potentially identifying data (see Chapter 7 for special ethical issues related to qualitative research).

It should be apparent from the preceding sections that although the need for guidelines for the use of human and animal subjects in research is evident and the principles themselves are clear, there are many instances when the nurse must use his or her best judgment both as a patient advocate and as a researcher when evaluating the ethical nature of a research project. In any research situation, the basic guiding principle of protecting the patient's human rights must always apply. When conflicts arise, the nurse must feel free to raise suitable questions with appropriate resources and personnel. In an institution these may include contacting the researcher first and then, if there is no resolution, the director of nursing research and the chairperson of the IRB. In cases when ethical considerations in a research article are in question, clarification from a colleague, agency, or IRB is indicated. The nurse should pursue his or her concerns until satisfied that the patient's rights and his or her rights as a professional nurse are protected.

Critical Thinking Challenges

- A state government official is interested in determining the number of infants infected with the human immunodeficiency virus (HIV) and has approached your hospital to participate in a state-wide--funded study. The protocol will include the testing of all newborns for HIV, but the mothers will not be told that the test is being done, nor will they be told the results. Using the basic ethical principles found in Box 13-2, defend or refute this practice. How will the findings of the proposed study be affected if the protocol is carried out? What threats to evidence do you see?
- The IRB of your health care agency does not include a nurse and you think it should. You discuss this with your supervisor, and she states that it really isn't necessary because the IRB uses strict guidelines. What essential arguments and explanations should you include in your proposal for including a nurse on your institution's IRB?
- A qualitative researcher intends to conduct a phenomenological study on caring and will sample informants who attend an outpatient clinic and who are severely and persistently mentally ill. The IRB denies the study indicating that informed consent cannot be obtained and that these patients will not be able to tolerate an interview. What assumptions have the members of this IRB made? If you were the researcher and you were given the opportunity to address their concerns, what would you say? Include information from Table 13-2.

KEY POINTS

- Ethical and legal considerations in research first received attention after World War II during the Nuremberg Trials, from which developed the Nuremberg Code. This became the standard for research guidelines protecting the human rights of research subjects.
- The National Research Act, passed in 1974, created the National Commission for the Protection of Human Subjects of Biomedical and Behavioral Research. The findings, contained in the Belmont Report, discuss three basic ethical principles (respect for persons, beneficence, and justice) that underlie the conduct of research involving human subjects. Federal regulations developed in response to the Commission's report provide guidelines for informed consent and IRB protocols.
- The ANA's Commission on Nursing Research published *Human Rights Guidelines for Nursing in Clinical and Other Research* in 1985, for protection of human rights of research subjects. It is relevant to nurses as researchers as well as caregivers. The ANA's *Code for Nurses* (ANA, 2001) is integral with the research guidelines.
- The Health Insurance Portability and Accountability Act (HIPPA), implemented in 2003, includes privacy rules to protect an individual's health information that affect health care organizations and the conduct of research.
- Protection of human rights includes (1) right to self-determination, (2) right to privacy and dignity, (3) right to anonymity and confidentiality, (4) right to fair treatment, and (5) right to protection from discomfort and harm.
- Procedures for protecting basic human rights include gaining informed consent, which illustrates the ethical principle of respect, and obtaining IRB approval, which illustrates the ethical principles of respect, beneficence, and justice.
- Special consideration should be given to studies involving vulnerable populations, such as children, the elderly, prisoners, and those who are mentally or physically disabled.
- Scientific fraud or misconduct represents unethical conduct and must be monitored as part of professional responsibility. Informal, ad hoc, or unauthorized research may expose patients to unwarranted risk and may not protect subject rights adequately.
- Nurses who are asked to be involved in product testing should be aware of FDA guidelines and regulations for testing medical devices before becoming involved in product testing and, perhaps, violating guidelines for ethical research.
- Animal rights need to be protected, and regulations for animal research have evolved over time. Nurses who encounter the use of animals in research should be alert to their rights.
- Nurses as consumers of research must be knowledgeable about the legal and ethical components of a research study so they can evaluate whether a researcher has ensured appropriate protection of human or animal rights.

REFERENCES

Altman LK: A flaw in the research process: uncorrected errors in journals. Medical science, *New York Times*, May 31, 1988.

American Geriatrics Society Ethics Committee: Informed consent for research on human subjects with dementia, *J Am Geriatric Soc* 46(10): 1308-1310, 1998.

American Nurses Association (ANA): *Human rights guidelines for nurses in clinical and other research,* Kansas City, Mo, 1985, ANA.

American Nurses Association (ANA): *Code for nurses with interpretive statements,* Kansas City, Mo, 2001a, ANA.

Andrews LB: Legal, ethical, and social concerns in the debate over stem-cell research, *Chronicle of Higher Education,* B4-5, January 29, 1999.

Baskin SA et al.: Barriers to obtaining consent in dementia research: implications for surrogate decision-making, *J Am Geriatric Soc* 46(3): 287-290, 1998.

Brainard J: Stem cell research moves forward, *Chronicle of Higher Education,* A22-25, October 1, 2004.

Brainard J, Miller DW: U.S. regulators suspend medical studies at two universities, *Chronicle of Higher Education,* A30, February 4, 2000.

Brink PJ: Autonomy versus do no harm, *West J Nurs Res* 14(3): 264–266, 1992.

Clinical Research Resources: *Regulations & guidance on clinical investigator & IRB responsibilities* Philadelphia, 2004, Clinical Research Resources.

Code of Federal Regulations: Protection of human subjects, 45 CFR 46, *OPRR Reports,* Revised March 8, 1983.

Commission on Research Integrity: Integrity and misconduct in research, Washington, DC, 1995, USDHHS.

Crane PB, Letvak S, Lewallen L, Hu J, and Jones E: Inclusion of women in nursing research 1995-2001, *Nurs Res* 53(4): 237-242, 2004.

Creighton H: Legal concerns of nursing research, *Nurs Res* 26(4): 337-340, 1977.

Davis A: Ethical issues in gerontological nursing research, *Geriatr Nurs* 2: 267-272, 1981.

Department of Health and Human Services: Department of Health and Human Services rules and regulations, 45CF46, Title 45, Part 46, *Fed Regul,* March 8, 1983.

Department of Health and Human Services: Standards for privacy of individually identifiable health information: final rule, *Code Fed Regul,* Title 45, Parts 160 and 164, Retrieved January 3, 2005a, from www.hhs.gov/ocr/hippa/finalreg.html (April 17, 2003).

Department of Health and Human Services: *Institutional review boards and the HIPPA privacy rule: information for researchers,* Retrieved January 3, 2005b, from http://privacy rule and research.nih.gov/irbandprivacyrule.asp (September 25, 2003).

Dobratz MC: Issues and dilemmas in conducting research with vulnerable home hospice patients, *J Nurs Scholarship* 35(4): 371-376, 2003.

Dubler NN: Personal communication, 1993.

Dubler NN, Post LF: Truth telling and informed consent. In Holland JC, editor: *Textbook of psycho-oncology,* New York, 1998, Oxford Press.

Federal Drug Administration: A guide to informed consent, *Code Fed Regul,* Title 21, Part 50, Retrieved January 3, 2005, from www.fda.gov/oc/ohrt/irbs/informedconsent.html (1998a).

Federal Drug Administration: Institutional review boards, *Code Fed Regul,* Title 21, Part 56, Retrieved January 6, 2005, from www.fda.gov/oc/ohrt/irbs/appendixc.html (1998b).

Flaskerud JH, Winslow BJ: Conceptualizing vulnerable populations health-related research, *Nurs Res* 47(2): 69-78, 1998.

French HW: AIDS research in Africa: juggling risks and hopes, *New York Times,* A1 and A12, October 9, 1997.

Haggerty LA, Hawkins J: Informed consent and the limits of confidentiality, *West J Nurs Res* 22(4): 508-514, 2000.

Hershey N, Miller RD: *Human experimentation and the law,* Germantown, Md, 1976, Aspen.

Hilts PJ: Agency faults a UCLA study for suffering of mental patients, *New York Times,* A1, 11, March 9, 1995.

Julion W, Gross D, Barclay-McLaughlin R: Recruiting families of color from the inner city: insights from the recruiters, *Nurs Outlook* 48(5): 230-237, 2000.

Kevles DJ: An injustice to a scientist is reversed and we learn some lesions, *Chronicle of higher Education,* B1-2, July 5, 1996.

Koenes SG, Karshmer JF: Depression: a comparison study between blind and sighted adolescents, *Issues Ment Health Nurs* 21: 269-279, 2000.

Levine RJ: Clarifying the concepts of research ethics, *Hastings Cent Rep* 93(3): 21-26, 1979.

Levine RJ: *Ethics and regulation of clinical research,* ed 2, Baltimore-Munich, 1986, Urban and Schwartzenberg.

Levine RJ: Consent for research on children, *Chronicle of Higher Education,* B1-2, November 10, 1995.

LoBiondo-Wood G et al.: Family adaptation to a child's transplant: pretransplant phase, *Prog Transplant* 10(2): 1-6, 2000.

Mallory C, Miles MS, and Holditch-Davis D: Reciprocity and retaining African-American women with HIV in research, *Appl Nurs Res* 15(1): 35-41, 2002.

McDonald KA: Studies on women's health produce a wealth of knowledge on the biology of gender differences, *Chronicle of Higher Education,* A19-22, June 25, 1999.

Melkus GD, Spollett G, Jefferson V, Chyun D, Tuohy B, Robinson T, and Kaisen A: A culturally competent intervention of education and care for Black women with Type 2 diabetes, *Appl Nurs Res* 17(1): 10-20, 2004.

Mitchell K: Protecting children's rights during research, *Pediatr Nurs* 10: 9-10, 1984.

Monaghan P: The Gods of very small things, *Chronicle of Higher Education,* A19-21, December 15, 2000.

National Bioethics Advisory Commission: Report and recommendations on research involving persons with mental disorders that may affect decisional capacity, 1998.

National Commission for the Protection of Human Subjects of Biomedical and Behavioral Research: *Belmont report: ethical principles and guidelines for research involving human subjects,* DHEW Pub No 05, Washington, DC, 1978, US Government Printing Office, 78-0012.

Office of Research Integrity Website: http://ori.dhhs.gov, 2000.

Olson DP: HIPPA privacy regulations and nursing research, *Nurs Res* 52(5): 344-348, 2003.

Pallikkathayll L, Crighton F, and Aaronson LS: Balancing ethical quandries with scientific rigor: Part I, *West J Nurs Res* 20(3): 388-393, 1998.

Pruchino RA, Hayden JM: Interview modality: effects on costs and data quality in a sample of older women, *J Aging Health* 12(1): 3-24, 2000.

Public Health Service Policy on Humane Care in Use of Lab Animals by Awardee Institution: *NIH Guidelines for Grants and Contracts,* 14(8), 1985.

Rankin M, Esteves MD: Perceptions of scientific misconduct in nursing, *Nurs Res* 46: 270-276, 1997.

Raybuck JA: The clinical nurse specialist as research coordinator in clinical drug trials, *Clin Nurse Specialist* 11(1): 15-19, 1997.

Reverby SM: History of an apology: from Tuskegee to the White House, *Res Pract* (8): 1-12, 2000.

Robb IH: *Nursing ethics: for hospital and private use,* Milwaukee, Wi, 1900, GN Gaspar.

Rothman DJ: Were Tuskegee and Willowbrook studies in nature? *Hastings Cent Rep* 12(2): 5-7, 1982.

Ryan K: Scientific misconduct in perspective: the need to improve accountability, *Chronicle of Higher Education,* B1-2, July 19, 1996.

Sailer GR et al.: Nurses' unique roles in randomized clinical trials, *J Prof Nurs* 15(6): 106-115, 1999.

Tigges BB: Parental consent and adolescent risk behavior research, *J Nurs Scholarship* 35(3): 283-289, 2003.

Tilden VP: Preventing scientific misconduct—times have changed, *Nurs Res* 49(5): 243, 2000.

Ulrich CM, Wallen GR, and Grady C: Research vulnerability and patient advocacy, *Nurs Res* 51(2): 71, 2002.

Ward LS: Race as a variable in cross-cultural research, *Nurs Outlook* 51(3): 120-125, 2003.

Wheeler DL: Three medical organizations embroiled in controversy over use of placebos in AIDS studies abroad, *Chronicle of Higher Education,* A15-16, August 13, 1997.

FOR FURTHER STUDY

Go to your Companion CD for review activities for this chapter.

evolve Go to Evolve at http://evolve.elsevier.com/LoBiondo/ for WebLinks, Content Updates, and additional research articles, for practice in reviewing and critiquing.

14

ROBIN WHITTEMORE

MARGARET GREY

Data-Collection Methods

KEY TERMS

biological measurement
close-ended items
concealment
consistency
content analysis
debriefing
external criticism
internal criticism
interrater reliability

intervention
intervention fidelity
interviews
Likert-type scales
measurement
objective
open-ended items
operational definition
operationalization

physiological measurement
questionnaires
reactivity
records or available data
scale
scientific observation
social desirability
systematic

LEARNING OUTCOMES

After reading this chapter, the student should be able to do the following:

- Define the types of data-collection methods used in nursing research.
- List the advantages and disadvantages of each data-collection method.
- Compare how specific data-collection methods contribute to the strength of evidence in a research study.
- Critically evaluate the data-collection methods used in published nursing research studies.

STUDY RESOURCES

Go to your Companion CD for review activities for this chapter.

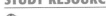 Go to Evolve at http://evolve.elsevier.com/LoBiondo/ for Weblinks, Content Updates, and additional research articles for practice in reviewing and critiquing.

As nurses, we use all of our senses when collecting data from the patients to whom we provide care. Nurse researchers also have available many ways to collect information about their research subjects. The major difference between the data collected when performing patient care and the data collected for the purpose of research is that the data-collection methods employed by researchers need to be objective and systematic. By **objective,** we mean that the data must not be influenced by another who collects the information; by **systematic,** we mean that the data must be collected in the same way by everyone who is involved in the collection procedure.

317

The methods that researchers use to collect information about subjects are the identifiable and repeatable operations that define the major variables being studied.

Operationalization is the process of translating the variables of interest to a researcher into observable and measurable phenomena. There may be a number of ways to collect the same information. For example, a researcher interested in measuring blood pressure (BP) could do so by measuring blood pressure using an ambulatory BP monitor or using an automated oscillometric BP monitor (Yucha et al., 2003). The method chosen by the researcher would depend on a number of decisions regarding the problem being studied, the nature of the subjects, and the relative costs and benefits of each method.

This chapter's purpose is to familiarize you with the various ways that researchers collect information from and about subjects. The chapter provides you as a nursing research consumer with the tools for evaluating the selection, utilization, and practicality of the various ways of collecting data.

MEASURING VARIABLES OF INTEREST

To a large extent, the success of a study depends on the quality of the data-collection methods chosen and employed. Researchers have many types of methods available for collecting information from subjects in research studies. Determining what measurement to use in a particular investigation may be the most difficult and time-consuming step in study design. In addition, as nursing research develops, researchers are beginning to have an array of quality instruments with adequate reliability and validity (see Chapter 15) from which to choose. Thus the process of evaluating and selecting the available instruments to measure variables of interest is of critical importance to the potential success of the study. In this section the selection of measures and the implementation of the data-collection process are discussed. An algorithm that influences a researcher's choice of data-collection methods is diagrammed in the Critical Thinking Decision Path.

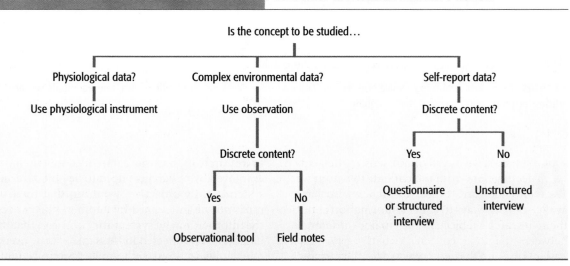

CRITICAL THINKING DECISION PATH | Consumer of Research Literature Review

Is the concept to be studied...

Physiological data? → Use physiological instrument

Complex environmental data? → Use observation → Discrete content?
- Yes → Observational tool
- No → Field notes

Self-report data? → Discrete content?
- Yes → Questionnaire or structured interview
- No → Unstructured interview

There are many different ways to collect information about variables of interest to nurses. Nurses are interested in physiological indicators of health (e.g., blood pressure and heart rates) but are also interested in psychosocial indicators of health (e.g., anxiety and quality of life). Psychosocial variables, such as anxiety, hope, social support, and quality of life, may be measured by several different techniques, such as observation of behavior or self-reports of feelings or attitudes by means of interviews or questionnaires. Researchers also may use data that have already been collected for another purpose, such as records, diaries, or other media, to study variables of interest.

As you can surmise, choosing the most appropriate method and instrument is difficult. The method must be appropriate to the problem, the hypothesis, the setting, and the population. For example, in the study of pain experiences of children, the researchers (Van Cleve et al., 2004, Appendix B) were interested in studying the pain experiences of children across multiple age groups. Because they were measuring children from ages 4 to 17, the same type of instrument could not be used. To deal with the reading and development levels of the children, they used tested age-appropriate instruments. For example, the children who were 4 to 13 years of age used the poker chip tool, in which the child chooses from one to four red chips, where each additional chip represents pain that ranges from "a little bit" to "the most pain" the child can experience. The older children, however, used the adolescent pediatric pain tool, which uses words and graphics to rate the pain experience.

Selection of the data-collection method begins during the literature review. In Chapter 4 it was noted that one purpose of the literature review is to provide clues to instrumentation. As the literature review is conducted, the researcher begins to explore how previous investigators defined and operationalized variables similar to those of interest in the current study. The researcher uses this information to define conceptually the variables to be studied. Once a variable has been defined conceptually, the researcher returns to the literature to define the variable operationally. This **operational definition** translates the conceptual definition into behaviors or verbalizations that can be measured for the study. In this second literature review the researcher searches for **measurement** instruments that might be used "as is" or adapted for use in the study. If instruments are available, the researcher needs to obtain permission for their use from the author.

An example may illustrate the relationship of the conceptual and operational definitions. Quality of life research is popular with researchers from many disciplines, including nursing. Definitions of quality of life may be related to health functioning, life satisfaction, or well-being. Quality of life may also be interpreted in a general way (well-being) or be related specifically to a type of illness. Therefore if a researcher is interested in studying quality of life, the researcher needs first to define what he or she means by the concept of quality of life. For example, Grey and colleagues (2000) defined quality of life in youth with type 1 diabetes as satisfaction with life that potentially is impacted by self-management of diabetes. According to this conceptual definition, the researcher would use a quality of life instrument specific to living with diabetes (operational definition) to determine the perceived quality of life of participants in the study. If another researcher disagreed with this definition or was more interested in general quality of life or quality of life in adults, a different instrument that measures overall or adult well-being may be more appropriate.

It is sometimes the case that no suitable way to measure a variable of interest exists, so the researcher needs to decide whether the variable is important to the study and whether a new instrument should be constructed. The construction of new instruments for data collection that have reasonable reliability and validity (see Chapter 15) is a most challenging task. Sometimes researchers decide not to study a variable if no suitable instrument exists; at other times the researcher may decide to invest time and energy into instrument development. Either decision is acceptable, depending on the goals of the study and the goals of the researcher.

Whether the researcher uses available methods or creates new ones, once the variables have been operationally defined in a manner consistent with the aims of the study, the population to be studied, and the setting, the researcher will determine how the data-collection phase of the study will be implemented. This decision deals with how the instruments for data collection will be given to the subjects. Consistency is the most important issue in this phase.

Consistency means that the data are collected from each subject in the study in exactly the same way or as close to the same way as possible. Consistency can minimize the bias introduced when more than one person collects the data. Data collectors must be carefully trained and supervised. To ensure consistency in data collection, sometimes referred to as **intervention fidelity** (Santacroce SJ, Maccarelli LM, Grey M, 2004), researchers must train data collectors in the methods to be used in the study so that each person collects the information in the same way. Information about how to observe, ask questions, and collect data often is included in a kind of "cookbook" protocol or manual for the research project. A researcher needs to spend time developing the protocol and training research assistants to collect data systematically and reliably. If data collectors are used, comments about their training and the consistency with which they collected data for the study should be provided by the researcher. For example, in the study by Koniak-Griffin and colleagues (2003) (see Appendix A), the procedure by which consistency of measurement was ensured is clearly presented. The authors state that all interviews were conducted by trained public health nurses who were not involved in the intervention and were blind to participant group assignment. Another example of the importance of training data collectors is pro-

vided by Schnell and colleagues (2003) in their study to evaluate a standardized protocol to assess and score urinary incontinence in nursing homes. These researchers needed to be accurate in their retrieval of data from existing medical records. Therefore they had two individuals collect data from medical records and they subsequently calculated the level of interrater agreement. In this study the index of agreement ranged from 0.75 to 1.0 using the kappa statistic. This demonstrates a high level of interrater agreement between the two observers. **Interrater reliability** (see Chapter 15) is the consistency of observations between two or more observers; it is often expressed as a percentage of agreement among raters or observers or as a coefficient of agreement that considers the element of chance (coefficient kappa). Bias is minimized when efforts are made by the researcher to ensure treatment fidelity, which, in turn, contributes to the strength of evidence provided by the findings of a research study.

 HELPFUL H I N T

Remember that the researcher may not always present complete information about the way the data were collected, especially when established tools were used. To learn about the tool that was used, the reader may need to consult the original article describing the tool.

 EVIDENCE-BASED PRACTICE TIP

It is difficult to place confidence in a study's findings if the data-collection methods are not consistent.

DATA-COLLECTION METHODS

In general, data-collection methods can be divided into the following five types: physiological, observational, interviews, questionnaires, and records or available data. Each of these methods has a specific purpose, as well as certain pros and cons inherent in its use. Each type of data-collection method is discussed, and then its respective uses and problems are discussed.

Physiological or Biological Measurements

In everyday practice, nurses collect physiological or biological data about patients such as their temperature, pulse rate, blood pressure, blood glucose levels, urine specific gravity, and pH of bodily fluids. Such data are frequently useful to nurse researchers. For example, Giuliano and colleagues (2003) examined the effect of varying degrees of backrest elevation on cardiac output and blood pressure in critically ill adults. Because cardiac output and blood pressure can be measured several different ways, it was important for the researchers to measure these outcomes at similar intervals and in similar ways for all participants of the study. In this study, cardiac output was measured using a continuous cardiac output pulmonary artery catheter with an attached heat exchange filament while blood pressure was measured using an indwelling arterial catheter connected to a continuous monitoring system.

 Physiological or biological measurement involves the use of specialized equipment to determine the physical and biological status of subjects. Frequently such measures also require specialized training. Such measures can be *physical,* such as weight or temperature; *chemical,* such as blood glucose level; *microbiological,* as with cultures; or *anatomical,* as in radiological examinations. What separates these measurements from others used in research is that they require the use of special equipment to make the observation. We can say, "This subject feels warm," but to determine how warm the subject is requires the use of a sensitive instrument, a thermometer.

Physiological or biological measurement is particularly suited to the study of several types of nursing problems. The aforementioned example is typical of studies dealing with ways to improve the performance of certain nursing actions, such as measuring and recording of patients' physiological data. Physiological measures may yield important criteria for determining the effectiveness of certain nursing interventions. In the aforementioned study of the effect of positioning on cardiac output and blood pressure, Giuliano and colleagues (2003) reported no significant differences in cardiac output or blood pressure with varying degrees of backrest elevation up to 45 degrees. These data indicate that in daily clinical practice, it may be unnecessary to reposition patients solely for the purpose of obtaining continuous cardiac output measurements.

The advantages of using physiological data-collection methods include their objectivity, precision, and sensitivity. Such methods are generally quite objective because unless there is a technical malfunction, two readings of the same instrument taken at the same time by two different nurses are likely to yield the same result. Because such instruments are intended to measure the variable being studied, they offer the advantage of being precise and sensitive enough to pick up subtle variations in the variable of interest. It is also unlikely that a subject in a study can deliberately distort physiological information.

Physiological measurements are not without inherent disadvantages, however. Some instruments may be quite expensive to obtain and use. In addition, such instruments often require specialized knowledge and training to be used accurately. Another problem with such measurements is that simply by using them, the variable of interest may be changed. Although some researchers think of these instruments as being nonintrusive, the presence of some types of devices might change the measurement. For example, the presence of a heart rate monitoring device might make some patients anxious and increase their heart rate. In addition, nearly all types of measuring devices are affected in some way by the environment. Even a simple thermometer can be affected by the subject drinking something hot immediately before the temperature is taken. Thus it is important to consider whether the researcher controlled such environmental variables in the study. Finally, there may not be a physiological way to measure the variable of interest. Occasionally researchers try to force a physiological parameter into a study in an effort to increase the precision of measurement. If the device does not really measure the variable of interest, however, the validity of its use is suspect.

Observational Methods

Sometimes nurse researchers are interested in determining how subjects behave under certain conditions. For example, the researcher might be interested in how children respond to painful situations. We might ask children how painful an experience was, but they may not be able to answer the question or to quantify the amount of pain, or they may distort their responses to please the researcher. Therefore sometimes observing the subject may give a more accurate picture of the behavior in question than asking the subject.

Although observing the environment is a normal part of living, **scientific observation** places a great deal of emphasis on the objective and systematic nature of the observation. The researcher is not merely looking at what is happening, but rather is watching with a trained eye for certain specific events. To be scientific, observations must fulfill the following four conditions:

1. The observations undertaken are consistent with the study's specific objectives.
2. There is a standardized and systematic plan for the observation and the recording of data.
3. All of the observations are checked and controlled.
4. The observations are related to scientific concepts and theories.

Observation is particularly suitable as a data-collection method in complex research situations that are best viewed as total entities and that are difficult to measure in parts, such as studies dealing with the nursing process, parent-child interactions, or group processes. In addition, observational methods can be the best way to operationalize some variables of interest in

nursing research studies, particularly individual characteristics and conditions, such as traits and symptoms, verbal and nonverbal communication behaviors, activities and skill attainment, and environmental characteristics.

Zimmerman and colleagues (2002) conducted a study on the relationship between nursing home environments and resident infections. Because asking either nursing home staff or nursing home residents to describe the nursing home environment may miss some important information or may be biased, the researchers used two observation tools to collect data on the environments. One observation instrument assessed environmental domains such as maintenance, cleanliness, odors, lighting, homelikeness, and noise; and the other observation instrument assessed the social environment by observing resident, staff, and visitor interactions. The researchers noted that there was consistency in recording of these observations between observers because the interrater reliability ranged from 95% to 100%.

Observational methods can be distinguished also by the role of the observer. This role is determined by the amount of interaction between the observer and those being observed. Each of the following four basic types of observational roles is distinguishable by the amount of concealment or intervention implemented by the observer:

1. Concealment without intervention
2. Concealment with intervention
3. No concealment without intervention
4. No concealment with intervention

These methods are illustrated in Figure 14-1, and examples are given later. **Concealment** refers to whether the subjects know they are being observed, and **intervention** deals with whether the observer provokes actions from those who are being observed. When a researcher is concerned that a subject's behavior will change as a result of being observed (**reactivity**), the type of observation most commonly employed is that of concealment without intervention. In this case, the researcher watches the subjects without their knowledge of the observation, and he or she

Concealment

		Yes	No
Intervention	**Yes**	Researcher hidden An intervention	Researcher open An intervention
	No	Researcher hidden No intervention	Researcher open No intervention

Figure 14-1. Types of observational roles in research.

does not provoke them into action. Often such concealed observations use hidden television cameras, audiotapes, or one-way mirrors. Concealment without intervention is often used in observational studies of children. You may be familiar with rooms with one-way mirrors in which a researcher can observe the behavior of the occupants of the room without being observed by them. Such studies allow for the observation of children's natural behavior and are often used in developmental research.

No concealment without intervention also is commonly used for observational studies. In this case, the researcher obtains informed consent from the subject to be observed and then simply observes his or her behavior. This was the type of observation done in the Koniak-Griffin (2003) study (Appendix A) in which data collectors videotaped and then observed mothers and infants interacting in a structured play episode. While this study included an intervention provided to some of the participants, the intervention did not occur within the context of the observation.

Observing subjects without their knowledge may violate assumptions of informed consent, and therefore researchers face ethical problems with this type of approach. However, sometimes there is no other way to collect such data, and the data collected are unlikely to have negative consequences for the subject; in these cases, the disadvantages of the study are outweighed by the advantages. Further, the problem is often handled by informing subjects after the observa-tion, allowing them the opportunity to refuse to have their data included in the study, and discussing any questions they might have. This process is called **debriefing.**

When the observer is neither concealed nor intervening, the ethical question is not a problem. Here the observer makes no attempt to change the subject's behavior and informs them that they are to be observed. Because the observer is present, this type of observation allows a greater depth of material to be studied than if the observer is separated from the subject by an artificial barrier, such as a one-way mirror. Participant observation is a commonly used observational technique in which the researcher functions as a part of a social group to study the group in question. The problem with this type of observation is reactivity (also referred to as the Hawthorne effect), or the distortion created when the subjects change behavior because they are being observed.

No concealment with intervention is employed when the researcher is observing the effects of some intervention introduced for sci-entific purposes. Because the subjects know they are participating in a research study, there are few problems with ethical concerns, but reactivity is also a problem with this type of study. The study by Bryan (2000) of the effect of prenatal couple invervention on enhancing parent-child interac-tion is an excellent example of no concealment with intervention. The researcher was not con-cealed in postnatal observations of parent-child teaching interactions and, if necessary, provided information on how to better interact with the infant after the observation.

Concealed observation with intervention involves staging a situation and observing the behaviors that are evoked in the subjects as a result of the intervention. Because the subjects are unaware of their participation in a research study, this type of observation has fallen into dis-favor and rarely is used in nursing research.

Observational methods may be structured or unstructured. Unstructured observational methods are not characterized by a total absence of structure but usually involve collecting descriptive information about the topic of interest. In participant observation, the observer keeps field notes that record the activities, as well as the observer's interpretations of these activities. *Field notes* usually are not restricted to any particular type of action or behavior; rather, they intend to paint a picture of a social situation in a more general sense. Another type of unstructured observation is the use of anecdotes. *Anecdotes* are not necessarily funny but usually focus on the behaviors of interest and frequently add to the richness of research reports by illustrating a particular point. On the other hand, structured observations, such as the standardized tools used to evaluate mother and infant interaction in the Koniak-Griffin (2003) study, require formal training and competence of the evaluators. The use of structured observations involves specifying in advance what behaviors or events are to be observed and using standardized tools or preparing forms for record keeping, such as categorization systems, checklists, and rating scales. Whichever system is employed, the observer watches the subject and then marks on the recording form what was seen. In any case, the observations must be similar among the observers (see earlier discussion and Chapter 15 for an explanation of interrater reliability). Thus it is important that observers be trained to be consistent in their observations and ratings of behavior.

 EVIDENCE-BASED PRACTICE TIP

When reading a research report that uses observation as a data-collection method, research consumers want to note evidence of consistency across data collectors through use of internal consistency reliability data. When that is present, it increases your confidence that the data were collected systematically.

Scientific observation has several advantages as a data-collection method, the main one being that observation may be the only way for the researcher to study the variable of interest. For example, what people say they do often is not what they really do. Therefore if the study is designed to obtain substantive findings about human behavior, observation may be the only way to ensure the validity of the findings. In addition, no other data-collection method can match the depth and variety of information that can be collected when using these techniques. Such techniques also are quite flexible in that they may be used in both experimental and nonexperimental designs and in laboratory and field studies.

 HELPFUL HINT

Sometimes a researcher may carefully train observers or data collectors, but the research report does not address this. Often the length of research reports dictates that certain information cannot be included. Readers can often assume that if reliability data are provided, then appropriate training occurred.

As with all data-collection methods, observation also has its disadvantages. We mentioned the problems of reactivity and ethical concerns when we discussed the concealment and intervention dimensions. In addition, data obtained by observational techniques are vulnerable to the bias of the observer. Emotions, prejudices, and values all can influence the way that behaviors and events are observed. In general, the more the observer needs to make inferences and judgments about what is being observed, the more likely it is that distortions will occur. Thus in judging the adequacy of observational methods, it is important to consider how observational tools were constructed and how observers were trained and evaluated.

Interviews and Questionnaires

Subjects in a research study often have information that is important to the study and that can be obtained only by asking the subject. Such questions may be asked orally by a researcher in person or over the telephone in an interview, or they may be asked in the form of a paper-and-pencil test. Both interviews and questionnaires have the purpose of asking subjects to report data for themselves, but each has unique advantages and disadvantages. **Interviews** are a method of data collection where a data collector questions a subject verbally. Interviews may be face-to-face or performed over the telephone, and they may consist of open-ended or close-ended questions. On the other hand, **questionnaires** are paper-and-pencil instruments designed to gather data from individuals about knowledge, attitudes, beliefs, and feelings. Survey research relies almost entirely on questioning subjects with either interviews or questionnaires, but these methods of data collection also can be used in many other types of research.

Individual items in an interview or questionnaire must be clearly written so that the intent of the question and the nature of the information sought are clear to the respondent. Although items must ask only one question, be free of suggestions, and use correct grammar, they may be either open-ended or close-ended. **Open-ended items** are used when the researcher wants the subjects to respond in their own words or when the researcher does not know all of the possible alternative responses. Open-ended questions are commonly used in qualitative research studies (see Chapters 6, 7, and 8). **Close-ended items** are used when there is a fixed number of alternative responses. Structured, fixed-response items are best used when the question has a finite number of responses and the respondent is to choose the one closest to the correct response. Fixed-response items have the advantage of simplifying the respondent's task and the researcher's analysis, but they may miss some important information about the subject. Unstructured or open-ended response formats allow more varied information to be collected and require a qualitative or **content analysis** method to analyze responses and accurately report combined subject responses.

When items of interviews and questionnaires are able to be combined mathematically to obtain an overall score, the measurement instrument is called a **scale.** An intelligence test is an example of a scale that combines individual item responses to determine an overall quantification of intelligence. A common scale used in nursing research is a Likert-type scale. **Likert-type scales** are lists of statements on which respondents indicate, for example, whether they "strongly agree," "agree," "disagree," or "strongly disagree." Sometimes finer distinctions are given or there may be a neutral category. The use of the neutral category, however, sometimes creates problems because it often is the most frequent response and this response is difficult to interpret.

> ☀ **EVIDENCE-BASED PRACTICE TIP**
>
> Scales used in nursing research should have evidence of adequate reliability and validity so that research consumers feel confident that the findings reflect what the researcher intended to measure (see Chapter 15).

Figure 14-2 shows a few items from a fictional survey of pediatric nurse practitioners. The first items are close-ended items and of a Likert-type format. Note that respondents are asked to choose how strongly they agree with each item. In using these questions in the survey, respondents are forced to choose from only these answers because it is thought that these will be the only responses. The only possible alternative response is to skip the item and leave it blank. On the other hand, sometimes researchers have no idea or have only a limited idea of what the respondent will say, or researchers want the answer in the respondent's own words, as with the second set of items. Here, respondents may also leave the item blank but are not forced to make a particular response.

Interviews and questionnaires are used commonly in nursing research. Both are strong approaches to gathering information for research, because they approach the task directly. In addition, both have the ability to obtain certain kinds of information, such as the subject's

Close-Ended (Likert-Type Scale)

A. How satisfied are you with your current position?
   1. Very satisfied
   2. Moderately satisfied
   3. Undecided
   4. Moderately dissatisfied
   5. Very dissatisfied

B. To what extent do the following factors contribute to your current level of positive satisfaction?

	Not at all	Very little	Somewhat	Moderate amount	A great deal
1. % of time in patient care	1	2	3	4	5
2. Types of patients	1	2	3	4	5
3. % of time in educational activity	1	2	3	4	5
4. % of time in administration	1	2	3	4	5

Close-Ended

A. On an average, how many clients do you see in one day?
   1. 1 to 3
   2. 4 to 6
   3. 7 to 9
   4. 10 to 12
   5. 13 to 15
   6. 16 to 18
   7. 19 to 20
   8. More than 20

B. How would you characterize your practice?
   1. Too slow
   2. Slow
   3. About right
   4. Busy
   5. Too busy

Open-Ended

A. Are there incentives that the National Association of Pediatric Nurse Associates and Practitioners ought to provide for members that are currently not being done?

_____
_____
_____
_____

Figure 14-2. Examples of close-ended and open-ended questions.

attitudes and beliefs, which would be difficult to obtain without asking the subject directly. All methods that involve verbal reports, however, share a problem with accuracy. There is often no way to know whether what the researcher is told is indeed true. For example, people are known to respond to questions in a way that makes a favorable impression. This response style is known as **social desirability.** Because there is no way to tell whether the respondent is telling the truth or responding in a socially desirable way, the researcher usually is forced to assume that the respondent is telling the truth (see Chapter 9).

Questionnaires and interviews also have some specific purposes, advantages, and disadvantages. Questionnaires and paper-and-pencil tests are most useful when there is a finite set of questions to be asked and the researcher can be assured of the clarity and specificity of the items. Questionnaires are desirable tools when the purpose is to collect information. If questionnaires are too long, they are not likely to be completed. Face-to-face techniques or interviews are best used when the researcher may need to clarify the task for the respondent or is interested in obtaining more personal information from the respondent. Telephone interviews allow the researcher to reach more respondents than face-to-face interviews, and they allow for more clarity than questionnaires.

> ### 💡 HELPFUL HINT
>
> Remember, sometimes researchers make trade-offs when determining the measures to be used. For example, a researcher may want to learn about an individual's attitudes regarding job satisfaction; practicalities may preclude using an interview, so a questionnaire may be used instead.

Koniak-Griffin and associates (2003, Appendix A) used a combination of interview, questionnaire, and observational data-collection methods to study the effects of an early intervention program for pregnant adolescents on infant and maternal outcomes. Interviews by trained public health nurses assessed maternal

health behaviors, complications of pregnancy, substance use, community resource use, employment status, and infant health status. In addition, questionnaires were administered to participants to evaluate social competence. Lastly, mother-infant interactions during a play episode were videotaped and evaluated using a structured observation method. Thus the researchers were able to evaluate both infant and maternal outcomes. This use of multiple measures gives a more complete picture than the use of just one measure.

Researchers face difficult choices when determining whether to use interviews or questionnaires. The final decision is often based on what instruments are available and their relative costs and benefits.

Both face-to-face and telephone interviews offer some advantages over questionnaires. All things being equal, interviews are better than questionnaires because the response rate is almost always higher and this helps eliminate bias in the sample (see Chapter 12). Respondents seem to be less likely to hang up the telephone or to close the door in an interviewer's face than to throw away a questionnaire. Another advantage of the interview is that some people, such as children, the blind, and the illiterate, could not fill out a questionnaire, but they could participate in an interview. With an interview, the data collector knows who is giving the answers. When questionnaires are mailed, for example, anyone in the household could be the person who supplies the answers.

Interviews also allow for some safeguards to be built into the interview situation. Interviewers can clarify misunderstood questions and observe the level of the respondent's understanding and cooperativeness. In addition, the researcher has strict control over the order of the questions. With questionnaires, the respondent can answer questions in any order. Sometimes changing the order of the questions can change the response. Finally, interviews allow for richer and more complex data to be collected. This is particularly so when open-ended responses are sought. Even when close-ended response items are used, interviews can probe to understand why a respondent answered in a particular way.

Interviews can also be conducted in a group setting, which is called a focus group interview. Wilson, Pittman, and Wold (2000) used an unstructured focus group interview method to study Hispanic migrant children's health experiences. These unstructured interviews occurred in small groups (4 to 8 in each group) with children 8 to 14 years of age. These small group interviews allow the participants to freely explain and share information individually and collectively. Agreement and disagreement among participants may be elicited. This allows the researchers to efficiently obtain specific information from a number of subjects simultaneously.

Questionnaires also have certain advantages. They are much less expensive to administer than interviews because interviews may require the hiring and training of interviewers. Thus if a researcher has a fixed amount of time and money, a larger and more diverse sample can be obtained with questionnaires. Questionnaires also allow for complete anonymity, which may be important if the study deals with sensitive issues. Finally, the fact that no interviewer is present assures the researcher and the reader that there will be no interviewer bias. Interviewer bias occurs when the interviewer unwittingly leads the respondent to answer in a certain way. This problem is especially pronounced in studies that use unstructured interview formats. A subtle nod of the head, for example, could lead a respondent to change an answer to correspond with what the researcher wants to hear.

Records or Available Data

All of the data-collection methods discussed thus far concern the ways that nurse researchers gather new data to study phenomena of interest. Not all studies, though, require a researcher to acquire new information. Sometimes existing information can be examined in a new way to study a problem. The use of records and available data sometimes is considered to be primarily the province of historical research, but hospital records, care plans, and existing data sources, such as the census, are frequently used for collecting information relevant to answering research questions about clinical problems. **Records or available data,** therefore, are forms of information that are collected from existing materials, such as hospital records, historical documents, or national databases, and are used to answer research questions in a new manner.

The use of available data has certain advantages. Because the data-collection step of the research process often is the most difficult and time-consuming step, the use of available records often allows for a significant saving of time. If the records have been kept in a similar manner over time, as with the National Health and Examination Surveys, analysis of these records allows for the examination of trends over time. In addition, the use of available data decreases problems of reactivity and response set bias. The researcher also does not have to ask individuals to participate in the study.

On the other hand, institutions are sometimes reluctant to allow researchers to have access to their records. If the records are kept so that an individual cannot be identified, this is usually not a problem. However, the Health Insurance Portability and Accountability Act (HIPPA), a federal law, protects the rights of individuals who may be identified in records (see Chapter 14). Another problem that affects the quality of available data is that the researcher has access only to those records that have survived. If the records available are not representative of all of the possible records, the researcher may have a problem with bias. Often there is no way to tell whether the records have been saved in a biased manner, and the researcher has to make an intelligent guess as to their accuracy. For example, a researcher might be interested in studying socioeconomic factors associated with the suicide rate. These data frequently are underreported because of the stigma attached to suicide, and so the records would be biased. Recent interest in computerization of health records has led to an increase in discussion about the desirability of access to such records for research. At this point, it is not clear how much computerized health data will continue to be readily available for research without consent.

Another problem is related to the authenticity of the records. The distinction of primary and secondary sources is as relevant here as it was in discussing the literature review (see Chapter 4). A book, for example, may have been ghostwritten but credit accorded to the known author. It may be difficult for the researcher to ferret out these types of subtle biases. Lastly, existing records may have a significant amount of missing data. For example, years of education may only be recorded on a portion of the sample records.

Nonetheless, records and available data constitute a rich source of information for study. The previously mentioned study by Schnell and colleagues (2003), whereby the implementation of a nursing protocol to assess urinary incontinence was evaluated by examining existing medical records, is an example of using available data to answer research questions of interest to nurses.

 EVIDENCE-BASED PRACTICE TIP

A critical evaluation of any data-collection method includes evaluating the appropriateness, objectivity, and consistency of the method employed.

CONSTRUCTION OF NEW INSTRUMENTS

As already mentioned in this chapter, researchers sometimes cannot locate an instrument or method with acceptable reliability and validity to measure the variable of interest. This often is the case when testing a part of a nursing theory or when evaluating the effect of a clinical intervention. Instrument development is complex and time consuming. It consists of the following steps:

- Define the concept to be measured
- Clarify target population
- Formulate the items
- Assess the items for content validity
- Develop instructions for respondents and users
- Pretest and pilot test the items
- Estimate reliability and validity

Defining the concept to be measured requires that the researcher develop an expertise in the concept. This requires an extensive review of the literature and of all existing tests and measurements that deal with related concepts. The researcher will use all of this information to synthesize the available knowledge so that the construct can be defined.

Once defined, the individual items measuring the concept can be developed. The researcher will develop many more items than are needed to address each aspect of the concept or components or subcomponents of the concept. The items are evaluated by a panel of experts in the field so that the researcher is assured that the items measure what they are intended to measure (content validity; see Chapter 15). Eventually the number of items will be decreased because some items will not work as they were intended and they will be eliminated from the study. In this phase, the researcher needs to ensure consistency among the items, as well as consistency in testing and scoring procedures.

Finally, the researcher administers or pilot tests the new instrument by giving it to a group of people who are similar to those who will be studied in the larger investigation. The purpose of this analysis is to determine the quality of the instrument as a whole (reliability and validity), as well as the ability of each item to discriminate individual respondents (variance in item response). Pilot testing a new instrument also yields important evidence about the reading level (too low or too high), length of the instrument (too short or too long), directions (clear or not clear), and return rate. Pilot testing also allows one to assess if the instrument is appropriate for the target population in terms of cultural or ethnic issues. The researcher also may administer a related instrument to see if the new instrument is sufficiently different from the older one.

It is important that researchers who invest significant amounts of time in tool development publish those results. This type of research serves not only to introduce other researchers to the tool but also to ultimately enhance nursing science because our ability to conduct meaningful research is limited only by our ability to measure important phenomena.

CRITIQUING GUIDE   *Data-Collection Methods*

Evaluating the adequacy of data-collection methods from written research reports is often problematic for new nursing research consumers. This is because the tool itself is not available for inspection and the reader may not feel comfortable judging the adequacy of the method without seeing it. All sections of a research article that address data-collection methods should provide evidence of consistency in the form of instrument reliability and validity and interrater reliability across data collectors. When reviewing data-collection methods, a number of questions can be asked to judge the method chosen by the researcher. These questions are listed in the Critiquing Criteria box.

All studies should have clearly identified data-collection methods. The conceptual and operational definitions of each important variable should be present in the report. Sometimes it is useful for the researcher to explain why a particular method was chosen. For example, if the study dealt with young children, the researcher may explain that a questionnaire was deemed to be an unreasonable task, so an interview was chosen.

Once you have identified the method chosen to measure each variable of interest, you should decide if the method used was the best way to measure the variable. If a questionnaire was used, for example, you might wonder why the decision was made not to use an interview. In addition, consider whether the method was appropriate to the clinical situation. Does it make sense to interview patients in the recovery room, for example?

Once you have decided whether all relevant variables are operationalized appropriately, you can begin to determine how well the method was carried out. For studies using physiological measurement, it is important to determine whether the instrument was appropriate to the problem and not forced to fit it. The rationale for selecting a particular instrument should be given. For example, it may be important to know that the study was conducted under the auspices of a manufacturing firm that provided the measuring instrument. In addition, provision should be made to evaluate the accuracy of the instrument and those who use it.

Several considerations are important when reading studies that use observational methods. Who were the observers, and how were they trained? Is there any reason to believe that different observers saw events or behaviors differ-

CRITIQUING CRITERIA   *Data-Collection Methods*

1. Are all of the data-collection instruments clearly identified and described?
2. Is the rationale for their selection given?
3. Is the method used appropriate to the problem being studied?
4. Were the methods used appropriate to the clinical situation?
5. Are the data-collection procedures similar for all subjects?
6. Were efforts made to ensure intervention fidelity through the data-collection protocol?

Physiological Measurement

1. Is the instrument used appropriate to the research problem and not forced to fit it?
2. Is a rationale given for why a particular instrument was selected?
3. Is there a provision for evaluating the accuracy of the instrument and those who use it?

Observational Methods

1. Who did the observing?
2. Were the observers trained to minimize any bias?
3. Was there an observational guide?
4. Were the observers required to make inferences about what they saw?
5. Is there any reason to believe that the presence of the observers affected the behavior of the subjects?
6. Were the observations performed using the principles of informed consent?

Interviews

1. Is the interview schedule described adequately enough to know whether it covers the subject?
2. Is there clear indication that the subjects understood the task and the questions?
3. Who were the interviewers, and how were they trained?
4. Is there evidence of any interviewer bias?

Questionnaires

1. Is the questionnaire described well enough to know whether it covers the subject?
2. Is there evidence that subjects were able to perform the task?
3. Is there clear indication that the subjects understood the questionnaire?
4. Are the majority of the items appropriately close-ended or open-ended?

Available Data and Records

1. Are the records used appropriate to the problem being studied?
2. Are the data examined in such a way as to provide new information and not summarize the records?
3. Has the author addressed questions of internal and external criticism?
4. Is there any indication of selection bias in the available records?

---

ently? Remember that the more inferences the observers are required to make, the more likely there will be problems with biased observations. Also consider the problem of reactivity; in any observational situation, the possibility exists that the mere presence of the observer could change the behavior in question. What is important here is not that reactivity could occur, but rather how much reactivity could affect the data. Finally, consider whether the observational procedure was ethical. The reader needs to consider whether subjects were informed that they were being observed, whether any intervention was performed, and whether subjects had agreed to be observed. Clearly, it is not difficult for data-collection bias to be introduced in a study, thereby decreasing the strength of the evidence provided by the findings.

Interviews and questionnaires should be clearly described to allow the reader to decide whether the variables were adequately operationalized. Sometimes the researcher will reference the original report about the tool, and the reader may wish to read this study before deciding if the method was appropriate for the present study. The respondent's task should be clear. Thus provision should be made for the subjects to understand both their overall responsibilities and the individual items. Who were the interviewers in the interview situation? Does the researcher explain how they were trained to decrease any interviewer bias?

Available data are subject to internal and external criticism. **Internal criticism** deals with the evaluation of the worth of the records. Internal criticism primarily refers to the accuracy of the data. The researcher should present evidence that the records are genuine. **External criticism** is concerned with the authenticity of the records. Are the records really written by the first author? Finally, the reader should be aware of the problems with selective survival. The researcher may not have an unbiased sample of all of the possible records in the problem area, and this may have a profound effect on the validity of the results.

Finally, the reader should consider the data-collection procedure. Is any assurance provided that all of the subjects received the same information? In addition, it is important to try to determine whether all of the information was collected in the same way for all of the subjects in the study.

Once you have decided that the data-collection method used was appropriate to the problem and the procedures were appropriate to the population studied, the reliability and validity of the instruments themselves need to be considered. These characteristics are discussed in the next chapter.

Critical Thinking Challenges

- Physiological measurements are objective, precise, and sensitive. Discuss factors that might impact on their validity and feasibility. How does this affect the study's strength and quality of the evidence provided by the findings and their applicability to practice?
- A student in research class asks why nurses who participate in a clinical research study in the role of a data collector, or perform a "treatment intervention," need to be trained. What important factors or rationale would you offer to support the establishment of interrater reliability? How does failure to establish interrater reliability affect the overall outcome of the study findings?
- Observational methods are a frequent data-collection method in nursing research. Discuss what makes nurses perfect potential candidates for this role and what the disadvantages are of using this method.
- Studies often use a survey to collect data. How can researchers increase their return rate of the survey, and how is it determined if the survey return is adequate?

KEY POINTS

- Data-collection methods are described as being both objective and systematic. The data-collection methods of a study provide the operational definitions of the relevant variables.
- Types of data-collection methods include physiological, observational, interviews, questionnaires, and available data or records. Each method has advantages and disadvantages.
- Physiological measurements are those methods that use technical instruments to collect data about patients' physical, chemical, microbiological, or anatomical status. They are suited to studying how to improve the effectiveness of nursing care. Physiological measurements are objective, precise, and sensitive, but they may be very expensive and may distort the variable of interest.
- Observational methods are used in nursing research when the variables of interest deal with events or behaviors. Scientific observation requires preplanning, systematic recording, controlling the observations, and providing a relationship to scientific theory. This method is best suited to research problems that are difficult to view as a part of a whole. Observers may be passive or active as well as concealed or obvious. Observational methods have several advantages: they provide flexibility to measure many types of situations, and they allow for a great depth and breadth of information to be collected. Observation has disadvantages as well: (1) data may be distorted as a result of the observer's presence (reactivity), (2) concealment requires the consideration of ethical issues, and (3) observations may be biased by the person who is doing the observing.
- Interviews are commonly used data-collection methods in nursing research. Items on interview schedules may be of direct or indirect interest. Either open-ended or close-ended questions may be used when asking the subject questions. The form of the question should be clear to the respondent, free of suggestion, and grammatically correct.
- Questionnaires, or paper-and-pencil tests, are useful when there are a finite number of questions to be asked. Questions need to be clear and specific. Questionnaires are less costly in time and money to administer to large groups of subjects, particularly if the subjects are geographically widespread. Questionnaires also can be completely anonymous and prevent interviewer bias.
- Interviews are best used when a large response rate and an unbiased sample are important because the refusal rate for interviews is much less than that for questionnaires. Interviews allow for portions of the population such as children and the illiterate, who would otherwise be omitted by the use of a questionnaire, to participate in the study. An interviewer can clarify and maintain the order of the questions for all participants.
- Records and available data also are an important source for research data. The use of available data may save the researcher considerable time and money when conducting a study. This method reduces problems with both reactivity and ethical concerns. However, records and available data are subject to problems of availability, authenticity, and accuracy.

REFERENCES

Bryan AA: Enhancing parent-child interaction with a prenatal couple intervention, *Matern Child Nurs* 25(3): 139-144, 2000.

Giuliano KK et al.: Backrest angle and cardiac output measurement in critically ill patients, *Nurs Res* 52: 242-248, 2003.

Grey M et al.: Coping skills training for youth with diabetes mellitus has long-lasting effects on metabolic control and quality of life, *J Pediatr* 137: 107-113, 2000.

Koniak-Griffin et al.: Nurse visitation for adolescent mothers, *Nurs Res* 52(2): 127-136, 2003.

Santacroce SJ, Maccarelli LM, and Grey M: Intervention fidelity, *Nurs Res* 53: 63-66, 2004.

Schnell JF et al.: A standardized quality assessment system to evaluate incontinence in the nursing home, *J Am Geriatr Soc* 51: 1754-1761, 2003.

Van Cleve L, Bossert E, Beecroft P, Adlard K, Alvarez O, and Savedra MC: The pain experience of children with leukemia during the first year after diagnosis, *Nurs Res* 53: 1-10, 2004.

Whittemore R, Grey M: The systematic development of nursing interventions, *J Nurs Scholarship* 34: 115-120, 2002.

Wilson AH, Pittman K, Wold, JL: Listening to the quiet voices of Hispanic migrant children about health, *J Pediatr Nurs* 15: 137-147, 2000.

Yucha CB, Yang MCK, Tsai PS, and Calderon KS: Comparison of blood pressure measurement consistency using tonometric and oscillometric instruments, *J Nurs Measurement* 11: 73-86, 2003.

Zimmerman S et al.: Nursing home facility risk factors for infection and hospitalization: importance of registered nurse turnover, administration, and social factors, *J Am Geriatr Soc* 50: 1987-1995, 2002.

WEB SITE READINGS

Kennedy C et al.: Interactive data collection: benefits of integrating new media into pediatric research, *Comput Inform Nurs* 21: 120-127, 2003.

Olsen DP: HIPPA privacy regulations and nursing research, *Nurs Res* 52: 344-348, 2003.

Read CY: Conducting a client-focused survey using e-mail, *Comput Inform Nurs* 22: 83-89, 2004.

FOR FURTHER STUDY

Go to your Companion CD for review activities for this chapter.

evolve Go to Evolve at http://evolve.elsevier.com/LoBiondo/ for WebLinks, Content Updates, and additional research articles, for practice in reviewing and critiquing.

15

JUDITH HABER

GERI LOBIONDO-WOOD

Reliability and Validity

KEY TERMS

chance (random) errors
concurrent validity
construct validity
content validity
contrasted-groups (known-groups)
   approach
convergent validity
criterion-related validity
Cronbach's alpha
divergent/discriminant validity
equivalence

error variance
face validity
factor analysis
homogeneity
hypothesis-testing approach
internal consistency
interrater reliability
item to total correlations
Kappa
Kuder-Richardson coefficient
multitrait-multimethod approach

observed test score
parallel or alternate form reliability
predictive validity
reliability
reliability coefficient
split-half reliability
stability
systematic (constant) error
test-retest reliability
validity

LEARNING OUTCOMES

After reading this chapter, the student should be able to do the following:

- Discuss how measurement error can affect the outcomes of a research study.
- Discuss the purposes of reliability and validity.
- Define reliability.
- Discuss the concepts of stability, equivalence, and homogeneity as they relate to reliability.
- Compare and contrast the estimates of reliability.
- Define validity.
- Compare and contrast content, criterion-related, and construct validity.
- Identify the criteria for critiquing the reliability and validity of measurement tools.
- Use the critiquing criteria to evaluate the reliability and validity of measurement tools.
- Discuss how evidence related to reliability and validity contributes to clinical decision making.

STUDY RESOURCES

Go to your Companion CD for review activities for this chapter.

evolve Go to Evolve at http://evolve.elsevier.com/LoBiondo/ for Weblinks, Content Updates, and additional research articles for practice in reviewing and critiquing.

Measurement of nursing phenomena is a major concern of nursing researchers. Unless measurement instruments validly and reliably reflect the concepts of the theory being tested, conclusions drawn from a study will be invalid and will not advance the development of nursing theory and evidence-based practice. Issues of reliability and validity are of central concern to the researcher as well as to the critiquer of research. From either perspective, the measurement instruments that are used in a research study must be evaluated. Many new constructs are relevant to nursing theory, and a growing number of established measurement instruments are available to researchers. Researchers often face the challenge of developing new instruments, however, and as part of that process, establishing the reliability and validity of those tools. The growing importance of measurement issues, tool development, and related issues (e.g., reliability and validity) is evident in the issues of the *Journal of Nursing Measurement* and other nursing research journals.

Nurse investigators use instruments that have been developed by researchers in nursing and other disciplines. The critiquer of research, when reading research studies and reports, must assess the reliability and validity of the instruments used in the study to determine the soundness of these selections in relation to the concepts or variables under investigation. The appropriateness of the instruments and the extent to which reliability and validity are demonstrated have a profound influence on the findings and the internal and external validity of the study. Invalid measures produce invalid estimates of the relationships between variables, thus affecting internal validity. The use of invalid measures produces inaccurate generalizations to the populations being studied, thus affecting external validity and the ability to apply or not apply research findings in clinical practice. As such, the assessment of reliability and validity is an extremely important skill for critiquers of nursing research to develop.

Regardless of whether a new or already developed measurement tool is used in a research study, evidence of reliability and validity is of crucial importance. Box 15-1 identifies several computer resources that research consumers can use to access and evaluate the reliability and validity of the measurement instruments used in research studies. This chapter examines the major types of reliability and validity and demonstrates the applicability of these concepts to the development, selection, and evaluation of measurement tools in nursing research.

RELIABILITY, VALIDITY, AND MEASUREMENT ERROR

Researchers may be concerned about whether the scores that were obtained for a sample of subjects were consistent, true measures of the behaviors and thus an accurate reflection of the differences between individuals. The extent of variability in test scores that is attributable to error rather than a true measure of the behaviors is the **error variance.**

An **observed test score** that is derived from a set of items actually consists of the true score plus error (Figure 15-1). The error may be either chance error or random error, or it may be systematic error. Validity is concerned with systematic error, whereas reliability is concerned with random error. **Chance** or **random errors** are errors that are difficult to control (e.g., a respondent's anxiety level at the time of testing). Random errors are unsystematic in nature. Random errors are a result of a transient state in the subject, the context of the study, or the administration of the instrument (Waltz, Strickland, and Lenz, 1991). For example, perceptions or behaviors that occur at a specific point in time (e.g., anxiety) are known as a state or transient characteristic and are often beyond the awareness and control of the examiner. Another example of random error is in a study that measures blood pressure. Random error could occur by misplacement of the cuff, not waiting for a specific time period before taking the blood pressure, or placing the arm randomly in relationship to the heart while measuring blood pressure.

BOX 15-1 COMPUTER RESOURCES FOR ACCESSING AND EVALUATING THE VALIDITY AND RELIABILITY OF MEASUREMENT INSTRUMENTS*

- Mental Measurements Year Book—Test Reviews Online
  To subscribe, visit
    http://buros.unl.edu/buros/jsp/search.jsp
  These are online abstracts of 4000 commercially available tests, over 2000 of which have been critically appraised by the Buros Institute. These are the same reviews that appear in the print version of the Mental Measurement Yearbook Series. Searches can be conducted by author or by using the 18 search categories.
- 1997 Guide to Behavioral Resources on the Internet
  To subscribe, visit http://www.faulknergray.com
  Faulkner and Gray, Inc.
  11 Penn Plaza
  New York, NY 10001
  1-800-535-8403
  This is a print guide to more than 500 Internet resources devoted to mental health and behavioral research, including research tools.
- On-line Journal of Knowledge Synthesis for Nursing
  To subscribe, visit www.nursingsociety.org

  This provides full-text articles and searches, hypertext navigation, links to CINAHL and MEDLINE, tables, and figures.
- Virginia Henderson International Nursing Library
  To subscribe, visit www.nursingsociety.org
  This includes the following databases: registry of nurse researchers, registry of research projects, and registry of research results.
- Sigma Theta Tau International Nursing Honor Society
  550 West North Street
  Indianapolis, IN 46202
  317-634-8171
  www.nursingsociety.org
- CINAHL CD-ROM or On-line Services
  This provides access to searches in nursing and 17 allied health disciplines.
  CINAHL Information Systems
  1509 Wilson Terrace
  Glendale, CA 91206
  1-800-959-7167
  http://www.cinahl.com/

*See Chapter 4 for detailed information about computer resources.

Observed score (X_O)	=	True variance (X_T)	+	Error variance (X_E)
Actual score obtained		Consistent, hypothetical stable or true score		CHANCE/RANDOM ERROR — Transient subject factors — Instrumentation variations — Transient environmental factors SYSTEMATIC ERROR — Consistent instrument, subject or environmental factors

Figure 15-1. Components of observed scores.

Systematic or **constant error** is measurement error that is attributable to relatively stable characteristics of the study population that may bias their behavior and/or cause incorrect instrument calibration. Such error has a systematic biasing influence on the subjects' responses and thereby influences the validity of the instruments. For instance, level of education, socioeconomic status, social desirability, response set, or other characteristics may influence the validity of the instrument by altering measurement of the "true" responses in a systematic way.

For example, a subject is completing a survey about attitudes about caring for HIV/AIDS patients. If he or she wants to please the investigator, items may constantly be answered in a socially desirable way, thus making the estimate of validity inaccurate. Systematic error occurs also when an instrument is improperly calibrated. Consider a scale that consistently gives a person's weight at 2 pounds less than the actual body weight. The scale could be quite reliable (i.e., capable of reproducing the precise measurement), but the result is consistently invalid.

 HELPFUL H I N T

Research articles vary considerably in the amount of detail included about reliability and validity. When the focus of a study is tool development, psychometric evaluation—including extensive reliability and validity data—is carefully documented and appears throughout the article rather than briefly in the "Instruments" section, as in other research studies.

VALIDITY

Validity refers to whether a measurement instrument accurately measures what it is supposed to measure. When an instrument is valid, it truly reflects the concept it is supposed to measure.

A valid instrument that is supposed to measure anxiety does so; it does not measure some other construct, such as stress. A reliable measure can consistently rank participants on a given construct (e.g., anxiety), but a valid measure correctly measures the construct of interest. A measure can be reliable but not valid. Let us say that a researcher wanted to measure anxiety in patients by measuring their body temperatures. The researcher could obtain highly accurate, consistent, and precise temperature recordings, but such a measure could not be a valid indicator of anxiety. Thus the high reliability of an instrument is not necessarily congruent with evidence of validity. A valid instrument, however, is reliable. An instrument cannot validly measure the attribute of interest if it is erratic, inconsistent, and inaccurate.

There are three major kinds of validity that vary according to the kind of information provided and the purpose of the investigator (i.e., *content, criterion-related,* and *construct validity*). A critiquer of research articles will want to evaluate whether sufficient evidence of validity is present and whether the type of validity is appropriate to the design of the study and instruments used in the study.

 EVIDENCE-BASED PRACTICE TIP

Selecting measurement instruments that have strong evidence of validity increases the reader's confidence in the study findings—that the researcher actually measured what she or he intended to measure.

Content Validity

Content validity represents the universe of content, or the domain of a given construct. The universe of content provides the framework and basis for formulating the items that will adequately represent the content. When an investigator is developing a tool and issues of content validity arise, the concern is whether the measurement tool and the items it contains are representative of the content domain that the researcher intends to measure. The researcher begins by defining the concept and identifying the dimensions that are the components of the concept. The items that reflect the concept and its dimensions are formulated.

When the researcher has completed this task, the items are submitted to a panel of judges considered to be experts about this concept. Researchers typically request that the judges indicate their agreement with the scope of the items and the extent to which the items reflect the concept under consideration.

Fowles and Feucht (2004) developed the Barriers to Healthy Eating Scale (BHES), an instrument for measuring real or imagined barriers to healthy eating in pregnant women. Based on Pender's Health Promotion Model (HPM), the investigators suggest that clarifying barriers to healthy dietary intake may assist in identifying factors that place pregnant women and their unborn babies at risk. The BHES consisted of 18 items divided into 5 theoretically derived subscales: perception of unavailability (3 items), inconvenience (3 items), expense (3 items), preferences (6 items), and difficulty in engaging in healthy eating (3 items). Content validity was assessed by a panel of two experts with graduate training in the field of nutrition to review the scale items and rate each item on how relevant the items were to barriers to healthy eating in pregnancy. A Content Validity Index (CVI) was calculated to determine the extent of agreement between the two content experts who assessed the relevance (1 = not relevant, 2 = somewhat relevant, 3 = quite relevant, 4 = very relevant) of the instrument items to the objectives that guided tool construction and the degree to which the items represent the content domain. A CVI of .72 was obtained.

A subtype of content validity is **face validity,** which is a rudimentary type of validity that basically verifies that the instrument gives the appearance of measuring the concept. It is an intuitive type of validity in which colleagues or subjects are asked to read the instrument and evaluate the content in terms of whether it appears to reflect the concept the researcher intends to measure. This procedure may be useful in the tool development process in relation to determining readability and clarity of content. It should in no way, however, be considered a satisfactory alternative to other types of validity.

Bull, Luo, and Maruyama (2000) developed a 12-item questionnaire designed to measure continuity of care. The conceptualization of care continuity was derived from qualitative interviews with elders and family caregivers and focused on continuity of information. The scale was composed of two subscales: information on care management and information on continuity of services. Face validity was developed by having elders and their family caregivers review the items for clarity and relevance.

> ### EVIDENCE-BASED PRACTICE TIP
>
> If face and/or content validity, the most basic types of validity, was (were) the only type(s) of validity reported in a research article, the research consumer would not appraise the measurement tool(s) as having strong psychometric properties, which would negatively influence confidence about the study findings.

Criterion-Related Validity

Criterion-related validity indicates to what degree the subject's performance on the measurement tool and the subject's actual behavior are related. The criterion is usually the second measure, which assesses the same concept under study.

Two forms of criterion-related validity are concurrent and predictive. **Concurrent validity** refers to the degree of correlation of two measures of the same concept administered at the same time. A high correlation coefficient indicates agreement between the two measures. **Predictive validity** refers to the degree of correlation between the measure of the concept and some future measure of the same concept. Because of the passage of time, the correlation coefficients are likely to be lower for predictive validity studies.

Barnason and colleagues (2002) assessed concurrent validity of the Barnason Efficacy Expectation Scale (BEES), a 15-item instrument used to measure perceived self-efficacy in coronary artery bypass graft (CABG) patients. Items included in the measurement were confidence in physical functioning and psychosocial functioning, coronary artery disease risk factor modification (diet and exercise), and self-care management in the recovery and rehabilitation period following CABG surgery. In order to assess concurrent validity, convenience sampling was used to recruit subjects. The BEES tool and the Jenkins Self-Efficacy Expectation Scales for Selected Cardiac Recovery Behaviors tool were both administered to a total of 112 CABG patients before discharge from the hospital. Both instruments were intended to measure behaviors needed for recovery and rehabilitation of cardiac patients, with the BEES tool being more specific to CABG patients. The Pearson correlations between the BEES total score and the Jenkins scales were significant ($p<.01$), with correlations ranging from 0.19 to 0.47. A criterion correlation value of $r > .20$ was selected before analysis, as the Jenkins scales are not as behavior-specific as the BEES tool. All subscales met the criterion selected ($r = .20$) except the lifting subscale ($r = .19$). The authors note that the moderate correlations between the Jenkins subscales and the BEES tool are consistent with the findings of the noted psychologist Bandura (1997), as the BEES tool items are behavior-specific compared to Jenkin's tool items which were more generalized, thereby supporting concurrent validity of the BEES.

Knauth and Skowron (2004) evaluated the predictive validity of the Differentiation of Self Inventory for Adolescents, a 46-item self-report measure of an individual's ability to differentiate between emotional and intellectual functioning. It assesses four dimensions of differentiation: emotional reactivity (e.g., I am overly sensitive to criticism); I position (e.g., I usually do not change my behavior simply to please another person); emotional cutoff (e.g., I tend to distance myself when people get too close to me); and fusion with others (e.g., I usually need a lot of encouragement from others when starting a big

job or task). Higher scores reflect greater differentiation. Predictive validity was assessed by testing the relationship between the Trait Anxiety subscale of the State-Trait Anxiety Inventory (STAI) (Spielberger et al., 1983), a widely used adolescent self-report scale with established reliability and validity. A multiple regression on the predictor, Trait Anxiety and the Differentiation of Self scores, was significant ($F[1,355] = 174.73$; $p = .001$; $R2 = .33$). The results indicate that the greater chronic anxiety was significantly associated with lower differentiation of self scores. An additional test for predictive validity was carried out by a test of the additional variance accounted for by the ability of chronic anxiety (Trait Anxiety) to predict symptoms. This test was significant ($F[1,354] = 10.36$; $p = .001$; $R2 = .02$), indicating that greater differentiation of self predicted fewer symptoms over and above chronic anxiety, thereby lending support to the predictive validity of the Differentiation of Self Inventory for Adolescents.

Construct Validity

Construct validity is based on the extent to which a test measures a theoretical construct or trait. It attempts to validate a body of theory underlying the measurement and testing of the hypothesized relationships. Empirical testing confirms or fails to confirm the relationships that would be predicted among concepts and, as such, provides more or less support for the construct validity of the instruments measuring those concepts. The establishment of construct validity is a complex process, often involving several studies and approaches. The hypothesis-testing, factor analytical, convergent and divergent, and contrasted-groups approaches are discussed.

Hypothesis-Testing Approach

When the **hypothesis-testing approach** is used, the investigator uses the theory or concept underlying the measurement instruments to validate the instrument. The investigator does this by developing hypotheses regarding the behavior of individuals with varying scores on the measurement instrument, gathering data to test the hypotheses, and making inferences on the basis of the findings concerning whether the rationale underlying the instrument's construction is adequate to explain the findings.

For example, Barnason and colleagues (2002) used a hypothesis-testing approach to establish the construct validity of the Barnason Self-Efficacy Expectation Scale (BEES). Construct validity was tested based on the empirically supported hypothesis that individuals with better health status and functioning also would have higher levels of self-efficacy. To explore this hypothesis, correlations were made between the BEES total score and physiological behaviors of interest in this CABG population. Measures of physiological functioning used in this psychometric study were subscales of the Medical Outcomes Study Short-Form 36 (MOS SF-36), which has been used extensively in the literature as a measure of health status and functioning with established reliability and validity. The MOS SF-36 is a multidimensional scale measuring health concepts. However, in this study the physiological functioning sub-scales of physical functioning, role-physical functioning (role limitations due to physical problems), and general health were specifically used because those aspects of functioning were more closely related to the behaviors measured by the BEES.

The BEES mean score was correlated with aspects of physiological functioning (physical, role-physical, and general health), with significant weak to moderate correlations ranging from $r = .25$ to .41. These findings provide support for the hypotheses and therefore preliminary support for the theoretical basis, conceptual accuracy, and construct validity of the BEES in the CABG population: individuals with better health status have higher levels of self-efficacy. The homogeneous nature of the sample as well as the use of a convenience sampling strategy, however, suggests the need for further testing of the BEES with adults from varied age, gender, socioeconomic, and cultural groups.

Convergent and Divergent Approaches

Two strategies for assessing construct validity include convergent and divergent approaches.

Convergent validity refers to a search for other measures of the construct. Sometimes two or more tools that theoretically measure the same construct are identified, and both are administered to the same subjects. A correlational analysis (i.e., test of relationship; see Chapters 16 and 17) is performed. If the measures are positively correlated, convergent validity is said to be supported. Powers and colleagues (2004) evaluated the convergent validity of the Mobility Subscale of the Braden Scale for Predicting Pressure Sore Risk (Braden and Bergstrom, 1994), one of the most widely used tools for predicting pressure ulcer risk. It is one of only two existing pressure ulcer prediction tools recognized by the U.S. Agency for Health Care Policy and Research (DHHS, 1992). Immobility was identified as an important risk factor for the development of pressure ulcers, and the mobility subscale was predictive of skin breakdown. The mobility subscale of the Braden Scale was created to quantify levels of mobility on the basis of individual clinical observations. Convergent validity was assessed using actigraphy as a direct measure for frequency of movement. It was hypothesized that participants scoring low (score of 1) on the mobility subscale would have lower mean frequency of movement recorded by actigraphy than those with higher scores. It was further hypothesized that as the mobility subscale scores increased, the mean frequency of the movements recorded by actigraphy would increase. Two consecutive data-collection periods from 6 AM to 6 PM in a 48-hour interval were chosen for analysis. Only spontaneous patient movement was reflected in the data analysis of actigraph recordings. The statistically significant difference in the mean activity by subscale groups ($F[3,15] = 31.69; p = .001$) supported the hypothesis that the mean activity in each group increased as predicted, with the greatest amount of activity occurring in the group with the highest scores. The mean activity of mobility subscale Level 4 (no limitations in mobility) was significantly greater than that of the other three levels, thereby lending support to the convergent validity of the mobility subscale of the Braden Scale.

Divergent validity, sometimes called **discriminant validity,** uses measurement approaches that differentiate one construct from others that may be similar. Sometimes researchers search for instruments that measure the opposite of the construct. If the divergent measure is negatively related to other measures, validity for the measure is strengthened. Hess (1998) assessed the divergent validity of the IPNG by using a one-tailed *t* test to compare professional governance between aggregated scores of nurses from hospitals with and without shared governance. The two groups were similar in demographic characteristics, but nurses from hospitals with shared governance reported significantly higher scores on the IPNG than those nurses from hospitals without shared governance ($p = .0005$, one-tailed), thereby supporting the divergent validity of the IPNG. Singleton, Anderson, and Heishman (2003) examined the discriminant validity of the Tobacco Craving Questionnaire (TCQ) by comparing the effect of visual imagery scripts to elicit self-reported tobacco craving. While the craving scripts had a moderate to high effect on increased craving, which suggests evidence of convergent validity of the TCQ, there was no evidence either that the no-craving script affected craving scores ($p = .000$) or that the craving scripts affected positive mood ($p = .01$), thereby supporting the discriminant validity of the TCQ.

A specific method of assessing convergent and divergent validity is the **multitrait-multimethod approach.** Similar to the approach described, this method, proposed by Campbell and Fiske (1959), also involves examining the relationship between instruments that should measure the same construct and between those that should measure different constructs. A variety of measurement strategies, however, are used. For example, anxiety could be measured by the following:

- Administering the State-Trait Anxiety Inventory
- Recording blood pressure readings
- Asking the subject about anxious feelings
- Observing the subject's behavior

The results of one of these measures should then be correlated with the results of each of the others in a multitrait-multimethod matrix (Waltz, Strickland, and Lenz, 1991). In their classic study designed to develop, validate, and standardize a measure of dimensions of interpersonal relationships (including social support, reciprocity, and conflict), Tilden, Nelson, and May (1990) used the multitrait-multimethod approach to validity assessment. The two traits of social support and conflict of the Interpersonal Relationship Inventory (IPRI) were each measured with two different methods—a subject self-report tool and an investigator-observation visual analog rating. Reciprocity was not included because of its high correlation with social support.

The use of multiple measures of a concept decreases systematic error. A variety of data-collection methods (e.g., self-report, observation, interview, and collection of physiological data) will also diminish the effect of systematic error.

Contrasted-Groups Approach

When the **contrasted-groups approach** (sometimes called the **known-groups approach**) to the development of construct validity is used, the researcher identifies two groups of individuals who are suspected to score extremely high or low in the characteristic being measured by the instrument. The instrument is administered to both the high-scoring and the low-scoring group, and the differences in scores are examined. If the instrument is sensitive to individual differences in the trait being measured, the mean performance of these two groups should differ significantly and evidence of construct validity would be supported. A *t* test or analysis of variance is used to statistically test the difference between the two groups. In the study by Secco

(2002) that sought to develop and assess the psychometric properties of the Infant Care Questionnaire (ICQ), a self-report scale designed to measure a mother's perception of her abilities and competence as an infant care provider, the contrasted-groups approach was used to provide evidence of construct validity for the Mom and Baby dimension of the ICQ. The known groups were mothers of different parity (healthy low-risk primiparous versus multiparous mothers [$N = 164$] of term infants) and mothers with different amounts of past infant care experience. Multiparous mothers, those with higher ratings of past infant care experience, and those with greater time in the mothering role are expected to have significantly higher Mom and Baby scores than primiparous mothers with lower ratings of infant care experience. As illustrated in Table 15-1, repeated measures analysis of variance demonstrated significantly higher Mom and Baby scores for the multiparous mothers compared with primiparous mothers by time [$F(2, N = 140) = 21.78, p = .000$] and parity [$F(1, N = 140) = 10.78, p < .001$]. Trends observed with time in the infant care provider role were lower scores for primiparous mothers at all three measurement times and diminished mean differences between parity groups over time. The authors propose that these findings are associated with the maternal role attainment theory, which states that knowledge, skill, and competence perceptions are acquired during the postnatal period and that experience is a key factor in attainment of competence. The significantly higher scores on

the Mom and Baby means for the multiparous mothers suggest that the ICQ was sensitive enough to capture the differences between primiparous and multiparous mothers, thereby providing evidence of construct validity using the contrasted-groups approach.

Factor Analytical Approach

A final approach to assessing construct validity is **factor analysis.** This is a procedure that gives the researcher information about the extent to which a set of items measures the same underlying construct or dimension of a construct. Factor analysis assesses the degree to which the individual items on a scale truly cluster together around one or more dimensions. Items designed to measure the same dimension should load on the same factor; those designed to measure different dimensions should load on different factors (Anastasi, 1988; Nunnally and Bernstein, 1993). This analysis will also indicate whether the items in the instrument reflect a single construct or several constructs.

Gary and Yarandi (2004) carried out a factor analysis to determine the factor structure of the Beck Depression Inventory II (BDI-II), a 21-item well-known depression screening instrument, in a sample of rural Southern African-American women, a population for which the psychometric properties of the BDI-II are not known. The BDI-II is a self-report instrument used to measure depression in three dimensions: cognition, somatization, and motivation. Over the years it has been used to categorize people into depressed and nondepressed groups, with depression ranging from minimal to mild, moderate, and severe. The study sample consisted of 206 African-American women, none of whom self-reported receiving mental health care during the preceding year and at the time of data collection. An iterated principal-factor analysis was performed with a Promx (oblique) rotation used to identify the self-reported dimensions of depression. The analysis of the 21 items yielded a 2-factor solution; symptoms such as pessimism, worthlessness, punishment feelings,

TABLE **15-1** **Repeated Measures Analysis of Variance for Mean Mom and Baby Dimension Scores by Time [$F(2, N = 140) = 21.78, p < .001$] and Parity [$F(1, N = 140) = 10.78, p < .001$]**

	Primiparous (N = 97)	Multiparous (N = 43)	Mothers (N = 140)
Week 1	3.74	4.09	3.85
Week 2	4.00	4.23	4.10
Week 3	4.07	4.18	4.10

TABLE **15-2 Factor Matrix for a Sample (*N* = 206) of African-American Women**

Symptom	Factor I	Factor II
Pessimism	0.81	−0.22
Worthlessness	0.73	−0.10
Punishment feelings	0.65	0.03
Sadness	0.45	0.19
Self-dislike	0.44	0.15
Loss of interest	0.44	0.25
Indecisiveness	0.43	0.22
Past failure	0.40	0.12
Guilty feelings	0.35	0.28
Self-criticalness	0.34	0.28
Suicidal thoughts or wishes	0.28	0.17
Tiredness or fatigue	−0.03	0.76
Loss of energy	−0.06	0.63
Concentration difficulty	0.12	0.58
Irritability	0.15	0.55
Changes in appetite	−0.01	0.54
Changes in sleeping patterns	0.16	0.51
Loss of interest in sex	−0.07	0.48
Loss of pleasure	0.21	0.42
Crying	0.27	0.34
Agitation	0.28	0.34

symptoms of depression and were compared with two samples Beck et al. (1996) used for constructing the psychometric properties of the BDI-II. One sample involved patients from four different psychiatric clinics; the other sample included Canadian college students. It is interesting to note that the African-American women, a sample not in psychiatric treatment, had factor loadings more reflective of the Canadian college students than the outpatient psychiatric group although there were overlaps among the three samples. Such findings could suggest that the BDI-II is useful as a first-line screening instrument for African-American women. However, the authors offer a note of caution about widespread applicability because of the lack of scientific data about how depression manifests itself among African-Americans.

 HELPFUL H I N T

When validity data about the measurement instruments used in a study are not included in a research article, you have no way of determining whether the intended concept is actually being captured by the measurement tool. Before you use the results in such a case, it is important to go back to the original source to check the instrument's validity.

 EVIDENCE-BASED PRACTICE TIP

When the tools used in a study are presented, note whether the sample(s) used to develop the measurement instrument(s) is (are) similar to your patient population.

sadness, self-dislike, loss of interest, indecisiveness, and past failure were labeled Factor I. As indicated in Table 15-2, all of these symptoms were psychological and cognitive in nature, thereby contributing a cognitive dimension of self-reported depression. Factor II included somatic symptoms such as tiredness or fatigue, loss of energy, difficulty concentrating, changes in appetite, changes in sleeping patterns, irritability, loss of interest in sex, and loss of pleasure. Such factors were thought to represent a "somatic-affective" dimension of self-reported depression. The two factors clearly discriminate between the cognitive and somatic-affective

The Critical Thinking Decision Path will help you assess the appropriateness of the type of validity and reliability selected for use in a particular research study.

CRITICAL THINKING DECISION PATH | Determining the Appropriate Type of Validity and Reliability Selected for a Study

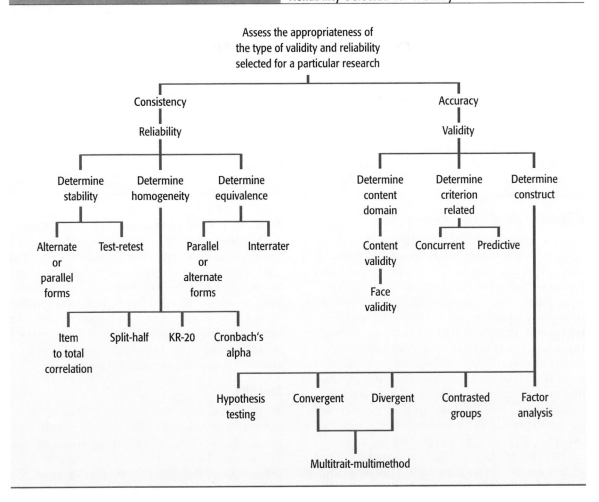

RELIABILITY

Reliable people are those whose behavior can be relied on to be consistent and predictable. Likewise, the **reliability** of a research instrument is defined as the extent to which the instrument yields the same results on repeated measures. Reliability is then concerned with consistency, accuracy, precision, stability, equivalence, and homogeneity. Concurrent with the questions of

validity or after they are answered, the researcher and the critiquer ask how reliable the instrument is. A reliable measure is one that can produce the same results if the behavior is measured again by the same scale. Reliability then refers to the proportion of accuracy to inaccuracy in measurement. In other words, if we use the same or comparable instruments on more than one occasion to measure a set of behaviors that ordinarily remains relatively constant, we would expect similar results if the tools are reliable. The three main attributes of a reliable scale are stability, homogeneity, and equivalence. The *stability* of an instrument refers to the instrument's ability to produce the same results with repeated testing. The *homogeneity* of an instrument means that all the items in a tool measure the same concept or characteristic. An instrument is said to exhibit *equivalence* if the tool produces the same results when equivalent or parallel instruments or procedures are used. Each of these attributes and the means to estimate them will be discussed. Before these are discussed, an understanding of how to interpret reliability is essential.

Reliability Coefficient Interpretation

Because all of the attributes of reliability are concerned with the degree of consistency between scores that are obtained at two or more independent times of testing, they often are expressed in terms of a correlation coefficient. The reliability coefficient ranges from 0 to 1. The **reliability coefficient** expresses the relationship between the error variance, the true variance, and the observed score. A zero correlation indicates that there is no relationship. When the error variance in a measurement instrument is low, the reliability coefficient will be closer to 1. The closer to 1 the coefficient is, the more reliable the tool. For example, a reliability coefficient of a tool is reported to be 0.89. This tells you that the error variance is small and the tool has little measurement error. On the other hand, if the reliability coefficient of a measure is reported to be 0.49, the error variance is high and the tool has a problem with measurement error. For a tool to be considered reliable, a level of 0.70 or higher is considered to be an acceptable level of reliability. The interpretation of the reliability coefficient, which is also called the alpha coefficient, depends on the proposed purpose of the measure. There are five major tests of reliability that can be used to calculate a reliability coefficient. The test(s) used depend(s) on the nature of the tool. They are known as **test-retest, parallel or alternate**

BOX 15-2 MEASURES USED TO TEST RELIABILITY

STABILITY
Test-retest reliability
Parallel or alternate form

HOMOGENEITY
Item to total correlation
Split-half reliability
Kuder-Richardson coefficient
Cronbach's alpha

EQUIVALENCE
Parallel or alternate form
Interrater reliability

---

form, item-total correlation, split-half, Kuder-Richardson (KR-20), Cronbach's alpha, and **interrater reliability.** These tests are discussed as they relate to the attributes of stability, equivalence, and homogeneity (Box 15-2). There is no best means to assess reliability in relationship to stability, homogeneity, and equivalence. The critiquer should be aware that the method of reliability that the researcher uses should be consistent with the investigator's aim.

Stability

An instrument is thought to be stable or to exhibit **stability** when the same results are obtained on repeated administration of the instrument. Researchers are concerned with an instrument's stability when they expect the instrument to measure a concept consistently over a period of time. Measurement over time is important when an instrument is used in a longitudinal study and therefore will be used on several occasions. Stability is also a consideration when a researcher is conducting an intervention study that is designed to effect a change in a specific variable. In this case, the instrument is administered once and then again later after the alteration or change intervention has been completed. The tests that are used to estimate stability are test-retest and parallel or alternate form.

Test-Retest Reliability

Test-retest reliability is the administration of the same instrument to the same subjects under similar conditions on two or more occasions. Scores from repeated testing are compared. This comparison is expressed by a correlation coefficient, usually a Pearson r (see Chapter 16). The interval between repeated administrations varies and depends on the concept or variable being measured. For example, if the variable that the test measures is related to the developmental stages in children, the interval between tests should be short. The amount of time over which the variable was measured should also be recorded in the report. An example of an instrument that was assessed for test-retest reliability is the Barriers to Healthy Eating Scale (BHES), a tool to assess barriers that may impede healthy eating in pregnant women and place them at risk for complications. Based on the Pender Health Promotion Model (HPM) (1996), the 18-item BHES was completed by 2 separate convenience samples ($n = 20$ for Phase I pilot; $n = 227$ for Phase II psychometric study) of pregnant women in their last trimester of pregnancy. Test-retest reliability was assessed by correlating BHES scores at Time 1 and Time 2 and by internal consistency testing. A strong positive correlation was noted for total BHES scores from Time 1 and 2 weeks later at Time 2 ($r = .79$; $p = .01$). Correlations between each of the five subscales at Time 1 to the same subscale at Time 2 ranged from .35 to .91, thus providing evidence of adequate test-retest reliability (Fowles and Feucht, 2004). Another example is provided by the Korean translation of the Exercise Self-Efficacy Scale (Shin, Jang, and Pender, 2001). The Exercise Self-Efficacy Scale was previously developed and tested for reliability and validity in other English-speaking populations, and the translated version was assessed for use in a Korean population. The concept of test-retest is illustrated by the following: "*Test-retest reliability* measures were performed as a measure of instrument *stability* on a sample of 14 participants who were comparable to the study population.

The *test-retest interval* was two weeks, and the *correlation coefficient* was .77" (Shin, Jang, and Pender, 2001). In this case, the interval was adequate (2 weeks) between testing and the coefficient was above .70 (Nunnally and Bernstein, 1993).

Parallel or Alternate Form

Parallel or alternate form reliability is applicable and can be tested only if two comparable forms of the same instrument exist. It is like test-retest reliability in that the same individuals are tested within a specific interval, but it differs because a different form of the same test is given to the subjects on the second testing. **Parallel forms** or tests contain the same types of items that are based on the same domain or concept, but the wording of the items is different. The development of parallel forms is desired if the instrument is intended to measure a variable for which a researcher believes that "test-wiseness" will be a problem. For example, the pilot study "Breast Cancer: Education, Counseling, and Adjustment" (Hoskins et al., 2001) studied the differential effect of a phase-specific standardized educational video intervention in comparison to a telephone counseling intervention on physical, emotional, and social adjustment in women with breast cancer and their partners. The use of repeated measures over the four data-collection points—"Coping With Your Diagnosis," "Recovering from Surgery," "Understanding Adjuvant Therapy," and "Ongoing Recovery"— made it appropriate to use two **alternate forms** of the Partner Relationship Inventory (Hoskins, 1988) to measure emotional adjustment in partners. An item on one scale ("I am able to tell my partner how I feel") is consistent with the paired item on the second form ("My partner tries to understand my feelings"). Practically speaking, it is difficult to develop alternate forms of an instrument when one considers the many issues of reliability and validity of an instrument. If alternate forms of a test exist, they should be highly correlated if the measures are to be considered reliable.

HELPFUL H I N T

When a longitudinal design with multiple data-collection points is being conducted, look for evidence of test-retest or parallel form reliability.

Internal Consistency/Homogeneity

Another attribute of an instrument related to reliability is the **internal consistency** or **homogeneity** with which the items within the scale reflect or measure the same concept. This means that the items within the scale correlate or are complementary to each other. This also means that a scale is unidimensional. A unidimensional scale is one that measures one concept, such as self-efficacy. The Barnason Efficacy Expectation Scale (BEES) is a 15-item tool designed to determine the coronary artery bypass graft (CABG) patient's self-efficacy related to the risk reduction related aspects of recovery and lifestyle adjustment following CABG surgery. The testing of the instrument revealed an overall alpha coefficient of 0.92 inclusive of all 20 items. Because the alpha was above .70, it was sufficient evidence for supporting the internal consistency of the BEES. Homogeneity can be assessed by using one of four methods: item to total correlations, split-half reliability, Kuder-Richardson (KR-20) coefficient, or Cronbach's alpha (Box 15-3).

 EVIDENCE-BASED PRACTICE TIP

When the characteristics of a study sample differ significantly from the sample in the original study, check to see if the researcher has reestablished the reliability of the instrument with the current sample.

Item to Total Correlations

Item to total correlations measure the relationship between each of the items and the total scale. When item to total correlations are calculated, a

BOX 15-3 EXAMPLES OF REPORTED CRONBACH'S ALPHA

- Cronbach's coefficient alpha was calculated as a measure of internal consistency for the scale. A standardized alpha of .94 was obtained (Shin, Jang, and Pender, 2001).
- "An alpha coefficient of .92 was sufficient evidence for the internal consistency of the Self-Efficacy for Exercise measure" (Resnick and Jenkins, 2000).
- "Internal consistency reliability using Cronbach's coefficient alpha was computed for this sample. Results for the composite sample (.91-boys and .93-girls) as well as subsamples by grade and sex, are presented . . ." (Weber, 2000).
- "The 38-item Professional Practice Environment (PPE) Scale had a standardized alpha coefficient of .93. The Cronbach's alpha coefficients for the eight subscales were: Handling disagreement/Conflict, 8-items, .88; Internal work motivation, 7-items, .86; Control over practice, 7-items, .82; Leadership and autonomy in clinical practice, 5-items, .83; Staff relationships with physicians, 2-items, .79; Teamwork, 2-items, .78; Cultural sensitivity, 3-items, .78; and Communication about patients, 2-items, .80" (Erickson et al., 2004).

correlation for each item on the scale is generated (Table 15-3). Items that do not achieve a high correlation may be deleted from the instrument. Usually in a research study, all of the item to total correlations are not reported unless the study is a report of a methodological study. The lowest and highest correlations are typically reported. An example of an item to total correlation report is illustrated in the study by Gary and Yarandi (2004) in which item to total correlations were computed for the 21-item Beck Depression Inventory II, which measures depression in three dimensions: cognition, somatization, and motivation. The corrected item-scale correlations and alpha are reported. The individual items range from .34 (loss of interest in sex) to .63 (sadness). The authors report that all of the corrected item-to-total correlations were significant after a "Bonferroni adjustment (alpha/21)

TABLE 15-3 **Means, Standard Deviations, and Corrected Item-Total Correlations (Cronbach's Alpha = 0.90)**

Variable	Mean	SD	Corr
Sadness	0.21	0.46	0.63
Pessimism	0.12	0.39	0.47
Past failure	0.25	0.57	0.44
Loss of pleasure	0.33	0.59	0.61
Guilty feelings	0.33	0.50	0.53
Punishment feelings	0.19	0.56	0.57
Self-dislike	0.17	0.54	0.51
Self-criticalness	0.30	0.63	0.52
Suicidal thoughts or wishes	0.05	0.28	0.40
Crying	0.38	0.89	0.52
Agitation	0.43	0.85	0.52
Loss of interest	0.26	0.57	0.58
Indecisiveness	0.24	0.58	0.54
Worthlessness	0.11	0.40	0.51
Loss of energy	0.62	0.58	0.47
Changes in sleeping patterns	0.84	0.95	0.58
Irritability	0.31	0.62	0.59
Changes in appetite	0.64	0.82	0.45
Concentration difficulty	0.54	0.75	0.60
Tiredness or fatigue	0.74	0.81	0.61
Loss of interest in sex	0.64	0.87	0.34

was used to control for the overall error rate." They also determined that the coefficient alpha of the BDI II for the current sample of rural Southern African-American women was 0.91, suggesting a high level of internal consistency for the study sample and thus supporting the reliability of the scale (Nunnally and Bernstein, 1993).

Split-Half Reliability

Split-half reliability involves dividing a scale into two halves and making a comparison. The halves may be odd-numbered and even-numbered items or may be a simple division of the first from the second half, or items may be randomly selected into halves that will be analyzed opposite one another. The split-half provides a

measure of consistency in terms of sampling the content. The two halves of the test or the contents in both halves are assumed to be comparable, and a reliability coefficient is calculated. If the scores for the two halves are approximately equal, the test may be considered reliable. A formula called the Spearman-Brown formula is one method used to calculate the reliability coefficient. In a study testing the Worry Interference Scale (WIS), a seven-item self-report measure was developed to assess the degree to which thoughts about breast cancer are perceived as interfering with the respondent's daily functioning. It is imbedded within a larger questionnaire that also assesses perceived risk, intention to undergo genetic testing, and frequency of worry about getting breast cancer. The WIS scale items assess disruptions in sleep, work, concentration, relationships, having fun, feeling sexually attractive, meeting family needs, and reproductive decisions. The author computed a Spearman-Brown split-half reliability and found a reliability coefficient that ranged from 0.83 to 0.92 for the first four items and from 0.75 to 0.83 where split-half reliabilities of at least 0.75 are considered internally consistent (Ibrahim, 2002).

Kuder-Richardson (KR-20) Coefficient

The **Kuder-Richardson (KR-20) coefficient** is the estimate of homogeneity used for instruments that have a dichotomous response format. A dichotomous response format is one in which the question asks for a "yes/no" or "true/false" response. The technique yields a correlation that is based on the consistency of responses to all the items of a single form of a test that is administered one time. In a study investigating the effectiveness of a randomized support group intervention for African-American women with breast cancer, breast cancer knowledge was assessed with a 25-item true/false scale developed for the study. Items were obtained from the American Cancer Society's publication entitled *Cancer Facts and Figures* and comprised the following categories: knowledge of risk factors for developing breast cancer (10 items, e.g., "Most women diagnosed with breast cancer have at least one known risk factor for the disease"); symptoms of breast cancer (5 items, e.g., "Women who have breast cancer never experience any symptoms of the disease"); side effects of treatment (3 items, e.g., "A common side effect of radiation is sunburn-like symptoms"); treatment efficacy (4 items, e.g., "For women with small tumors that may not have spread outside the breast, having either a mastectomy or lumpectomy with axillary lymph node dissection results in the same overall life expectancy"); and methods of treatment (3 items, e.g., "Hormone treatment is used only for premenopausal women"). Because the scale was a binary format (true/false), Kuder-Richardson reliability for the entire scale was calculated at 0.75, which is acceptable, having exceeded the minimum acceptable KR-20 score of 0.70; however, the magnitude of the correlation is not robust.

Cronbach's Alpha

The fourth and most commonly used test of internal consistency is **Cronbach's alpha.** Many tools used to measure psychosocial variables and attitudes have a Likert scale response format. A Likert scale format asks the subject to respond to a question on a scale of varying degrees of intensity between two extremes. The two extremes are anchored by responses ranging from "strongly agree" to "strongly disagree" or "most like me" to

"least like me." The points between the two extremes may range from 1 to 5 or from 1 to 7. Subjects are asked to circle the response closest to how they feel. Figure 15-2 provides examples of items from a tool that uses a Likert scale format. Cronbach's alpha simultaneously compares each item in the scale with the others. A total score is then used in the analysis of data. The School-Age Temperament Inventory (SATI) (McClowry, Halverson, and Sanson, 2003) was tested for internal consistency, as well as for construct validity. The testing of the instrument revealed alpha coefficients that ranged from .80 to .92 for the four dimensions, which supported internal consistency data from the original SATI reliability studies as illustrated in Table 15-4. Because the alphas were above .70, it was suffi-

TABLE **15-4 Cronbach's Alpha of the SATI Dimensions**

Dimensions	Original	Sample 1	Sample 2	Sample 3
Negative reactivity	.90	.89	.90	.92
Task persistence	.90	.89	.91	.92
Approach/ withdrawal	.88	.84	.86	.92
Activity	.85	.80	.86	.92

I trust that life events happen to fit a plan that is larger and more gentle than I can know.

```
        1       2       3       4       5
      Never                         Always
```

I am aware of an inner source of comfort, strength, and security.

```
        1       2       3       4       5
      Never                         Always
```

Figure 15-2. Examples of a Likert scale. (Redrawn from Roberts KT, Aspy CB: Development of the serenity scale, *J Nurs Measure* 1(2):145-164, 1993.)

cient evidence for supporting the internal consistency of the instrument. Examples of reported Cronbach's alpha are in Box 15-3.

 HELPFUL H I N T

If a research article provides information about the reliability of a measurement instrument but does not specify the type of reliability, it is probably safe to assume that internal consistency reliability was assessed using Cronbach's alpha.

Equivalence

Equivalence either is the consistency or agreement among observers using the same measurement tool or is the consistency or agreement between alternate forms of a tool. An instrument is thought to demonstrate equivalence when two or more observers have a high percentage of agreement of an observed behavior or when alternate forms of a test yield a high correlation. There are two methods to test equivalence: interrater reliability and alternate or parallel form.

Interrater Reliability

Some measurement instruments are not self-administered questionnaires but are direct measurements of observed behavior. Instruments that depend on direct observation of a behavior that is to be systematically recorded must be tested for **interrater reliability.** To accomplish interrater reliability, two or more individuals should make an observation or one observer should examine the behavior on several occasions. The observers should be trained or oriented to the definition and operationalization of the behavior to be observed. In the method of direct observation of behavior, the consistency or reliability of the observations between observers is extremely important. In the instance of interrater reliability, the reliability or consistency of the observer is tested rather than the reliability of the instrument. Interrater reliability is expressed as a percentage of agreement between scorers or as a correlation coefficient of the scores assigned to the observed behaviors.

In the study "Measurement of Activity in Older Adults: Reliability and Validity of the Step Activity Monitor (SAM)," Resnick and colleagues (2001) establish interrater reliability for the step activity monitor, a step counter developed for a wide variety of gait styles (ranging from a slow shuffle, such as a Parkinsonian-type gait, to a fast run) and used to measure activity in older adults. The authors note that while other tools are available to assess activity/exercise in older adults, they are generally self-report instruments that provide researchers or nurses with the individual's perception of the amount of activity performed rather than an objective accounting. In contrast, the SAM provides objective information about step activity (total number of steps taken over a period of time). Participants in the study ($N = 30$) were recruited from the outpatient office in a continuing care retirement community. Participants were asked to walk at their own speed on a carpeted level surface for 1 minute, rest for 2 minutes, and then ambulate over the same path for another minute. Two observers, observing at the same time, counted steps during both episodes of ambulation. The two observers, both advanced practice nurses, had prior experience in observational gait assessment of older adults and step counting. Interrater reliability was based on intraclass correlations of the two separate 1-minute readings of the SAM done 2 minutes apart. Statistically significant correlations of .80 or greater between the mean of the two observers and the results of the SAM at each testing interval (calculating the average deviation between the SAM and the mean of the two observers) produced an interrater reliability estimate of .98, indicating a high level of agreement between observers. Santacroce, Maccarelli, and Grey (2004) note that consistency in observation or intervention delivery is key to concluding that the evidence provided by the study findings is valid and reliable. Another type of interrater reliability is Cohen's Kappa, a coefficient of agreement between 2 raters that is considered to be a more precise estimate of interrater reliability. **Kappa** expresses the level of agreement that is observed beyond the level that would be expected by chance alone. Kappa K > .08 or better is generally taken to indicate good interrater reliability. K < 0.68 allows tentative conclusions to be drawn at times lower levels are accepted (McDowell and Newell, 1996).

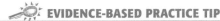

EVIDENCE-BASED PRACTICE TIP

Interrater reliability is an important approach to minimizing bias.

Parallel or Alternate Form

Parallel or alternate form was described in the discussion of stability in this chapter. Use of parallel forms is then a measure of stability and equivalence. The procedures for assessing equivalence using parallel forms are the same.

CRITIQUING GUIDE   *Reliability and Validity*

Reliability and validity are two crucial aspects in the critical appraisal of a measurement instrument. Criteria for critiquing reliability and validity are presented in the Critiquing Criteria box. The reviewer evaluates an instrument's level of reliability and validity, as well as the manner in which these were established. In a research report, the reliability and validity for each measure should be presented. If these data have not been presented at all, the reviewer must seriously question the merit and use of the tool and the evidence provided by the study's results.

If a study does not use reliable and valid questionnaires, the results of a study cannot be credible. It is very difficult to place confidence in the evidence generated by a study's findings if the measures used did not have established validity and reliability. It is the ethical responsibility of the critiquer to question the reliability and validity of instruments used in research studies and

examine the findings in light of the quality of the instruments used and the data presented. The following discussion highlights key areas related to reliability and validity that should be evident to the critiquer in a research article.

Appropriate reliability tests should have been performed by the developer of the measurement tool and should then have been included by the current user in the research report. If the initial standardization sample and the current sample have different characteristics, the reader would expect the following: (1) that a pilot study for the present sample would have been conducted to determine if the reliability was maintained, or (2) that a reliability estimate was calculated on the current sample. For example, if the standardization sample for a tool that measures "satisfaction in an intimate heterosexual relationship" comprises undergraduate college students and if an investigator plans to use the tool

1. Was an appropriate method used to test the reliability of the tool?
2. Is the reliability of the tool adequate?
3. Was an appropriate method(s) used to test the validity of the instrument?
4. Is the validity of the measurement tool adequate?
5. If the sample from the developmental stage of the tool was different from the current sample, were the reliability and validity recalculated to determine if the tool is still adequate?
6. Have the strengths and weaknesses of the reliability and validity of each instrument been presented?
7. Are strengths and weaknesses of the reliability and validity appropriately addressed in the "Discussion," "Limitations," or "Recommendations" sections of the report?
8. How do the reliability and/or validity affect the strength and quality of the evidence provided by the study findings?

with married couples, it would be advisable to establish the reliability of the tool with the latter group.

The investigator determines which type of reliability procedures are used in the study, depending on the nature of the measurement tool and how it will be used. For example, if the instrument is to be administered twice, the critiquer might determine that test-retest reliability should have been used to establish the stability of the tool. If an alternate form has been developed for use in a repeated-measures design, evidence of alternate form reliability should be presented to determine the equivalence of the parallel forms. If the degree of internal consistency among the items is relevant, an appropriate test of internal consistency should be presented. In some instances, more than one type of reliability will be presented, but the critiquer should determine whether all are appropriate. For example, the Kuder-Richardson formula implies that there is a single right or wrong answer, making it inappropriate to use with scales that provide a format of three or more possible responses. In such cases, another formula is applied, such as Cronbach's coefficient alpha formula. Another important consideration is the acceptable level of reliability, which varies according to the type of test. Coefficients of reliability of 0.70 or higher are desirable. The validity of an instrument is

limited by its reliability; that is, less confidence can be placed in scores from tests with low reliability coefficients.

Satisfactory evidence of validity is probably the most difficult item for the reviewer to ascertain. It is this aspect of measurement that is most likely to fall short of meeting the required criteria. Validity studies are time-consuming, as well as complex, and sometimes researchers will settle for presenting minimal validity data. Therefore the critiquer should closely examine the item content of a tool when evaluating its strengths and weaknesses and try to find conclusive evidence of content validity. In the body of a research article, however, it is most unusual to have more than a few sample items available for review. Because this is the case, the critiquer should determine whether the appropriate assessment of content validity was used to meet the researcher's goal. Such procedures provide the critiquer with assurance that the tool is psychometrically sound and that the content of the items is consistent with the conceptual framework and construct definitions. Construct validity and criterion-related validity are some of the more precise statistical tests of whether the tool measures what it is supposed to measure. Ideally, an instrument should provide evidence of content validity, as well as criterion-related or construct validity, before a reviewer invests a high level of confidence in the tool. You can expect to see evidence that the reliability and validity of a measurement tool is reestablished periodically as McClowry and colleagues (2003) did with the School-Age Temperament Inventory.

The reader would also expect to see the strengths and weaknesses of instrument reliability and validity presented in the "Discussion," "Limitations," and/or "Recommendations" sections of a research article. In this context, the reliability and validity might be discussed in relation to other tools devised to measure the same variable. The relationship of the study's findings to the strengths and weaknesses in instrument reliability and validity is another important discussion point. Finally, recommendations for improving future studies in relation to instrument reliability and validity should be proposed. For example, in the "Instruments" and "Discussion" sections of a study investigating examining relationships among spirituality, perceived social support, death anxiety, and nurses' willingness to care for AIDS patients, Sherman (1996) appropriately reports the weaknesses in the reliability of the TDAS. She states that although the TDAS is often cited in the literature, the low internal consistency reliability of the scale (0.76) supports the recommendation that the instrument be pilot-tested on the specific sample on which it will be administered. Because of the marginally acceptable reliability of the TDAS and because the study sample (i.e., registered nurses) differed

from the original sample (i.e., college students) used for establishing reliability, a pilot study, yielding a marginally acceptable reliability coefficient of 0.78, was conducted using a sample of 30 nurses enrolled in a doctoral course. Sherman continues, however, to comment that in the actual study, the TDAS's reliability coefficient of 0.63 was lower than anticipated, based on the results of the pilot study. Although Sherman appropriately addresses the low reliability of TDAS in relation to the psychometric properties of the tool and makes recommendations about revising the response format, she does not address this weakness in relation to the hypotheses and the findings of the study.

As you can see, the area of reliability and validity is complex. These aspects of research reports can be evaluated to varying degrees. The research consumer should not feel inhibited by the complexity of this topic but may use the guidelines presented in this chapter to systematically assess the reliability and validity aspects of a research study. Collegial dialogue is also an approach to evaluating the merits and shortcomings of an existing, as well as a newly developed, instrument that is reported in the nursing literature. Such an exchange promotes the understanding of methodologies and techniques of reliability and validity, stimulates the acquisition of a basic knowledge of psychometrics, and encourages the exploration of alternative methods of observation and use of reliable and valid tools in clinical practice.

Critical Thinking Challenges

- Discuss the three types of validity that must be established before a reviewer invests a high level of confidence in the measurement instrument. How does validity increase confidence in the study findings? Include examples of each type of validity.
- What are the major tests of reliability? Is it necessary to establish more than one measure of reliability for each instrument used in a study? Which do you think is the most essential measure of reliability? Include examples in your answer.
- Is it possible to have a valid instrument that is not reliable? Is the reverse possible? With each scenario explain how the study's findings are affected. Support your answer with instruments you might use in the clinical setting with your patients/clients.
- When a researcher does not report reliability or, more likely, validity data, which threat(s) to internal and external validity should the research consumer consider? How would these threats affect the strength and quality of the evidence provided by the findings of the study?

KEY POINTS

- Reliability and validity are crucial aspects of conducting and critiquing research.
- Validity refers to whether an instrument measures what it is purported to measure, and it is a crucial aspect of evaluating a tool.
- Three types of validity are content validity, criterion-related validity, and construct validity.
- The choice of a validation method is important and is made by the researcher on the basis of the characteristics of the measurement device in question and its utilization.
- Reliability refers to the accuracy/inaccuracy ratio in a measurement device.
- The major tests of reliability are as follows: test-retest, parallel or alternate form, split-half, item to total correlation, Kuder-Richardson, Cronbach's alpha, and interrater reliability.
- The selection of a method for establishing reliability depends on the characteristics of the tool, the testing method that is used for collecting data from the standardization sample, and the kinds of data that are obtained.

REFERENCES

Anastasi A: *Psychological testing,* ed 6, New York, 1988, Macmillan.

Bandura A: *The self-efficacy: the exercise of control,* New York, 1997, WH Freeman.

Barnason S, Zimmerman L, Atwood J, Nieveen J, and Schmaderer M: Development of a self-efficacy instrument for coronary artery bypass graft patients, *J Nurs Meas* 10(2): 123-133, 2002.

Braden B, Bergstrom N: Predictive validity of the Braden Scale for pressure sore risk in a nursing home population, *Res Nurs Health* 17: 459-470, 1994.

Bull MJ, Luo D, and Maruyama GM: Measuring continuity of elders' posthospital care, *J Nurs Meas* 8(1): 41-60, 2000.

Campbell D, Fiske D: Convergent and discriminant validation by the matrix, *Psychol Bull* 53: 273-302, 1959.

Erickson JI, Duffy ME, Gibbons MP, Fitzmaurice J, Ditomassi M, and Jones D: Development and psychometric evaluation of the professional practice environment scale, *J Nurs Schol* 36(3): 279-285, 2004.

Fowles ER, Feucht J: Testing the barriers to healthy eating scale, *West J Nurs Res* 26(4): 429-443, 2004.

Gary FA, Yarandi HN: Depression among southern rural African American women, *Nurs Res* 53(4): 251-259, 2004.

Hess RG: Measuring nursing governance, *Nurs Res* 47(1): 35-42, 1998.

Hoskins CN: *The partner relationship inventory,* Palo Alto, Calif, 1988, Consulting Psychologists Press.

Hoskins CN, Haber J, Budin WC, Cartwright-Alcarese F, Kowalsi MO, Panke J, and Maislin G: Breast cancer: education, counseling, and adjustment, *Psychol Rep* 89: 677-704, 2001.

Ibrahim SER: Rates of adherence to pharmacological treatment among children and adolesoents with attention deficit hyperactivity disorder, *Hum Psychopharm* 17: 225-231, 2002.

Knauth DG, Skowron EA: Psychometric evaluation of the differentiation of self inventory for adolescents, *Nurs Res* 53(3): 163-171, 2004.

McClowry SG, Halverson CF, and Sanson A: A re-examination of the validity and reliability of the school-age temperament inventory, *Nurs Res* 52(3): 176-182, 2003.

McDowell I, Newell C: *Measuring health: A guide to rating scales and questionnaires,* New York, 1996, Oxford Press.

Nunnally JC, Bernstein IH: *Psychometric theory,* ed 3, New York, 1993, McGraw-Hill.

Powers GC, Zentner T, Nelson F, and Bergstrom N: Validation of the mobility subscale of the Braden scale for predicting pressure sore risk, *Nurs Res* 53(5): 340-346, 2004.

Resnick B, Jenkins LS: Testing the reliability and validity of the self-efficacy for exercise scale, *Nurs Res* 49: 154-159, 2000.

Resnick B, Nahm ES, Orwig D, Zimmerman SS, and Magaziner J: Measurement of activity in older adults: reliability and validity of the step activity monitor, *J Nurs Meas* 9(3): 275-290, 2001.

Santacroce SJ, Maccarelli LM, and Grey M: Intervention fidelity, *Nurs Res* 53(1): 63-66, 2004.

Secco L: The infant care questionnaire: assessment of reliability and validity in a sample of healthy mothers, *J Nurs Meas* 10(2): 97-109, 2002.

Sherman DW: Nurses' willingness to care for AIDS patients and spirituality, social support, and death anxiety, *Image* 28(3): 205-213, 1996.

Shin YH, Jang HJ, and Pender N: Psychometric evaluation of the exercise self-efficacy scale among Korean adults with chronic illness, *Res Nurs Health* 24: 68-77, 2001.

Singleton EG, Anderson LM, and Heishman SJ: Reliability and validity of the tobacco craving questionnaire and validation of a craving-induction procedure using multiple measures of craving and mood, *Soc Study Addiction Alcohol Other Drugs* 98: 1537-1546, 2003.

Spielberger CD, Gorsuch RI, and Lushene RE: Manual for the State-Trait Anxiety Inventory, Palo Alto, California, *Consult Psychologists,* 1970.

Taylor KL, Lamdan RM, Siegal JE, Moran-Klimi K, Shelby R, and Hrywna M: Psychological adjustment among African-american breast cancer patients: one-year follow-up of a randomized psychoeducational group intervention, *Health Psychol* 22(3): 316-323, 2003.

Templer DI: The construction and validation of a death anxiety scale, *J Gen Psychol* 82: 165-177, 1970.

Tilden VP, Nelson CA, and May BA: The IPR inventory: development and psychometric characteristics, *Nurs Res* 39(6): 337-343, 1990.

Trask PC, Paterson AG, Wang C, Hayasaka S, Milliron KJ, Blumberg LR, Gonzalez R, Murray S, and Merajver SD: Cancer-specific worry interference in women attending a breast and ovarian cancer risk evaluation program: impact on emotional distress and health functioning, *Psycho-Oncology* 10: 349-360, 2001.

Waltz C, Strickland O, and Lenz E: *Measurement in nursing research,* ed 3, Philadelphia, 1991, FA Davis.

Weber S: Factor structure of the Reynolds adolescent depression scale in a sample of school-based adolescents, *J Nurs Meas* 8: 23-40, 2000.

US Department of Health and Human Services (USDHHS): Pressure ulcers in adults: Prediction and prevention, Rockville, Maryland, 1992, Public Health Service Agency for Health Care Policy and Research.

FOR FURTHER STUDY

🔘 Go to your Companion CD for review activities for this chapter.

evolve Go to Evolve at http://evolve.elsevier.com/LoBiondo/ for WebLinks, Content Updates, and additional research articles, for practice in reviewing and critiquing.

16

ROBIN WHITTEMORE

MARGARET GREY

Data Analysis: Descriptive and Inferential Statistics

KEY TERMS

analysis of covariance (ANCOVA)
analysis of variance (ANOVA)
chi-square (χ^2)
correlation
degrees of freedom
descriptive statistics
factor analysis
Fisher's exact probability test
frequency distribution
inferential statistics
interval measurement
kurtosis
levels of measurement
level of significance (alpha level)
linear structural relationships
    (LISREL)
mean
measurment

measures of central tendency
measures of variability
median
modality
mode
multiple analysis of variance
    (MANOVA)
multiple regression
nominal measurement
nonparametric statistics
nonparametric tests of
    significance
normal curve
null hypothesis
ordinal measurement
parameter
parametric statistics
path analysis

Pearson correlation coefficient
    (Pearson *r;* Pearson product
    moment correlation coefficient)
percentile
probability
range
ratio measurement
sampling error
scientific hypothesis
semiquartile range (semiinterquartile
    range)
standard deviation (SD)
standard error of the mean
t statistic
type I error
type II error
Z score

LEARNING OUTCOMES

After reading this chapter, the student should be able to do the following:
- Differentiate between descriptive and inferential statistics.
- State the purposes of descriptive statistics.
- Identify the levels of measurement in a research study.
- Describe a frequency distribution.
- List measures of central tendency and their use.
- List measures of variability and their use.
- Identify the purpose of inferential statistics.
- Distinguish between a parameter and a statistic.
- Explain the concept of probability as it applies to the analysis of sample data.

- Distinguish between type I and type II error and its effect on a study's outcome.
- Distinguish between parametric and nonparametric tests.
- List the commonly used statistical tests and their purposes.
- Critically analyze the statistics used in published research studies.

STUDY RESOURCES

Go to your Companion CD for review activities for this chapter.

evolve Go to Evolve at http://evolve.elsevier.com/LoBiondo/ for Weblinks, Content Updates, and additional research articles for practice in reviewing and critiquing.

The use of statistics pervades the nursing and health care literature. You will find that descriptive and inferential statistics are located in the "Methods" and/or "Results" section of a research article. Before you get overwhelmed by the complexity of the information, please realize that you will not have to be familiar with or be able to calculate a large number of complex statistical tests used to analyze data. An understanding of which tests are used with which kind of design and type of data is sufficient. This understanding is important because any time you use evidence from a research study to make clinical decisions, appraisal of the difference the evidence makes is essential to informing those decisions you make in your practice.

Even though as a research consumer you will not be performing the data analysis, it is important to understand the researcher's challenge in relation to data analysis. After carefully collecting data, the researcher is faced with the task of organizing and analyzing the individual pieces of information so that the meaning of study results is clear. The researcher must choose methods of organizing and analyzing the raw data based on the design, the type of data collected, and the

hypothesis or question that was tested. Statistical procedures are used to give organization and meaning to data.

As you read a research article and get to the "Results" section, you will find the data generated form the testing of the hypothesis or research questions. These data are the result of analysis using both **descriptive and inferential statistics.** An example of what is found is as follows: "Participants had a mean age of 16.70 (SD = 1.13) and were predominantly poor, unmarried and from ethnic groups of color (Table 1)" (Koniak-Griffin et al., 2003, Appendix A). The information found in this paragraph and in Table 1 is known as descriptive statistics. Procedures that allow researchers to describe and summarize data are known as **descriptive statistics.** Descriptive statistical techniques reduce data to manageable proportions by summarizing them, and they also describe various characteristics of the data under study. Descriptive techniques include measures of central tendency, such as mode, median, and mean; measures of variability, such as range and standard deviation (SD); and some correlation techniques, such as scatter plots.

Koniak-Griffin and colleagues (2003) also state: "The total of days for non-birth related infant hospitalizations during the first 24 months of life was significantly lower in the EIP (143 days) than the TPHNC group (21 days) ($x2 = 32.48$, $p < .001$) (Table 2)." This is an example of

The authors wish to acknowledge the contributions of Ann Bello who provided material for this chapter in the previous edition of this text.

analysis using inferential statistics. Procedures that allow researchers to estimate how reliably they can make predictions and generalize findings based on the data are known as **inferential statistics. Inferential statistics** are used to analyze the data collected, test hypotheses, and answer the research questions in a research study. With inferential statistics, the researcher is trying to draw conclusions that extend beyond the immediate data of the study.

The purpose of this chapter is to demonstrate how researchers use descriptive and inferential statistics in nursing research studies so that you, as a research consumer, are better able to determine the appropriateness of the statistics used and to interpret the strength and quality of the reported findings, as well as their clinical significance and applicability for practice. Basic concepts and terminology common in evidence-based practice publications are presented in Chapter 20. The information will help you to begin to make sense of the statistics used in research papers.

DESCRIPTIVE STATISTICS

Levels of Measurement

Measurement is the assignment of numbers to variables or events according to rules. Every variable in a research study that is assigned a specific number must be similar to every other variable assigned that number. For example, male subjects may be assigned the number 1 and female subjects the number 2. The measurement level is determined by the nature of the object or event being measured. **Levels of measurement** in ascending order are nominal, ordinal, interval, and ratio. The levels of measurement are the determining factors of the type of statistics to be used in analyzing data. The higher the level of measurement, the greater the flexibility the researcher has in choosing statistical procedures. Every attempt should be made to use the highest level of measurement possible so that the maximum amount of information will be obtained from the data as highlighted in Table 16-1. The following Critical Thinking Decision Path, titled "Descriptive Statistics," illustrates the relationship between levels of measurement and appropriate choice of specific descriptive statistics.

TABLE **16-1 Level of Measurement Summary Table**

Measurement	Description	Measures of Central Tendency	Measures of Variability
Nominal	Classification	Mode	Modal percentage, range, frequency distribution
Ordinal	Relative rankings	Mode, median	Range, percentile, semiquartile range, frequency distribution
Interval	Rank ordering with equal intervals	Mode, median, mean	Range, percentile, semiquartile range, standard deviation
Ratio	Rank ordering with equal intervals and absolute zero	Mode, median, mean	All

CRITICAL THINKING DECISION PATH Descriptive Statistics

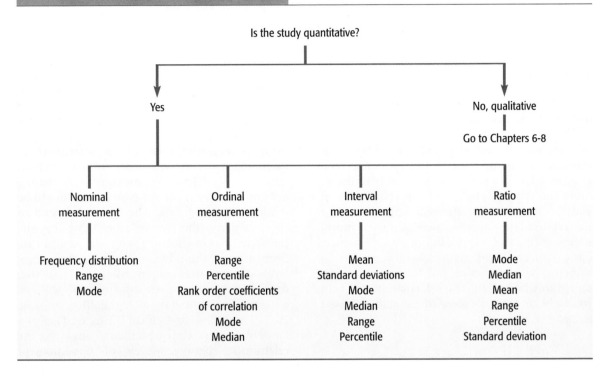

Is the study quantitative?

Yes

No, qualitative

Go to Chapters 6-8

Nominal measurement	Ordinal measurement	Interval measurement	Ratio measurement
Frequency distribution	Range	Mean	Mode
Range	Percentile	Standard deviations	Median
Mode	Rank order coefficients of correlation	Mode	Mean
	Mode	Median	Range
	Median	Range	Percentile
		Percentile	Standard deviation

Nominal measurement is used to classify variables or events into categories. The categories are mutually exclusive; the variable or event either has or does not have the characteristic. The numbers assigned to each category are nothing more than labels; such numbers do not indicate more or less of a characteristic. Nominal level measurement can be used to categorize a sample on such information as gender, hair color, marital status, or religious affiliation. The study by Koniak-Griffin and colleagues (2003) of nurse visitation for adolescent mothers includes several examples of nominal level measurement, including ethnic/racial background and marital status (see Appendix A). The nominal level of measurement allows the least amount of mathematical manipulation. Most commonly the frequency of each event is counted, as well as the percent of the total each category represents. A variable at

the nominal level can also be considered a *dichotomous* or a *categorical* variable. A dichotomous (nominal) variable is one that has only two true values such as true/false or gender (male/female) (See Chapter 20). Variables that are at the nominal level and categorical still have mutually exclusive categories but have more than two true values such as marital status (single, married, divorced, separate or widowed). In both cases, the nominal variables are mutually exclusive. For example in the Koniak-Griffin article, (2003) ethnic/racial background is nominal and categorical. Gender of the infant, though not included in the report would be considered a dichotomous nominal variable (male/female).

Ordinal measurement is used to show relative rankings of variables or events. The numbers assigned to each category can be compared, and a member of a higher category can be said to have more of an attribute than a person in a lower category. The intervals between numbers on the scale are not necessarily equal, and neither is zero an absolute zero. For example, ordinal measurement is used to formulate class rankings, where one student can be ranked higher or lower than another. However, the difference in actual grade point average between students may differ widely. Another example is ranking individuals by their level of wellness and by their ability to carry out activities of daily living. Using the New York Heart Association classification of cardiac failure, individuals can be assigned to one of four classifications. Classification I represents little disease or interference with activities of daily living, while classification IV represents severe disease and little ability to carry out the activities of daily living independently, but an individual in class IV cannot be said to be four times sicker than an individual in class I. A similar scale based on an individual's current health status is used to classify an individual's anesthesia risk.

Ordinal level data are limited in the amount of mathematical manipulation possible. In addition to what is possible with nominal data, medians, percentiles, and rank order coefficients of correlation can be calculated.

Interval measurement shows rankings of events or variables on a scale with equal intervals between the numbers. The zero point remains arbitrary and not absolute. For example, interval measurements are used in measuring temperatures on the Fahrenheit scale. The distances between degrees are equal, but the zero point is arbitrary and does not represent the absence of temperature. Test scores also represent interval data. The differences between test scores represent equal intervals, but a zero does not represent the total absence of knowledge.

In many areas in the social sciences, including nursing, the classification of the level of measurement of intelligence, aptitude, and personality tests is controversial, with some regarding these measurements as ordinal and others as

interval. The research consumer needs to be aware of this controversy and to look at each study individually in terms of how the data are analyzed (Knapp, 1990, 1993; Wang et al., 1999). Interval level data allow more manipulation of data, including the addition and subtraction of numbers and the calculation of means. This additional manipulation is why many argue for the higher classification level. The Spielberger State Anxiety Inventory and the Center for Epidemiologic Studies Depression Scale were used as interval measurements by Davison and associates (2003) to evaluate the effect of an individualized information session on psychological distress in men with prostate cancer and their partners (see Appendix D).

Ratio measurement shows rankings of events or variables on scales with equal intervals and absolute zeros. The number represents the actual amount of the property the object possesses. Ratio measurement is the highest level of measurement, but it is usually achieved only in the physical sciences. Examples of ratio level data are height, weight, pulse, and blood pressure. All mathematical procedures can be performed on data from ratio scales. Therefore the use of any statistical procedure is possible as long as it is appropriate to the design of the study.

 HELPFUL H I N T

Descriptive statistics assist in summarizing the data. The descriptive statistics calculated must be appropriate to both the purpose of the study and the level of measurement.

Frequency Distribution

One of the most basic ways of organizing data is in a frequency distribution. In a **frequency distribution** the number of times each event occurs is counted or the data are grouped and the frequency of each group is reported. An instructor reporting the results of an examination could report the number of students receiving each grade or could group the grades and report the

TABLE **16-2 Frequency Distribution**

	Individual			Group	
Score	**Tally**	**Frequency**	**Score**	**Tally**	**Frequency**
90	|	1	>89	|	1
88	|	1			
86	|	1	80-89	JHT JHT JHT	15
84	JHT |	6			
82	||	2	70-79	JHT JHT JHT JHT |||	23
80	JHT	5			
78	JHT	5			
76	|	1	60-69	JHT JHT	10
74	JHT ||	7			
72	JHT ||||	9	<59	||	2
70	|	1			
68	|||	3			
66	||	2			
64	||||	4			
62	|	1			
60		0			
58	|	1			
56		0			
54	|	1			
52		0			
50		0			
Total		51			51

Mean, 73.1; standard deviation, +12.1; median, 74; mode, 72; range, 36 (54-90).

number in each group. Table 16-2 shows the results of an examination given to a class of 51 students. The results of the examination are reported in several ways. The columns on the left give the raw data tally and the frequency for each grade, whereas the columns on the right give the grouped data tally and grouped frequencies.

When data are grouped, it is necessary to define the size of the group or the interval width so that no score will fall into two groups and each group will be mutually exclusive. The grouping of the data in Table 16-2 prevents overlap; each score falls into only one group. If the grouping had been 70 to 80 and 80 to 90, scores of 80 would have fallen into two categories. The grouping should allow for a precise presentation of the

data without serious loss of information. Very large interval widths lead to loss of data information and may obscure patterns in the data. If the test scores in Table 16-2 had been grouped as 40 to 69 and 70 to 99, the pattern of the scores would have been obscured.

Information about frequency distributions may be presented in the form of a table, such as Table 16-2, or in graphic form. Figure 16-1 illustrates the most common graphic forms: the histogram and the frequency polygon. The two graphic methods are similar in that both plot scores or percentages of occurrence against frequency. The greater the number of points plotted, the smoother the resulting graph. The shape of the resulting graph allows for observa-

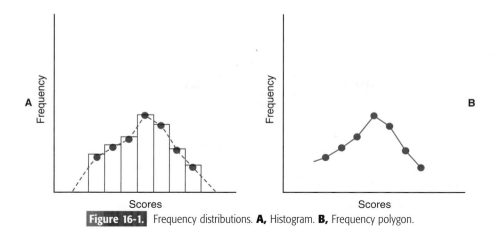

Figure 16-1. Frequency distributions. **A,** Histogram. **B,** Frequency polygon.

tions that further describe the data. In their study of risk factors for cardiovascular disease in children with type 1 diabetes, Lipman and associates (2000) report the number of children in each body mass percentile and the number of children in each grouping of cholesterol level using histograms (Figure 16-2).

Measures of Central Tendency

Measures of central tendency answer questions such as the following: "What does the average nurse think?" "What is the average temperature of patients on a unit?" They yield a single number that describes the middle of the group and summarize the members of a sample. In statistics there are three measures of central tendency: the mode, the median, and the mean. Depending on the distribution, these measures may not all give the same answer to the question: "What is the average?" Each measure of central tendency has a specific use and is most appropriate to specific kinds of measurement and types of distributions.

Mode   The **mode** is the most frequent score or result, and it can be obtained by inspection of the frequency distribution table or graph. It is important to note that a sample distribution can have more than one mode. The number of modes contained in a distribution is called the **modality** of the distribution. The mode is the

type of descriptive statistic most appropriately used with nominal data but can be used with all levels of measurement (see Table 16-1). The mode cannot be used for any subsequent calculations, and it is unstable; that is, the mode can fluctuate widely from sample to sample from the same population. A change in just one score in Table 16-2 would change the mode from 72.

Median   The **median** is the middle score or the score where 50% of the scores are above it and 50% of the scores are below it. The median is not sensitive to extremes in high and low scores. In the series of scores in Table 16-2, the twenty-sixth score will always be the median regardless of how much the high and low scores change. It is best used when the data are skewed (see Normal Distribution in this chapter), and the researcher is interested in the "typical" score. For example, if age is a variable and there is a wide range with extreme scores that may affect the mean, it would be appropriate to also report the median. The median is easy to find either by inspection or by calculation and can be used with ordinal or higher data as shown in Table 16-1.

Mean   The **mean** is the arithmetical average of all the scores and is used with interval or ratio data (see Table 16-1). It is what is usually thought of when the term average is used in general con-

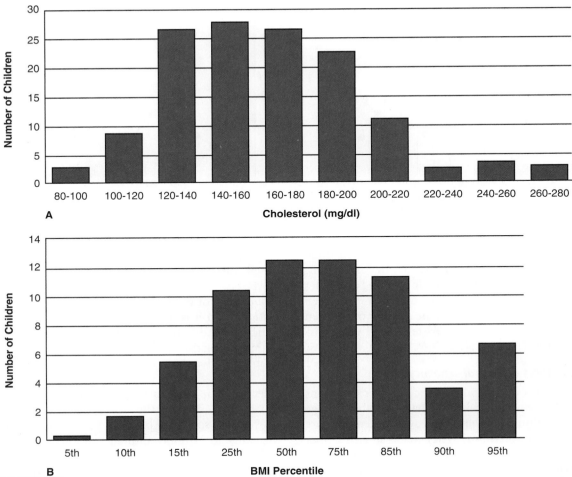

Figure 16-2. **A,** Total cholesterol levels in children with insulin-dependent diabetes mellitus ($n = 140$). **B,** Body mass index (BMI) of children with insulin-dependent diabetes mellitus ($n = 67$). (Reprinted from Lipman TH et al.: Risk factors for cardiovascular disease in children with type I diabetes, *Nurs Res* 49(3):164-165, 2000.)

versation and is the most widely used measure of central tendency. Most statistical tests of significance use the mean. The mean is affected by every score but is more stable than the median or mode, and of the three measures of central tendency, it is the most constant or least affected by chance. The larger the sample size, the less affected the mean will be by a single extreme score. The mean is generally considered the single best point for summarizing data.

 HELPFUL H I N T

Of the three measures of central tendency, the mean is the most stable, the least affected by extremes, and the most useful for other calculations. The mean can only be calculated with interval and ratio data.

Table 16-3 shows how Davison and colleagues (2003, Appendix D) in their study of an individualized information session for men with

TABLE 16-3 **Descriptive Statistics for Study Variables (*N* = 73)***

Variable	M	SD
MEN WITH PROSTATE CANCER		
State anxiety		
Pretest	41.92	12.03
Posttest	35.58	10.82
Depression		
Pretest	11.49	8.21
Posttest	9.21	7.93
PARTNERS OF MEN WITH PROSTATE CANCER		
State anxiety		
Pretest	45.10	12.23
Posttest	38.32	12.14
Depression		
Pretest	15.15	10.94
Posttest	11.04	9.58

*From Davison J, Goldenberg L, Gleave ME, Degner LF: Provision of individualized information to men and their partners to facilitate treatment decision making in prostate cancer, *Nurs Res* 30:107-114, 2003.

prostate cancer and their partners list the means (M) and standard deviations (SD) for the study variables of anxiety and depression (see Appendix D). These scores represent the average of each variable and the amount of variation in the scores before and after the intervention. For example, the state anxiety mean of men pretest was 41.92 with an SD (variation) of 12.03 and their state anxiety decreased posttest to 35.58 with a smaller variation of 10.82.

When one compares the measures of central tendency, the mean is the most stable and the median the most typical of these statistics. If the distribution of a sample is symmetrical and unimodal, the mean, median, and mode will coincide. If the distribution is skewed, the mean will be pulled in the direction of the long tail of the distribution. With a skewed distribution, all three statistics should be reported. For example, national income in the United States is skewed.

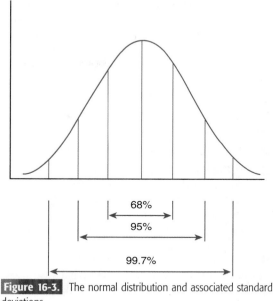

Figure 16-3. The normal distribution and associated standard deviations.

The mean wage differs from the median wage, because the high salaries are so much greater than the low salaries.

> 💡 **HELPFUL** H I N T
>
> Measures of central tendency are descriptive statistics that describe the characteristics of a sample.

Normal Distribution

The concept of the normal distribution is a theoretical one, based on the observation that data from repeated measures of interval or ratio level data group themselves about a midpoint in a distribution in a manner that closely approximates the normal curve illustrated in Figure 16-3. In addition, if the means of a large number of samples of the same interval or ratio data are calculated and plotted on a graph, that curve also approximates the normal curve. This tendency of the means to approximate the normal curve is termed the sampling distribution of the means. The mean of the sampling distribution of the means is the mean of the population.

The **normal curve** is one that is symmetrical about the mean and is unimodal. The mean, median, and mode are equal. An additional characteristic of the normal curve is that a fixed percentage of the scores falls within a given distance of the mean. As shown in Figure 16-3, about 68% of the scores or means will fall within 1 SD of the mean, 95% within 2 SD of the mean, and 99.7% within 3 SD of the mean.

Skewness   However, not all samples of data approximate the normal curve. Some samples are nonsymmetrical and have the peak off-center. For example, worldwide individual income has a positive skew, with most individuals in the low-to-moderate range and very few in the upper range. The mean in a positive skew is to the right of the median. In contrast, age of death in the United States has a negative skew because most deaths occur at older ages so the peak of the distribution curve would be to the right of a normal curve. In a negative skew, the mean is to the left of the median. Figure 16-4 illustrates positive and negative skew. In each diagram the peak is off-center and one tail is longer.

 EVIDENCE-BASED PRACTICE TIP

Inspection of descriptive statistics for the sample will indicate whether or not the sample data are skewed.

Interpreting Measures of Variability

Variability or dispersion is concerned with the spread of data. Measures of variability answer questions such as the following: "Is the sample homogeneous or heterogeneous?" "Is the sample similar or different?" If a researcher measures oral temperatures in two samples, one sample drawn from a healthy population and one sample from a hospitalized population, it is possible that the two samples will have the same mean. However, it is likely that there will be a wider range of temperatures in the hospitalized sample than in the healthy sample. Measures of variability are used to describe these differences in the dispersion of data. As with measures of central tendency, the various measures of variability are appropriate to specific kinds of measurement and types of distributions.

HELPFUL H I N T

Remember that descriptive statistics related to variability will enable you to evaluate the homogeneity or heterogeneity of a sample.

Range   The **range** is the simplest but most unstable measure of variability. Range is the difference between the highest and lowest scores. A change in either of these two scores would change the range. The range should always be reported with

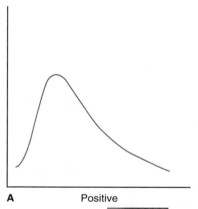

A   Positive

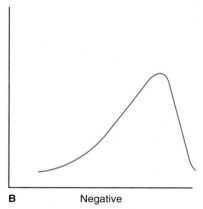

B   Negative

Figure 16-4. **A,** Positive skew. **B,** Negative skew.

other measures of variability. For example in the Davison et al. study (2003, Appendix D), the range of age in patients was 41 to 79 years, while the range of age in partners was 29 to 76 years. The range in patients thus was 38 years and in partners the range was 47 years. This range affects the standard deviation discussed below. The range in Table 16-2 is 36, but this could easily change with an increase or decrease in the high score of 90 or the low score of 54.

Semiquartile Range   The **semiquartile range (semiinterquartile range)** indicates the range of the middle 50% of the scores. It is more stable than the range, because it is less likely to be changed by a single extreme score. It lies between the upper and lower quartiles, the upper quartile being the point below which 75% of the scores fall and the lower quartile being the point below which 25% of the scores fall. The middle 50% of the scores in Table 16-2 lies between 68 and 78, and the semiquartile range is 10.

Percentile   A **percentile** represents the percentage of cases a given score exceeds. The median is the 50% percentile, and in Table 16-2 it is a score of 74. A score in the 90th percentile is exceeded by only 10% of the scores. The zero percentile and the 100th percentile are usually dropped.

Standard Deviation   The **standard deviation (SD)** is the most frequently used measure of variability, and it is based on the concept of the normal curve (see Figure 16-3). It is a measure of average deviation of the scores from the mean and as such should always be reported with the mean. The standard deviation takes all scores into account and can be used to interpret individual scores. Because the mean (X) and SD for the examination in Table 16-2 were 73.16+/−12.1, a student should know that 68% of the grades were between 85.1 and 61. If the student received a grade of 88, he would know he did better than most of the class, whereas a grade of 58 would indicate he did not do as well as most of the class. Table 16-3, from the study by Davison and

colleagues (2003), reports the mean and SD of the study variables of anxiety and depression. As illustrated in this table, the mean score for the variable "trait anxiety" for men was 41.92, and the SD was 12.03. This means that 68% of the men scored between 29.89 and 53.95 on the measure of state anxiety. This table allows the reader to inspect the data and get a feel for the variation the data contain (see Appendix C).

The SD is used in the calculation of many inferential statistics. One limitation of the SD is that it is expressed in terms of the units used in the measurement and cannot be used to compare means that have different units. If researchers were interested in the relationship between height measured in inches and weight measured in pounds, it would be necessary for them to convert the height and weight measurements to standard units or Z scores. The **Z score** is used to compare measurements in standard units. Each of the scores is converted to a Z score, and then the Z scores are used to examine the relative distance of the scores from the mean. A Z score of 1.5 means that the observation is 1.5 SD above the mean, whereas a score of −2 means that the observation is 2 SD below the mean. By using Z scores, a researcher can compare results from scales that use different measurement units, such as height and weight.

 HELPFUL H I N T

Many measures of variability exist. The SD is the most stable and useful because it helps you to visualize how the scores disperse around the mean.

INFERENTIAL STATISTICS

It can now be seen that descriptive statistics are the statistics used when the researcher needs to summarize the data. Next our attention turns to the use of inferential statistics. Inferential statistics combine mathematical processes and logic and allow researchers to test hypotheses about a population using data obtained from probability samples. Statistical inference is generally used for two purposes—to estimate the probability that statistics found in the sample accurately reflect the population parameter and to test hypotheses about a population.

In the first purpose, a **parameter** is a characteristic of a *population*, whereas a **statistic** is a characteristic of a *sample*. We use statistics to estimate population parameters. Suppose we randomly sample 100 people with chronic lung disease and use an interval level scale to study their knowledge of the disease. If the mean score for these subjects is 65, the mean represents the sample statistic. If we were able to study every subject with chronic lung disease, we also could calculate an average knowledge score and that score would be the parameter for the population. As you know, a researcher rarely is able to study an entire population, so inferential statistics provide evidence that allow the researcher to make statements about the larger population from studying the sample.

The example given alludes to two important qualifications of how a study must be conducted so that inferential statistics may be used. First, it was stated that the sample was selected using probability methods (see Chapter 12). Because you are already familiar with the advantages of probability sampling, it should be clear that if we wish to make statements about a population from a sample, that sample must be representative. All procedures for inferential statistics are based on the assumption that the sample was drawn with a known probability. Second, it was stated that the scale had to reach the interval level of measurement. This is because the mathematical operations involved in doing inferential statistics require this level of measurement. It should be noted that in studies that use nonprobability methods of sampling inferential statistics are also used. To compensate for the use of nonprobability sampling methods, researchers employ such techniques as sample size estimation using power analysis. The following two Critical Thinking Decision Paths examine inferential statistics and provide matrices that researchers use for statistical decision making.

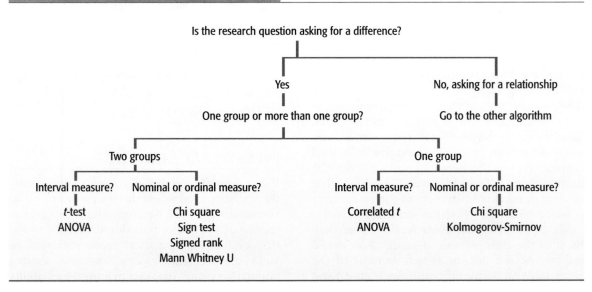

CRITICAL THINKING DECISION PATH | Inferential Statistics—Difference Questions

Is the research question asking for a difference?

Yes — No, asking for a relationship

One group or more than one group? — Go to the other algorithm

Two groups — One group

Interval measure? — Nominal or ordinal measure? — Interval measure? — Nominal or ordinal measure?

t-test
ANOVA

Chi square
Sign test
Signed rank
Mann Whitney U

Correlated *t*
ANOVA

Chi square
Kolmogorov-Smirnov

CRITICAL THINKING DECISION PATH | Inferential Statistics—Relationship Questions

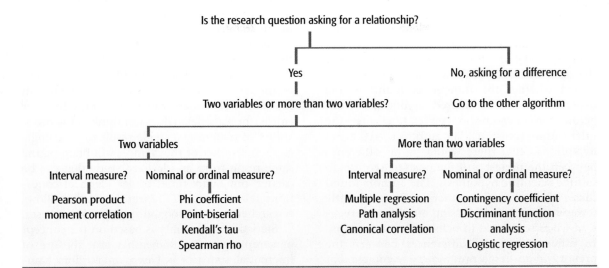

Is the research question asking for a relationship?

Yes — No, asking for a difference

Two variables or more than two variables? — Go to the other algorithm

Two variables — More than two variables

Interval measure? — Nominal or ordinal measure? — Interval measure? — Nominal or ordinal measure?

Pearson product moment correlation — Phi coefficient / Point-biserial / Kendall's tau / Spearman rho — Multiple regression / Path analysis / Canonical correlation — Contingency coefficient / Discriminant function analysis / Logistic regression

---

☼ EVIDENCE-BASED PRACTICE TIP

Try to figure out whether the statistical test chosen was appropriate for the design, the type of data collected, and the level of measurement.

Hypothesis Testing

The second and most commonly used purpose of inferential statistics is hypothesis testing. Statistical hypothesis testing allows researchers to make objective decisions about the outcome of their study. The use of statistical hypothesis testing allows researchers to answer such questions as the following: "How much of this effect is a result of chance?" "How strongly are these two variables associated with each other?" "What is the effect of the intervention?"

The procedures used when making inferences are based on principles of negative inference. In other words, if a researcher studied the effect of a new educational program for patients with chronic lung disease, the researcher would actu-

ally have two hypotheses—the scientific hypothesis and the null hypothesis. The research or **scientific hypothesis** is that which the researcher believes will be the outcome of the study. In our example, the scientific hypothesis would be that the educational intervention would have a marked impact on the outcome in the experimental group beyond that in the control group. The **null hypothesis,** which is the hypothesis that actually can be tested by statistical methods, would state that there is no difference between the groups. Inferential statistics use the null hypothesis to test the validity of a scientific hypothesis in sample data. The null hypothesis states that there is no actual relationship between the variables and that any observed relationship or difference is merely a function of chance fluctuations in sampling.

The concept of the null hypothesis is often confusing. An example may help clarify this concept. The study by Davison and colleagues (2003) (see Appendix D) provides a good example. The investigators were interested in determining if a computerized system to focus information counseling for men who are newly diagnosed with prostate cancer and their partners would lower levels of psychological distress and enable them to become more active participants in treatment decision making. One of the scientific hypotheses was that men and their partners would have lower levels of anxiety and depression at 4 months after the intervention. On the basis of this hypothesis, the authors determined whether the differences found in the dependent variables differed significantly from before the intervention (pretest) to after the intervention (posttest). The authors used the null hypothesis—that there would be no difference between the pretest and the posttest scores—to test the scientific hypothesis. The authors found that men and their partners had significantly lower anxiety and depression after the intervention when compared to before the intervention. In other words, the differences between the pretest and posttest scores were large enough that they were unlikely to be caused by chance. Thus the null hypothesis was rejected.

All statistical hypothesis testing is a process of disproof or rejection. It is impossible to prove that a scientific hypothesis is true, but it is possible to demonstrate that the null hypothesis has a high probability of being incorrect. To reject the null hypothesis, then, is considered to show support for the scientific hypothesis and is the desired outcome of most studies reporting inferential statistics.

 HELPFUL H I N T

Remember that most samples used in clinical research are samples of convenience, but most researchers use inferential statistics. Although such use violates one of the assumptions of such tests, the tests are robust enough to not seriously affect the results unless the data are skewed in unknown ways.

Probability

The researcher can never *prove* the scientific hypothesis but can show support for it by reject-ing the null hypothesis, that is, by showing that the null hypothesis has a high probability of being incorrect. We have now introduced the theory underlying all of the procedures discussed in this chapter—probability theory. Probability is a concept that we talk about all the time, such as the chance of rain today, but we have a difficult time defining it. The **probability** of an event is the event's long-run relative frequency in repeated trials under similar conditions. In other words, the statistician does not think of the probability of obtaining a single result from a single study but rather of the chances of obtaining the same result from an idealized study that can be carried out many times under identical conditions. It is the notion of repeated trials that allows researchers to use probability to test hypotheses.

Statistical probability is based on the concept of **sampling error.** Remember that the use of inferential statistics is based on random sampling. However, even when samples are randomly selected, there is always the possibility of some errors in sampling. Therefore the characteristics of any given sample may be different from those of the entire population. Suppose a group of researchers has at their disposal a large group of patients with decubitus ulcers and they wish to study the average length of time for ulcers to heal with the usual nursing care. If the researchers studied the entire population, they might obtain an average healing time of 50 days, with a standard deviation (SD) of 10 days. Now suppose that the researchers did not have the money necessary to study all of the patients but wished instead to do several consecutive studies of these patients. For this study, they first draw a sample of 25 patients, calculate the mean and SD, and replace the subjects in the population before drawing the next sample. If the researchers repeated this process many times in different samples, they would likely demonstrate a different mean for each sample. For example, the researchers might find that one sample's mean might be 50.5, the next 47.5, and the next 62.5. The tendency for statistics to fluctuate from one sample to another is known as sampling error.

Sampling distributions are theoretical. In practice, researchers do not routinely draw consecutive samples from the same population; usually they compute statistics and make inferences based on one sample. However, the knowledge of the properties of the sampling distribution—if these repeated samples are hypothetically obtained—permits the researcher to draw a conclusion based on one sample. This is possible because the sampling distribution of the means has certain known properties.

The sampling distribution of the means follows a normal curve, and the mean of the sampling distribution will be the mean of the population. As discussed in the previous section on normal distribution, the fact that the sampling distribution of the means is normal tells us several other important things. When scores are normally distributed, we know that 68% of the cases will fall between +1 SD and −1 SD, or that the probability is 68 out of 100 that any one randomly drawn sample mean will lie within the range of values between ±1 SD (see Figure 16-3). In the example given, if we drew only one sample, we would have a 68% chance of finding a sample mean that fell between 40 and 60. The SD of a theoretical distribution of sample means is called the **standard error of the mean.** The word error is used because the various means that make up the distribution contain some error in their estimates of the population mean. The error is considered to be standard because it implies the magnitude of the average error, just as a SD implies the average variation from one mean. The *smaller* the standard error, the *less* variable are the sample means and the *more accurate* are those means as estimates of the population value.

Although researchers rarely construct sampling distributions, standard error can be estimated because it bears a systematic relationship to the sample SD and the size of the sample. This tells us that increasing the size of the sample will increase the accuracy of our estimates of population parameters. It should make intuitive sense that to increase the size of a sample will decrease the likelihood that one outlying score will dramatically affect the sample mean (see Chapter 12). The other reason that the sampling distribution is so important is that there are sampling distributions for all statistics. Researchers consult these distributions when making determinations about rejecting the null hypothesis.

EVIDENCE-BASED PRACTICE TIP

Remember that the strength and quality of evidence are enhanced by repeated trials that have consistent findings, thereby increasing generalizability of the findings and applicability to clinical practice.

Type I and Type II Errors

The researcher's decision to accept or reject the null hypothesis is based on a consideration of how probable it is that the observed differences are a result of chance alone. Because data on the entire population are not available, the researcher can never flatly assert that the null hypothesis is or is not true. Thus statistical inference is always based on incomplete information about a population, and it is possible for errors to occur when making this decision. There are two types of errors in statistical inference—type I and type II.

Let us return to the example of the study by Davison and colleagues (2003) (see Appendix D) of men newly diagnosed with prostate cancer and their partners who received a focused information counseling intervention. Remember that one null hypothesis of the study was that there would be no differences in psychological outcomes between pretest and posttest scores. The authors reported a significant difference in anxiety and depression scores of both men and their partners before and after the intervention ($n = 74$). If the differences found were truly a function of chance (because this group of participants was unusual in some way) and if the number of participants was too small, a type I error would occur. A **type I error** is the researchers' rejection of the null hypothesis when

Conclusion of test of significance	REALITY	
	Null hypothesis is true	Null hypothesis is not true
Not statistically significant	Correct conclusion	Type II error
Statistically significant	Type I error	Correct conclusion

Figure 16-5. Outcome of statistical decision making.

it is actually true. If, on the other hand, the researchers had found that the groups did not differ but they had studied only a few patients, a type II error might occur. A **type II error** is the researchers' acceptance of a null hypothesis that is actually false. The relationship of the two types of errors is shown in Figure 16-5. When critiquing a study to see if there is a possibility of a type I error having occurred (rejecting the null hypothesis when it is actually true), one should consider the reliability and validity of the instruments used. For example, if the instruments did not accurately and precisely measure the intervention variables, one could conclude that the intervention made a difference when in reality it did not. It is critical to consider the reliability and validity of all the measurement instruments reported (see Chapter 15). In a practice discipline, type I errors usually are considered more serious because if a researcher declares that differences exist where none are present, the potential exists for patient care to be affected adversely. Type II errors (accepting the null hypothesis when it is false) may occur if the sample in the study is too small, thereby limiting the opportunity to measure *the treatment effect,* a true difference between two groups. A larger sample size improves the ability to *detect the treatment effect,* that is, differences between two groups. If no significant difference is found between two groups with a large sample, it provides stronger evidence (than with a small sample) not to reject the null hypothesis.

Level of Significance

The researcher does not know when an error in statistical decision making has occurred. It is possible to know only that the null hypothesis is indeed true or false if data from the total population are available. However, the researcher can control the risk of making type I errors by setting the level of significance before the study begins (a priori). The importance of setting the level of significance before the study is conducted is explained in detail by Slakter, Wu, and Suzuki-Slakter (1991). The **level of significance (alpha level)** is the probability of making a type I error, the probability of rejecting a true null hypothesis. The minimum level of significance acceptable for nursing research is 0.05. If the researcher sets alpha, or the level of significance, at 0.05, the researcher is willing to accept the fact that if the study were done 100 times, the decision to reject the null hypothesis would be wrong 5 times out of those 100 trials. If, as is sometimes done, the researcher wants to have a smaller risk of rejecting a true null hypothesis, the level of significance may be set at 0.01. In this case the researcher is willing to be wrong only once in 100 trials. The decision as to how strictly the alpha level should be set depends on how important it is to not make an error. For example, if the results of a study are to be used to determine whether a great deal of money should be spent in an area of nursing care, the researcher may decide that the accuracy of the results is so important that an alpha level of 0.01 is chosen. In most studies, however, alpha is set at 0.05.

Whatever level of significance is set, one either rejects or accepts the null hypothesis when comparing the statistical results to the preset alpha. For example, in the Davison study (2003) (see Appendix D), the null hypothesis regarding participants' (men with prostate cancer and their partners) psychological outcomes was rejected because the variables of the hypothesis were significant at the 0.05 level or less.

Perhaps you are thinking that researchers should always use the lowest alpha level possible because it makes sense that researchers would like to keep the risk of both types of errors at a minimum. Unfortunately, decreasing the risk of making a type I error increases the risk of making a type II error. What this means is that the stricter the researcher is in preventing the rejection of a true null hypothesis, the more likely is the possibility that a false null hypothesis will be accepted. Therefore the researcher always has to accept more of a risk of one type of error when setting the alpha level.

Another method of determining level of significance and whether to accept or reject the null hypothesis is called the *critical values method*. In this method, by calculating the estimates of population mean and SD, a range of values is determined from which one can compare the sample mean findings and decide whether or not to reject the null hypothesis. Let us use the example of a study in which we want to know the importance of support groups for caregivers of the elderly. We ask 100 caregivers to rate how important support groups are for them with an instrument that ranges from 0 (not important at all) to 100 (very important). If we use Figure 16-3 as the theoretical distribution for our study (a normal distribution with a mean of 50), 68% of the population would score between 40 and 60, and 95% would score between 30 and 70. Thus our null hypothesis would be that the mean scoring for the population of caregivers would be 50 and the scientific hypothesis would be greater or less than 50. After we complete our measurement with our sample, we find that the sample mean score is 75. This mean is consistent with the scientific hypothesis, and we can be 95% sure that most of the time our sample mean would fall under this cutoff, thus giving us confidence in rejecting our null hypothesis. In other words, only 5 out of 100 times would we obtain this result by chance alone.

HELPFUL HINT

Decreasing the alpha level acceptable for a study increases the chance that a type II error will occur. Remember that when a researcher is doing many statistical tests, the probability of some of the tests being significant increases as the number of tests increases. Therefore when a number of tests are being conducted, the researcher will often decrease the alpha level to 0.01.

Practical and Statistical Significance

The reader should realize that there is a difference between statistical significance and practical significance. When a researcher tests a hypothesis and finds that it is statistically significant, this means that the finding is unlikely to have happened by chance. In other words, if the level of significance has been set at 0.05, the odds are 19 to 1 that the conclusion the researcher makes on the basis of the statistical test performed on sample data is correct. The researcher would reach the wrong conclusion only 5 times in 100.

Suppose a researcher is interested in the effect of loud rock music on the behavior of laboratory mice. The researcher could design an experiment to study this question and find that loud music makes the mice act strangely. A statistical test suggests that this finding is not the result of chance. However, such a finding may or may not have practical significance, even though the finding has statistical significance. Although some would argue that this study might have relevance to understanding the behavior of teenagers, some would also argue that the study has no practical value. Thus the findings of a study may have statistical significance, but they may have no practical value or significance. Although researchers should consider the practicality of a problem in the early stages of a research project (see Chapter 3), a distinction between the statistical and practical significance of the findings also should be made when discussing the results of a study. Some people believe that if findings are not statistically significant, they have no practical value. Consider the Davison and associates study (2003), which determined whether providing individualized information to men who were newly diagnosed with prostate cancer and their partners would lower their levels of psychological distress and enable them to be more actively involved in treatment decision making. In this study several of the hypotheses were statistically supported and several were not. The nonsupported hypotheses provide as much information about the intervention as do the supported hypotheses. The data allowed the researchers to return to the previous literature in the area and draw from those findings both statistical and practical significance.

 EVIDENCE-BASED PRACTICE TIP

You will study the results to determine whether the new treatment is effective, the size of the effect, and whether the effect is clinically important.

Tests of Statistical Significance

Tests of significance may be parametric or nonparametric. Most of the studies in nursing research literature use parametric tests that have the following three attributes:

1. They involve the estimation of at least one **population** parameter.
2. They require measurement on at least an interval scale.
3. They involve certain assumptions about the variables being studied.

These assumptions usually include that the variable is normally distributed in the overall population. In contrast to parametric tests, **nonparametric tests of significance** are not based on the estimation of population parameters, so they involve less restrictive assumptions about the underlying distribution. Nonparametric tests usually are applied when the variables have been measured on a nominal or ordinal scale.

There has been some debate about the relative merits of the two types of statistical tests. The moderate position taken by most researchers and statisticians is that **nonparametric statistics** are best used when the data cannot be assumed to be at the interval level of measurement or when the sample is small and the normality of the underlying distribution cannot be inferred. If these assumptions can be made, however, most researchers prefer to use **parametric statistics** because they are more powerful and more flexible than nonparametric statistics.

Researchers use many different statistical tests of significance to test hypotheses. The procedure and the rationale for their use are similar from test to test. Once the researcher has chosen a significance level and collected the data, the data are used to compute the appropriate test statistic. For each test there is a related theoretical distribution that shows the probable and improbable values for that statistic. On the basis of the statistical result and the values in the distribution, the researcher either accepts or rejects the null hypothesis and then reports both the statistical result and its probability. Thus a researcher may perform a statistical test called a *t* test, obtain a value of 8.98, and report that it is statistically significant at the $p < .05$ level. This means that the researcher had 5 chances out of 100 to be wrong in concluding that this result could not have been obtained by chance. In addition, the likelihood of finding a statistic that is high enough to be statistically significant is increased as the sample size increases. This likelihood is indicated by the **degrees of freedom** that are often reported with the statistic and the probability value. Degrees of freedom is usually abbreviated as *df.*

Tables 16-4 and 16-5 show the most commonly used inferential statistics. The test used depends on the level of the measurement of the variables in question and the type of hypothesis being studied. Basically these statistics test two types of hypotheses—that there is a difference between groups (Table 16-4) or that there is a relationship between two or more variables (Table 16-5).

TABLE 16-4 **Tests of Differences between Means**

Level of Measurement	One Group	Two Groups		More Than Two Groups
		Related	Independent	
NONPARAMETRIC				
Nominal	Chi-square	Chi-square Fisher exact probability	Chi-square	Chi-square
Ordinal	Kolmogorov- Smirnov	Sign test	Chi-square	Chi-square
		Wilcoxon matched pairs Signed rank	Median test Mann-Whitney U	
PARAMETRIC				
Interval or ratio	Correlated *t* ANOVA (repeated measures)	Correlated *t*	Independent *t*	ANOVA
			ANOVA	ANCOVA MANOVA

HELPFUL HINT

Just because a researcher has used nonparametric statistics does not mean that the study is not useful. The use of nonparametric statistics is appropriate when measurements are not made at the interval level or the variable under study is not normally distributed.

EVIDENCE-BASED PRACTICE TIP

Try to discern whether the test chosen for analyzing the data was chosen because it gave a significant *p* value. A statistical test should be chosen on the basis of its appropriateness for the type of data collected, not because it gives the answer that the researcher hoped to obtain.

Tests of Difference

The type of test used for any particular study depends primarily on whether the researcher is examining differences in one, two, or three or more groups and whether the data to be analyzed

are nominal, ordinal, or interval (see Table 16-4). Suppose a researcher has done an experimental study using an after-only design (see Chapter 10). What the researcher hopes to determine is that the two randomly assigned groups are different after the introduction of the experimental treatment. If the measurements taken are at the interval level, the researcher would use the *t* test to analyze the data. If the *t* statistic was found to be high enough as to be unlikely to have occurred by chance, the researcher would reject the null hypothesis and conclude that the two groups were indeed more different than would have been expected on the basis of chance alone. In other words, the researcher would conclude that the experimental treatment had the desired effect.

The study discussed earlier by Davison and colleagues (2003) (Appendix D) illustrates the use of the *t* statistic. In this study, the *t* test was used to determine if there was a difference between the anxiety and depression scores of men newly diagnosed with prostate cancer and their partners before and after the information counseling intervention. They found that anxiety and depression scores were significantly lower 4 months after the intervention in both men with cancer and their partners compared to before the intervention.

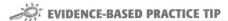

Parametric Tests   The *t statistic* is commonly used in nursing research. This statistic tests whether two group means are different. Thus this statistic is used when the researcher has two groups, and the question is whether the mean scores on some measure are more different than would be expected by chance. To use this test, the variables must have been measured at the interval or ratio level, and the two groups must be independent. By independent we mean that nothing in one group helps determine who is in the other group. If the groups are related, as when samples are matched (see Chapter 12), and the researcher also wants to determine differences between the two groups, a paired or correlated *t* test would be used.

The *t* statistic illustrates one of the major purposes of research in nursing—to demonstrate that there are differences between groups. Groups may be naturally occurring collections, such as age groups, or they may be experimentally created, such as the treatment and control groups. Sometimes a researcher has more than two groups, or measurements are taken more than once, as in the Koniak-Griffin and associates (2003) study (Appendix A). One research question that these authors wanted to answer was whether an early intervention program (**EIP**) for pregnant adolescents had an impact on the social competence of participants over a 2-year period of time. In this study, the researchers used **analysis of variance (ANOVA),** a test similar to the *t* test. Like the *t* statistic, the ANOVA statistic tests whether group means differ, but rather than testing each pair of means separately, ANOVA considers the variation between groups and within groups. Koniak-Griffin and associates (2003) found that participants in the treatment group had better social competence (i.e., self-esteem, perception of stress) that approached significance ($p = .057$) as compared to baseline and the control group. However, groups did not differ in external social competence (i.e., community life skills and social skills). This study used a variation of the ANOVA, the repeated measures ANOVA, because this statistic takes into account the fact that multiple measures at several points in time affect the potential range of scores.

In other cases, particularly in experimental work, the researchers use *t* tests or ANOVA to determine whether random assignment to groups was effective in creating groups that are equivalent before introduction of the experimental treatment. In this case the researcher wants to show that there is no difference among the groups. In the Koniak-Griffin and associates (2003) study mentioned previously, the authors reported that the intervention and control groups were comparable at baseline with respect to age, gestational age, socioeconomic status, ethnic/racial background, marital status, and educational level. These results suggested that if differences were found between the two groups at follow-up, they were likely due to the intervention. Suppose, however, that these groups had differed on educational level at baseline. For the researchers to conclude that their intervention program was effective, they would need to control statistically for educational level. This is done by using the technique of **analysis of covariance (ANCOVA)**. ANCOVA also measures differences among group means, and it uses a statistical technique to equate the groups under study on an important variable. Another expansion of the notion of analysis of variance is **multiple analysis of variance (MANOVA),** which also is used to determine differences in group means, but it is used when there is more than one dependent variable.

Nonparametric Tests   In the example from Koniak-Griffin and associates (2003), the researchers tested whether the subjects in the intervention and control groups were similar with respect to marital status and ethnic/racial background. These two variables are not interval level data, so the researchers could not test this difference with any of the tests discussed thus far. When data are at the nominal level and the researcher wants to determine whether groups are different, the researcher uses another commonly used statistic, the **chi-square (χ^2)**. Chi-square is a nonparametric statistic used to determine whether the frequency in each category is different from what would be expected by chance. As with the *t* test and ANOVA, if the calculated chi-square is high enough, the researcher would conclude that the frequencies found would not be expected on the basis of chance alone, and the null hypothesis would be rejected. Although this test is quite robust and can be used in many different situations, it cannot be used to compare frequencies when samples are small and expected frequencies are less than 6 in each cell. In these instances the **Fisher's exact probability test** is used.

When the data are ranks, or are at the ordinal level, researchers have several other nonparametric tests at their disposal. These include the *Kolmogorov-Smirnov test,* the *sign test,* the *Wilcoxon matched pairs test,* the *signed rank test for related groups,* the *median test,* and the *Mann-Whitney U test for independent groups.* Explanation of these tests is beyond the scope of this chapter;

those readers who desire further information should consult a general statistics book.

Nursing research studies often employ several different statistical tests. The randomized clinical trial by Koniak-Griffin and associates (2003) of the effects of an early intervention program for pregnant adolescents illustrates the use of several of these statistical tests. The researchers were interested in comparing the new program with usual public health nursing care on infant and maternal outcomes. Although the patients were randomly assigned to experimental and treatment groups, it was important to determine whether the random assignment procedure succeeded in creating equivalent groups. For data measured at the nominal level, such as marital status, the chi-square statistic was used as mentioned previously. For data measured at the interval level, such as age, the *t* test was used. Finally, to test the effect of the intervention, the chi-square method was used for nominal variables, such as infant hospitalizations, infant immunizations, and maternal repeat pregnancy, while the ANOVA method was used for measures of social competence.

Tests of Relationships

Researchers often are interested in exploring the *relationship* between two or more variables. Such studies use statistics that determine the **correlation,** or the degree of association, between two or more variables. Tests of the relationships between variables are sometimes considered to be descriptive statistics when they are used to describe the magnitude and direction of a relationship of two variables in a sample and the researcher does not wish to make statements about the larger population. Such statistics also can be inferential when they are used to test hypotheses about the correlations that exist in the target population.

Null hypothesis tests of the relationships between variables assume that there is no relationship between the variables. Thus when a researcher rejects this type of null hypothesis, the conclusion is that the variables are in fact related.

Suppose a researcher is interested in the relationship between the age of patients and the length of time it takes them to recover from surgery. As with other statistics discussed, the researcher would design a study to collect the appropriate data and then analyze the data using measures of association. In the example, age and length of time until recovery can be considered interval level measurements. The researcher would use a test called the **Pearson correlation coefficient, Pearson r,** or **Pearson product moment correlation coefficient.** Once the Pearson r is calculated, the researcher consults the distribution for this test to determine whether the value obtained is likely to have occurred by chance. Again, the research reports both the value of the correlation and its probability of occurring by chance.

Correlation coefficients can range in value from −1.0 to +1.0 and also can be zero. A zero coefficient means that there is no relationship between the variables. *A perfect positive correlation* is indicated by a +1.0 coefficient, and a *perfect negative correlation* by a −1.0 coefficient. We can illustrate the meaning of these coefficients by using the example from the previous paragraph. If there were no relationship between the age of the patient and the time required for the patient to recover from surgery, the researcher would find a correlation of zero. However, if the correlation was +1.0, this would mean that the older the patient, the longer the recovery time. A negative coefficient would imply that the younger the patient, the longer the recovery time. Figure 16-6 illustrates a perfect positive correlation, a perfect negative correlation, and no correlation.

Of course, relationships are rarely perfect. The magnitude of the relationship is indicated by how close the correlation comes to the absolute value of 1. Thus a correlation of −0.76 is just as strong as a correlation of +0.76, but the direction of the relationship is opposite. In addition, a correlation of 0.76 is stronger than a correlation of 0.32. When a researcher tests hypotheses about the relationships between two variables, the test considers whether the magnitude of the correlation is large enough not to have occurred by chance. This is the meaning of the probability value or the *p* value reported with correlation coefficients. As with other statistical tests of significance, the larger the sample, the greater the likelihood of finding a significant correlation. Therefore researchers also report the degrees of freedom associated with the test performed.

Pender and colleagues (2002) conducted a cross-sectional study to determine if preexercise self-efficacy predicted girls' (8 to 17 years of age) perceptions of exertion during exercise. The authors found that higher preexercise self-efficacy was associated with lower perceptions of exertion during exercise (20 minutes on a cycle ergometer at 60% of each girl's peak oxygen uptake), with a correlation coefficient of −0.41.

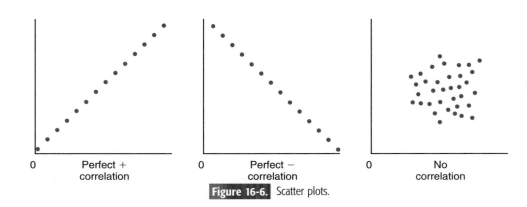

0   Perfect +   0   Perfect −   0   No
     correlation   correlation   correlation

Figure 16-6. Scatter plots.

This reflects a moderate correlation, and it indicates that approximately 17% (0.41×0.41) of the variability in perceived exercise exertion is explained by exercise self-efficacy in this sample.

Nominal and ordinal data also can be tested for relationships by nonparametric statistics. When two variables being tested have only two levels (e.g., male/female; yes/no), the phi coefficient can be used to express relationships. When the researcher is interested in the relationship between a nominal variable and an interval variable, the point-biserial correlation is used. Spearman rho is used to determine the degree of association between two sets of ranks, as is *Kendall's tau.* All of these correlation coefficients may range in value from -1.0 to $+1.0$. These tests are shown in Table 16-5.

Nursing problems are rarely so simple that they can be explained by only two variables. When researchers are interested in studying complex relationships among more than two variables, they use techniques other than those we have discussed thus far. When researchers are interested in understanding more about a problem than just the relationship between two variables, they often use a technique called **multiple regression,** which measures the relationship between one interval level dependent variable and several independent variables. Multiple regression is the expansion of correlation to include more than two variables, and it is used when the researcher wants to determine what variables contribute to the explanation of the dependent variable and to what degree. For example, a researcher may be interested in determining what factors help women decide to breastfeed their infants. A number of variables, such as the mother's age, previous experience with breastfeeding, number of other children, and knowledge of the advantages of breastfeeding, might be measured and then analyzed to see whether they, separately and together, predict the length of breastfeeding. Such a study would require the use of multiple regression. The results of a study such as this might help nurses know that a younger mother with only one other child might be more likely to benefit from a teaching program about breastfeeding than an older mother with several other children.

The reader of research reports often will see multiple regression techniques described as *forward solution, backward solution,* or *stepwise solution.* These are techniques used in multiple regression to find the smallest group of variables that will account for the greatest proportion of variance in the dependent variable. In the forward solution the independent variable with the highest correlation with the dependent variables is entered first, and the next variable is the one that will increase the explained variance the most. In the backward solution all variables are entered into the solution, and each variable is

TABLE 16-5 **Tests of Association**

Level of Measurement	Two Variables	More Than Two Variables
NONPARAMETRIC		
Nominal	Phi coefficient	Contingency coefficient
	Point-biserial	
Ordinal	Kendall's tau	Discriminant function analysis
	Spearman rho	
PARAMETRIC		
Interval or ratio	Pearson *r*	Multiple regression
		Path analysis
		Canonical correlation

deleted to see whether the explained variance drops significantly. The stepwise solution is a combination of the two approaches. In general, all of the approaches give similar, although not identical, results.

Suppose the individual who was researching breastfeeding was interested in not just breastfeeding but also maternal satisfaction. *Canonical correlation* is used when there is more than one dependent variable. If the data are nominal or ordinal, the contingency coefficient or discriminant function analyses are used. These last tests are beyond the scope of this text; further information can be found in the "Additional Readings" section.

Zalon (2004) was interested in understanding the correlates (pain, depression, fatigue) of recovery (functional status and self-perception of recovery) among older adults after major abdominal surgery at different time points. To assess these factors, she needed to needed to go beyond the analysis of relationships between and among the variables (correlation analysis). Using multivariate regression, the author found that pain, depression, and fatigue explained significant and different amounts of the variation in functional status and self-perception at the different time periods in the study. These data allowed her to build on the past research that she reviewed as well as to suggest both future descriptive and intervention research, thus moving the data toward evidence-based practice.

☼ EVIDENCE-BASED PRACTICE TIP

Tests of relationship are usually associated with nonexperimental designs that provide Level IV evidence. Establishment of a strong statistically significant relationship between variables often lends support for replicating the study to increase the consistency of the findings and provide a foundation for developing an intervention study.

Advanced Statistics

Sometimes researchers are interested in even more complex problems. For example, Bezanson and associates (2004) conducted a study that would develop and validate a probability model for prolonged mechanical ventilation (MV) using selected presurgical patient characteristics in older age groups (Medicare recipients 65 years and older). The ventilatory support model provided the framework for the research team to test the model. Data were provided by the existing coronary artery surgery database. The team selected key variables based on literature and past research that would potentially affect MV. On the basis of a proposed model, the relationships between the independent and dependent variables were tested using logistic regression analysis. Logistic regression is a form of advanced statistics used when a researcher wishes to confirm the relationship of a set of categorical data (data that have a discrete value). In this study the researchers were able to identify factors that place Medicare recipients at risk for late extubation.

This notion of testing specific relationships in a specific order can be extended further to test hypothesized variables that are made up of several measures. A technique called the analysis of **linear structural relationships (LISREL)** tests path models made up of variables that are not actually measured. For example, a researcher might study the concept of self-esteem and use three different measures to determine subjects' levels of self-esteem. The researcher would test how carefully these three measures actually gauge self-esteem by testing a measurement model using LISREL. Because many of the variables of interest to nursing are not easily defined and measured and because we are ultimately interested in causal models, LISREL and other advanced statistics are more commonly used in nursing studies. For examples, in the studies by Uphold, Lenz, and Soeken (2000) and by Gigliotti (2002), the researchers were testing theories about complex problems, and the LISREL technique allowed them the opportunity to study complex interactions among variables simultaneously.

Another advanced technique often used in nursing research is factor analysis. Factor analysis helps us understand concepts more fully and contributes to our ability to measure concepts reliably and validly (see Chapter 15). **Factor analysis** takes a large number of variables and groups them into a smaller number of factors. It is used to reduce a set of data so that it may be easily described and used. In addition, factor analysis is used for instrument development and theory development. In instrument development, factor analysis is used to group individual items on a scale into meaningful factors or subscales. Secco (2002), for example, was interested in assessing perceptions of competence in the maternal role function of infant care providers. She developed the Infant Care Questionnaire (ICQ) and tested it for reliability and validity in a sample of healthy low-risk primiparous and multiparous mothers of term infants. *Factor analysis* was used to determine whether the scale actually measured the concepts that they intended the instrument to measure. Many other statistical techniques are available to nurse researchers. Consult any of the sources listed in the "Additional Readings" section if further information is desired or if a test not discussed here is included in a study of interest to you.

The Use of Statistics

In conclusion, statistics are used in nursing research to describe the samples of research studies and to test for hypothesized differences or associations in the sample. Knowing the characteristics of the sample of a research study allows for determining the population for whom the results will be generalized. For example, if a study sample was primarily Caucasian with a mean age of 42 years (SD 2.5), the findings may not be applicable to elderly African-Americans. Cultural, demographic, or clinical factors of an elderly population of a different ethnic group may contribute to different results. Thus understanding the descriptive statistics of a study assists in determining the applicability of findings to different practice settings.

Statistics are also used to test hypotheses proposed by the researchers. Inferential statistics used to analyze data (i.e., t test, F test, r coefficient) and the associated significance level (p values) indicate the likelihood that the association or difference found in any study is due to chance or to a true difference between groups. The closer the p value is to zero, the less likely the association or difference of a study is due to chance. Thus inferential statistics provide an objective way to determine if the results of the study are likely to be a true representation of reality (Brown, 1999; Munro, 2001).

EVIDENCE-BASED PRACTICE TIP

A basic understanding of statistics will improve your ability to think about the effect of the independent variable (IV) on the dependent variable (DV) and related patient outcomes for your patient population and practice setting.

Many students who have not had a course in statistics think they cannot critique the statistics of research. However, students should be able to critically analyze the use of statistics even if they do not understand the derivation of the numbers presented. What is most important in critiquing this aspect of a research study is that the procedures for summarizing and analyzing the data make sense in light of the purpose of the study (see Critiquing Criteria box).

Before a decision can be made as to whether the statistics employed make sense, it is important to return to the beginning of the paper and determine the purpose of the study. Although all studies use descriptive statistics to summarize the data obtained, many studies go on to use inferential statistics to test specific hypotheses. If a study is an exploratory one, it is possible that

only descriptive statistics will be presented because their purpose is to describe the characteristics of a population.

Just as the hypotheses or research questions should flow from the purpose of a study, so should the hypotheses or research questions suggest the type of analysis that will follow. The hypotheses or the research questions should indicate the major variables that are expected to be presented in summary form. Each of the variables in the hypotheses or research questions should be followed in the "Results" section with appropriate descriptive information.

After studying the hypotheses or research questions, the reader should proceed to the "Methods" section. Using the operational definition provided, the levels of measurement employed to measure each of the variables listed

---

CRITIQUING CRITERIA *Descriptive and Inferential Statistics*

1. Were appropriate descriptive statistics used?
2. What level of measurement is used to measure each of the major variables?
3. Is the sample size large enough to prevent one extreme score from affecting the summary statistics used?
4. What descriptive statistics are reported?
5. Were these descriptive statistics appropriate to the level of measurement for each variable?
6. Are there appropriate summary statistics for each major variable?
7. Does the hypothesis indicate that the researcher is interested in testing for differences between groups or in testing for relationships? What is the level of significance?
8. Does the level of measurement permit the use of parametric statistics?
9. Is the size of the sample large enough to permit the use of parametric statistics?
10. Has the researcher provided enough information to decide whether the appropriate statistics were used?
11. Are the statistics used appropriate to the problem, the hypothesis, the method, the sample, and the level of measurement?
12. Are the results for each of the hypotheses presented clearly and appropriately?
13. If tables and graphs are used, do they agree with the text and extend it, or do they merely repeat it?
14. Are the results understandable?
15. Is a distinction made between practical significance and statistical significance? How is it made?

in the hypotheses or research questions need to be identified. From this information it should be possible to determine the measures of central tendency and variability that should be employed to summarize the data. For example, you would not expect to see a mean used as a summary statistic for the nominal variable of gender. In all likelihood, gender would be reported as a frequency distribution. The means and SD should be provided for measurements performed at the interval level. The sample size is another aspect of the "Methods" section that is important when evaluating the researcher's use of descriptive statistics. The larger the sample, the less chance that one outlying score will affect the summary statistics.

If tables or graphs are used, they should agree with the information presented in the text. The tables and charts should be clearly and completely labeled. If the researcher presents grouped frequency data, the groups should be logical and mutually exclusive. The size of the interval in grouped data should not obscure the pattern of the data, nor should it create an artificial pattern. Each table and chart should be referred to in the text, but each should add to the text—not merely repeat it. Each table or graph should have an obvious connection to the study being reported.

In reading a table such as Table 16-3, the reader should first look at the heading. The title should give a valid indication of the information contained in the table. Next, the reader should review the column headings. Do these headings follow from the title? Is each heading clear and are any nonstandard abbreviations explained? Are the statistics contained in the table appropriate to the level of measurement used? In Table 16-3, the column heading follows from the title. Each study variable is listed along with its mean and SD. Mean and SD are appropriate statistics because these data were regarded as interval data.

After evaluating the descriptive statistics, inferential statistics can then be evaluated. The first place to begin critiquing the inferential statistical analysis of a research report is with the

hypothesis or research question. If the hypothesis or research question indicates that a relationship will be found, you should expect to find indices of correlation. If the study is experimental or quasiexperimental, the hypothesis would indicate that the author is looking for differences between the groups studied, and you would expect to find statistical tests of differences between means that test the effect of the intervention.

Then as you read the "Methods" section of the paper, again consider what level of measurement the author has used to measure the important variables. If the level of measurement is interval or ratio, the statistics most likely will be parametric statistics. On the other hand, if the variables are measured at the nominal or ordinal level, the statistics used should be nonparametric. Also consider the size of the sample, and remember that samples have to be large enough to permit the assumption of normality. If the sample is quite small, for example, 5 to 10 subjects, the researcher may have violated the assumptions necessary for inferential statistics to be used (see Chapter 12). Thus the important question is whether the researcher has provided enough justification to use the statistics presented.

Finally, consider the results as they are presented. There should be enough data presented for each hypothesis or research question studied to determine whether the researcher actually examined each hypothesis or research question. The tables should accurately reflect the procedure performed and be in harmony with the text. For example, the text should not indicate that a test reached statistical significance while the tables indicate that the probability value of the test was above 0.05. If the researcher has used analyses that are not discussed in this text, you may want to refer to a statistics text to decide whether the analysis was appropriate to the hypothesis or research question and the level of measurement.

There are two other aspects of the data analysis section that the reader should critique. The paper should not read as if it were a statistical textbook. The results of the study in the text of the paper should be clear enough to the average reader so that the reader can determine what was done and what the results were. In addition, the author should attempt to make a distinction between practical and statistical significance of the evidence related to the findings. Some results may be statistically significant, but their practical importance may be doubtful in terms of applicability for a patient population or clinical setting. If this is so, the author should note it. Alternatively, you may find yourself reading a research report that is elegantly presented, but you come away with a "so what?" feeling. Such a feeling may indicate that the practical significance of the study and its findings has not been adequately explained in the report. From an evidence-based practice perspective, a significant hypothesis or research question should contribute to improving patient care and clinical outcomes.

Note that the critical analysis of a research paper's statistical analysis is not done in a vacuum. It is possible to judge the adequacy of the analysis only in relationship to the other important aspects of the paper: the problem, the hypotheses, the research question, the design, the data-collection methods, and the sample. Without consideration of these aspects of the research process, the statistics themselves have very little meaning. Statistics can lie; thus it is most important that the researcher use the appropriate statistic for the problem. For example, a researcher may sometimes use a nonparametric statistic when it appears that a parametric statistic is appropriate. Because parametric statistics are more powerful than nonparametric, the result of the parametric analysis may not have been what the researcher expected. However, the nonparametric result might be in the expected direction, so the researcher reports only that result.

Example of the Use and Critique of Statistics

The purpose of the study by Koniak-Griffin and colleagues (2003) (see Appendix A) was to evaluate the 2-year postbirth infant health and maternal outcomes of an early and intense program of home visitation by public health nurses compared to standard public health nursing care in a sample of Latina and African-American adolescent mothers. The statement of purpose implies that the investigators were interested in looking at differences between groups, thereby suggesting an experimental design that provides Level II evidence. Therefore, the reader should expect that the analysis will consist of statistical tests that examine differences between means, such as t tests or ANOVA.

Sample characteristics were adequately described. In this difficult to reach and follow-up sample, there was high attrition ($n = 43$ out of 144 initially recruited). The final sample size was 101. If the participants who did not complete the study were different than those who completed the study, findings of the study would be difficult to interpret (i.e., those who completed the program had less problems). Therefore the investigators compared mother and infant characteristics such as socioeconomic status, substance abuse, and length of gestation of the dropouts and the completers. The results of statistical tests comparing these groups revealed no significant group differences, a fact that suggests that sampling bias has been minimized.

Dependent variables consisted of a variety of maternal (i.e., substance abuse, social competence) and infant outcomes (i.e., hospitalizations, immunizations) and were measured over time at 6 weeks and at 6, 12, 18, and 24 months after birth. The investigators were interested in looking at differences between the early intervention program group and the standard care control group that received traditional public health nursing care. Various statistical tests were used to examine differences depending on the level of measurement. Dependent variables calculated as proportions, such as infant hospitalizations and change in maternal substance abuse over time, were compared using the nonparametric chi-square test. Dependent variables calculated at the interval level were compared using repeated measures ANOVA.

These tests are appropriate to the study design and the hypotheses because the researchers were interested in differences between the two groups. Results for each of the hypotheses are presented, and they suggest that there are differences in some of the outcomes between the two groups. Tables agree with the text, and the results are understandable to the reader. The discussion points out limitations to the study. Clear implications for practice are found, and they support the practical significance of the study. The statistical level of significance was set at 0.05 and is consistent throughout the paper. Therefore the researchers' statistics were appropriate to the study's purpose, design, method, sample, and levels of measurement.

Critical Thinking Challenges

- Discuss the ways a researcher might use the computer in analyzing data and presenting descriptive statistical results of a study.
- What is the relationship between the level of measurement a researcher uses and the choice of a statistical procedure? How is this level of measurement associated with the level of evidence in the study design?
- What type of visual representation can be used to demonstrate the use of correlations? Use examples from clinical practice to illustrate the difference between positive and negative correlations.
- A classmate from research class tells you that she thinks it is ridiculous for the instructor to ask the students to critique the descriptive statistics used in a study when none of the students have taken a statistics course. Would you agree or disagree with her claim? Defend your position.
- What assumptions are violated when a clinical research study uses a convenience sample and applies inferential statistics?
- What are the advantages and disadvantages of decreasing the alpha level for a study? What is the relationship between setting an alpha level and type I and type II errors?
- Discuss the parameters for using nonparametric statistics in a study and its impact on the usefulness of applying the evidence provided by the findings in practice.
- A research study's findings are not considered significant at the 0.05 level; are this study's findings deemed to provide evidence that is applicable to practice? Justify your answer.

KEY POINTS

- Descriptive statistics are a means of describing and organizing data gathered in research.
- The four levels of measurement are nominal, ordinal, interval, and ratio. Each has appropriate descriptive techniques associated with it.
- Measures of central tendency describe the average member of a sample. The mode is the most frequent score, the median is the middle score, and the mean is the arithmetical average of the scores. The mean is the most stable and useful of the measures of central tendency, and with the standard deviation it forms the basis for many of the inferential statistics.
- The frequency distribution presents data in tabular or graphic form and allows for the calculation or observations of characteristics of the distribution of the data, including skewness, symmetry, modality, and kurtosis.
- In nonsymmetrical distributions, the degree and direction of the pull of the peak off-center are described in terms of skew.
- The ranges reflect differences between high and low scores.
- The standard deviation is the most stable and useful measure of variability. It is derived from the concept of the normal curve. In the normal curve, sample scores and the means of large numbers of samples group themselves around the midpoint in the distribution, with a fixed percentage of the scores falling within given distances of the mean. This tendency of means to approximate the normal curve is called the sampling distributions of the means. A Z score is the standard deviation converted to standard units.
- Inferential statistics are a tool to test hypotheses about populations from sample data.
- Because the sampling distribution of the means follows a normal curve, researchers are able to estimate the probability that a certain sample will have the same properties as the total population of interest. Sampling distributions provide the basis for all inferential statistics.
- Inferential statistics allow researchers to estimate population parameters and to test hypotheses. The use of these statistics allows researchers to make objective decisions about the outcome of the study. Such decisions are based on the rejection or acceptance of the null hypothesis, which states that there is no relationship between the variables.
- If the null hypothesis is accepted, this result indicates that the findings are likely to have occurred by chance. If the null hypothesis is rejected, the researcher accepts the scientific hypothesis that a relationship exists between the variables that is unlikely to have been found by chance.
- Statistical hypothesis testing is subject to two types of errors—type I and type II.
- Type I error occurs when the researcher rejects a null hypothesis that is actually true.
- Type II error occurs when the researcher accepts a null hypothesis that is actually false.
- The researcher controls the risk of making a type I error by setting the alpha level, or level of significance. Unfortunately, reducing the risk of a type I error by reducing the level of significance increases the risk of making a type II error.
- The results of statistical tests are reported to be significant or nonsignificant. Statistically significant results are those whose probability of occurring is less than 0.05 or 0.01, depending on the level of significance set by the researcher.
- Commonly used parametric and nonparametric statistical tests include those that test for differences between means, such as the t test and ANOVA, and those that test for differences in proportions, such as the chi-square test.
- Tests that examine data for the presence of relationships include the Pearson r, the sign test, the Wilcoxon matched pairs, signed rank test, and multiple regression.
- Advanced statistical procedures include path analysis, LISREL, and factor analysis.

- The most important aspect of critiquing statistical analyses is the relationship of the statistics employed to the problem, design, and method used in the study. Clues to the appropriate statistical test to be used by the researcher should stem from the researcher's hypotheses. The reader also should determine if all of the hypotheses have been presented in the paper.
- A basic understanding of statistics will improve your ability to think about the level of evidence provided by the study design and findings and their relevance to patient outcomes for your patient population and practice setting.

REFERENCES

Bezanson JL, Weaver M, Kinney MR, Waldrum M, and Weintraub WS: Presurgical risk factors for late extubation in Medicare recipients after cardiac surgery, *Nurs Res* 53: 46-52, 2004.

Brown SJ: *Knowledge for health care practice: a guide to using research evidence,* Philadelphia, 1999, WB Saunders.

Davison BJ et al.: Provision of individualized information to men and their partners to facilitate treatment decision making in prostate cancer, *Oncol Nurs Forum* 30(1): 107-114, 2003.

Gigliotti E: A confirmation of the factor structure of the Norbeck Social Support Scale, *Nurs Res* 51: 276-284, 2002.

Knapp TR: Treating ordinal scales as interval scales: an attempt to resolve the controversy, *Nurs Res* 39(2): 121-123, 1990.

Knapp TR: Treating ordinal scales as ordinal scales, *Nurs Res* 42(3): 184-186, 1993.

Koniak-Griffin et al.: Nurse visitation for adolescent mothers, *Nurs Res* 52(2): 127-136, 2003.

Lipman TH et al.: Risk factors for cardiovascular disease in children with type 1 diabetes, *Nurs Res* 49(3): 160-166, 2000.

Munro BH: *Statistical methods for health care research,* ed 4, 2001, Philadelphia, Lippincott.

Pender NJ et al.: Self-efficacy and perceived exertion of girls during exercise, *Nurs Res* 51: 86-91, 2002.

Secco L: The Infant Care Questionnaire: assessment of reliability and validity in a sample of healthy mothers, *J Nurs Measurement* 10: 97-110, 2002.

Slakter MJ, Wu YWB, and Suzuki-Slakter NS: [:statistical nonsense at the .00000 level], *Nurs Res* 40: 248-249, 1991.

Uphold CR, Lenz ER, and Soeken KL: Social support transactions between professional and nonprofessional women and their mothers, *Res Nurs Health* 23: 447-460, 2000.

Wang S et al.: Bridging the gap between the pros and the cons in treating ordinal scales as interval scales from an analysis point of view, *Nurs Res* 48(4): 226-229, 1999.

Zalon ML: Correlates of recovery among older adults after abdominal surgery, *Nurs Res* 53: 99-106, 2004.

FOR FURTHER STUDY

Go to your Companion CD for review activities for this chapter.

evolve Go to Evolve at http://evolve.elsevier.com/LoBiondo/ for WebLinks, Content Updates, and additional research articles, for practice in reviewing and critiquing.

17

GERI LOBIONDO-WOOD

Analysis of Findings

KEY TERMS

confidence interval
findings
generalizability

limitations
recommendations

LEARNING OUTCOMES

After reading this chapter, the student should be able to do the following:

- Discuss the difference between the "Results" section of a study and the "Discussion of the Results" section.
- Identify the format of the "Results" section.
- Determine if both statistically supported and statistically unsupported findings are discussed.
- Determine whether the results are objectively reported.
- Describe how tables and figures are used in a research report.
- List the criteria of a meaningful table.
- Identify the format and components of the "Discussion of the Results" section.
- Determine the purpose of the "Discussion" section.
- Discuss the importance of including generalizations and limitations of a study in the report.
- Determine the purpose of including recommendations in the study report.
- Discuss how the strength, quality, and consistency of evidence provided by the findings are related to a study's limitations, generalizability and applicability to practice.

STUDY RESOURCES

Go to your Companion CD for review activities for this chapter.

Go to Evolve at http://evolve.elsevier.com/LoBiondo/ for Weblinks, Content Updates, and additional research articles for practice in reviewing and critiquing.

The ultimate goals of nursing research are to develop nursing knowledge and evidence-based nursing practice, thereby supporting the scientific basis of nursing. From the viewpoint of the research consumer, the analysis of the results, interpretations, and generalizations that a researcher generates from a study becomes a highly important piece of the research project. After the analysis of the data, the researcher puts the final pieces of the jigsaw puzzle together to view the total picture with a critical eye. This process is analogous to evaluation, the last step in the nursing process. The research consumer may view these last sections as an easier step for the investigator, but it is here that a most critical and creative process comes to the forefront. In the final sections of the report, after the statistical procedures have been applied, the researcher relates the statistical or numerical findings to the research question, hypotheses, theoretical framework, literature, methods, and analyses and begins the task of formulating the application of the study's findings to practice.

The final sections of published research reports are generally titled "Results" and "Discussion," but other topics, such as limitations of findings, implications for future research and nursing practice, recommendations, conclusions, and application to practice, may be separately addressed or subsumed within these sections. The presentation format of these areas is a function of the author's and the journal's stylistic considerations. The function of these final sections is to relate all aspects of the research process, as well as to discuss, interpret, and identify the limitations and generalizations relevant to the investigation, thereby furthering evidence-based practice. The process that both an investigator and the research consumer use to assess the results of a study is depicted in the following Critical Thinking Decision Path.

CRITICAL THINKING DECISION PATH   Assessing Study Results

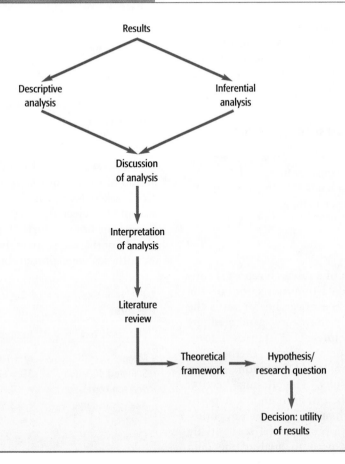

The goal of this chapter is to introduce the purpose and content of the final sections of a research investigation where data are presented, interpreted, discussed, and generalized. An understanding of what an investigator presents in these sections will help the research consumer to critically analyze an investigator's findings.

FINDINGS

The **findings** of a study are the results, conclusions, interpretations, recommendations, generalizations, and implications for future research and nursing practice, which are addressed by separating the presentation into two major areas. These two areas are the results and the discussion of the results. The "Results" section focuses on the results or statistical findings of a study, and the "Discussion of the Results" section focuses on the remaining topics. For both sections, the rule applies—as it does to all other sections of a report—that the content must be presented clearly, concisely, and logically.

 EVIDENCE-BASED PRACTICE TIP

Evidence-based practice is an active process that requires you to consider how, and if, research findings are applicable to your patient population and practice setting.

Results

The "Results" section of a research report is considered to be the data-bound section of the report and is where the researcher presents the quantitative data or numbers generated by the descriptive and inferential statistical tests. The results of the data analysis set the stage for the interpretations or "Discussion" section that follows the "Results." The "Results" section should then reflect the question and/or hypothesis tested. The information from each hypothesis or research question should be sequentially presented. The tests used to analyze the data

should be identified. If the exact test that was used is not explicitly stated, then the values obtained should be noted. The researcher does this by providing the numerical values of the statistics and stating the specific test value and probability level achieved (see Chapter 16). Examples of these statistical results can be found in Table 17-1. These numbers and their signs should not frighten the novice. The numbers are important, but there is much more to the research process than the numbers. They are one piece of the whole. Chapter 16 conceptually presents the meanings of the numbers found in studies. Whether the consumer only superficially understands statistics or has an in-depth knowledge of statistics, it should be obvious that the results are clearly stated, and the presence or lack of statistically significant results should be noted.

 HELPFUL HINT

In the "Results" section of a research report, the descriptive statistics results are generally presented first; then the results of each of hypothesis or research question that was tested are presented.

The researcher is bound to present the data for all of the hypotheses posed or research questions asked (e.g., whether the hypotheses were accepted, rejected, supported, partially supported, or not supported). If the data supported the hypotheses, it may be assumed that the hypotheses were *proven*, but this is not true. It

TABLE **17-1 Examples of Reported Statistical Results**

Statistical Test	Examples of Reported Results
Mean	$m = 118.28$
Standard deviation	$SD = 62.5$
Pearson correlation	$r = 0.49, P < 0.01$
Analysis of variance	$F = 3.59, df = 2, 48, P < 0.05$
t test	$t = 2.65, P < 0.01$
Chi-square	$X^2 = 2.52, df = 1, P < 0.05$

does not necessarily mean that the hypotheses were proven; it only means that the hypotheses were supported and the results suggest that the relationships or differences tested, which were derived from the theoretical framework, were probably logical in that study's sample. Novice research consumers may think that if a researcher's results are not supported statistically or are only partially supported, the study is irrelevant or possibly should not have been published, but this also is not true. If the data are not supported, the research consumer should not expect the researcher to bury the work in a file. It is as important for a research consumer to review and understand unsupported studies as it is for the researcher. Information obtained from unsupported studies can often be as useful as data obtained from supported studies.

Unsupported studies can be used to suggest **limitations** (weaknesses of a study) of particular aspects of a study's design and procedures. Data from unsupported studies may suggest that current modes of practice or current theory in an area may not be supported by research evidence and therefore must be reexamined and researched further. Data help generate new knowledge and evidence, as well as prevent knowledge stagnation. Generally, the results are interpreted in a separate section of the report. At times, the research critiquer may find that the "Results" section contains the results and the researcher's interpretations, which are generally found in the "Discussion" section. Integrating the results with the discussion in a report is the author's or journal editor's decision. Both sections may be integrated when a study contains several segments that may be viewed as fairly separate subproblems of a major overall problem.

The investigator should also demonstrate objectivity in the presentation of the results. For example, a quote by Van Cleve et al. (2004, Appendix B) is the appropriate means to express results: "The older children (self-report) showed a significant relation between pain intensity and management effectiveness in interviews 2 ($r = -.651$; $p = .009$), 5 ($r = -.574$; $p = .025$), and 7

($r = -.656$; $p = .008$); there was no significant relation between management effectiveness and pain intensity afterward." The investigators would be accused of lacking objectivity if they had stated the results in the following manner: "The results were not surprising as we found a significant relationship between pain intensity and pain management, as we expected." Opinions or reactionary statements about the data in the "Results" section are therefore avoided. Box 17-1 provides examples of objectively stated results. The critiquer of a study should consider the following points when reading a "Results" section:

- The investigators responded objectively to the results in the discussion of the results.
- In the discussion of the results, the investigator interpreted the evidence provided by the results, with a careful reflection on all aspects of the study that preceded the results.
- The data presented are summarized. Much data are generated, but only the critical summary numbers for each test are pre-

---

BOX 17-1   EXAMPLES OF RESULTS SECTION

"Mothers reported significantly lower levels of total mood disturbance after transplantation than at the pretransplantation evaluation (t [3.07], df = .14, $p < .01$)" (LoBiondo-Wood et al., 2004).

"For depression the predictor variables (resources and appraisal) accounted for 30% of the variance (F = 8.45, $p < .001$)" (Lee et al., 2001).

"Results of t-tests on the 2-week data indicated that caregivers in the intervention cohort reported higher scores on continuity of information about the elder's condition ($t = 2.28$, $p = .026$) and about services available ($t = 2.19$, $p = .03$)" (Bull, Hansen, and Gross, 2000).

"Abused women reported a higher previous incidence of STD than did nonabused women, primarily trichomonas (16.5% vs. 6.2%, $p < .001$) and chlamydia (24.2% vs. 16.35, $p < .02$)" (Dimmitt Champion et al. 2001).

sented. Examples of summarized data are the means and standard deviations of age, education, and income. Including all data is too cumbersome. The results can be viewed as a summation section.

- The condensation of data is done both in the written text and through the use of tables and figures. Tables and figures facilitate the presentation of large amounts of data.
- Results for the descriptive and inferential statistics for each hypothesis or research question are presented. No data should be omitted even if they are not significant.
- Any untoward events during the course of the study should be reported.

In their study Van Cleve and associates (2004) developed tables to present the results visually. Table 17-2 provides descriptive results about the subjects' location of pain for all age groups and for the total sample. Table 17-3 provides partial

results of testing for differences in pain intensity before and after management and also coping differences between age groups (for complete results, see Appendix B). Tables allow researchers to provide a more visually thorough explanation and discussion of the results. Van Cleve et al. (2004) also use figures to show the children's use of analgesics over time. If tables and figures are used, they must be concise. Although the text is the major mode of communicating the results, the tables and figures serve a supplementary but independent role. The role of tables and figures is to report results with some detail that the investigator does not explore in the text. This does not mean that tables and figures should not be mentioned in the text. The amount of detail that the author uses in the text to describe the specific tabled data varies with the needs of the researcher. A good table is one that meets the following criteria:

- Supplements and economizes the text
- Has precise titles and headings
- Does not repeat the text

Another example of a table that meets these criteria can be found in the study by Koniak-Griffin and associates (2003; see Appendix A). The research team wanted to report the outcomes related to infant health and repeat childbearing during the first 24-months postpartum. Because of the number of variables, it is much easier for the reader to have a table that simply and clearly summarizes the results, as seen in

TABLE 17-2 **Pain Location**

	4-7 Years n (%)	8-17 Years n (%)	Total Sample n (%)
Legs	240 (29.1)	159 (23.4)	399 (26.4)
Abdomen	149 (18.0)	106 (15.6)	255 (16.6)
Head/neck	102 (12.4)	147 (20.6)	249 (16.4)
Back	116 (14.1)	104 (15.3)	220 (14.5)

From Van Cleve L, Bossert E, Beecroft P, Adlard K, Alvarea O, and Savedra MC: The pain experience of children with leukemia during the first year after diagnosis, *Nurs Res* 53: 1-10, 2004.

TABLE 17-3 **Intensity Before and After Management and Coping Differences in Pain**

Age/Interview	Before X̄ (SD)	After X̄ (SD)	Percent Change	t	p
Interview 1 ($n = 36$)	1.86 (1.22)	1.33 (0.99)	13.25	−2.574	.014*
Interview 2 ($n = 30$)	1.60 (1.48)	1.03 (1.13)	14.25	−1.979	.057
Interview 3 ($n = 26$)	1.62 (1.39)	1.46 (1.33)	4.0	−0.537	.596
Interview 4 ($n = 25$)	2.16 (1.43)	1.16 (1.11)	25.0	−2.887	.008**
Interview 5 ($n = 27$)	1.93 (1.38)	1.37 (1.18)	14.0	−1.922	.066
Interview 6 ($n = 22$)	1.91 (1.48)	0.91 (0.92)	25.0	−2.925	.008***
Interview 7 ($n = 23$)	1.91 (1.59)	1.26 (1.21)	16.25	−1.845	.079

*$P < .05$; **$P < .01$; ***$P < .001$
From Van Cleve L, Bossert E, Beecroft P, Adlard K, Alvarea O, and Savedra MC: The pain experience of children with leukemia during the first year after diagnosis, *Nurs Res* 53: 1-10, 2004.

this table. To describe each one of these variables in the text of the article would not have economized space and would have been difficult to visualize. The table developed by the researchers (Table 17-4) allows the readers not only to visualize the variables quickly but also to assess the results.

 HELPFUL H I N T

A well-written "Results" section is systematic, logical, concise, and drawn from all of the analyzed data. All that is written in the "Results" section should be geared to letting the data reflect the testing of the problems and hypotheses. The length of this section depends on the scope and breadth of the analysis.

 EVIDENCE-BASED PRACTICE TIP

As you reflect upon the results of a study think about how the results fit with previous research on the topic and the strength and quality of available evidence on which to base clinical practice decisions.

Discussion of the Results

In the final section of the report, the investigator interprets and discusses the results of the study. In the "Discussion" section, a skilled researcher makes the data come alive. The researcher gives the numbers in quantitative studies or the concepts in qualitative studies meaning and interpretation. The reviewer may ask where the investigator extracted the meaning that is applied in this section. If the researcher does the job properly, the reviewer will find a return to the beginning of the study. The researcher returns to the earlier points in the study where a problem statement was identified and independent and dependent variables were related on the basis of a theoretical framework (Chapter 5) and literature review (Chapter 4). It is in this section that the researcher discusses the following:

- Both the supported and nonsupported data
- The limitations or weaknesses of a study in light of the design, the sample, instruments, or data-collection procedures
- How the theoretical framework was supported
- How the data may suggest additional or previously unrealized relationships

TABLE **17-4** **Infant Health Outcomes and Repeat Childbearing During the First 24 Months Postpartum**

Measure	Early Intervention Program (*n* = 56)	Traditional Public Health Nursing Care (*n* = 45)	Total (*N* = 101)
Inpatient hospitalizations (exclude birth-related hospitalizations***)	143	211	354
Episodes of hospitalizations**	19	36	55
Children hospitalized	12 (21%)	16 (36%)	28 (28%)
Emergency room visits			
Total number of ER visits	149	118	267
Number of children with ER visits	36 (64%)	40 (89%)	76 (75%)
Number of children with no ER visits within 24 months*	20 (36%)	5 (11%)	25 (25%)
Immunization status			
Children adequately immunized	77%	87%	82%

*$p < .05$; **$p < .01$; ***$p < .001$.
Note: ER = emergency room.
Koniak-Griffin D, Verzemnieks IL, Anderson NLR, Brecht ML, Lesses J, Kim S, and Turner-Pluts C: Nurse visitation for adolescent mothers: two-year infant health and maternal outcomes, *Nurs Res* 52:127-136, 2003.

- The strength and quality of the evidence provided by the study and its findings interpreted in relation to its applicability to practice

Even if the data are supported, the reviewer should not believe it to be the final word. It is important to remember that statistical significance is not the end point of a researcher's thinking and low *p* values may not be indicative of research breakthroughs. To the research critiquer, this means that statistical significance in a research study does not always indicate that the results of a study are clinically significant. As the body of nursing research grows, so does the profession's ability to critically analyze beyond the test of significance and assess a research study's applicability to practice. Chapters 19 and 20 review methods used to analyze the usefulness and applicability of research findings. Within the nursing literature, discussion of clinical significance and evidence-based practice has also emerged (Melnyk and Fineout-Overholt, 2002; Goode, 2000; Ingersoll, 2000). As indicated throughout this text, many important pieces in the research puzzle must fit together for a study to be evaluated as a well-done project. The evidence generated by the findings of a research study is appraised in order to validate current practice and/or support the need for a change in practice. Therefore researchers and reviewers should accept statistical significance with prudence. Statistically significant findings are not the sole means of establishing the study's merit. Remember that accepting statistical significance solely means that one is accepting that the sample mean is the same as the population mean, which may not be true (see Chapters 12 and 17). Another method to assess if the findings from one study can be generalized is to calculate a **confidence interval.** A confidence interval quantifies the uncertainty of a statistic or the probable value range within which a population parameter is expected to lie (see Chapter 20). The process used to calculate a confidence interval is beyond the scope of this text, but references are provided for further explanation (Gardner and Altman, 1986, 1989; Wright, 1997). Other aspects, such as

theory, sample, instrumentation, and methods, should also be considered.

When the results are not statistically supported, the researcher also returns to the theoretical framework and analyzes the earlier thinking process. Results of nonsupported hypotheses do not require the investigator to go on a fault-finding tour of each piece of the project. Such a course can become an overdone process. All research has weakness. This analysis is an attempt to identify the weaknesses and to suggest what the possible or actual problems were in the study. At times, the theoretical thinking is correct, but the researcher finds that the strength of the evidence offered is affected by problems or limitations that could be attributed to the instruments (see Chapters 14 and 15), the sampling methods (see Chapter 12), the design (see Chapters 9 to 11), or the analysis (see Chapter 16). Therefore when results are not supported, the investigator attempts to go on a fact-finding tour rather than a fault-finding one. The purpose of the discussion, then, is not to show humility or one's technical competence but rather to enable the reviewer to judge the validity of the interpretations drawn from the data and the general worth of the study. It is in the "Discussion" section of the report that the researcher ties together all the loose ends of the study and returns to the beginning to assess if the findings support, extend, or counter the theoretical framework of the study. It is from this point that reviewers of research can begin to think about clinical relevance, the need for replication, or the germination of an idea for further research study. Finally, the reviewer of a research project should find this section either in separate sections or subsumed within the "Discussion" section, and it should include generalizability and recommendations for future research, as well as a summary or a conclusion.

Generalizations **(generalizability)** are inferences that the data are representative of similar phenomena in a population beyond the study's sample. Reviewers of research are cautioned not to generalize beyond the population on which a study is based. Rarely, if ever, can one study be a recommendation for action. Beware of research studies that may overgeneralize. Generalizations that draw conclusions and make inferences within a particular situation and at a particular time are appropriate. An example of such a generalization is drawn from the study conducted by Lee and associates (2001) that was designed to study the relationship between empathy and caregiving appraisal and outcomes in informal caregivers of older adults. The researchers, when discussing the sample in light of the results, appropriately noted the following:

"Several limitations can be noted in this study. First, the results are drawn from a sample of primarily white caregivers with relatively high educational levels. Therefore, the results are only generalizable to those with similar backgrounds. . . . Suggestions for future research would be to include subjects from varied ethnic backgrounds and to recruit subjects randomly from the community . . ."

This type of statement is important for reviewers of research. It helps to guide thinking in terms of a study's clinical relevance and also suggests areas for further research (see Chapters 19 and 20). One study does not provide all of the answers, nor should it. The final steps of evaluation are critical links to the refinement of practice and the generation of future research. Evaluation of research, like evaluation of the nursing process, is not the last link in the chain but a connection between findings that may serve to improve nursing theory and nursing practice.

BOX 17-2   EXAMPLES OF RESEARCH RECOMMENDATIONS AND PRACTICE IMPLICATIONS

RESEARCH RECOMMENDATIONS

"Further investigation is needed to incorporate fathers' views. Also lacking are the children's views. These children are difficult to study because the majority undergo surgery before 5 years of age. The study's findings emphasize the importance of exploring over time how families are affected by long term needs" (LoBiondo-Wood et al., 2004).

"Further directions for research are to determine whether the influences on fatigue supported in the trimmed models continue at later points in the treatment protocol and whether they are apparent in treatment for other cancer diagnoses" (Berger and Walker, 2001).

"Suggestions for future research would be to include subjects from varied ethnic backgrounds and to recruit subjects randomly from the community so that caregivers who do not have access to social services can be included. This sampling approach would increase the generalizability of the findings" (Lee et al., 2001).

PRACTICE IMPLICATIONS

"One consistent finding was noted when women with higher baseline role/physical function reported higher fatigue at the first two cycle midpoints. Perhaps these women pushed themselves to continue to perform usual daily activities at pretreatment levels, leading to higher fatigue. Education on the use of energy conservation techniques may assist women of all lifestyles during chemotherapy" (Berger and Walker, 2001).

"The findings lead to the conclusion that interventions with the parents of this vulnerable group should focus not only on improving parenting quality, but also on promoting the physical and emotional health of mothers so as to reduce the frequency of caregiver changes. However, interventions need to be ethnically appropriate and include support, as well as education, for mothers" (Holditch-Davis et al., 2001).

"The study's findings suggest that as nurses teach and support mothers prior to the transplant surgery, they need to take into account the uncertainty and stress that mothers feel early in the process. A great deal of information and teaching are provided prior to the transplant. The stress perceived early in the process may mask coping skills. In light of the high stress levels, use of fewer coping mechanisms and uncertainty suggests the need for follow-up and teaching reinforcement" (LoBiondo-Wood et al., 2004).

HELPFUL H I N T

It has been said that a good study is one that raises more questions than it answers. So the research consumer should not view an investigator's review of limitations, generalizations, and implications of the findings for practice as lack of research skills but as the beginning of the next step in the research process.

The final area that the investigator integrates into the "Discussion" section is the recommendations. The **recommendations** are the investigator's suggestions for the study's application to practice, theory, and further research. This requires the investigator to reflect on the following questions:

- "What contribution to nursing does this study make?"
- "What is the strength, quality, and consistency of the evidence provided by the findings?"
- "Does the evidence provided in the findings validate current practice or support the need for change in practice?"

Box 17-2 provides examples of recommendations for future research and implications for nursing practice. This evaluation places the study into the realm of what is known and what needs to be known before being utilized. Nursing knowledge and practice have grown tremendously over the last century through the efforts of many nursing researchers and scholars. This thought is critical and has been reaffirmed by many nurse researchers in the past decade, such as Hinshaw (2000) and Gortner (2000).

CRITIQUING GUIDE *Results and Discussion*

The results and the discussion of the results are the researcher's opportunity to examine the logic of the hypothesis(es) or research question(s) posed, the theoretical framework, the methods, and the analysis (see the following Critiquing Criteria box). This final section requires as much logic, conciseness, and specificity as employed in the preceding steps of the research process. The consumer should be able to identify statements of the type of analysis that was used and whether the data statistically supported the hypothesis(es) or research question(s). These statements should be straightforward and not reflect bias (see Tables 17-3 and 17-4). Auxiliary data or serendipitous findings also may be pre-

sented. If such auxiliary findings are presented, they should be as dispassionately presented as were the hypothesis and research question data. The statistical test used also should be noted. The numerical value of the obtained data also should be presented (see Tables 17-1, 17-3, and 17-4). The presentation of the tests, the numerical values found, and the statements of support or nonsupport should be clear, concise, and systematically reported. For illustrative purposes that facilitate readability, the researchers should present extensive findings in tables.

The "Discussion" section should interpret the data for further research, including its strength and quality, gaps, limitations, and conclusions of

1. Are the results of each of the hypotheses presented?
2. Is the information regarding the results concisely and sequentially presented?
3. Are the tests that were used to analyze the data presented?
4. Are the results presented objectively?
5. If tables or figures are used, do they meet the following standards?
   a. They supplement and economize the text.
   b. They have precise titles and headings.
   c. They are not repetitious of the text.
6. Are the results interpreted in light of the hypotheses and theoretical framework and all of the other steps that preceded the results?
7. If the data are supported, does the investigator provide a discussion of how the theoretical framework was supported?
8. If the data are not supported, does the investigator attempt to identify the study's weaknesses and strengths, as well as suggest possible solutions for the research area?
9. Does the researcher discuss the study's clinical relevance?
10. Are any generalizations made, and if so are they within the scope of the findings or beyond the findings?
11. Are any recommendations for future research stated or implied?
12. What is the study's strength of evidence?

the study, as well as give recommendations in tables. If the study is related to a larger program of research, the investigator can discuss the relationship of this study to the program of research. For example, Hoskins and colleagues (2001) report the findings of a pilot study designed to test the differential effectiveness of a phase-specific educational video intervention in comparison to a telephone counseling intervention on emotional, social, and physical adjustment of women with breast cancer and their partners. The "Discussion" section identifies this pilot study as phase III of this program of research and sets the stage for phase IV, a randomized clinical trial. Drawing these aspects into the study should give the consumer a sense of the relationship of the findings to the theoretical framework as well as the larger context of the research. Statements reflecting the underlying theory are necessary, whether or not the hypotheses were supported.

If the findings were not supported, the consumer should—as the researcher did—attempt to identify, without finding fault, possible methodological problems (e.g., sample too small to detect a treatment effect). Finally, a concise presentation of the study's generalizability and the implications of the findings for practice and research should be evident. The last presentation can help the research consumer begin to rethink clinical practice, provoke discussion in clinical settings (see Chapters 19 and 20), and find similar studies that may support or refute the phenomena being studied to more fully understand the problem.

One study alone does not lead to a practice change. Evidence-based practice requires the research consumer to critically read and understand each study, that is, the quality of the study, the strength of the evidence generated by the findings and its consistency with other studies in the area, and the number of studies that were conducted in the area. This assessment along with the active use of clinical judgment and patient preference leads to evidence-based practice.

Critical Thinking Challenges

- Defend or refute the following statement: "All results should be reported and interpreted whether or not they support the hypothesis." If all the findings are not reported, would this affect the applicability to your patient population and practice setting?
- What type of knowledge does the researcher draw on to interpret the results of a study? Is the same type of knowledge used when the results of a study are not statistically significant?
- Do you agree or disagree with the statement that "a good study is one that raises more questions than it answers"? Support your view with examples.
- How is it possible for research consumers to critique the findings and recommendations of a reported study? How could you use the internet for critiquing the findings of a study?
- Now that nurses and nursing students have access to the Cochrane Library database or *Evidence-Based Nursing* (both critique multiple studies available on a clinical topic), as well as published meta-analyses on clinical research topics, why is it still necessary to learn how to critically read and critique research studies? Justify your response.

KEY POINTS

- The analysis of the findings is the final step of a research investigation. It is in this section that the consumer will find the results printed in a straightforward manner.
- All results should be reported whether or not they support the hypothesis. Tables and figures may be used to illustrate and condense data for presentation.
- Once the results are reported, the researcher interprets the results. In this presentation, usually titled "Discussion," the consumer should be able to identify the key topics being discussed. The key topics, which include an interpretation of the results, are the limitations, generalizations, implications, and recommendations for future research.
- The researcher draws together the theoretical framework and makes interpretations based on the findings and theory in the section on the interpretation of the results. Both statistically supported and unsupported results should be interpreted. If the results are not supported, the researcher should discuss the results, reflecting on the theory, as well as possible problems with the methods, procedures, design, and analysis.

- The researcher should present the limitations or weaknesses of the study. This presentation is important because it affects the study's generalizability. The generalizations or inferences about similar findings in other samples also are presented in light of the findings.
- The research consumer should be alert for sweeping claims or overgeneralizations that a researcher may state. An overextension of the data can alert the consumer to possible researcher bias.
- The recommendations provide the consumer with suggestions regarding the study's application to practice, theory, and future research. These recommendations furnish the critiquer with a final perspective from the researcher on the utility of the investigation.
- The strength, quality, and consistency of the evidence provided by the findings are related to the study's limitations, generalizability, and applicability to practice.

REFERENCES

Berger AN, Walker SN: An exploratory model of fatigue in women receiving adjuvant breast cancer chemotherapy, *Nurs Res* 50: 42-52, 2001.

Bull MJ, Hansen HE, and Gross CR: A professional-patient partnership model of discharge planning with elders hospitalized with heart failure, *Nurs Res* 13(1): 19-28, 2000.

Dimmitt Champion J et al.: Minority women with sexually transmitted diseases: sexual abuse and risk for pelvic inflammatory disease, *Res Nurs Health* 24: 38-43, 2001.

Gardner MJ, Altman DG: Confidence intervals rather than p values: estimation rather than hypothesis testing, *Brit Med J Clin Res* 292: 746-750, 1986.

Gardner MJ, Altman DG, editors: Statistics with confidence, *Brit Med J*, 255: 659, 1989.

Goode CJ: What constitutes the "evidence" in evidence-based practice, *Appl Nurs Res* 13(4): 222-225, 2000.

Gortner S: Knowledge development in nursing: our historical roots and future opportunities, *Nurs Outlook* 48: 60-67, 2000.

Hinshaw AS: Nursing knowledge for the 21st century: opportunities and challenges, *J Nurs Scholarship* 32(2): 117-123, 2000.

Holditch-Davis D et al.: Parental caregiving and developmental outcomes of infants of mothers with HIV, *Nurs Res* 50: 5-14, 2001.

Hoskins CN, Haber J, Budin WC, Cartwright-Alcarese F, Kowalski MO, Panke J, and Maislin G: Breast cancer: education, counseling, and adjustment—a pilot study, *Psychol Rep* 89: 677-704, 2001.

Ingersoll GL: Evidence-based nursing: what it is and what it isn't, *Nurs Outlook* 48: 151, 2000.

Koniak-Griffin D, Verzemnieks IL, Anderson NLR, Brecht ML, Lesses J, Kim S, and Turner-Pluts C: Nurse visitation for adolescent mothers: two-year infant health and maternal outcomes, *Nurs Res* 52: 127-136, 2003.

Lee HS, Brennan PF, and Daly BJ: Relationship of empathy to appraisal, depression, life satisfaction, and physical health in informal caregivers of older adults, *Res Nurs Health* 24: 44-56, 2001.

LoBiondo-Wood G et al.: The impact of transplantation on quality of life: a longitudinal perspective, *J Spec Ped Nurs* 9: 59-66, 2004.

Melnyk BM, Fineout-Overholt E: Key steps in evidence based practice: asking compelling questions and searching for the best evidence, *Ped Nurs* 28: 262, 263,266, 2002.

Van Cleve L, Bossert E, Beecroft P, Adlard K, Alvarea O, and Savedra MC: The pain experience of children with leukemia during the first year after diagnosis, *Nurs Res* 53: 1-10, 2004.

Wright DB: *Understanding statistics: an introduction for the social sciences*, London, 1997, Sage Publications.

FOR FURTHER STUDY

⊙ Go to your Companion CD for review activities for this chapter.

evolve Go to Evolve at http://evolve.elsevier.com/LoBiondo/ for WebLinks, Content Updates, and additional research articles, for practice in reviewing and critiquing.

18

JUDITH A. HEERMANN

BETTY J. CRAFT

Evaluating Quantitative Research

KEY TERMS

evidence-base
replication

scientific merit

LEARNING OUTCOMES

After reading this chapter, the student should be able to do the following:
- Identify the purpose of the critiquing process.
- Describe the criteria for each step of the critiquing process.
- Evaluate the strengths and weaknesses of a research report.
- Apply levels of evidence to evaluation of a quantitative research report.
- Discuss the implications of the findings of a research report for evidence-based nursing practice.
- Construct a critique of a research report.

STUDY RESOURCES

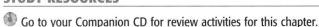 Go to your Companion CD for review activities for this chapter.

evolve Go to Evolve at http://evolve.elsevier.com/LoBiondo/ for Weblinks, Content Updates, and additional research articles for practice in reviewing and critiquing.

As reinforced throughout each chapter of this book, it is not just important to do and read research but to use research actively for evidence-based practice. As nurse researchers increase the depth (quality) and breadth (quantity) from descriptive research designs to randomized clinical trials, the data to support clinical interventions and quality outcomes are becoming more readily available. Each published study, no matter which design used, reflects a *level of evidence*, but the critique of each study goes well beyond the level of evidence produced by the design used. The strength of the evidence that each study produces individually and collectively is key. This chapter presents a critique of two studies that each test questions with different quantitative designs using the critiquing criteria.

Each component of a research study is examined to determine the merit of a research report.

Criteria designed to assist you in judging the relative value of a research report are found in previous chapters. An abbreviated set of questions summarizing the more detailed criteria, found at the end of each chapter, is used in this chapter as a framework for two sample research critiques (Table 18-1). These critiques are included to exemplify the process of evaluating reported research for potential application to practice, thus extending the evidence-base for nursing. For clarification, you are encouraged to refer to the earlier chapters for the detailed presentation of the critiquing criteria and explanations of the research process. The criteria and examples in this chapter apply to quantitative studies using experimental, quasiexperimental, and nonexperimental research designs that provided Level II, III, and IV evidence.

STYLISTIC CONSIDERATIONS

As an evaluator you should realize several important aspects related to the world of publishing before beginning to critique research studies. First, different journals have different publication goals and target specific professional markets. For example, *Nursing Research* is a journal that publishes articles on the conduct or results of research in nursing. Although *The Journal of Obstetric, Gynecologic, and Neonatal Nursing* publishes research articles, it also includes articles related to the knowledge, experience, trends, and policies in obstetrical, gynecological, and neonatal nursing. The emphasis in the latter journal is broader in that it contains clinical and theoretical articles, as well as research articles. Consequently, the style and content of a manuscript vary according to the type of journal to which it is being submitted.

Second, the author of a research article prepares the manuscript using both personal judgment and specific guidelines. *Personal judgment* refers to the researcher's expertise that is developed in the course of designing, executing, and analyzing the study. As a result of this expertise, the researcher is in the position to judge which content is most important to communicate to the profession. The decision is a function of the following:

- The research design: experimental or nonexperimental
- The focus of the study: basic or clinical
- The audience to which the results will be most appropriately communicated

Guidelines are provided by each journal for preparing research manuscripts for publication. The following major headings are essential sections in the research report:

- Introduction
- Methodology
- Results
- Discussion

Depending on stylistic considerations related to author's preferences and the publishing journal requirements, specific content is included in each section of the research report. Stylistic variations (as factors influencing the presentation of the research study) are distinct from the focus of evaluating the reported research for **scientific merit.** Constructive evaluation is based on objective, unbiased, and impartial appraisal of the evidence provided by the study findings in relation to the strengths and limitations. This is a step that precedes consideration of the relative worth (e.g., strength, quality, and consistency of evidence) of the findings for clinical application to nursing practice. Such judgments are the hallmark of promoting a sound evidence-base for quality nursing practice.

TABLE **18-1** **Major Content Sections of a Research Report and Related Critiquing Guidelines**

Section	Questions to Guide Evaluation
Problem statement and purpose (see Chapter 3)	1. What is the problem and/or purpose of the research study? 2. Does the problem or purpose statement express a relationship between two or more variables (e.g., between an independent and a dependent variable)? If so, what is/are the relationship(s)? Are they testable? 3. Does the problem statement and/or purpose specify the nature of the population being studied? What is it? 4. What significance of the problem—if any—has the investigator identified?
Review of literature and theoretical framework (see Chapters 4 and 5)	1. What concepts are included in the review? Of particular importance, note those concepts that are the independent and dependent variables and how they are conceptually defined. 2. Does the literature review make the relationships among the variables explicit or place the variables within a theoretical/conceptual framework? What are the relationships? 3. What gaps or conflicts in knowledge of the problem are identified? How is this study intended to fill those gaps or resolve those conflicts? 4. Are the references cited by the author mostly primary or secondary sources? Give an example of each. 5. What are the operational definitions of the independent and dependent variables? Do they reflect the conceptual definitions?
Hypothesis(es) or research question(s) (see Chapter 3)	1. What hypothesis(es) or research questions are stated in the study? Are they appropriately stated? 2. If research questions are stated, are they used in addition to hypotheses or to guide an exploratory study? 3. What are the independent and dependent variables in the statement of each hypothesis/research question? 4. If hypotheses are stated, is the form of the statement statistical (null) or research? 5. What is the direction of the relationship in each hypothesis, if indicated? 6. Are the hypotheses testable?
Sample (see Chapter 12)	1. How was the sample selected? 2. What type of sampling method is used in the study? Is it appropriate to the design? 3. Does the sample reflect the population as identified in the problem or purpose statement? 4. Is the sample size appropriate? How is it substantiated? 5. To what population may the findings be generalized? What are the limitations in generalizability?
Research design (see Chapters 9 to 11)	1. What type of design is used in the study? 2. What is the rationale for the design classification? 3. Does the design seem to flow from the proposed research problem, theoretical framework, literature review, and hypothesis?
Internal validity (see Chapter 9)	1. Discuss each threat to the internal validity of the study. 2. Does the design have controls at an acceptable level for the threats to internal validity?
External validity (see Chapter 9)	1. What are the limits to generalizability in terms of external validity?

TABLE **18-1** **Major Content Sections of a Research Report and Related Critiquing Guidelines—cont'd**

Section	Questions to Guide Evaluation
Research approach	
Methods (see Chapter 14)	1. What type(s) of data-collection method(s) is/are used in the study? 2. Are the data-collection procedures similar for all subjects?
Legal-ethical issues (see Chapter 13)	1. How have the rights of subjects been protected? 2. What indications are given that informed consent of the subjects has been ensured?

Instruments (see Chapter 14)	1. Physiological measurement
	   a. Is a rationale given for why a particular instrument or method was selected? If so, what is it?
	   b. What provision is made for maintaining the accuracy of the instrument and its use, if any?
	2. Observational methods.
	   a. Who did the observing?
	   b. How were the observers trained to minimize bias?
	   c. Was there an observational guide?
	   d. Were the observers required to make inferences about what they saw?
	   e. Is there any reason to believe that the presence of the observers affecte the behavior of the subjects?
	3. Interviews
	   a. Who were the interviewers? How were they trained to minimize bias?
	   b. Is there evidence of any interview bias? If so, what is it?
	4. Questionnaires
	   a. What is the type and/or format of the questionnaire(s) (e.g., Likert, open-ended)? Is(Are) it(they) consistent with the conceptual definition(s)?
	5. Available data and records
	   a. Are the records that were used appropriate to the problem being studied?
	   b. Are the data being used to describe the sample or to test the hypothesis?

Reliability and validity (see Chapter 15)	1. What type of reliability is reported for each instrument? 2. What level of reliability is reported? Is it acceptable? 3. What type of validity is reported for each instrument? 4. Does the validity of each instrument seem adequate? Why?

Analysis of data (see Chapter 16)	1. What level of measurement is used to measure each of the major variables?
	2. What descriptive or inferential statistics are reported?
	3. Were these descriptive or inferential statistics appropriate to the level of measurement for each variable?
	4. Are the inferential statistics used appropriate to the intent of the hypothesis(es)?
	5. Does the author report the level of significance set for the study? If so, what is it?
	6. If tables or figures are used, do they meet the following standards?
	   a. They supplement and economize the text.
	   b. They have precise titles and headings.
	   c. They do not repeat the text.

TABLE **18-1** **Major Content Sections of a Research Report and Related Critiquing Guidelines—cont'd**

Section	Questions to Guide Evaluation
Conclusions, implications, and recommendations (see Chapter 17)	1. If hypothesis(es) testing was done, was/were the hypothesis(es) supported or not supported?
	2. Are the results interpreted in the context of the problem/purpose, hypothesis, and theoretical framework/literature reviewed?
	3. What does the investigator identify as possible limitations and/or problems in the study related to the design, methods, and sample?
	4. What relevance for nursing practice does the investigator identify, if any?
	5. What generalizations are made?
	6. Are the generalizations within the scope of the findings or beyond the findings?
	7. What recommendations for future research are stated or implied?
Application and utilization for nursing practice (see Chapter 17)	1. Does the study appear valid? That is, do its strengths outweigh its weaknesses?
	2. Are there other studies with similar findings?
	3. What risks/benefits are involved for patients if the research findings would be used in practice?
	4. Is direct application of the research findings feasible in terms of time, effort, money, and legal/ethical risks?
	5. How and under what circumstances are the findings applicable to nursing practice?
	6. Should these results be applied to nursing practice?
	7. Would it be possible to replicate this study in another clinical practice setting?
	8. What is the study's level of evidence?
	9. What is the study's strength of evidence?

CRITIQUE *of a Quantitative Research Study*

SAMPLE #1

The study *An Exercise Program to Improve Fall-Related Outcomes in Elderly Nursing Home Residents* by Schoenfelder and Rubenstein (2004) is critiqued. The article is presented in its entirety and is followed by the critique on p. 000. (From *Applied Nursing Research* 17:21-31, 2004.)

AN EXERCISE PROGRAM TO IMPROVE FALL-RELATED OUTCOMES IN ELDERLY NURSING HOME RESIDENTS

Deborah Perry Schoenfelder and Linda M. Rubenstein

This study tested a 3-month ankle-strengthening and walking program designed to improve or maintain the fall-related outcomes of balance, ankle strength, walking speed, risk of falling, fear of falling, and confidence to perform daily activities without falling (falls efficacy) in elderly nursing home residents. Nursing home residents ($N = 81$) between the ages of 64 and 100 years participated in the study. Two of the fall-related outcomes, balance and fear of falling, were maintained or improved for the exercise group in comparison to the control group.

© 2004 Elsevier Inc. All rights reserved.

OLDER ADULTS WHO RESIDE in nursing homes often have multiple health risks, including the risk of falling with the resultant potential for injury. Frail elders who fall are likely to fall repeatedly, further increasing their risk for serious injury. Fractures, soft-tissue injury and immobility may lead to long-term disability or death. The fear of falling again may inhibit physical activities necessary for good health and can compromise quality of life when older people restrict their activities beyond what is necessary for safety (Lachman, et al., 1998: Mustard & Mayer, 1997).

There is promise that exercise can improve fall-related outcomes. Results of a pilot study suggested that a walking and ankle-strengthening program could improve fall-related outcomes and prevent or slow physical deterioration in elderly nursing home residents (Schoenfelder, 2000). This follow-up study investigated the effectiveness of an ankle-strengthening and walking program for elderly nursing home residents in improving balance, ankle strength, and walking speed; decreasing risk of falling and fear of falling; and improving confidence in performing daily activities without falling (falls efficacy).

BACKGROUND

Incidence

Falls are the most frequently reported adverse incident in long-term care facilities (Gurwitz, Sanchez-Cross, Eckler, & Matulis, 1994). A fall can be defined as any event in which a person inadvertently or intentionally comes to rest on the ground or another low level (Tideiksaar, 1998). At least 40% of older nursing home residents fall annually, with a mean incidence rate of 1.5 falls per bed per year (Nygaard, 1998).

Risk Factors

Risk factors for falling are classified as intrinsic or extrinsic. Intrinsic factors are internal to the individual. Increased age, a history of falls, impaired balance, poor muscle strength including ankle strength, and slow walking speed are examples of intrinsic risk factors (Davis, Ross, Nevitt, & Wasnich, 1999; Mustard & Mayer, 1997). Other intrinsic risk factors include age-related physiologic changes and chronic conditions of various body systems, particularly cardiovascular, neurologic, musculoskeletal, and urologic conditions

Deborah Perry Schoenfelder, PhD, RN. *Clinical Associate Professor, College of Nursing, The University of Iowa, Iowa City, IA, USA.* Linda M. Rubenstein, PhD. *Assistant Research Scientist, Department of Epidemiology, College of Public Health. The University of Iowa, Iowa City, IA, USA.*

Supported by grant # 1 R15 NR04220-01A1 through the National Institutes of Health.

Address reprint requests to Deborah Perry Schoenfelder, PhD, RN, College of Nursing, The University of Iowa, 378 Nursing Building, University of Iowa, Iowa City, IA 52242. E-mail: deborah-schoenfelder@uiowa.edu

0897-1897/04/1701-0004$30.00/0
doi:10.1016/j.apnr.2003.10.008

(Edwards & Lee, 1998; Tinetti & Williams, 1998). Gait and balance impairments are strong predictors for falling, and walking velocity has been found to be slower for older adults who fall than for older nonfallers (Cho & Kamen, 1998; Davis, Ross, Nevitt, Wasnich, 1999; Edwards & Lee, 1998). Acute health status changes also put older adults at risk for falling (Kuehn & Sendelweck, 1995), as does adverse reactions to medications (Leipzig, Cumming, & Tinetti, 1999; Mustard & Mayer, 1997). In addition to being a consequence of falling, fear of falling has been identified as a risk factor for falling (Baloh, Jacobson, Enrietto, Corona, & Honrubia, 1998). There is evidence that falls efficacy, the confidence that an individual has to do daily activities without falling, is an important factor to consider in fall prevention efforts (Tinetti, Richman, & Powell, 1990).

Extrinsic risk factors for falling are those environmental hazards that increase the chances of falling such as the presence of throw rugs, low lighting, and slippery floors (North American Nursing Diagnosis Association, 2001; Schoenfelder, 2000). The way older persons function in and interact with their environments also affects their safety. One study suggested that those who are distracted by doing a familiar, manual task along with functional maneuvers are more apt to fall (Lundin-Olsson, Nyberg, & Gustafson, 1998).

Exercise Studies

Older adults benefit from exercise of various types, including muscle strengthening exercises, flexibility training, aerobic exercises, and walking to offset declining strength or to increase muscle strength and to improve balance and gait velocity (Chandler & Hadley, 1996). There is evidence that exercise can also reduce falling and risk of falling in older people. A review of controlled clinical trials reported that studies successfully reduced falls or risk of falls when strength and balance retraining, endurance training, and Tai Chi were used (Gardner, Robertson, & Campbell, 2000).

The bulk of the research that tests the effects of exercise on fall-related outcomes for older adults has been done with community-dwelling elders. For example, in a study that used strength and balance exercises for older women living in the community, participants in the exercise group had improved balance

and had a lower fall rate than the control group. The proportion of participants who were injured from a fall was lower in the exercise group (26.2%) than in the control group (39.1%) (Campbell et al., 1997). Buchner and colleagues (1997) tested the effect of strength and endurance training for older community-dwelling adults and found there was a significant beneficial effect of exercise on time to first fall and on the overall fall rate for exercisers that was not present for those in the control group.

Walking is a common form of exercise and can be highly beneficial for older adults. Older nursing home residents who participated in a walking program showed improvement in their ambulatory status (measured on a seven point scale ranging from "independence" to "complete dependence") and a decrease in falls after participating in the program (Koroknay, Werner, Cohen-Mansfield, & Braun, 1995).

Walking is a common form of exercise and can be highly beneficial for older adults.

Although elderly nursing home residents are at a great risk for falling and deterioration of physical and functional abilities, this population has not been studied extensively to test the effects of exercise on fall-related outcomes. Keeping an exercise program uncomplicated and yet effective is key for beginning or sustaining a program so that nursing home staff will include a regularly scheduled program into their busy work days and elders will be more apt to exercise consistently. A simple program was chosen that included an ankle strengthening exercise followed by up to 10 minutes of supervised walking, so that equipment needs and time commitment for subjects and research staff were at a minimum. In addition, the combination of an ankle-strengthening exercise and walking program has not been reported in the literature.

Although elderly nursing home residents are at a great risk for falling and deterioration of physical and functional abilities, this population has not been studied extensively to test the effects of exercise on fall-related outcomes.

The researchers hypothesized that the proportion of elders with consistent or improved fall-related outcomes would be significantly higher for those individuals participating in the ankle strengthening and

Independent Variable	3 mos post intervention	6 mos post intervention
Exercise Program	Physiological Domain	Physiological Domain
– Ankle strengthening	↑ Balance	≈↓ Balance
– Walking	↑ Ankle strength	≈↓ Ankle strength
	↑ Walking speed	≈↓ Walking speed
	↓ Falls risk	≈↑ Falls risk
	Psychological Domain	Psychological Domain
	↓ Fear of failing	≈↑ Fear of failing
	↑ Falls Efficacy Scale	≈↓ Falls Efficacy Scale
↑ = increase	↓ = dectease	≈ = stay the same or worsen

Figure 1. Relationship of independent variables and outcome variables.

walking program than for those elders who did not participate. The fall-related outcomes for this study were balance, ankle strength, walking speed, falls risk, fear of falling, and confidence to perform daily activities without falling (falls efficacy). The predicted relationship of the exercise program and the fall-related outcomes is depicted in Figure 1.

METHODS

Setting and Participants

The study was conducted in 10 private, urban nursing homes in eastern Iowa, ranging in size from 68 beds to 178 beds. The procedures to protect human subjects in this study were reviewed and approved by The University of Iowa Institutional Review Board. Nursing home residents were recruited who (1) were at least 65 years old; (2) were able to ambulate independently or with an assistive device so that they could take part in the ankle-strengthening and walking program; (3) were able to speak English; (4) did not have an unstable physical condition, evidence of an end-stage terminal illness, or a history of acting-out or abusive behavior, and (5) had a score of 20 or above on the Mini-Mental State Examination to be able to answer the interview questions and to understand and follow directions for the ankle strengthening and walking program. After obtaining signed informed consent, chart reviews were conducted by research team members to ascertain any chronic conditions. Physicians were contacted and asked to indicate potential participants who might have physical conditions that would contraindicate taking part in the exercise program.

Procedure

Participants were matched in pairs by Risk Assessment for Falls Scale II scores (RAFS II) and randomly assigned within each pair to the intervention or control group. When subjects were roommates or spouses, those individuals were assigned to the same group to lessen the possibility of contamination between the intervention and control groups.

Subjects assigned to the intervention group participated in a 3-month ankle-strengthening and walking program and had data collected on demographics, mobility/activity information, balance, ankle strength, walking speed, fall risk data, fear of falling, and falls efficacy before the intervention and at 3 months (completion of the intervention) and 6 months after initiation of the intervention.

Subjects in the control group were assessed for the same baseline data as the intervention group subjects. Data were gathered again at 3 and 6 months with no exercise intervention by the research team. The group did, however, receive an attention placebo to control for the effects of attention and motivational strategies. Subjects in the control group were visited weekly by the same research team member that conducted the exercise program. About 30 minutes was devoted each time to an activity such as book reading or "friendly visiting."

For all assessments conducted at 3 and 6 months, examiners doing the assessments had no contact with the participants other than the assessments once group assignments were made. The examiners were graduate and undergraduate students who were trained by the principal investigator to accurately collect the data and correctly and safely perform the exercise intervention.

Intervention

The 3-month supervised exercising was done three times weekly for about 15 to 20 minutes each time. The ankle-strengthening exercise was done first followed by the supervised walking. The training program was tailored to individual's ability to do the ankle exercise at the beginning of the program and the distance and time the subject was able to walk for the timed 6-meter walk at pretest. The program was advanced as strength and endurance increased and the exercises were mastered. Equipment necessary for the exercise program included any assistive device the subject used and a straight chair. A research team member closely supervised subjects as they exercised. Team members were graduate and undergraduate students who were trained by the principal investigator to safely supervise correct performance of the exercise intervention.

Ankle-strengthening exercise. In addition to strengthening the ankles, this exercise served as a warmup for the walking program. The ankle strengthening exercise consisted of (1) standing upright with knees straight, slowly raise both heels until weight is on balls of the feet doing up to three sets of 10 to 15 repetitions, while holding onto the back of a straight chair, and then when able progressing to (2) bilateral heel raises (as described earlier) with ankle weights attached, increasing the weight when the subject is able to complete three sets of 10 to 15 repetitions.

Walking program. Subjects walked for 10 minutes, if tolerated. Time was increased until 10 minutes of sustained walking was reached. If and when that goal was reached, subjects were encouraged to walk at a faster (yet safe and functional) pace for 10 uninterrupted minutes.

Variables/Instruments

Demographic information. Age, sex, marital status, race, education, and length of residence at the nursing home were collected.

Mobility/activity information. Level of mobility was ascertained by asking participants whether they ambulate unassisted, with an assistive device, or with an

assistive device and another person. Subjects were also observed for their mobility level when walking speed was measured. In addition, subjects were asked how often they walked, attended group exercise classes, and other activities/exercises in which they participated.

Fear of falling. Subjects were asked "How concerned are you about falling?" to which they could respond "not at all concerned," "somewhat concerned," "fairly concerned," or "very concerned." If subjects responded somewhat, fairly, or very concerned, the follow-up question "Do you think this concern has made you cut down on the activities that you used to do?" was asked to which the subject could respond with a "yes" or "no." Test-retest reliability for the first question was acceptable (Kappa = 0.66) and lower for the second question (Kappa = 0.36) (Tinetti, Richman, & Powell, 1990).

Balance. Balance was measured by a stopwatch for up to 10 seconds in three stances: (1) parallel stance ("Classic Romberg" with feet together, side by side), (2) semitandem stance (toe of one foot beside heel of other foot), and (3) tandem stance ("Sharpen Romberg" stance, with heel of one foot touching and in a straight line with the toe of the other). No assistive devices were allowed, eyes were open during the stances, and arms could be in any position. Pearson correlation coefficients reported by Graybiel and Fregly (1966) for the parallel and tandem stances ranged from 0.57 to 0.96.

Ankle strength. Ankle plantar flexion strength was measured by having subjects place their dominant foot on a mechanical force transducer. The foot and upper leg were contained in an apparatus to stabilize the foot and leg and keep the knee flexed at a 90° angle and to keep the plantar surface of the foot at a 90° angle with the lower leg. Then when seated, subjects attempted to plantar flex their foot against the mechanical force transducer, a spring gauge was moved, giving a measure of maximal ankle plantar flexion strength. Three trials were conducted, and the greatest movement was recorded in newtons. Strength was corrected for body size by dividing the measure by the height of the subject (Lord, Caplan, & Ward, 1993). The mechanical force transducer was calibrated for accuracy by a technical expert from The University of Iowa Medical

Instrument Shop who built the transducer and stabilizer.

Walking speed. The time to walk six meters was measured in seconds with a stopwatch. Although the intent of the exercise program was not to walk at an exceedingly fast or unsafe pace, walking at a moderate or moderately fast pace was a reasonable goal for functional purposes.

Cognition. The Mini-Mental State Examination (Folstein, Folstein, & McHugh, 1975) is an 11-item screening test of cognitive function. Scores range from 0 (severe dementia) to 30 (normal). The scale was used as one factor to determine inclusion in the study, using 20 as the cutoff score. A score of 23 or below has been established as indicative of cognitive impairment (Cockrell & Folstein, 1988). Test-retest reliability over a 24-hour period was at least 0.89 in a psychiatric and neurologic population and interrater reliability was at least .82.

Fall Risk Assessment. The RAFS II (Ross, Watson, Gyldenvand, & Reinboth, 1991) is a 13-item tool that provides an indication of the risk of falling. The scale was used for assigning subjects in matched pairs to the intervention or control groups and to assess the outcome variable of risk for falls. Items assessed are length of time since admission, age, history of falling, balance, mental status, agitation, depression, anxiety, vision, communication, medications, chronic diseases, and urinary function. Total scores range from 1 to 39 with a score of 14 or greater indicating a high risk for potential of trauma by falling. The RAFS II was used in an acute care hospital and three extended care facilities and found to be 90% accurate for predicting falls (Gyldenvand, 1984).

Falls efficacy. Falls efficacy was measured by using a modified Falls Efficacy Scale (FES). The Falls Efficacy Scale (Tinetti, Richman, & Powell, 1990) is a 10-item tool designed to assess the degree of perceived self-confidence for avoiding a fall during each of 10 relatively nonhazardous activities of daily living routinely performed by community dwelling elders. Expert validation was accomplished by reaching consensus among therapists, nurses, and physicians concerning the activities to include in the FES. Test-retest reliability revealed a Pearson's correlation of 0.71 for a sample of community elders and residents of an intermediate care facility (Tinetti, Richman, & Powell, 1990). Internal consistency was shown with a Cronbach's alpha coefficient of 0.89 for a sample of community-dwelling older adults (Dayhoff, Baird, Bennett, & Backer, 1994). In consultation with a nursing home director of nursing and two gerontological nursing experts, the tool was modified so that the list of activities were appropriate for elderly nursing home residents and still measured the concept of falls efficacy (Schoenfelder, 2000). The items "prepare meals not requiring carrying heavy or hot objects" and "answer the door or telephone" were deleted because these items did not make sense for most residents within their nursing home settings. The two deleted items were replaced with the items "do 'light' housekeeping in your room" (e.g., clean up your nightstand or dresser) and "get up at night to go to the bathroom." The item "reach into cabinets or closets" was modified to "reach into closets" and the item "walk around the house" was changed to "walk around the nursing home" to better fit typical activities for nursing home residents. Internal consistency was maintained in the modified version (Cronbach's alpha = 0.99).

Data Analysis

The main study outcomes were balance, ankle strength, walking speed, risk of falling, fear of falling, and falls efficacy. Data were collected for all variables at baseline, 3 months, and 6 months. Comparisons were made between the intervention and control groups based on the proportion of elders who remained the same or improved versus those who declined by 3 and 6 months. Descriptive statistics were generated for the intervention and control groups at baseline. Tests for group differences used the Pearson's chi square test or Fisher's Exact test for categorical data and either a t test (normal distributions) or Kruskal-Wallace (non-normal distribution) test for continuous data. Exact nonparametric tests were used to assess variables with small cell sizes and for repeated measured analyses.

RESULTS

Sample Characteristics

The initial sample ($N = 81$) consisted of 62 women and 19 men between the ages of 64 and 100 years (mean = 84.1). The demographic, mobility, and activity characteristics for the entire sample at pretest are summarized in Table 1. Fifty-three percent of the participants had fallen in the past year.

Mobility status was significantly associated with age but not gender.

Baseline mean scores for selected sample characteristics and fall-related variables are reported in Table 2. There were no significant baseline differences between the intervention and control groups for all outcome measures, also shown in Table 2.

Study Results

Mobility status at baseline was significantly associated with balance, walking time, falls efficacy, and risk of falling (chi-square p values ≤.05). Because of this association, all group and repeated measures analyses controlled for baseline mobility status. Mobility status was significantly associated with age but not gender. The mean age for independent walkers was 5 to 7 years younger than the mean ages for the assistance groups.

Means for selected sample characteristics at the 3- and 6-month follow-ups are shown in Table 3, and the results for change at the two follow-ups are listed in Table 4. Most elders were able to complete the parallel stance for 10 seconds at baseline, and there was no significant change within or between groups over time. Among those who used assistive devices and for all mobility levels combined, a significantly larger proportion of the intervention group showed maintenance or improvement over time with the semitandem stance compared with the control group at the completion of the exercise program at 3 months. This finding also remained significant at 6 months, even though the intervention group had not done the supervised exercise program for 3 months.

In the time period from 3 to 6 months, among those who used an assistive device, a significantly larger proportion of the intervention group exhibited the same or improvement in fear of falling compared with the control group.

Most other outcome variables exhibited nonsignificant changes over time in the predicted direction (indicated in bold in Table 3). Lack of significance was most likely related to the small numbers of respondents in each mobility group.

DISCUSSION

There were significant changes as hypothesized for semitandem stance. The exercise program emphasized balance and did indeed improve balance as measured by the semitandem stance. Not only was balance maintained or improved at the completion of the supervised exercise program, the effect remained significant 3 months after completion of the program. This finding suggests that interruption in an exercise program does not mean the positive effects are immediately lost. Reestablishing the exercise program after an illness or injury or hospitalization would therefore be warranted for elderly nursing home residents. The tandem stance was too difficult for most subjects to do and therefore did not show significant maintenance or improvement.

Fear of falling was significantly affected, specifically from 3 to 6 months for intervention subjects who required an assistive device to ambulate. It is likely that concern for falling was raised during the exercise program for subjects who were increasing their level of exercise, having been more accustomed to a less active lifestyle. However, as time progressed, it may have been that exercise subjects became less fearful of falling after they saw that they could exercise and move about safely. It is difficult to know why fear of falling did not significantly improve for the independent group and the device and person group. The results may be partially explained by the small numbers in each group (independent: device and person) as compared with the device-only group.

It was expected that ankle strength would be significantly affected by the exercise program because there was an exercise specifically targeted at strengthening ankles. Although the results were not significant, the results for all mobility levels were in the predicted direction ($p = .08$). Larger sample sizes would most likely show a significant effect for this important fall-related outcome. Lower strength gain (knees and ankles) was significantly associated with increase in gait speed and improved falls efficacy (Chandler, Duncan, Kochersberger, and Studenski, 1998), two of the fall-related outcomes in this study. Although ankle range of motion (ROM) was not measured in this study, the ankle exercise would probably increase dorsiflexion and plantar flexion ROM. Recent findings suggest that

TABLE 1 **Demographic, Mobility, and Activity Characteristics at Baseline**

	Total Sample (N = 81)		Intervention Group (N = 42)		Control Group (N = 39)	
	Frequency	**Percent**	**Frequency**	**Percent**	**Frequency**	**Percent**
Demographic Variables						
Gender						
Female	62	76.5	30	71.4	32	82.1
Male	19	23.5	12	28.6	7	17.9
Age						
64-69	6	7.4	4	9.5	2	5.1
70-79	16	19.8	6	14.3	10	25.6
80-89	39	48.1	22	52.4	17	43.6
90 and older	20	24.7	10	23.8	10	25.6
Marital Status						
Windowed	60	74.1	34	81.0	26	66.7
Married	6	7.4	2	4.8	4	10.3
Divorced/separated	7	8.6	3	7.1	4	10.3
Never married	8	9.9	3	7.1	5	12.8
Menetal status (MMSE)						
20-23	20	24.7	7	16.7	13	33.3
24-30	61	75.3	35	83.3	26	66.7
Education	(N = 79)				(N = 38)	
Less than high school	24	30.0	15	35.7	9	23.7
High school graduate/trade school	34	42.5	16	38.1	18	47.4
Beyond high school and other than trade school	21	27.5	11	26.2	11	28.9
Mobility	(N = 80)				(N = 38)	
Walks independently	14	17.5	10	23.8	4	10.5
Uses assistive device	51	63.8	25	59.5	26	68.4
Assistive device–person	15	18.8	7	16.7	8	21.1
Activity						
Walking	(N = 80)		(N = 41)			
3 or more times/week	67	83.8	35	85.4	32	82.1
1 or 2 times/week	11	13.8	6	14.6	5	12.8
Does not walk weekly	2	2.5	0	0	2	5.1
Exercise Class						
3 or more times/week	10	12.4	6	14.3	4	10.3
1 or 2 times/week	20	24.7	9	21.4	11	28.2
Does not attend exercise classes	51	63.0	27	64.3	24	61.5

Abbreviation: *MMSE*, Mini-Mental State Examination.

TABLE 2 Baseline Mean Scores for Selected Sample Characteristics

Variable	*Total Sample* N	Mean Score (*SD*)	*Intervention Group* N	Mean Score (*SD*)	*Control Group* N	Mean Score (*SD*)	Difference in Intervention and Control Group mean scores (*p* level, Wilcoxon Rank-Sum Test)
Age (in years)	81	84.1 (7.7)	42	83.9 (7.9)	39	84.3 (7.5)	0.91
Mental status (MMSE score, range 0-30)	81	25.6 (2.9)	42	25.9 (2.5)	39	25.3 (3.3)	0.49
Balance (up to 10 seconds)							
Parallel	81	9.2 (2.5)	42	9.4 (2.2)	39	8.9 (2.8)	0.33
Semi-tandem	81	8.4 (3.7)	42	8.7 (2.9)	39	8.0 (4.5)	0.29
Tandem	81	2.6 (3.5)	42	3.3 (4.0)	39	1.9 (2.7)	0.50
Ankle strength (n/m)	81	27.3 (16.4)	42	28.6 (16.9)	39	25.9 (15.9)	0.50
Walking speed (in seconds)	76	20.7 (14.7)	40	20.4 (16.4)	36	20.9 (12.8)	0.33
Falls Risk (RAFS II score, range 1-39, 14 & above indicates high risk)	81	15.3 (3.3)	42	15.3 (3.3)	39	15.4 (3.3)	0.83
Falls Efficacy Scale (range 0-100)	81	77.8 (21.2)	42	78.1 (20.3)	39	77.5 (22.4)	0.94 0.12 (*p* level, Cochran-Mantel-Haenszel methods)
Fear of Falling (range 1-4)	81	2.4 (1.3)	42	2.2 (1.2)	39	2.5 (1.3)	

Abbreviation: *MMSE*, Mini-Mental State Examination.

interventions for increasing ankle ROM may increase balance and reduce falls in older adults (Mecagni, Smith, Roberts, & O'Sullivan, 2000).

Walking speed, falls risk, and falls efficacy also showed change over time in the predicted direction for some of the mobility levels.

Walking speed, falls risk, and falls efficacy also showed change over time in the predicted direction for some of the mobility levels. Again, having small numbers in each cell made it difficult to obtain significant findings. Nevertheless, the authors believe that walking speed, falls risk, and falls efficacy are important outcomes for evaluating the effectiveness of programs to prevent falls or stop the cycle of falling. Regarding walking speed, it would seem that frail elders might be more apt to walk on a routine basis (e.g., to the bathroom and to the dining area) rather than propel themselves in a wheelchair if they were able to walk at a more "functional" speed. In addition, walking requires balance and the act of walking regularly probably improves balance as it did in this study. Reducing the risk for falling and increasing falls efficacy are also important outcomes to measure. Several of the risk factors in the RAFS II are modifiable by health care intervention, and having confidence in being able to perform activities without falling would likely lead to more active participation in those daily activities.

Major strengths of this study were the use of a control group, excellent adherence to the exercise program and no reported adverse effects to the exercise program. No doubt adherence was at a high level because the exercises were supervised, conducted on a one-on-one basis, simple to do, and not time consuming. Also, no falls or injuries occurred while exer-

TABLE 3 Means (*SD*) for 3 Months and 6 Months Follow-up for Selected Sample Characteristics

	Total Sample						Intervention Group						Control Group					
	3 months			6 months			3 months			6 months			3 months			6 months		
Variable	N	Mean	(SD)	N	Mean	(SD)	N	Mean	(SD)	N	Mean	(SD)	N	Mean	(SD)	N	Mean	(SD)
MMSE Score (range 0-30)	66	23.5	(3.8)	58	22.9	(4.6)	33	24.5	(3.3)	30	24.0	(4.1)	33	22.6	(4.2)	28	21.8	(4.9)
Balance																		
Parallel	67	9.2	(2.7)	58	9.2	(2.6)	33	9.6	(1.8)	30	9.0	(2.7)	34	8.8	(3.3)	28	9.3	(2.6)
Semitandem	67	8.5	(3.2)	58	7.5	(3.9)	33	9.0	(2.7)	30	8.2	(3.5)	34	8.0	(3.6)	28	6.8	(4.3)
Tandem	67	3.7	(3.9)	58	3.0	(3.6)	33	4.6	(3.9)	30	3.6	(4.1)	34	2.7	(3.6)	28	2.4	(3.0)
Ankle strength (Newton/meters)	67	29.7	(20.2)	58	30.2	(17.9)	33	33.8	(21.0)	30	36.2	(19.0)	34	25.7	(18.9)	28	23.8	(14.5)
Walking speed in seconds	67	19.6	(17.7)	58	19.5	(17.6)	33	20.6	(19.1)	30	20.5	(19.4)	34	18.7	(16.3)	28	18.5	(15.7)
Fall risk (RAFSII, rang 1-39)*	67	15.7	(3.8)	58	15.3	(3.8)	33	15.2	(3.8)	30	15.3	(3.7)	34	16.3	(3.8)	28	15.3	(3.9)
Falls efficacy scale (range 1-100)	66	76.8	(23.2)	58	79.3	(24.1)	33	79.6	(22.3)	30	78.6	(26.4)	33	74.0	(24.1)	28	80.1	(21.9)
Fear of falling (range 1-4)	66	2.4	(1.3)	58	2.5	(1.2)	33	2.6	(1.4)	30	2.5	(1.3)	33	2.3	(1.2)	28	2.5	(1.2)

Abbreviation: *MMSE*, Mini-Mental State Examination.
*Fourteen and above indicates high risk.

413

TABLE 4 **Results for Change Over Time**

Variable, Group, and Mobility Class	Stay the Same or Improve versus Decline from Pretest to 3-Month Posttest			Stay the Same or Improve versus Decline from 3-Month to 6-Month Posttest		
	Intervention	Control	p Value	Intervention	Control	p Value
	% (frequency)	% (frequency)	(Chi-square or Fisher's Exact tests)	% (frequency)	% (frequency)	(Chi-square or Fisher's Exact tests)
Semitandem						
Device and Person	80.0 (4)	60.0 (3)	0.417	20.0 (1)	40.0 (2)	0.487
Device Only	100 (15)	73.9 (14)	**0.053***	**86.7 (13)**	**47.4 (9)**	**0.030***
Independent	88.9 (6)	100 (3)	0.436	**89.0 (8)**	33.3 (1)	0.127
All Levels	**93.1 (25)**	**74.1 (20)**	**0.057***	**75.9 (22)**	**44.4 (12)**	**0.028***
Tandem						
Device and Person	50.0 (2)	100 (3)	NA	**25.0 (1)**	**0 (3)**	**NA**
Device Only	55.6 (5)	60.0 (6)	0.845	**66.7 (6)**	30 (3)	0.179
Independent	50.0 (2)	100 (1)	NA	None	None	NA
All Levels	53.0 (9)	71.4 (10)	0.461	**41.2 (7)**	**21.4 (3)**	**0.076**
Walking Speed						
Device and Person	**60.0 (3)**	**50.0 (5)**	**0.740**	20.0 (1)	33.3 (2)	NA
Device Only	**50.0 (8)**	**38.1 (8)**	**0.520**	**68.8 (11)**	**38.1 (8)**	**0.099**
Independent	22.2 (2)	100.0 (3)	NA	**66.7 (6)**	**33.3 (1)**	**0.523**
All Levels	43.3 (13)	46.7 (14)	0.795	**60.0 (18)**	**36.7 (11)**	**0.121**
Ankle Strength						
Device and Person	33.3 (2)	75 (6)	0.277	66.7 (4)	37.5 (3)	0.592
Device Only	**52.9 (9)**	**36.4 (8)**	**0.345**	41.2 (7)	31.8 (7)	0.738
Independent	**55.6 (5)**	**33.3 (1)**	**0.502**	66.7 (6)	None	0.182
All Levels	**50 (16)**	**45.5 (15)**	**0.806**	**53.1 (17)**	**30.3 (10)**	**0.080**
Fear of Falling						
Device and Person	66.7 (4)	75.0 (6)	0.733	50.0 (3)	87.5 (7)	0.249
Device Only	**76.5 (13)**	**59.1 (13)**	**0.318**	**88.2 (15)**	**44.5 (10)**	**0.008***
Independent	100 (9)	75.0 (3)	0.853	**66.7 (6)**	**50.0 (2)**	**0.571**
All Levels	**81.3 (26)**	**64.7 (22)**	**0.171**	**75.0 (24)**	**55.9 (19)**	**0.126**
FES Total						
Device and Person	50.0 (3)	62.5 (5)	0.529	50.0 (3)	75.0 (6)	0.580
Device Only	**64.7 (11)**	**54.6 (12)**	**0.744**	**58.8 (10)**	**54.6 (12)**	**0.789**
Independent	**55.6 (5)**	**50 (2)**	**0.853**	**66.7 (9)**	**50.0 (2)**	**0.571**
All Levels	**59.4 (19)**	**55.9 (19)**	**0.808**	**69.4 (19)**	**58.2 (20)**	**0.964**
RAFS						
Device and Person	100.0 (5)	100 (8)	NA	100.0 (4)	100.0 (8)	NA
Device Only	**93.3 (14)**	**70.0 (14)**	**0.198**	100.0 (10)	100.0 (10)	NA
Independent	**78.8 (6)**	**66.7 (2)**	**0.785**	100.0 (6)	100.0 (2)	NA
All Levels	**89.5 (25)**	**77.4 (24)**	**0.306**	100.0 (20)	100.0 (20)	NA

NOTE. p Values are generated from chi-square tests, Fisher's Exact tests, and likelihood ratio tests.
Abbreviation: NA, not applicable.
*bold print: p ≤ .054.
bold print only: change in predicted direction.

cising in this study and no physical complaints were expressed by the intervention subjects.

There were limitations with this research. A major challenge is encountered any time researchers are attempting to obtain large sample sizes with very old adults who are frail. Recruitment was somewhat difficult in that some potential subjects were hesitant to start an exercise program. Attrition was also a limitation in this study that reduced the sample size to 67 at the 3-month follow-up and to 58 at the 6-month follow-up. Most of the attrition was due to extended illness or death. Another possible limitation that was anticipated was that subjects might tend to respond to certain questions according to how they believed the examiner would want them to respond (e.g., confidence levels on the FES). Subjects were instructed to respond according to how they truly felt rather than how they thought the examiner would want them to respond so as to minimize this potential limitation. In general, subjects voiced difficulty responding to the FES 100-point scale. This difficulty might be caused by having response labels only at the two ends of the scale, or the difficulty might be caused by having too large of a scale (i.e., 100 point) to conceptualize and translate into a confidence level. Finally, because a large majority of older Iowans are white, it was expected that the study sample would not vary in ethnic or racial composition and that was the case. This needs to be considered when discussing generalizability of the results. Nevertheless, this study can be replicated in settings with more diverse populations in the future.

The findings in this study have implications for nursing research. The results show promise that a simple exercise plan can have positive effects on fall-related outcomes, especially balance and fear of falling as indicated by this study. The tests and instruments used in this research were, for the most part, easy to administer and score. The exception, as noted earlier, was the FES. Based on the difficulty that subjects had responding to this instrument, the authors recommend using a tool to measure falls efficacy that has few numbered points and has descriptors for each of those points.

Recommendations can be made for nursing practice based on this research. Nursing home staff can easily be trained to use the exercise program. Depending on the mobility of residents, the exercises can be done individually or in groups of two or more residents while maintaining safety. Along with implementing the exercise program, walking in general should be emphasized for residents, offering both tangible and intangible incentives for walking. The use of standardized nursing language for preventing falls is essential. By using the nursing diagnosis Risk for Falls (North American Nursing Diagnosis Association, 2001), risk factors can be linked with relevant nursing interventions to achieve the desired outcome of not falling in the first place or not having a repeat fall, therefore avoiding possible injury. Correctly identifying risk factors will facilitate accurate selection of outcomes and interventions to address the diagnosis. For example, the Nursing Outcomes Classification outcomes Risk Control and Safety Behavior: Fall Prevention may be appropriate choices depending on the identified risk factors (Johnson, Maas, & Moorhead, 2000). Examples of Nursing Interventions Classification interventions that address falling include Environmental Management: Safety; Fall Prevention; and Surveillance: Safety (McCloskey & Bulechek, 2000). The outcome indicators and intervention activities focus on decreasing or controlling the specific risk factors identified for individuals who are vulnerable to falling.

The occurrence of falling in elderly nursing home residents is unfortunately not uncommon and of great concern to nurses and other health professionals caring for older nursing home residents. Interventions to decrease the chances of falling need to be identified through research efforts and applied in nursing practice. There is mounting evidence that exercise can improve fall-related outcomes for older adults, even frail elders. And there is promise that exercise, especially exercise to improve balance, can prevent or stop the cycle of falling.

REFERENCES

Baloh, R.W., Jacobson, K.M., Enrietto, J.A., Corona, S., and Honrubia, V. (1998). Balance disorders in older persons: Quantification with posturography. *Otolaryngology, Head and Neck Surgery, 119,* 89-92.

Buchner, D.M., Cress, M.E., de Lateur, B.J., Esselman, P.C., Margherita, A.J., Price, R., & Wagner, E.H. (1997). The effect of strength and endurance training on gait, balance, fall risk, and health services use in community-living older adults. *Journal of Gerontology: Medical Sciences, 52A,* M218-M224.

Campbell, A.J., Robertson, M.C., Gardner, M.M., Norton, R.N., Tilyard, M.W., & Buchner, D.M. (1997). Randomised controlled trial of a general practice programme of home based exercise to prevent falls in elderly women. *British Medical Journal, 315,* 1065-1069.

Chandler, J.M., Duncan, P.W., Kochersberger, G., & Studenski, S. (1998). Is lower extremity strength gain associated with improvement in physical performance and disability in frail, community-dwelling elders? *Archives of Physical Medical Rehabilitation, 79,* 24-30

Chandler, J.M., & Hadley, E.C. (1996). Exercise to improve physiologic and functional performance in old age. *Clinics in Geriatric Medicine, 12(4),* 761-784.

Cho, C., & Kamen, G. (1998). Detecting balance deficits in frequent fallers using clinical and quantitative evaluation tools. *Journal of the American Geriatrics Society, 46,* 426-430.

Cockrell, J.R., & Folstein, M.F. (1988). Mini-Mental State Examination (MMSE). *Psychopharmacology Bulletin, 24(4),* 689-692.

Davis, J.W., Ross, P.D., Nevitt, M.C., & Wasnich, R.D. (1999). Risk factors for falls and for serious injuries on falling among older Japanese women in Hawaii. *Journal of the American Geriatrics Society, 47,* 792-798.

Dayhoff, N.E., Baird, C., Bennett, S., & Backer, J. (1994). Fear of falling: measuring fear and appraisals of potential harm. *Rehabilitation Nursing Research, 3,* 97-104.

Edwards, B.J., & Lee, S. (1998). Gait disorders and falls in a retirement home: A pilot study. *Annals of Long-Term Care, 6,* 140-143.

Folstein, M.F., Folstein, S.E., & McHugh, P.R. (1975). Mini-Mental State: A practical method for grading the cognitive state of patients for the clinician. *Journal of Psychiatric Research, 12,* 189-198.

Gardner, M.M., Robertson, M.C., & Campbell, A.J. (2000). Exercise in preventing falls and fall related injuries in older people: A review of randomised controlled trials. *British Journal of Sports Medicine, 34,* 7-17.

Graybiel, A. & Fregly, A. (1966). A new quantitative ataxia test battery. *Acta Otolaryngology, 61,* 292-312.

Gurwitz, J.H., Sanchez-Cross, M.R., Eckler, M.A., & Matulis, J. (1994). The epidemiology of adverse and unexpected events in the long-term care setting. *Journal of the American Geriatrics Society, 42,* 33-38.

Gyldenvand, T. (1984). Falls: The construction and validation of the Risk Assessment for Full Scale II (RAFS II). (Thesis). University of Iowa, Iowa City, IA.

Johnson, M., Maas, M., & Moorhead, S. (2000). *Nursing outcomes classification (NOC).* (2nd ed.). St. Louis: Mosby.

Koroknay, V.J., Werner, P., Cohen-Mansfield, J., & Braun, J.V. (1995). Maintaining ambulation in the frail nursing home resident: A nursing administered walking program. *Journal of Gerontological Nursing, 21,* 18-24.

Kuehn, A.F., & Sendelweck, S. (1995). Acute health status and its relationship to falls in the nursing home. *Journal of Gerontological Nursing, 21,* 41-49.

Lachman, M.E., Howland, J., Tennstedt, S., Jette, A., Assmann, S., & Peterson, E.W. (1998). Fear of falling and activity restriction: The survey of activities and fear of falling in the elderly (SAFE). *Journal of Gerontology: Psychological Sciences, 53B,* P43-P50.

Leipzig, R.M., Cumming, R.G., & Tinetti, M.E. (1999). Drugs and falls in order people: A systematic review and meta-analysis: I. Psychotropic drugs. *Journal of the American Geriatrics Society, 47,* 30-39.

Lord, S.R., Caplan, G.A., & Ward, J.A. (1993). Balance, reaction time, and muscle strength in exercising and nonexercising older women: A pilot study. *Archives of Physical Medicine Rehabilitation, 74,* 837-839.

Lundin-Olsson, L., Nyberg, L., & Gustafson, Y. (1998). Attention, frailty, and falls: The effect of a manual task on basic mobility. *Journal of the American Geriatrics Society, 43,* 1198-1206.

McCloskey, J.C., & Bulechek, G.M. (2000). *Nursing interventions classification (NIC).* (3rd ed.). St. Louis: Mosby.

Mecagni, C., Smith, J.P., Roberts, K.E., & O'Sullivan, S.B. (2000). Balance and ankle range of motion in community-dwelling women aged 64 to 87 years: A correlational study. *Physical Therapy, 80,* 1004-1011.

Mustard, C.A., & Mayer, T. (1997). Case-control study of exposure to medication and the risk of injurious falls requiring hospitalization among nursing home residents. *American Journal of Epidemiology, 145,* 738-745.

North American Nursing Diagnosis Association (2001). Nursing diagnoses: Definitions and classification 2001-2002. Philadelphia: Author.

Nygaard, H.A. (1998). Falls and psychotropic drug consumption in long-term care residents: Is there an obvious association? *Gerontology, 44,* 46-50.

Ross, J.E., Watson, C.A., Gyldenvand, T.A., & Reinboth, J. (1991). Potential for trauma: Falls. In Maas M., Buckwalter K.C., & Hardy M. (Eds.). *Nursing diagnosis and interventions for the elderly.* (18-31). Redwood City, CA: Addison-Wesley.

Schoenfelder, D.P. (2000). A fall prevention program for elderly individuals. *Journal of Gerontological Nursing, 26,* 43-51.

Tideiksaar, R. (1998). *Falls in older persons: Prevention and management.* (2nd ed.). Baltimore: Health Professions Press.

Tinetti, M.E., Richman, D., & Powell, L. (1990). Falls efficacy as a measure of fear of falling. *Journal of Gerontology, 45(6),* P239-243.

Tinetti, M.E., & Williams, C.S. (1998). The effect of falls and fall injuries on functioning in community-dwelling older persons. *Journal of Gerontology: Medical Sciences, 53A,* M112-M119.

INTRODUCTION TO CRITQUE #1

The article *An Exercise Program to Improve Fall-Related Outcomes in Elderly Nursing Home Residents* is examined in terms of its quality and the potential usefulness of the findings for application to nursing practice.

PROBLEM AND PURPOSE

The authors specify the aim or purpose of the study as investigation of "the effectiveness of an ankle-strengthening and walking program for elderly nursing home residents in improving balance, ankle strength, and walking speed; decreasing risk of falling and fear of falling; and improving confidence in performing daily activities without falling (falls efficacy)." The independent variable is the ankle strengthening and walking program that affects the dependent variables, i.e., balance, ankle strength, walking speed, risk of falling, fear of falling, and falls efficacy. The purpose specifies a population of elderly nursing home residents, is appropriately stated, and provides direction for statistical analyses. The significance of the problem is to test the effectiveness of a nursing intervention to establish evidence-based recommendations for use of an exercise program to improve fall-related outcomes and minimize physical deterioration in elderly nursing home residents.

REVIEW OF LITERATURE AND DEFINITIONS

Schoenfelder and Rubenstein (2004) specify the relationships of the study variables included in the study in Figure 1. Thus, if an exercise program is implemented with elderly nursing home residents, improvements are predicted in balance, ankle strength, and walking speed (physiological indicators) and fall efficacy (psychological domain) along with decreases in risk of falls (physiological) and fear of falling (psychological) at the 3-month data-collection point. Potential declines in benefits were predicted at the 6-month data-collection point. The literature review does not address why losses are anticipated after stopping the intervention at 3 months. This limitation identified in the background literature review likely reflects the journal's directions for authors, which asks for a brief description of the study background with emphasis on applications for nursing practice (*Applied Nursing Research*: Information for Contributors, 2004).

The concepts include falls, risk factors for falling, strengthening, and walking. Conceptual definitions are provided for falls and falls efficacy but not for the other variables depicted in Figure 1. The definition provided for fall is "any event in which a person inadvertently or intentionally [*sic*] comes to rest on the ground or another low level." Falls efficacy is said to be "the confidence that an individual has to do daily activities without falling." The limitation or gap specified in the literature review was lack of studies testing the efficacy of exercise on fall-related outcomes in nursing home populations. The present study examined a simple ankle strengthening exercise and walking program that is feasible in the busy work day schedules in nursing home settings.

The majority of references used appear to be primary sources. The reference to Campbell et al. (cited by Schoenfelder and Rubenstein, 2004) is an example of a primary source because it is a report of a randomized controlled trial. The reference selected to illustrate the use of a secondary source is the Gardner, Robertson, and Campbell publication, which is a review of randomized controlled trials (cited by Christman et al., 2000).

The independent variable of the exercise program included ankle strengthening and walking. Ankle strengthening was operationalized by describing the standing position, movements, and the number of repetitions included in the intervention. Both exercising and walking were closely supervised by a research team member. Walking was operationalized as 10 minutes of walking, with individual subjects progressing toward this goal as tolerated. Once 10 minutes of sustained walking was reached, additional speed was encouraged with consideration for a safe and functional pace. The dependent variables were fear of falling, balance, ankle strength, walking speed, falls risk, and falls efficacy. Fear of falling was operationalized as two questions designed by the investigators to measure concern for falling and decrease in activities due to concerns. Balance was measured using a stopwatch to time 10 seconds in 3 stances: parallel, semi-tandem, and tandem with no assistive devices allowed. Ankle plantar flexion strength was measured by placing the foot on a mechanical force transducer built by a technical expert with details of the procedure provided in the article. Walking speed was determined using a stopwatch to ascertain the number of seconds taken to walk 6 m. Falls risk assessment was measured by the Risk Assessment for Falls Scale II (RAFS II). Falls efficacy was measured using a modifiied Falls Efficacy Scale.

HYPOTHESES AND/OR RESEARCH QUESTIONS

A research hypothesis is used to guide this experimental study. The investigators "hypothesized that the proportion of elders with consistent or improved fall-related outcomes would be significantly higher for those individuals participating in the ankle strengthening and walking program than for those elders who did not participate. The fall-related outcomes . . . were balance, ankle strength, walking speed, falls risk, fear of falling, and confidence to perform daily activities without falling (falls efficacy)." The predicted direction of the relationships of the independent variables (ankle strengthening exercise and walking program) and the dependent variables (fall-related outcomes) was provided by Schoenfelder and Rubenstein (2004) in Figure 1. The relationships are testable.

SAMPLE

The convenience sample consisted of 81 nursing home residents (62 women and 19 men) aged 64 to 100 years who agreed to participate and who met the selection criteria. The sample size dropped to 67 at 3 months and 58 at 6 months due to prolonged illness or death. The sampling method is acceptable for the experimental research design although the use of a nonprobability sample limits generalizability to the sample itself, thereby decreasing external validity. The sample selected for inclusion in the study matches the population proposed in the purpose statement, which specifies elders. Using a mean age of 84.1 years and including those elders residing in nursing homes are consistent with the intent to fill the gap in study of nursing home residents. The range of ages, 64 to 100 years, includes one or more individuals 1 year younger than the stated criteria of 65 or older. Justification of the sample size using power analysis is not provided. Schoenfelder and Rubenstein acknowledge that lack of significance of the findings is likely due to the small sample size. Small sample size may contribute to limitations in accurately testing the effect of the intervention.

RESEARCH DESIGN

The three criteria for an experimental design, often called a randomized clinical trial (RCT) that provides Level II evidence (see Table 2-1), are met in this study as follows: (1) the residents who signed informed consent were matched in pairs based on RADS II scores and were "randomly assigned within each pair to intervention or control group"; (2) there was a separate control group; and (3) manipulation of the independent variable was met by providing the intervention group subjects 3 months of ankle strengthening exercise and walking program while the control group subjects received an attention placebo. The choice of an experimental design flows from the purpose and compares the effects of the intervention with an attention control placebo on fall-related outcomes. The design allows for testing the hypothesis that postulates more consistent or improved fall-related outcomes in the intervention group than in the control group. The limited literature review did not include a theoretical framework nor provide comprehensive explanation of the relationship of the variables and predicted changes.

Internal Validity

Examination of threats to internal validity reveals no indication of difficulty associated with the history of this adult population of nursing home residents during this 3-month intervention study. The threat due to mortality is recognized by the authors in the discussion of attrition. This loss of participants to follow-up (see Chapter 20), which occurred primarily because of extended illness or death, also reflects a threat due to maturation with this paricular aging population. Since the loss is relatively equivalent between the intervention and control groups, the threat is limited to that of decreased sample size due to subject mortality and testability of hypothesis. These threats to internal validity decrease the probability of detecting accurately the effect of the intervention. Selection bias is controlled by inclusion and exclusion criteria as well as use of matching pairs followed by random assignment to groups within each pair. Potential threats due to instrumentation and testing appear controlled through use of a standardized procedure to ensure consistency in observation and measurement of variables. The threats identified seem minimal.

External Validity

Generalizability of findings is limited by the use of a nonprobability sampling technique. The findings may be generalized only to the sample.

RESEARCH APPROACH

Methods

Data-collection methods include a physiological measure, structured interviews, observation, and chart reviews. The data collectors were trained by the principle investigator; evidence of interrater reliability was reported, and thus a strength of the study is that data collection appears consistent and systematic throughout the study.

Legal-Ethical Issues

The study was approved by the University Institutional Review Board. Signed informed consent was obtained prior to chart review and physician contact.

Instruments

A mechanical force transducer was a physiological measure used to determine ankle strength. The use of the measure was adapted to ensure safety for the elderly participants, and calibration for accuracy was provided by a technical expert from the authors' university. Observation was used to gather data about balance and walking strength. Some items in the falls risk assessment may have been gathered by observation, but the details on ascertaining the data used to complete this RAFS II are not delineated. Observations were made by undergraduate and graduate student data gatherers trained by the principal investigator "to accurately collect data." Stopwatches were used to time walking and balance, and the stances for balance determinations were clearly specified so that inferences would not seem to be necessary. The presence of observers for these measures supported attaining best performance and also provided for safety of participants. The same data gatherers were trained to do the interviews about mobility and activity information, falls efficacy, and falls risk. Schoenfelder and Rubenstein (2004) discuss the possibility of bias due to wish to please the interviewer data gatherers. Fear of falling questions asked by interviewers consisted of two questions. The first question addressed whether the subject was concerned about falling and was rated on a four-point Likert scale ranging from not at all concerned to very concerned. If the individual was concerned, the second question was asked: "Do you think this concern has made you cut down on the activities that you used to do?" They answered yes or no. Consistency with conceptualization of fear of falling seems self-evident.

Available data and records used were referred to in chart reviews for demographics and risk fall assessment. The data selected were appropriate. The demographic data were used to describe the sample, and risk falls assessment was used for hypothesis testing.

Reliability and Validity

Test-retest reliability for the first question on the Fear of Falling instrument is reported as a kappa = 0.66, which the authors refer to as an acceptable level. The kappa for the second item is reported as only 0.36. Correlation coefficients ranging from 0.57 to 0.96 are reported by Graybiel and Fregly (as cited in Schoenfelder and Rubenstein, 2004) for the balance measure, but the type of reliability or vailidity being addressed cannot be ascertained without reviewing the original work. Test-retest reliability of 0.89 and interrater reliability of 0.82 reported for the Mini-Mental State Examination are acceptable. The only reliability validity reported for the RAFS II is a predictive validity score of 90%. Test-retest reliability of 0.71 and internal consistency with a Cronbach's alpha of 0.89 were reported for the Falls Efficacy Scale (FES) with community dwelling elders in previous work. The tool was modified for use with nursing home residents in consultation with two gerontological nursing experts and a nursing home director to establish content validity for use with the nursing home population included in this study. The internal consistency in the modified version is reported as 0.99, raising the possibility of item redundancy. No other reports of reliability or validity for the instruments were identified, but overall it appears that the majority of measures used were adequate.

ANALYSIS OF DATA

Schoenfelder and Rubenstein treat the data for the dependent measures as intervals or ratios when means and standard deviations are used. Balance, ankle strength, and walking speed are ratio levels of measure since an absolute zero exists. Scores for FES (1-100), RAFS II (1-39), and Fear of Falling (1-4) measures are treated as intervals. Descriptive statistics include frequencies, means, standard deviations, and percentages. The inferential statistics are Chi-square and Fisher's Exact tests, which are appropriate for hypothesis testing. To determine comparability of groups, the Wilcoxin Rank-Sum test was used for examining the difference in control and intervention group baseline mean scores for selected sample characteristics. The inferential and descriptive statistics used are appropriate for the level of measurement and for hypothesis testing. The level of significance set for the study is specified as equal to or less than 0.054.

Four tables are used to present additional information. The tables are precisely titled and headed. Unnecessary repetition is avoided.

CONCLUSIONS, IMPLICATIONS, AND RECOMMENDATIONS

The authors reported significant changes in semi-tandem stance, fear of falling for the 3 to 6 month period for the group of individuals with assistive devices to ambulate but not for the independent or the device and person groups.

The strength of the experimental design, in this case the RCT, lies in its ability to help the researcher control the effects of any extraneous variables that offer competing explanations or present threats to internal validity. These are important to consider when interpreting the findings of an RCT where you want to determine the true effect of an intervention so you can determine its potential applicability for practice. The authors appropriately interpret the findings in relation to the study hypothesis. The lack of significance is discussed in relation to limitations in sample size. Continued inclusion of the variables as outcome measures for fall prevention programs is encouraged since changes were in the anticipated direction, though not significant. The major limitation of sample size is acknowledged as a common challenge in this population as is recruitment of frail elders hesitant to start an exercise program. Additional limitations included the difficulty subjects experienced in responding to the FES 100-point scale. The lack of diversity in the population in the largely white Midwest is appropriately identified as an additional limit to generalizability to be addressed in future studies.

Schoenfelder and Rubenstein (2004) identify the relevance for nursing practice when they discuss the importance of reestablishing an exercise program following illness or hospitalization based on findings that balance improved (as indicated by the measure of semi-tandom stance) and that the improvement remained significant 3 months after completion of the exercise program. Recommendations for nursing practice include the feasibility of training nursing home staff to use the exercise program with individuals or groups safely; this is congruent with the report of no subject loss due to injury. Implications for research include additional study of the promising findings that support the use of a simple exercise plan to improve fall-related outcomes, and continued use of instruments that are viewed as easy to use and score. However, it is recommended that the FES be replaced with a measure using fewer numbered points and having descriptors for each point, enabling the respondent to more readily identify the appropriate response for him/her.

APPLICATION TO NURSING PRACTICE

This study provides Level II evidence because it utilizes an experimental design. Validity of the study is supported by the strengths that are evident in the design and conduct of the research, outweighing its weaknesses. The results provide further support to the findings of a pilot study that suggested improved fall-related outcomes resulting from an ankle strengthening and walking program. The benefits would outweigh the risks for the nursing home resident assuming that the exercise program is implemented with carefully selected residents for whom the exercise would be appropriate and that trained personnel are used who adhere to the safety guidelines of the exercise program.

Feasibility of direct application would need to be determined in the context of each nursing home based on the contraints discussed above. The time, effort, and cost of incorporating information on the use of exercise could be substantial in this time of limited budgets and staffing shortages. Legal and ethical concerns exist both for implementing and for failing to implement an exercise program that provides benefits to residents. Failing to adequately screen for inclusion and adhere closely to safety precautions could have legal as well as ethical implications. Failure to provide care with established benefits for residents also suggests potential legal and ethical ramifications. The study needs to be replicated in other nursing homes and with more diverse populations to provide a solid base of evidence for changing practice.

CRITIQUE *of a Quantitative Research Study*

SAMPLE #2

The study *Quality of Life in Hospice Patients With Terminal Illness* by Woung-Ru Tang, Lauren S. Aaronson, and Sarah A. Forbes, published in *Western Journal of Nursing Research* (2004), is critiqued. The article is presented first and followed by the critique on p. 000. (From *Western Journal of Nursing Research* 26:113-128, 2004.)

QUALITY OF LIFE IN HOSPICE PATIENTS WITH TERMINAL ILLNESS

Woung-Ru Tang, Lauren S. Aaronson, Sarah A. Forbes

To better understand quality of life (QOL) and its important correlates among patients with terminal illness, a cross-sectional correlational design was used in a study based on Stewart, Teno, Patrick, and Lynn's conceptual model of factors affecting QOL of dying patients and their families. Sixty participants were recruited from two local hospice programs in the midwestern region of the United States. Data were collected at the participants' homes. The participants had an above average QOL. Living with the caregiver, spirituality, pain intensity, physical performance status, and social support as a set explained 38% of the variance in their QOL. Among these five predictors, living with the caregiver, spirituality, and social support statistically were significant predictors of the QOL of these participants. Participants who did not live with their caregivers experienced less pain intensity, perceived higher spirituality, had more social support, and had a significantly better QOL. Important contributions of these findings are discussed.

Keywords: *patients with terminal illness; quality of life; spirituality*

Death and dying are inevitable events in a human's life. Although no one can escape this experience, death rarely receives attention from scientists and society as a whole. By 2020, 2.5 million persons will die annually in the United States (Brock & Foley, 1998). Advanced technology and modern medicine have increased the length of life; however, quality of life (QOL) at the end of life remains relatively unexplored.

RESEARCH ON END OF LIFE

Although hospice care is believed to foster QOL while dying, little research has assessed QOL in hospice patients. Only a few studies in the United States have evaluated hospice care outcomes (Kane, Klein, Bernstein, Rothenberg, & Wales, 1985; Kane, Wales, Bernstein, Leibowitz, & Kaplan, 1984; Kidder, 1992; Mor, Greer, & Kastenbaum, 1988; Morris et al., 1986; Wallston, Burger, Smith, & Baugher, 1988), and most of these have concentrated on cost-effectiveness. Although Mor et al. (1998) measured QOL as one of the important hospice outcomes, their study used the family caregivers' proxy measure of the patients' QOL. Others have found a discrepancy between patients' rating of their QOL and proxy measures and caution against using such proxy measures (Bretscher et al., 1999; Brunelli et al., 1998; Clipp & George, 1992; Ganzini, Johnston, & Hoffman, 1999; Hardy, Edmonds, Turner, Rees, & A'Hern, 1999; Higginson & McCarthy, 1993; Maguire, Walsh, Jeacock, & Kingston, 1999; McMillan, 1996; Weitzner, Meyers, Steinbruecker, Saleeba, & Sandifer, 1997). Still other studies either focused on physical and psychological symptoms or on satisfaction with care, failing to capture all of the domains of QOL for patients with terminal illness (e.g., Kane et al., 1984, 1985; Peruselli, Paci, Franceschi, Legori, & Mannucci, 1997).

QOL

QOL is believed to be the most important outcome of care at the end of life (Stewart, Teno, Patrick, & Lynn, 1999). QOL has been conceptualized in two ways: global QOL and health-related QOL (HRQOL). Global QOL is defined as an individual's subjective well-being (Cella, 1994; Cohen, Hassan, Lapointe, & Mount,

Woung-Ru Tang, R.N., Ph.D., Assistant Professor, Graduate Institute of Nursing, Chang Gung University; *Lauren S. Aaronson*, R.N., Ph.D., FAAN, Professor, School of Nursing, University of Kansas; *Sarah A. Forbes*, R.N., Ph.D., Associate Professor, School of Nursing, University of Kansas

1996; Cohen & Mount, 1992; Cohen, Mount, & Mac-Donald, 1996), or a global evaluation of satisfaction with one's life (Cooley, 1998; Nuamah, Cooley, Fawcett, & McCorkle, 1999). HRQOL, on the other hand, is "a more focused concept related to the impact of a medical condition or the impact of specific medical interventions on a person's physical, psychological, and social well-being" (Skeel, 1998, p. 876). HRQOL is relevant for patients receiving active treatment for disease (Choe, Padilla, Chae, & Kim, 2001). For individuals at the end of life, however, when the focus of treatment changes from curing disease to preserving QOL, global QOL becomes more relevant (Clinch, Dudgeon, & Schipper, 1998; Cohen et al., 1996; Houck, Avis, Gallant, Fuller, & Goodman, 1999; Lynn, 1997; McMillan, 1996; Stewart et al., 1999).

In general, there are several domains that contribute to an individual's global QOL. These are physical, psychological, social, and existential well-being (Cohen, Hassan, et al., 1996; Ferrell, 1995; Ferrell, Grant, Funk, Otis-Green, & Garcia, 1998). Physical well-being captures the individuals' perceptions of their physical condition including symptoms; psychological well-being taps emotional responses, such as depression and anxiety; existential well-being embodies the individual's ability to find meaning and purpose in life and to transcend difficult life circumstances; and social well-being focuses on individuals' perceptions of their support from others. Because QOL is considered to be one of the most important outcomes for end-of-life care, surprisingly few studies have examined important correlates of global QOL for a patient with terminal illness.

Stewart et al. (1999) presented a conceptual framework for evaluating quality of care for patients who were seriously ill and dying and their families. This framework is based on Donabedian's (1992) formulation of structure, process, and outcomes. The structure (e.g., access to hospice, provider skills) and process (e.g., physical care, attention to emotional needs) of care influence desired outcomes, including global QOL. Being mindful of the response burden for hospice patients, four key variables (i.e., spirituality, pain, physical performance, social support) were selected from Stewart et al.'s (1999) conceptual framework for investigation.

Spirituality, Pain, Physical Performance, and Social Support

Spirituality is the interconnectedness between self, others, nature, and Ultimate Other (God) (Clark & Heidenreich, 1995; Floriani, 1999; Hood Morris, 1996; Hungelmann, Kenkel-Rossi, Klassen, & Stollenwerk, 1996). Spirituality provides a sense of meaning and purpose, enables transcendence, and empowers individuals to be whole and to live life fully. Spirituality has two components, religious well-being (i.e., a relationship with God or Higher Being) and existential well-being (i.e., a sense of purpose and meaning in life; Moberg, 1979). Reed (1987) found that adults with terminal illness have greater religiousness when compared to other adults and that these adults' spirituality was positively correlated with psychological well-being. At this point, little is known about the relationship between spirituality and other aspects of QOL, such as physical and social well-being.

Pain is the most debilitating and frequently reported symptom of patients with terminal illness (Dahl, 1996; Hall, Schroder, & Weaver, 2002). Pain interferes with psychological and existential well-being and diminishes social relationships (Easley & Elliott, 2001; Ferrell, Rhiner, Cohen, & Grant, 1991). Although the relationship between physical pain and QOL has been empirically demonstrated (Ferrell et al., 1991), relatively little research has evaluated the relationship of pain to all aspects of QOL in a hospice setting, where there often is greater attention to pain management.

According to Stewart et al.'s (1999) framework, physical performance status is another factor that influences patients' QOL. Many patients are completely dependent in activities of daily living before death (McCarthy, 1990; Peruselli et al., 1997). Researchers and clinicians often place emphasis on the physical domain of QOL, assuming one's QOL decreases as disease and physical disability progress. Some researchers, however, have documented that other aspects of QOL gain importance as one approaches death. For example, the existential domain has been demonstrated to increase in importance as one approaches death and becomes increasingly physically debilitated (Cohen, Mount, Tomas, & Mount, 1996). The interplay between physical performance status and other factors on QOL at the end of life remains unclear.

Social support is a key element in how people manage and cope with illness (Lamendola & Newman, 1994; Smith, Fernengel, Holcroft, Gerald, & Marien, 1994). Focusing on the patients with terminal illness, Stewart et al. (1999) identified emotional and tangible supports as important to QOL. Hospice, by the very nature of its focus, offers emotional and tangible support to patients who are dying. Social support has been found to have a significant relationship with QOL for patients with terminal illness (Cohen, Hassan, et al., 1996), to be associated with less distress due to pain (Rosenfeld et al., 1996), and to have a positive relationship with spirituality (Reed, 1994). The relationship of social support to QOL in a hospice population also warrants further investigation.

PURPOSE

The purpose of the present study was to fill the gaps in current end-of-life research by examining important correlates of QOL of participants. The following research question was addressed: What is the relationship among spirituality, pain, physical performance status, social support, and QOL of patients receiving hospice care?

DESIGN

To study the relationship between these important factors and QOL of participants among those who receive in-home hospice care, a cross-sectional, correlational design with a convenience sample was used.

SAMPLE

A convenience sample ($N = 60$) of participants was obtained through two local hospice programs. During the 4-month period of data collection, 95 participants received invitation letters from the directors of the hospice programs. Nine patients died, and one moved to a nursing home setting before the follow-up phone call. Among the 85 potential participants, 63 agreed to participate in the study, and 60 participants completed the questionnaires. The effective response rate for the present study was 71%.

Participants' mean age was 73 years ($SD = 11$). The median length of stay (LOS) in a hospice program until data collection day was 28.8 days. The majority of the participants were Caucasian (95%), 55% were married (32% widowed, 10% divorced, and one each were single or separated), and 43% were men. More than one half (63%) of the participants indicated their religious affiliation as Protestant, 20% were Catholic, and 8% each indicated either "other" or "none." Of the participants, 25 (42%) had more than 12 years of education, and 22% did not complete high school. All participants lived in a home setting; the majority cohabited with a caregiver (78%). Most (82%) had a cancer diagnosis, especially lung cancer (23%). Of the participants, 39 (65%) had agreed to forgo cardiopulmonary resuscitation (CPR). The mortality rate during the data collection period was 53%. For those who died during the data collection process, 91% of the participants died at their homes with family members present. In addition, one participant died in a nursing home during a respite care period, and two others died in the hospital after receiving CPR.

MEASURES

For this investigation, five instruments, each measuring one study variable, were used. Psychometric properties for each questionnaire are described.

McGill Quality of Life Questionnaire (MQOL)

QOL of participants was measured using Cohen, Hassan, et al.'s (1996). Cohen, Mount, Tomas, et al.'s (1996), and Cohen et al.'s (1997) 16-item MQOL (plus one single-item global measure of QOL-SIS). There are five subscales within this instrument: Physical Symptoms, Physical Well-Being, Psychological Symptoms, Existential Well-Being, and Social Well-Being. Each MQOL item is scored ranging from 0 to 10, 0 = *the worst situation* and 10 = *the best*. The MQOL total score is the mean of the scores of the five subscales.

Reliability as estimated by Cronbach's alpha ranged from .83 to .89. Convergent and construct validity has been supported in a comparison study on cancer patients (Cohen, Mount, Tomas, et al., 1996).

Spiritual Well-Being Scale (SWBS)

The spirituality of participants was measured using Paloutzian and Ellison's (1982) 20-item SWBS. There are two subscales within the SWBS: Religious and Existential Well-Being. Higher scores represent higher levels of spirituality. National norms were obtained on this instrument across a variety of samples (Bufford, Paloutzian, & Ellison, 1991). Reliability, as measured by Crobach's alpha, ranged from .82 to .86. Construct validity was supported by its positive relationship with self-transcendence (Walton, Schultz, Beck, & Walls, 1991), religiousness and hope (Mickley, Soeken, & Belcher, 1992), mental health, and QOL (Riley et al., 1998); and its negative relationship with loneliness (Walton et al., 1991) and demands of illness (Fernsler, Klemm, & Miller, 1999).

American Pain Society Patient Outcome Questionnaire (APS-POQ)

The APS-POQ was developed by the American Pain Society Quality of Care Committee (McNeill, Sherwood, Starck, & Thompson, 1998). Because pain intensity was our major interest and we wanted to reduce response burden on participants, only the Pain Intensity subscale of APS-POQ was used in the present study. First, participants were asked if they have had any pain in the last 24 hr. Those who indicated that they were in pain rated how much discomfort or pain they were having at that time on a scale ranging from 0 (*no pain*) to 10 (*worst pain possible*). They also indicated the worst pain and the average level of pain they have had in the last 24 hr. Internal consistency reliability was .75 for the Pain Intensity subscale (McNeill et al., 1998).

Eastern Cooperative Oncology Group Performance Status Rating (ECOG-PSR)

The ECOG-PSR (Zubrod et al., 1960) is a single-item measure of physical performance status that indicates overall physical status and ambulatory ability. The total score of ECOG-PSR ranges from 0 (*fully active*) to 4 (*completely disabled*). Because ECOG-PSR is a single-item instrument, internal consistency reliability cannot be assessed. Concurrent validity of the ECOG-PSR was demonstrated by correlating the ECOG-PSR score with the total Edmonton Functional Assessment Tool (Kaasa, Loomis, Gillis, Bruera, & Hanson, 1997) score ($r = .85$, $p < .0001$).

The Medical Outcomes Study Social Support Survey (MOS-SS)

The MOS-SS was developed by Sherbourne and Stewart (1991) to measure multidimensional aspects of social support. There are five subscales within this instrument: Emotional, Informational, Tangible, Positive Social Interaction, and Affectionate Social Support. Respondents are asked to indicate how often each kind of support is available to them if they need it. For the purpose of this investigation, we used only the Emotional, Informational, and Affectionate Support subscales to measure the participants' social support to reduce participant burden and because they receive tangible support from their caregivers. Internal consistency reliability was reported as .97 for the total score of MOS-SS (Sherbourne & Stewart, 1991). Construct validity was supported by its negative relationship with loneliness ($r = -.67$), and positive relationships with family functioning ($r = .53$), marital functioning ($r = .56$), mental health ($r = .45$), and current health ($r = 2.2$) (Sherbourne & Stewart, 1991).

Procedure

Participants' approvals were obtained prior to data collection. All data were collected at participants' homes by the first author. Times to meet with participants were arranged for their convenience. After explaining the purpose of the present study and obtaining informed consent, each question was read verbatim to the participants, and responses were immediately recorded. Although this procedure might have resulted in more socially acceptable responses, it was necessary to limit respondent burden.

Data Analysis

To examine the relationship between the independent variables and the dependent variable, Pearson correlations and regression analysis were conducted. Because of the exploratory nature of the present study, in addition to the independent variables addressed in the research question, demographic and health care utilization information were evaluated to determine if they might be relevant to include or control in the regression analysis.

RESULTS

In the present study, spirituality, pain, physical performance status, and social support were the independent variables used to predict the dependent variable—patients' QOL. The means and standard deviations of the study variables, including total scores and subscales, are presented in Table 1. The three most frequent complaints of troublesome symptoms were pain (55.7%), fatigue (47.5%), and shortness of breath (26.2%).

Living with the caregiver was the only demographic variable associated with QOL. Those who lived with their caregiver had a lower QOL than those who did

TABLE 1 **Means and Standard Deviations of Study Variables (N = 60)**

Study Variables (Possible Range)	M (SD)
Dependent variable	
Quality-of-life total score (0-10)	6.7 (1.3)
Social well-being (0-10)	8.3 (1.5)
Psychological well-being (0-10)	6.8 (2.4)
Existential well-being (0-10)	6.5 (2.1)
Physical symptoms (0-10)	6.3 (2.1)
Physical well-being (0-10)	5.3 (2.2)
Independent variables	
Spirituality total score (20-120)	95.8 (18.0)
Religious well-being (10-60)	51.0 (9.1)
Existential well-being (10-60)	44.8 (9.7)
Pain intensity (0-10)	4.2 (1.8)
63.9% had pain	
Physical performance (0-4)	2.9 (.83)
Social support	
Emotional support (4-20)	16.8 (3.2)
Informational support (4-20)	16.5 (3.1)
Affectionate support (3-15)	13.1 (2.6)

NOTE: Quality of life was measured with the McGill Quality of Life Questionnaire (Cohen et al., 1997); spirituality was measured with the Spiritual Well-Being Scale (Paloutzian & Ellison, 1982); pain was measured with the Pain Intensity subscale of the American Pain Society Patient Outcome Questionnaire (McNeill, Sherwood, Starck, & Thompson, 1998); physical performance was measured with the Eastern Cooperative Oncology Group Performance Status Rating (Zubrod et al., 1960); social support was measured with the Medical Outcomes Study Social Support Survey (Sherbourne & Stewart, 1991).

not live with their caregiver (6.28 vs. 7.69, $t = 3.34$, $p < .01$). This variable, therefore, was included in the regression equation for participants' QOL.

Correlation coefficients among the study variables are presented in Table 2. Participants' QOL correlated significantly with pain intensity ($r = -.31$), spirituality ($r = .42$), and social support ($r = .34$). In the present study, physical performance status did not have a significant correlation with participants' QOL ($r = -.06$, $p = .32$).

Results of the multiple regression analysis showed that the five independent variables entered as a set were significantly related to participants' QOL, $R^2 = .38$, $F(5, 54) = 6.66$, $p = .001$ (see Table 3). The unstandardized regression coefficients (b weight) indicated that living with the caregiver ($b = -1.13$, $t = -2.6$, $p = .01$), spirituality ($b = .02$, $t = 2.6$, $p = .01$), and social support ($b = .04$, $t = 2.1$, $p = .04$) were statistically significant contributors to participants' QOL.

DISCUSSION

The hospice patients in the present study had an above average QOL. When compared to national norms on the SWBS (Bufford et al., 1991), participants in the present study had a moderate level of spirituality, a very positive view of their relationship with God, and a moderate level of life satisfaction and purpose. Patients with terminal illness who select hospice care may have greater spiritual and existential well-being than those who do not seek or accept hospice care. Acceptance of hospice care may reflect a greater acknowledgement of their approaching death. When patients accept approaching death, they tend to re-evaluate their purpose and meaning of life. The high QOL in this sample may be because of their higher spiritual and existential well-being. Whether this is because of hospice care, or a function of pre-existing beliefs that led to selecting hospice care, cannot be determined from the present study. The high correlation between religious and existential well-being ($r = .79$), however, coupled with the fact that only 8% ($n = 5$) did not identify with a religion, suggests there were high pre-existing beliefs among this sample. Although some researchers have suggested that individuals do not have to practice or believe in a particular religion to have spiritual well-being (Hatch, Burg, Naberhaus, &

TABLE 2 **Correlations Among Independent and Dependent Variables (N = 60)**

Variable	1	2	3	4	5
1. Quality of life	1.00	−0.31**	−0.06	0.42***	0.34**
2. Pain intensity		1.00	−0.17	−0.15	−0.15
3. Physical performance			1.00	0.01	0.13
4. Spirituality				1.00	0.24*
5. Social support					1.00

NOTE: Quality of life was measured with the McGill Quality of Life Questionnaire (Cohen et al., 1997); spirituality was measured with the Spiritual Well-Being Scale (Paloutzian & Ellison, 1982); pain was measured with the Pain Intensity subscale of the American Pain Society Patient Outcome Questionnaire (McNeill, Sherwood, Starck, & Thompson, 1998); physical performance was measured with the Eastern Cooperative Oncology Group Performance Status Rating (Zubrod et al., 1960); social support was measured with the Medical Outcomes Study Social Support Survey (Sherbourne & Stewart, 1991).
*$p < .05$, **$p < .01$, ***$p < .001$.

TABLE 3 **Results of Multiple Regression Analysis for Quality of Life of Patients with Terminal Illness (N = 60)**

Variable	b	SE	t	Total R^2	F
Living with the caregiver	−1.13	0.43	−2.61**		
Pain intensity	−0.10	0.07	−1.47		
Physical performance	−0.002	0.21	−0.01	0.38	6.66***
Spirituality	0.02	0.01	2.64**		
Social support	0.04	0.02	2.07*		

NOTE: Quality of life was measured with the McGill Quality of Life Questionnaire (Cohen et al., 1997); spirituality was measured with the Spiritual Well-Being Scale (Paloutzian & Ellison, 1982); pain was measured with the Pain Intensity subscale of the American Pain Society Patient Outcome Questionnaire (McNeill, Sherwood, Starck, & Thompson, 1998); physical performance was measured with the Eastern Cooperative Oncology Group Performance Status Rating (Zubrod et al., 1960); social support was measured with the Medical Outcomes Study Social Support Survey (Sherbourne & Stewart, 1991).
*$p < .05$, **$p < .01$, ***$p < .001$.

Hellmich, 1998; Thomas & Retsas, 1999), others have suggested that individuals who have a strong religious belief are more likely to have strong psychological and spiritual well-being (Bufford et al., 1991; Hermann, 2001; Mickley & Soeken, 1993). Spiritual well-being may support patients selecting hospice care and thus account for their having greater QOL than those who do not seed or accept hospice care.

Although others (Cohen, Mount, & MacDonald, 1996; Ferrell et al., 1991; Ganzini et al., 1999; Houck et al., 1999; Riley et al., 1998; Skevington, 1998; Zacharias, Gilg, & Foxall, 1994) have found spirituality and social support to be important predictors of QOL in patients with terminal illness, this is the first study to look at this relationship in a hospice population. In addition to relatively high spirituality, the majority of the participants in the present study also reported a high level of social support. Most indicated that their support came from their primary caregivers or other family members. Some patients who lived alone referred to their pets (e.g., cat, dog, bird) as the source of their social support, which raises an interesting issue on the value of pets for social support of patients with terminal illness. Other sources of contact, such as hospice personnel, may also be important for those patients who lived alone, thus contributing to their QOL through this enhanced social support.

According to findings from an independent t test and the regression analysis, participants who lived alone had a significantly better QOL than those who lived with their caregivers. This was somewhat surprising. Of the 47 participants who lived with their caregivers, 10 (21%) needed to move to the caregivers' houses. Change in living environment (i.e., having to move to the caregiver's home) and fear of becoming a burden may have contributed to this unexpected finding. Besides existing stress from the challenge of death and dying, change in the living environment may be a tremendous adjustment process for patients with terminal illness and may become an important factor that hinders their QOL. That patients who live with their caregivers fear becoming a burden to their caregivers was also evident from numerous comments by participants. For example, patients said, "All I want to do is die. I want to end this as soon as possible because I don't want to see my family suffer with me. I don't want to become a burden on them." "If the Lord wants me, please just take me as soon as possible. I don't want to wear them out." That being afraid to be a burden is one of the major concerns for patients with terminal illness has been identified by others (Singer, Martin, & Kelner, 1999; Steinhauser et al., 2000).

Pain intensity was not a significant predictor of QOL, which also was a surprising finding. According to the literature, researchers found that QOL is relatively unimpaired when patients have mild pain (Serlin, Mendoza, Nakamura, Edwards, & Cleeland, 1995). Of participants in the present study, 63% experienced only mild pain in the last 24 hr, providing supporting evidence for the common belief that hospice care may provide better pain management. All patients in the present study were in hospice care. The QOL of the patients in the present study may not be altered by their pain intensity, not only because of their lower levels of pain but also because of the concomitant reduced variability in pain in the present study.

Participants' physical performance status also did not have a significant relationship with their QOL. Elderly people with a terminal illness may value different aspects of their life. For example, participants may value spiritual well-being more than their functional ability in activities of daily living as they face the challenge of death and dying. On the other hand, there may not have been sufficient variation in this indicator to detect a significant influence on participants' QOL.

The majority (77%) of patients in the present study had ECOG-PSR scores of 3 or 4.

A major strength of the present study was the collection of QOL data directly from participants through in-home visits. The method of data collection also resulted in little missing data. There were some limitations, however, that may have affected the results of the study. The strength of collecting data directly from participants also meant that this sample was limited to those who were well enough to be interviewed. Most participants were White, and all came from two local hospice programs in a single metropolitan area. Findings, therefore, may not be generalizable across different cultural and ethnic groups, to the entire hospice population, or across different care settings. As one of the first studies to focus on end of life among hospice patients, and to gather data directly from patients with terminal illness, the present study makes an important contribution to better understanding hospice patients and their needs and concerns.

REFERENCES

Bretscher, M., Rummans, T., Sloan, J., Kaur, J., Bartlett, A., Borkenhagen, L., et al. (1999). Quality of life in hospice patients. *Psychosomatics, 40,* 309-313.

Brock, D. B., & Foley, D. J. (1998). Demography and epidemiology of dying in the U.S. with emphasis on deaths of older persons. *Hospice Journal, 13*(1/2), 49-60.

Brunelli, C., Costantini, M., Giulio, P. D., Gallucci, M., Fusco, F., Miccinesi, G., et al. (1998). Quality of life evaluation: When do terminal cancer patients and health care providers agree? *Journal of Pain and Symptom Management, 15,* 151-158.

Bufford, R. K., Paloutzian, R. F., & Ellison, C. W. (1991). Norms for the Spiritual Well-Being Scale. *Journal of Psychology and Theology, 19*(1), 56-70.

Cella, D. F. (1994). Quality of life: Concepts and definition. *Journal of Pain and Symptom Management, 9,* 186-192.

Choe, M. A., Padilla, G. V., Chae, Y. R., & Kim, S. (2001). The meaning of health-related quality of life in a Korean sample. *International Journal of Nursing Studies, 38,* 557-566.

Clark, C., & Heidenreich, T. (1995). Spiritual care for the critically ill. *American Journal of Critical Care, 4,* 77-81.

Clinch, J. J., Dudgeon, D., & Schipper, H. (1998). Quality of life assessment in palliative care. In D. Doyle, G.W.C. Hanks, & N. MacDonald (Eds.), *Oxford textbook of palliative medicine* (2nd ed., pp. 83-94). New York: Oxford University Press.

Clipp, E. C., & George, L. K. (1992). Patients with cancer and their spouse caregivers: Perceptions of the illness experience. *Cancer, 69,* 1074-1079.

Cohen, S. R., Hassan, S. A., Lapointe, B. J., & Mount, B. M. (1996). Quality of life in HIV disease as measured by the McGill Quality of Life Questionnaire. *AIDS, 10,* 1421-1427.

Cohen, S. R., & Mount, B. (1992). Quality of life in terminal illness: Defining and measuring subjective well-being in the dying. *Journal of Palliative Care, 8*(3), 40-45.

Cohen, S. R., Mount, B. M., Bruera, E., Provost, M., Row, J., & Tong, K. (1997). Validity of the McGill Quality of Life Questionnaire in the palliative care setting: A multi-centre Canadian study demonstrating the importance of the existential domain. *Palliative Medicine, 11,* 3-20.

Cohen, S. R., Mount, B. M., & MacDonald, N. (1996). Defining quality of life. *European Journal of Cancer, 32A*(5), 753-754.

Cohen, S. R., Mount, B. M., Tomas, J. N., & Mount, L. F. (1996). Existential well-being is an important determinant of quality of life: Evidence from the McGill Quality of Life Questionnaire. *American Cancer Society, 77,* 576-586.

Cooley, M. E. (1998). Quality of life in persons with non-small cell lung cancer: A concept analysis. *Cancer Nursing, 21,* 151-161.

Dahl, J. L. (1996). Effective pain management in terminal care. *Clinics in Geriatric Medicine, 12,* 279-300.

Donabedian, A. (1992). The role of outcomes in quality assessment and assurance. *Quality Review Bulletin, 18,* 356-360.

Easley, M. K., & Elliott. S. (2001). Managing pain at the end of life. *Nursing Clinics of North America, 36,* 779-794.

Fernsler, J. I., Klemm, P., & Miller, M. A. (1999). Spiritual well-being and demands of illness in people with colorectal cancer. *Cancer Nursing, 22,* 134-140.

Ferrell, B. R. (1995). The impact of pain on quality of life: A decade of research. *Nursing Clinics of North America, 30,* 609-624.

Ferrell, B. R., Grant, M., Funk, B., Otis-Green, S., & Garcia, N. (1998). Quality of life in breast cancer: Part I: Physical and social well-being. *Cancer Nursing, 20,* 398-408.

Ferrell, B. R., Rhiner. M., Cohen, M. Z., & Grant, M. (1991). Pain as a metaphor for illness: Part I: Impact of cancer pain on family caregivers. *Oncology Nursing Forum, 18,* 1303-1309.

Floriani, C. M. (1999). The spiritual side of pain: Hospice caregivers help a suffering patient make peace with two religions. *American Journal of Nursing, 99,* 24pp-24rr.

Ganzini, L., Johnston, W. S., & Hoffman, W. F. (1999). Correlates of suffering in amyotrophic lateral sclerosis. *American Academy of Neurology, 52,* 1434-1440.

Hall, P., Schroder, C., & Weaver, L. (2002). The last 48 hours in long-term care: A focused chart audit. *Journal of the American Geriatrics Society, 50,* 501-506.

Hardy, J. R., Edmonds, P., Turner, R., Rees, E., & A'Hern, R. (1999). The use of the Rotterdam Symptom Checklist in palliative care. *Journal of Pain and Symptom Management, 18,* 79-84.

Hatch, R. L., Burg, M. A., Naberhaus, D. S., & Hellmich, L. K. (1998). The spiritual involvement and testing of a new instrument. *Journal of Family Practice, 46,* 476-486.

Hermann, C. P. (2001). Spiritual needs of dying patients: A qualitative study. *Oncology Nursing Forum, 28,* 67-72.

Higginson, I., & McCarthy, M. (1993). Validity of the support team assessment schedule: Do staffs' ratings reflect those made by patients or their families? *Palliative Medicine, 7,* 219-228.

Hood Morris, L. E. (1996). A spiritual well-being model: Use with older women who experience depression. *Issues in Mental Health Nursing, 17,* 439-455.

Houck, K., Avis, N. E., Gallant, J. M., Fuller, A. F., & Goodman, A. (1999). Quality of life in advanced ovarian cancer: Identifying specific concerns. *Journal of Palliative Medicine, 2,* 397-402.

Hungelmann, J., Kenkel-Rossi, E., Klassen, L., & Stollenwerk, R. (1996). Focus on spiritual well-being: Harmonious interconnectedness of mind-body-spirit—Use of the JAREL Spiritual Well-Being Scale. *Geriatric Nursing, 17,* 262-266.

Kaasa, T., Loomis, J., Gillis, K., Bruera, E., & Hanson, J. (1997). The Edmonton Functional Assessment Tool: Preliminary development and evaluation for use in palliative care. *Journal of Pain and Symptom Management, 13,* 10-19.

Kane, R. L., Klein, S. J., Bernstein, L., Rothenberg, R., & Wales. J. (1985). Hospice role in the alleviating emotional stress of terminal patients and their families. *Medical Care, 23,* 189-197.

Kane, R. L., Wales, J., Bernstein, L., Leibowitz, A., & Kaplan, S. (1984). A randomized controlled trial of hospice care. *Lancet, 1*(8382), 890-894.

Kidder, D. (1992). The effects of hospice coverage on Medicare expenditures. *Health Service Research, 27,* 195-217.

Lamendola, F. P., & Newman, M. A. (1994). The paradox of HIV/AIDS as expanding consciousness. *Advances in Nursing Science, 16,* 13-24.

Lynn. J. (1997). Measuring quality of care at the end of life: A statement of principles. *Journal of American Geriatrics Society, 45,* 526-527.

Maguire, P., Walsh, S., Jeacock, J., & Kingston, R. (1999). Physical and psychological needs of patients dying from colorectal cancer. *Palliative Medicine, 13,* 45-50.

McCarthy, M. (1990). Hospice patients: A pilot study in 12 services. *Palliative Medicine, 4,* 93-104.

McMillan, S. C. (1996). The quality of life of patients with cancer receiving hospice care. *Oncology Nursing Forum, 23,* 1221-1228.

McNeill, J. A., Sherwood, G. D., Starck, P. L., & Thompson, C. J. (1998). Assessing clinical outcomes: Patient satisfaction with pain management. *Journal of Pain and Symptom Management, 16*, 29-40.

Mickley, J., & Soeken, K. (1993). Religiousness and hope in Hispanic and Anglo-American women with breast cancer. *Oncology Nursing Forum, 20*, 1171-1177.

Mickley, J. R., Soeken, K., & Belcher, A. (1992). Spiritual well-being, religiousness, and hope among women with breast cancer. *Image: Journal of Nursing Scholarship, 24*, 267-272.

Moberg, D. O. (1979). *Spiritual well-being: Sociological perspectives.* Washington, DC: University Press of America.

Mor, V., Greer, D. S., & Kastenbaum, R. (1988). *The hospice experiment.* Baltimore: Johns Hopkins University Press.

Morris, J. N., Mor, V., Goldberg, R. J., Sherwood, S., Greer, D. S., & Hiris, J. (1986). The effect of treatment setting and patient characteristics on pain in terminal cancer patients: A Report from the National Hospice Study. *Journal of Chronic Disease, 39*, 27-35.

Nuamah, I. F., Cooley, M. E., Fawcett, J., & McCorkle, R. (1999). Testing a theory for health-related quality of life in cancer patients: A structural equation approach. *Research in Nursing and Health, 22*, 231-242.

Paloutzian, R. F., & Ellison, C. W. (1982). Loneliness, spiritual well-being, and quality of life. In A. Peplau & D. Porlman (Eds.) *Loneliness: A sourcebook of current theory, research and theory* (pp. 224-237). New York: Wiley InterScience.

Peruselli, C., Paci, E., Franceschi, P., Legori, T., & Mannucci, F. (1997). Outcome evaluation in a home palliative care service. *Journal of Pain and Symptom Management, 13*, 158-165.

Reed, P. (1987). Spirituality and well-being in terminally ill hospitalized adults. *Research in Nursing and Health, 10*, 335-344.

Reed, P. (1994). Response to "The relationship between spritiual perspecitive, social support, and depression in caregiving and noncaregiving wives." *Scholarly Inquiry for Nursing Practice: An International Journal, 8*, 391-396.

Riley, B. B., Perna. R., Tate, D. G., Forchheimer, M., Anderson, C., & Luera, G. (1998). Types of spiritual well-being among persons with chronic illness: Their relation to various forms of quality of life. *Archives of Physical Medicine and Rehabilitation, 79*, 258-264.

Rosenfeld, B., Breitbart, W., McDonald, M. V., Passik, S. D., Thaler, H., & Portenoy, R. K. (1996). Pain in ambulatory AIDS patients II: Impact of pain on psychological functioning and quality of life. *Pain, 68*, 328-328.

Serlin, R. C., Mendoza, T. R., Nakamura, Y., Edwards, K. R., & Cleeland, C. S. (1995). When is cancer pain mild, moderate, or severe? Grading pain severity by its interference with function. *Pain, 61*, 277-284.

Sherbourne, C., & Stewart, A. (1991). The MOS Social Support Survey. *Social Science and Medicine, 32*, 705-714.

Singer, P. A., Martin, D. K., & Kelner, M. (1999). Quality end of life care: Patients' perspectives. *Journal of the American Medical Association, 281*, 163-168.

Skeel, R. T. (1998). Measurement of outcomes in supportive oncology: Quality of life. In A. M. Berger, R. K. Portenoy, & D. E. Weissman (Eds.), *Principles and practice of supportive oncology* (pp. 875-888). New York: Lippincott-Raven.

Skevington, S. M. (1998). Investigating the relationship between pain and discomfort and quality of life, using the WHOQOL. *Pain, 76*, 395-406.

Smith, C. E., Fernengel, K., Holcroft, C., Gerald, K., & Marien, L. (1994). Meta-analysis of the associations between social support and health outcomes. *Annual Behavioral Medicine, 16*, 352-362.

Steinhauser, K. E., Christakin, N. A., Clipp, E. C., McNeilly, M., McIntyre, L., & Tulsdy, J. A. (2000). Factors considered important at the end of life by patients, family, physicians, and other care providers. *Journal of the American Medical Association, 284*, 2476-2482.

Stewart, A. L., Teno, J., Patrick, D. L., & Lynn. J. (1999). The concept of quality of life of dying patients in the context of health care. *Journal of Pain and Symptom Management, 17*, 93-108.

Thomas, J., & Retsas, A. (1999). Transacting self-preservation: A grounded theory of the spiritual dimensions of people with terminal cancer. *International Journal of Nursing Studies, 36*, 191-201.

Wallston, K. A., Burger, C., Smith, R. A., & Baugher, R. J. (1988). Comparing the quality of death for hospice and non-hospice cancer patients. *Medical Care, 26*, 177-182.

Walton, C. G., Shultz, C. M., Beck, C. M., & Walls, R. C. (1991). Psychological correlates of loneliness in the older adult. *Archives of Psychiatric Nursing, 5*, 165-170.

Weitzner, M. A., Meyers, C. A., Steinbruecker, S., Saleeba, A. K., & Sandifer, S. D. (1997). Developing a caregiver quality of life instrument: Preliminary steps. *Cancer Practice, 5*, 25-31.

Zacharias, D. R., Gilg, C. A., & Foxall, M. G. (1994). Quality of life and coping in patients with gynecologic cancer and their spouses. *Oncology Nursing Forum, 21*, 1699-1706.

Zubrod, C. G., Schneiderman, M., Frei, E., Brindley, C., Gold, G. L., Shnider, B., et al. (1960). Appraisal of methods for the study of chemotherapy of cancer in man: Comparative therapeutic trial of nitrogen mustard and triethylene thiophosphoramide. *Journal of Chronic Disease, 11*, 7-33.

INTRODUCTION TO CRITIQUE #2

This critique examines the research reported by Tang, Aaronson, and Forbes (2004) that examined the quality of life (QOL) of hospice patients with terminal illness. The purpose of this critique is to determine the quality of the research on the basis of the information provided in the report, as well as its potential usefulness for nursing practice.

PROBLEM AND PURPOSE

The identified purpose is "to fill gaps in current end-of-life research question by examining important correlates of QOL of participants." The statement in conjunction with the research appropriately suggests testing relationships among the identified variables in a population of patients receiving hospice care. The authors identify the significance of the problem as lack of information on QOL at the end of life despite the fact that QOL is identified as an important outcome variable of care in the terminally ill. Furthermore, sources are incorporated that urge caution in use of family caregivers' proxy measures of patient QOL in lieu of patients' ratings.

REVIEW OF LITERATURE AND DEFINITIONS

Tang, Aaronsen, and Forbes (2004) limit the number of variables included from Stewart, Teno, Patrick, and Lynn's conceptual framework to QOL, spirituality, pain, physical performance, and social support in order to minimize response burden. Spirituality, pain, physical performance, and social support are the independent variables used to predict QOL (the dependent variable). Global QOL "is defined as an individual's subjective well-being, or a global evaluation of satisfaction with one's life." "Spirituality is the interconnectiveness between self, others, nature, and Ultimate Other (God)." Religious well-being and spiritual well-being are identified as two components of spirituality. Pain is not specifically defined. Physical performance is referred to as the performance of activities of daily living.

Emotional support and tangible support are identified as the types of social support particularly relevant for this population.

A number of gaps in the literature are appropriately identified in support of the study of the QOL of terminally ill patients in hospice care. Little is known about the relationship among the correlates and the QOL, particularly in this population and setting. This study proposes obtaining information on all the variables from the patients receiving hospice care and examining the relationships among the variables included. Most sources cited by these authors are primary. For example, the reference by Clipp and George reports a study of perceptions of illness experience in patients with cancer and their spouse caregivers (cited in Tang, Aaronson, and Forbes, 2004). This source is referenced as a study in the body of the literature review. The article by Ferrell is a review of literature on the impact of pain on the QOL (cited in Tang, Aaronson, and Forbes, 2004) and provides an example of a secondary source.

Measurement or operationalization of the variables is accomplished as follows: the McGill Quality of Life Questionnaire (MQOL) is used to measure quality of life; the Spiritual Well-Being Scale (SWBS) is used to measure spirituality; the Pain Intensity subscale of the American Pain Society Patient Outcome Questionnaire (APS-POQ) is used for pain measurement; the Eastern Cooperative Oncology Group Performance Status Rating (ECOG-PSR) is used to measure physical performance; and the Emotional, Informational and Affectionate Support subscales from the Medical Outcomes Study Social Support Survey (MOS-SS) are used to measure social support. The operational definitions are congruent with conceptual definitions.

HYPOTHESES AND/OR RESEARCH QUESTIONS

A research question from Tang, Aaronson, and Forbes (2004) is stated as follows: "What is the relationship among spirituality, pain, physical performance status, social support, and QOL of patients receiving hospice care?" A research question rather than a hypothesis is appropriately used to guide the study because of its exploratory nature. The dependent variable is QOL; the independent variables are spirituality, pain, physical performance status, and social support.

SAMPLE

The convenience sample of 63 participants was obtained from 2 hospice programs. A total of 95 potential participants were invited to participate via letters from the directors of the hospice programs; 9 of these died or moved before the follow-up phone call. Among the 85 potential participants, 63 agreed to participate but 60 completed the study. This is a nonprobability convenience sample, necessitating caution in generalizing beyond the sample. No justification is provided for the sample size (e.g., power analysis), but the authors used all individuals who agreed to participate. There were no specific inclusion or exclusion criteria mentioned, only that subjects were obtained from two local hospice programs. The sample is appropriate to the design because it reflects the population of interest, i.e., patients receiving hospice care. The type of nonprobability sampling strategy is appropriate given the exploratory nature of the design. The size is adequate for a pilot study that includes five variables.

RESEARCH DESIGN

Tang, Aaronson, and Forbes (2004) use a nonexperimental correlational cross-sectional design that provides Level IV evidence. Correlational designs are nonexperimental because there is no manipulation of an independent variable, no randomization, and no control group to serve as a comparison. This type of design permits examining the relationship of the variables included in the study; it does not test cause and effect relationships. The design is consistent with the purpose of exploring the relationship of spirituality, physical performance status, pain, and social support to QOL. The relationships are

those proposed in the literature review and the research question. The strength of evidence provided by nonexperimental designs is not as strong as experimental designs because there is a different level of control, thereby changing the risk of bias.

Internal Validity

Although the threats to internal validity are most clearly applicable to experimental research designs, attention to the relationships among the identified variables and rival interpretations that might potentially compromise the study is necessary for nonexperimental designs as well. No possible threats due to history, maturation, or mortality are identified for this study. Testing is not a problem because measures are taken only once. Potential bias associated with instrumentation exists due to differences in verbal administration of the instruments. However, this is probably minimized by having all interviews completed by one of the investigators for the study. Selection bias is noted as the major threat to internal validity because of the use of a convenience sample. The lack of random selection negates control for variables such as differences in subjects' life experiences. Overall, few threats to internal validity are identified that would inordinately decrease confidence in the results.

External Validity

Generalizability is limited to the sample because of the effect of sample selection (lack of specific inclusion and exclusion criteria listed).

RESEARCH APPROACH

Methods

Tang, Aaronson, and Forbes (2004) used structured interviews; that is, the researcher read each question verbatim from the questionnaires being used and recorded the responses immediately. It is assumed that the data collection was similar for all subjects because of this method of interviewing.

Legal-Ethical Issues

The rights of the subjects appear to have been well protected. Initially potential subjects were invited to participate by the directors of the hospice programs. After indicating an interest in participating, the purpose of the study was explained and informed consent was obtained from the subjects.

Instruments

Data-collection methods were limited to questionnaires used as interview guides. The items were read to the subjects by the investigator, who recorded their responses at that time. The investigator is reported as collecting data with no description of training before conducting the interviews. The authors identify the possibility of bias due to social desirability of responses when the questions are asked by interview rather than read by the respondent but deemed this approach necessary in order to limit subject burden.

Reliability and Validity

Tang, Aaronson, and Forbes (2004) report an adequate internal consistency reliability for MQOL estimated by a Cronbach's alpha of 0.83 to 0.89. The authors report establishment of construct and convergent validity with a comparison study of cancer patients completed by Cohen, Mount, Tomas, and Mount. Based on the instrument's description, the instrument has adequate reliability and validity. The SWBS is reported to have a Cronbach's alpha ranging from 0.82 to 0.86, which is considered adequate. Construct validity is supported by reports of positive relationships with self-transcendence, religiousness and hope, mental health, and QOL; and negative relationships with loneliness and demands of illness.

The APS-POQ has an internal consistency reliability of 0.75 for the pain intensity subscale. The consistency level of 0.75 is appropriate given the questions asked: present level of pain, worst pain, and average pain over the last 24 hours. No information is provided for the validity of the pain measure but face validity is apparent.

The ECOG-PSR is a single-item measure for which internal consistency is inappropriate since it is a single item. Concurrent validity is demonstrated by a significant correlation of 0.85 with the Edmonton Functional Assessment Tool. The validity for the ECOG-PSR seems adequate.

The MOS-SS total score internal consistency reliability of 0.97 is reported, but no reliability information is provided for the three subscales included in the study. Construct validity is supported by negative correlations with loneliness and positive relationships with family functioning, marital functioning, mental health, and current health. The correlation coefficients range from 0.22 to −0.67 and would seem adequate for validity determinations assuming they reached a level of significance.

ANALYSIS OF DATA

Each of the major variables is treated as an interval level of measure. Descriptive statistics used include frequencies, means, standard deviations, percentages, and correlations. These statistics are appropriate based on the assumption of interval level data. Inferential statistics used are t-tests, multiple regression analysis, and bivariate correlations. These statistical tests are appropriate to use with interval level data. The inferential test, multiple regression, is appropriate to the research question, which asks for the relationship of spirituality, social support, pain, and physical performance to QOL. Level of significance set for the study is not reported, but the significant results reported use 0.05.

Three tables were used to summarize information. The tables have precise titles and headings with little repetition of the text. The footnotes of the three tables are, however, repetitious.

CONCLUSIONS, IMPLICATIONS, AND RECOMMENDATIONS

Given the level of evidence provided by the findings of this study, the results are interpreted in the context of the research question. The results are discussed in terms of the relationships of variables drawn from the framework. The authors identify significant limitations as the following: restricting the subjects to those well enough to be interviewed, having only white individuals in the sample, and drawing from only two hospice programs.

The relevance for nursing practice from this study is the contribution to better understanding the needs and concerns of terminally ill patients receiving hospice care. These authors clearly identify limitations in terms of external validity, that is, the inability to generalize to other groups (cultural or ethnic), to the entire hospice population, or to different care settings other than hospice due to the convenience sample. Specific recommendations are implied in the discussion of unexpected findings and the recognition that this study is one of the first to focus on hospice patients and gather data directly from them.

APPLICATION TO NURSING PRACTICE

The study has merit given the stage of the research program. Nonexperimental studies that provide Level IV evidence often precede and provide the foundation for building a program of research that leads to experimental designs that test the effectiveness of nursing interventions. The study appears valid in that the strengths outweigh the weaknesses. Measures have established reliability and/or validity sup-

porting their use in this study. However, bias in relation to instrumentation is an issue given the reported reliability and validity data. The type of research design is appropriate given the initial stage of this line of investigation and the need to build a knowledge base for evidence-based practice. The level of evidence of this study would be Level IV. The major limitations of a convenience sample and limited representativeness of the sample are acknowledged and serve to direct future research.

Although direct application is not appropriate given the strength and quality of the evidence and the exploratory nature of the research, conceptual or cognitive application of the results from this correlational study to clinical practice is legitimate from the perspective of the Iowa model (Titler et al., 2001). Replication of the study is feasible and necessary.

REFERENCES

Schoenfelder DP, Rubenstein LM: An exercise program to improve fall-related outcomes in elderly nursing home residents, *Appl Nurs Res* 17:21-31, 2004.

Tang WR, Aaronson LS, Forbes SA: Quality of life in hospice patients with terminal illness, *West J Nurs Res* 26:113-128, 2004.

Titler MG, Kleiber C, Steelman VJ, Rake BA, Budreau G, Buckwalter KC, Tripp-Reimer T, Goode CJ: The Iowa model of evidence-based practice to promote quality care, *Crit Care Nurs Clin North Am* 13(4):497-509, 2001.

Critical Thinking Challenges

- Discuss how the stylistic considerations of a journal impact on the researcher's ability to present the research findings of a quantitative report.
- Are critiques of quantitative research reports by consumers of research, either in the role of student or practicing nurse, valid? Support your position.
- Should the various levels of quantitative evidence require different critiquing methods? What assumptions did you use to make this determination?

FOR FURTHER STUDY

Go to your Companion CD for review activities for this chapter.

evolve Go to Evolve at http://evolve.elsevier.com/LoBiondo/ for WebLinks, Content Updates, and additional research articles, for practice in reviewing and critiquing.

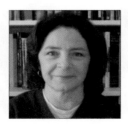

Beth Norman
Elizabeth Norman, PhD, RN, FAAN
Professor, College of Nursing,
New York University, New York,
New York.

I never intended to become a researcher specializing in military nursing history, but I thoroughly enjoyed teaching nursing students and I knew I would need a doctoral degree to succeed in a higher-education career. In 1980 I began my studies at New York University without a dissertation topic. After reading a popular book on Vietnam War veterans that contained stories from nurses who had served overseas, I went to the library to gather more material on these nurse-veterans whose stories I had never known. I found nothing in NYU's library, or through phone calls to the Pentagon, Veterans' Administration, and other agencies. I was not even able to learn how many military nurses had served in Vietnam. The thought that their intriguing experiences would soon be forgotten was so troublesome that I decided to record and analyze these nurses' experiences for my dissertation. And like so many other nurse-researchers, this study changed my life.

I quickly learned that you do not decide to conduct oral history interviews one week and go to talk with someone in your study soon afterwards. I was fortunate to find a mentor at NYU, a professor who spent 7 months working with me on my interview technique and questions. We also developed an extensive reading list. A historian has to be as fully informed as possible before sitting down with a subject. Nothing will make an interview fail quicker than when a person senses an interviewer is disorganized or unprepared. This fact is especially true with war veterans who are about to share the most intense times of their lives with you.

Using a snowball sampling technique, I readily found 50 women who agreed to be interviewed either in their homes or at their workplace. Armed with a map of Vietnam, two tape recorders (in case one broke), and questions, I began the work. Speaking with these women, some of whom were still in uniform, others who had become civilians, was interesting and often exhilarating. Their deep commitment to their patients, their courage under fire, and their compassion made me prouder to be a nurse than at any other time in my career. I remember thinking that if people such as these were nurses, I was in the right profession.

Speaking with these veterans was also stressful and, many times, very sad. I came to see that nurses truly see the consequences of war. The combat soldier is too busy fighting and trying to stay alive to recognize the true extent of the slaughter. It is the nurse standing by the bloody gurneys who knows war like no one else. Their stories of loss—youth, health, naiveté—were hard to hear over and over again. Many women cried as they recalled particular patients or the less than warm welcome our country gave the Vietnam veterans when they came home. They made me look at the world and at war in a much more meaningful way than I ever had.

I transcribed each tape and used an early word processing program to do content analysis; however, I collected so much information that I used only about one fourth of my data in my dissertation. After I graduated in 1986, I decided to write a book, and in 1990 published *Women at War: The Story of Fifty Military Nurses who Served in Vietnam 1965-1973* (University of Pennsylvania Press). To celebrate I had a party for these nurses. We had a grand time and several of them have become good friends. There is a bond that can develop between oral historian and subject as you share these war experiences. Many scholars are not aware of these friendships, but they are a nice reward for this type of research.

About the time my book was published, I decided to organize another wartime nursing study. Only this time I wanted to research the 77 military nurses who were captured in the Philippines in 1942 and became the largest group of female POWs in the history of our country. I felt that the prison experience would add another dimension to my wartime study. Using a contact I had made during the Vietnam study, I found these women and began the process again: reading, organizing my questions, and reviewing archival material. (As an aside, another secret to historical work is that archivists in private and federal libraries are the most friendly and helpful resource people you will ever meet in your work.)

Several of the WWII former POWs, like their Vietnam counterparts, only agreed to speak with me because I was a nurse. They felt that I would understand the difficult decisions they often had to make in a way that a non-nurse would not. These interviews took on a familiar pattern. War veterans almost always begin the interviews by asking you a few personal questions; then they tell you one or two funny stories from the war. I begin my formal interview with general questions about their youth, a time period that is generally easy to discuss. Slowly we work our way to the difficult questions about fear, death, triage, courage, and cowardice. The process is similar to peeling an onion, but I always end the sessions in the present time, not only to get important data but also to help them recover from their intense memories. Rarely do I conduct only one interview; usually I return many times over the course of the study. The multiple interviews combined with photos, diaries, and letters the veterans share provide rich data sources.

The WWII veterans taught me something else about nursing. For them, the ability to keep working, whether on the battlefield or in prison camp, was life-sustaining. Nursing gave them a reason to get up every morning. The women became a family and this family supported one another through the despair and loneliness of prison camp. Once again, I found myself proud to be a nurse.

During the course of this study, which took 8 years, I often experienced another joy of historical work—the hunt for long-lost but important material. Historians can spend weeks going through archival boxes or calling relatives of deceased subjects looking for a particular piece of information. When you find it, there is a feeling of "eureka" and a moment to be savored. This reaction happened when I found a diary on microfilm that no one knew existed or a series of essential memorandum in a box stored in a garage. The "hunt" is time consuming but it can be fun.

The story of this group was so compelling that I decided to write a book for the general public, and in 1999 Random House published the hardcover and in 2000 Pocket Books the paperback of *We Band of Angels: The Untold Story of American Nurses Trapped on Bataan by the Japanese*. My current project is a book about the men who served on Bataan. I became so absorbed with their story and plight that I wanted to study them before they were all gone. I am working with a coinvestigator for the first time, and together with Michael Norman I have traveled to Asia four times to interview former Filipino and Japanese soldiers and across our country to speak with American veterans for a book we call *Tears in the Darkness*. Spending time on Bataan in the Philippines allowed me to see where the nurses from *We Band of Angels* served, and where the men fought and suffered an died. Much of Bataan is unchanged; it is easy to imagine the noise and dust and to imagine the terror of combat. We are completing our manuscript, and I now can see the value of looking at historical experiences through the lens of three different cultures.

We all have much to learn about war and its aftermath. I hope that researchers just starting their careers will consider historical work so more of our past does not vanish before we learn its valuable secrets and lessons.

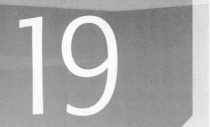

MARITA G. TITLER*

Developing an Evidence-Based Practice

KEY TERMS

conduct of research
diffusion
dissemination
evaluation
evidence-based guidelines

evidence-based practice
integrative research review
knowledge-focused triggers
learning outcomes
opinion leaders

problem-focused triggers
research utilization
translation science

LEARNING OUTCOMES

After reading this chapter, the student should be able to do the following:
- Differentiate among conduct of nursing research, research utilization, and evidence-based practice.
- Describe the steps of evidence-based practice.
- Identify three barriers to evidence-based practice and strategies to address each barrier.
- List three sources for finding evidence.
- Describe strategies for implementing evidence-based practice changes.
- Identify steps for evaluating an evidence-based change in practice.
- Use research findings and other forms of evidence to improve the quality of care.

STUDY RESOURCES

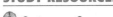 Go to your Companion CD for review activities for this chapter.

evolve Go to Evolve at http://evolve.elsevier.com/LoBiondo/ for Weblinks, Content Updates, and additional research articles for practice in reviewing and critiquing.

*The author would like to acknowledge Kim Jordan for her superb assistance in preparing this manuscript for publication.

"The stark reality [is] that we invest billions in research to find appropriate treatments, we spend more than $1 trillion on health care annually, we have extraordinary capacity to deliver the best care in the world, but we repeatedly fail to translate that knowledge and capacity into clinical practice" (Institute of Medicine, 2003) (p. 2). For example, fewer than half of adults over 50 years of age received recommended screening tests for colorectal cancer; inadequate care after a heart attack results in 18,000 unnecessary deaths per year; and 17 million people were informed by their pharmacist that the drugs they were prescribed could cause an interaction. Failure to rescue, decubitus ulcers, and postoperative sepsis account for 60% of all patient safety incidents among Medicare patients hospitalized from 2000 through 2002; decubitus ulcers account for $2.57 billion in excess inpatient costs to Medicare over 3 years (2000-2002); and postoperative pulmonary embolism or deep vein thrombosis (DVT) accounts for $1.4 billion in excess inpatient costs to Medicare over 3 years (2000-2002) (Health Grades Inc., 2004).

Conduct of research is only the first step in improving practice through the use of research (Titler and Everett, 2001). Because of the gap between discovery and use of knowledge in practice (Farquhar, Stryer, and Slutsky, 2002; Feldman and Kane, 2003; Lavis et al., 2003), concentrated efforts must focus on methods to speed translation of research findings into practice. Development and dissemination of evidence-based practice guidelines are essential steps, but alone do little to promote knowledge uptake by direct care providers. Promoting use of evidence in practice is an active process that is facilitated, in part, by modeling and imitation of others who have successfully adopted the innovation, an organizational culture that values and supports use of evidence, and by localization of the evidence for use in a specific health care setting (Berwick, 2003; Gillbody et al., 2003; Rogers, 2003a).

Translation of research into practice (TRIP) is a multifaceted, systemic process of promoting adoption of evidence-based practices (EBPs) in delivery of health care services that goes beyond dissemination of evidence-based guidelines (Farquhar et al., 2002). Dissemination activities take many forms including publications, conferences, consultations, and training programs, but promoting knowledge uptake and changing practitioner behaviors require active interchange with those in direct care. Although the science of translation is young, the effectiveness of interventions for promoting adoption of EBPs is being studied, and federal funding is supporting research in this area (Agency for Healthcare Research and Quality, 2003; Demakis et al., 2000; Farquhar et al., 2002). Additionally, more evidence is available to guide selection of strategies for translating research into practice than was available 5 years ago (Doebbeling et al., 2002; Dykes, 2003; Eisenberg and Kamerow, 2001; Katz et al., 2002). This chapter presents an overview of EBP—the process of implementing evidence into practice to improve patient outcomes—and a description of translation science.

OVERVIEW OF EVIDENCE-BASED PRACTICE

The relationships among conduct, dissemination, and utilization of research are illustrated in Figure 19-1. **Conduct of research** is the analysis of data collected from a homogenous group of subjects who meet study inclusion and exclusion criteria for the purpose of answering specific research questions or testing specified hypotheses. Research design, methods, and statistical analyses are guided by the state of the science in the area of investigation. Traditionally, conduct of research has included **dissemination** of findings via research reports in journals and at scientific conferences. In comparison, **research utilization** is the process of using *research findings* to improve patient care. It encompasses dissemination of scientific knowledge; critique of studies; synthesis of research findings; determining applicability of findings for practice; developing an evidence-based standard or guideline; implementing the standard; and evaluating the

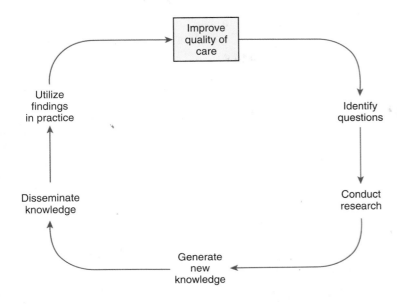

Figure 19-1. Model of the relationship between conduct, dissemination, and use of research. (Redrawn from Weiler K, Buckwalter K, Titler M: Debate: Is nursing research used in practice? In McCloskey J, Grace H, editors: *Current issues in nursing,* ed 4, St Louis, 1994, Mosby.)

practice change with respect to staff, patients, and cost/resource utilization (Titler et al., 2001). **Evidence-based practice** (EBP) has been defined by some experts as the synthesis and use of scientific findings from randomized clinical trials only (Estabrooks, 2004), while others define EBP more broadly to include use of empirical evidence from other scientific methods (e.g., descriptive studies) and use of information from case reports and expert opinion (Cook, 1998; Sackett et al., 2000). The definition used in this book is offered by Sackett and colleagues (2000) who define evidence-based practice as "the integration of best research evidence with clinical expertise and patient values." As illustrated in the knowledge generation and use cycle (Figure 19-1), application of research findings in practice may not only improve quality care but also create new and exciting questions to be addressed via conduct of research.

The terms *research utilization* and *evidence-based practice* are sometimes used interchangeably (Jennings and Loan, 2001). Although these two terms are related, they are not "one and the same." Adopting the definition of EBP as the conscious and judicious use of the current "best" evidence in the care of patients and delivery of

health care services, research utilization is a subset of EBP that focuses on the application of *research* findings. **Evidence-based practice** is a broader term that not only encompasses research utilization but also includes use of case reports and expert opinion in deciding the practices to be used in health care. When enough research evidence is available, it is recommended that the evidence base for practice be based on the research. In some cases, a sufficient research base may not be available, and the health care provider may need to supplement research findings with other types of evidence such as expert opinion and case reports when developing an EBP guideline. As more research is done in a specific area, the research evidence can be used to update and refine the guideline.

 EVIDENCE-BASED PRACTICE TIP

Remember that registered nurses (RNs) are expected to access, appraise, and incorporate research evidence into their professional judgment and decision-making as well as to consider preferences and values of their patient population.

Use of Evidence in Practice

Nursing has a rich history of using research in practice, pioneered by Florence Nightingale who used data to change practices that contributed to high mortality rates in hospitals and communities (Nightingale, 1858, 1859, 1863a, 1863b). Although during the early and mid 1900s, few nurses built on the solid foundation of research utilization exemplified by Nightingale, the nursing profession has provided major leadership for improving care through application of research findings in practice (Kirchhoff, 2004). Today nurses are being prepared as scientists in nursing, leading the way in translation science, and, as a result, the scientific body of nursing knowledge is growing. It is now every nurse's responsibility to facilitate the use of nursing knowledge in practice.

Cronenwett (1995) and others (Estabrooks, 2004) describe two forms of using research evidence in practice: conceptual and decision driven. Conceptually-driven forms influence the thinking of the health care provider, not necessarily action. Exposure to new scientific knowledge occurs, but the new knowledge may not be used to change or guide practice. An integrative review of the literature, formulation of a new theory, or generating new hypotheses may be the result. Use of knowledge in this way is referred to as knowledge creep or cognitive application. It is often used by individuals who read and incorporate research into their critical thinking. Decision-driven forms of using evidence in practice encompass application of scientific knowledge as part of a new practice, policy, procedure, or intervention. In this type of application of research findings, a critical decision is reached to change or endorse current practice based on review and critique of studies applicable to that practice. Examples of decision-driven models of using research in practice are the Iowa Model of Evidence-Based Practice to Promote Quality Care (Titler et al., 2001), the Promoting Action on Research Implementation in Health Services (PARIHS) model (Rycroft-Malone et al., 2002), and the Conduct and Utilization of Research in Nursing (CURN) model (Haller, Reynolds, and Horsley, 1979; Horsley et al., 1983).

Multifaceted active dissemination strategies are needed to promote use of research evidence in clinical and administrative health care decision-making, and they need to address *both* the individual practitioner and the organizational perspective. When nurses decide individually what evidence to use in practice, considerable variability in practice patterns results, potentially resulting in adverse patient outcomes. For example, a solely "individual" perspective of evidence-based practice would leave the decision about use of evidence-based endotracheal suctioning techniques to each nurse. Some nurses may be familiar with the research findings for endotracheal suctioning while others may not. This is likely to result in different and conflicting practices being used as nurses change shifts every 8 to 12 hours. From an organizational perspective, policies and procedures are written that are based on research, and then adoption of these practices by nurses is systematically promoted in the organization.

Models of Evidence-Based Practice

Multiple models of EBP and translation science are available (Berwick, 2003; Dufault, 2001, 2004; Olade, 2004; Rosswurm and Larrabee, 1999; Rycroft-Malone et al., 2002; Soukup, 2000; Stetler, 2003; Titler and Everett, 2001; Titler et al., 2001; Wagner et al., 2001). Common elements of these models are syntheses of evidence, implementation, evaluation of the impact on patient care, and consideration of the context/setting in which the evidence is implemented.

Although review of these models is beyond the scope of this chapter, implementing evidence in practice must be guided by a conceptual model to organize the strategies being used, and to elucidate the extraneous variables (e.g., behaviors and facilitators) that may influence adoption of EBPs (e.g., organizational size, characteristics of users). Conceptual models used in the TRIP I and TRIP II studies, funded by AHRQ, were adult learning , health education, social influence, marketing, and organizational and behavior theories (Farquhar et al., 2002). Investigators (Jones, 2000; Titler and Everett, 2001; Titler et al., 2003) have used E. Rogers' Diffusion of Innovation model (1995, 2004), the PARIHS (Promoting Action on Research Implementation in Health Services) model (Rycroft-Malone et al., 2002), the "push/pull framework" (Lavis et al., 2003; Nutley, Davies, and Walter, 2003; Nutley and Davies, 2000), the decision-making framework (Lomas et al., 1991), and the IHI model (Berwick, 2003) in translation science and EBP.

Of particular note in recent publications (Redfern and Christian, 2003; Rycroft-Malone et al., 2002) is the dialogue regarding use of linear conceptual models in contrast to those that are more dynamic and interactive. "Some early conceptual models of the implementation of evidence into practice advocated a linear and logical process where the emphasis was on informing and monitoring with a view to changing practice. More recent experience via projects such as the Promoting Action on Clinical Effectiveness (PACE) program and the STEP project indicate that the reality is messy and challenging and not easily represented by rational models" (Rycroft-Malone et al., 2002) (p. 174). Emerging from the EBP literature is an analytical dialogue regarding the type of models that should guide implementing evidence in practice. The *rational linear approach* to change management typifies the planned mode of change because it assumes the process of change will proceed through a logical step-by-step progression from one stage to the next. Within the *transitional tradition* is Lewin's force-field theory of change with its unfreezing, moving, and refreezing stages that strive to maintain equilibrium between forces driving and resisting change. Transitional change tends to be episodic, planned, and radical, as occurs when a new state replaces an old one over a controlled period of time. *Transformational change* is also radical but emergent in that the new state takes shape following the chaotic demise of the old and the period of time taken is uncontrolled. Redfern and Christian (2003) note, "oversimplified models of impact applied to innovation requires a dynamic, interactive and nonlinear process." Because Rogers' model discusses knowledge uptake as the process of first acquiring the knowledge through persuasion and confirmation, his framework has been, by some authors, categorized as linear and nondynamic. Rogers is very clear that his model of innovation diffusion is anything but linear, with empirical evidence to demonstrate that the characteristics of the innovation or EBP, and how it is communicated to users within a social system, affect the rate and extent of adopting the EBPs (Rogers, 2003a).

EVIDENCE-BASED PRACTICE TIP

Think about whether the EBP model you choose as your framework for guiding your EBP projects focuses on individual or organizational change.

The Iowa Model of Evidence-Based Practice

The Iowa Model of Evidence-Based Practice is overviewed here as an example of an EBP *practice* model (Figure 19-2). This model has been widely disseminated and adopted in academic and clinical settings (Titler et al., 2001). Since the original publication of this model in 1994 (Titler et al., 1994), the authors have received 152 written requests to use the model for publications, presentations, graduate and undergraduate research courses, and clinical research programs. It has been cited 44 times in nursing journal articles (Social Science Citation Index 2003). It is an organizational, collaborative model that incorporates conduct of research, use of research evidence, and other types of evidence (Titler et al., 2001). Authors of the Iowa model adopted the definition of EBP as the conscientious and judicious use of current best evidence to guide health care decisions (Sackett et al., 1996). Levels of evi-

**The Iowa Model of
Evidence-Based Practice to Promote Quality Care**

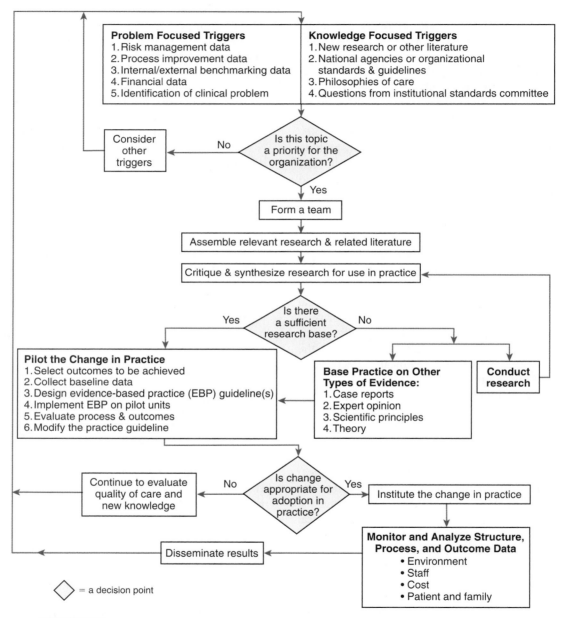

Figure 19-2. The Iowa Model of Evidence-Based Practice to Promote Quality Care. (Redrawn from Titler et al., 2001b.)

dence range from meta-analysis and randomized clinical trials to case reports and expert opinion (also see Table 2-1 in Chapter 2). In this model, knowledge-focused and problem-focused "trigger(s)" lead staff members to question current nursing practice and whether patient care can be improved through the use of research findings. If through the process of literature review and critique of studies it is found that there is not a sufficient number of scientifically sound studies to use as a base for practice, consideration is given to conducting a study. Nurses in practice collaborate with scientists in nursing and other disciplines to conduct clinical research that addresses practice problems encountered in the care of patients. Findings from such studies are then combined with findings from existing scientific knowledge to develop and implement these practices. If there is insufficient research to guide practice, and conducting a study is not feasible, other types of evidence (e.g., case reports, expert opinion, scientific principles, theory) are used and/or combined with available research evidence to guide practice. Priority is given to projects in which a high proportion of practice is guided by research evidence. Practice guidelines usually reflect research and nonresearch evidence and therefore are called EBP guidelines.

An EBP guideline is developed from the available evidence. The recommended practices, based on the relevant evidence, are compared to current practice, and a decision is made about the necessity for a practice change. If a practice change is warranted, changes are implemented using a process of planned change. The practice is first implemented with a small group of patients, and an evaluation is carried out. The EBP is then refined on the basis of evaluation data, and the change is implemented with additional patient populations for which it is appropriate. Patient/family, staff, and fiscal outcomes are monitored. Organizational support and administrative support are important factors for success in using evidence in care delivery.

 EVIDENCE-BASED PRACTICE TIP

Knowledge-focused and problem-focused triggers that represent information needs from clinical practice are converted into focused, structured clinical questions.

STEPS OF EVIDENCE-BASED PRACTICE

The Iowa Model of Evidence-Based Practice to Promote Quality Care (Titler et al., 2001) (see Figure 19-2) in conjunction with Rogers' diffusion of innovation model (Rogers, 1995, 2003b; Titler and Everett, 2001) provide guiding steps in actualizing EBP. A team approach is most helpful in fostering a specific EBP, with one person in the group providing the leadership for the project.

Selection of a Topic

The first step in carrying out an EBP project is to select a topic. Ideas for EBP come from several sources categorized as problem-focused and knowledge-focused triggers. **Problem-focused triggers** are those identified by staff through quality improvement, risk surveillance, benchmarking data, financial data, or recurrent clinical problems. An example of a problem-focused trigger is increased incidence of deep venous thrombosis and pulmonary emboli in trauma and neurosurgical patients. **Knowledge-focused triggers** are ideas generated when staff read research, listen to scientific papers at research conferences, or encounter EBP guidelines published by federal agencies or specialty organizations. Examples initiated from knowledge-focused triggers include pain management, prevention of skin breakdown, assessing placement of nasogastric and nasointestinal tubes, and use of saline to maintain patency of arterial lines. Sometimes topics arise from a combination of problem- and knowledge-focused triggers such as the length of bed rest time after femoral artery catheterization. In selecting a topic, it is essential that nurses consider how the topic and formulating a clinical question fit with organization, department, and unit priorities in order to garner support from leaders within the organization and the necessary resources to successfully complete the project.

Individuals should work collectively to achieve consensus in topic selection. Working in groups to review performance improvement data, brainstorm about ideas, and achieve consensus about the final selection is helpful. For example, a unit staff meeting may be used to discuss ideas for EBP, quality improvement committees may identify three to four practice areas in need of attention (e.g., urinary tract infections in the elderly, preventing constipation in the elderly), an EBP task force may be appointed to select and address a clinical practice issue (e.g., pain management), or a Delphi survey technique may be used to prioritize areas for EBP. Criteria to consider when selecting a topic are outlined in Box 19-1. Table 19-1 shows a helpful chart for selecting a topic.

 HELPFUL H I N T

No matter what method is used to select an EBP topic, it is critical that the staff members who will implement the potential practice changes are involved in selecting the topic and view it as contributing significantly to the quality of care and patient outcomes.

Forming a Team

A team is responsible for development, implementation, and evaluation of the EBP. The team or group may be an existing committee such as the quality improvement committee, the practice council, or the research committee. A task force approach also may be used, in which a group is appointed to address a specific practice issue and use research findings or other evidence to improve practice. The composition of the team is directed by the topic selected and should include interested stakeholders in the delivery of care. For example, a team working on EBP pain management should be interdisciplinary and include pharmacists, nurses, physicians, and psychologists. In contrast, a team working on the EBP of bathing might include a nurse expert in skin care, assistive nursing personnel, and staff nurses. In addition to forming a team, key stakeholders who can facilitate the EBP project or put up barriers against successful implementation should be identified. A stakeholder is a key individual or group of individuals who will be directly or indirectly affected by the implementation of the EBP. Some of these stakeholders are likely to be members of your team. Others may not be team members but are key individuals within the organization or unit that can adversely or positively influence the adoption of the EBP. Examples of key stakeholders are chief nursing officers, nursing directors of clinical services or divisions, medical directors, quality improvement chairpersons, nurse managers, nurse educators, researchers, nursing supervisors, chairs of committees or councils that must approve system changes (e.g., policy/procedure revisions; changes

BOX 19-1 SELECTION CRITERIA FOR AN EVIDENCE-BASED PRACTICE PROJECT

1. The priority of this topic for nursing and for the organization
2. The magnitude of the problem (small, medium, large)
3. Applicability to several or few clinical areas
4. Likelihood of the change to improve quality of care, decrease length of stay, contain costs, or improve patient satisfaction
5. Potential "landmines" associated with the topic and capability to diffuse them
6. Availability of baseline quality improvement or risk data that will be helpful during evaluation
7. Multidisciplinary nature of the topic and ability to create collaborative relationships to effect the needed changes
8. Interest and commitment of staff to the potential topic
9. Availability of a sound body of evidence, preferably research evidence

TABLE 19-1 **Tool to Use in Selecting a Topic for Evidence-Based Practice**

| Topic Ideas | Priority for: | | Magnitude of Problem (1 = small; 5 = large) | Applicability (1 = narrow; 5 = broad) | Likelihood to: | | | |
	Nursing (1 = low; 5 = high)	Organization (1 = low; 5 = high)			Improve Quality of Care (1 = low; 5 = high)	Decrease Length of Stay/Contain Costs (1 = low; 5 = high)	Improve Satisfaction (1 = low; 5 = high)	Body of Science (1 = little; 5 = multiple studies)

Each topic should be rated by using the scoring criteria and a 1-to-5 scale.
The topic(s) receiving the higher score(s) should be considered for selection.
Adapted from Titler M: *Toolkit for promoting evidence-based practice,* 2002.

in documentation forms), and patients/families. Questions to consider in identification of key stakeholders include the following:

- How are decisions made in the practice areas where the EBP will be implemented?
- What types of system changes will be needed?
- Who is involved in decision-making?
- Who is likely to lead and champion implementation of the EBP?
- Who can influence the decision to proceed with implementation of an EBP?
- What type of cooperation do you need from which stakeholders to be successful?

Failure to involve or keep supportive stakeholders informed may place the success of the EBP project at risk because they are unable to anticipate and/or defend the rationale for changing practice, particularly with resistors (nonsupportive stakeholders) who have a great deal of influence among their peer group. Use Figure 19-3 to think about the status of key stakeholders, and to strategize about interventions to engage various types of stakeholders for your EBP project.

An important early task for the EBP team is to formulate the evidence-based practice question (see Chapters 3 and 21). This helps set boundaries around the project and assists in retrieval of the evidence. A clearly defined question should specify the types of people/patients, interventions or exposures, outcomes, and relevant study designs (Alderson, Green, and Higgins, 2003). For types of people, one should specify the diseases or conditions of interest, the patient population (e.g., age, gender, educational status), and the setting. For example, if the topic for the EBP project is pain, the group needs to specify the type of pain (e.g., acute, persistent, cancer), the age of the population (e.g., children, neonates, adults, older adults), and the setting (e.g., inpatient, outpatient, ambulatory care, homecare, primary care). For intervention, specify the types of interventions of interest to the project, and the comparison interventions (e.g., standard care, alternative treatments). For the pain example, the interventions of interest might include pharma-

cological treatment, analgesic administration methods (e.g., patient-controlled analgesia, epidural, intravenous), pain assessment, non-pharmacological treatment, and/or patient/family education regarding self-care pain management. For outcomes, select those outcomes of primary importance, and consider the type of outcome data that will be needed for decision-making (e.g., benefits, harm, cost). Avoid including outcomes that may be interesting but of little importance to the project. Finally consider the types of study designs that are likely to provide reliable data to answer the question, and search for the highest level of evidence available. A similar type of approach to formulating the practice question is PICO: *P*atient, population or problem; *I*ntervention/treatment; *C*omparison intervention/treatment, and *O*utcome(s) (University of Illinois at Chicago, 2003) This approach is illustrated in Table 19-2.

 EVIDENCE-BASED PRACTICE TIP

The PICO approach is very helpful in formulating the clinical question. It is also a helpful format to use in organizing written documentation of the findings related to your EBP project.

Evidence Retrieval

Once a topic is selected, relevant research and related literature need to be retrieved and should include clinical studies, meta-analyses, integrative literature reviews, and existing EBP guidelines. Use the rating systems in Table 2-1 or Table 19-3 to help you think about the level of evidence provided by the relevant research and related literature. As more evidence is available to guide practice, professional organizations and federal agencies are developing and making available EBP guidelines. It is important that these guidelines are accessed as part of the literature retrieval process. The Agency for Healthcare Research and Quality (AHRQ) funds 13 Evidence-Based Prac-

High – Stakeholder Influence-Low	
• Can positively affect dissemination and adoption • Need information to gain their buy-in *Strategies:* • Collaborate • Involve and/or provide opportunities where they can be supportive • Encourage feedback • Empower	• Can positively affect dissemination and adoption if given attention • Need attention to maintain buy-in and prevent development of ambivalence *Strategies:* • Collaborate • Encourage feedback • Elicit support via their professional status • Encourage participation, prn • Involve at some level
High support High influence	High support Low influence
Low support High influence	Low support Low influence
• Can negatively affect dissemination and adoption • Need great amount of attention and information to obtain and maintain neutrality and work towards buy-in *Strategies:* • Consensus • Build relationships • Detail benefits for them • Involve some (1 or 2) of these individuals on team • Monitor their support	• Least able to influence dissemination and adoption • May have some negative impact • Some attention to obtain neutrality and to work towards buy-in *Strategies:* • Consensus • Build relationships • Involve at some level – team member

Left axis: Low – Stakeholder Support-High

Figure 19-3. Stakeholders (resistors and facilitators). (Redrawn from Titler, 2002.)

TABLE **19-2 Using PICO to Formulate the EBP Question**

	Patient/Population/ Problem	Intervention/Treatment	Comparison Intervention	Outcome(s)
Tips for building question	How would we describe a group of patients similar to ours?	Which main intervention are we considering?	What is the main alternative to compare with the intervention?	What can we hope to accomplish?
Example 1	Pain management for elders admitted to hospital with hip fracture	Pain assessment—pain tool; patient-controlled analgesia	Standard of care Nurse-administered analgesic	Regular (e.g., every 4 hr) pain assessment Less pain intensity Earlier mobility Decreased LOS
Example 2	Pain assessment of cognitively impaired elders	Pain assessment tool designed for assessing pain in cognitively impaired elders in long-term care setting	No pain assessment Yes/no question	Regular pain assessment with treatment of pain Fewer residents in pain

Adapted from University of Illinois at Chicago: *P.I.C.O. model for clinical questions,* http://www.uic.edu/depts/lib/lhsp/resources/pico.shtml.

BOX **19-2** AGENCY FOR HEALTHCARE RESEARCH AND QUALITY EVIDENCE-BASED PRACTICE CENTERS*

1. Blue Cross and Blue Shield Association, Technology Evaluation Center (TEC), Chicago, IL
2. Duke University, Durham, NC
3. ECRI, Plymouth Meeting, PA
4. Johns Hopkins University, Baltimore, MD
5. McMaster University, Hamilton, Ontario, Canada
6. Oregon Evidence-Based Practice Center, Portland, OR
7. RTI International—University of North Carolina at Chapel Hill, Chapel Hill, NC
8. Southern California Evidence-Based Practice Center—RAND, Santa Monica, CA
9. Stanford University, Stanford, CA, and University of California, San Francisco, CA
10. Tufts—New England Medical Center (formerly New England Medical Center), Boston, MA
11. University of Alberta, Edmonton, Alberta, Canada
12. University of Minnesota, Minneapolis, MN
13. University of Ottawa, Ottawa, Canada

*http://www.ahrq.gov/clinic/epc/

---

tice Centers (Box 19-2) that develop evidence reports in selected clinical topics. AHRQ also sponsors a National Guideline Clearinghouse where abstracts of EBP guidelines are published on a website (http://www.guideline.gov). Other professional organizations that have EBP guide-lines available are the American Pain Society (http://www.ampainsoc.org); the Oncology Nursing Society (http://www.ons.org); the American Association of Critical-Care Nurses (http://www.aacn.org); the Association for Women's Health, Obstetrics, and Neonatal

TABLE 19-3 **Summary of Evidence-Based Practice Rating Systems**

Guideline for Management of Acute and Chronic Pain in Sickle-Cell Disease (APS, 1999b)	ACCP/AACVPR Pulmonary Rehabilitation Guideline Panel (ACCP/AACVPR, 1997)	U.S. Preventative Services Task Force (Harris et al., 2001)
Type of Evidence I. Meta-analysis of multiple well-designed controlled studies II. At least one well-designed experimental study III. Well-designed, quasiexperimental studies, such as nonrandomized controlled, single-group prepost, cohort, time series, or matched-case controlled studies IV. Well-designed nonexperimental studies such as comparative and correlational descriptive and case studies V. Case reports and clinical examples **Strength and Consistency of Evidence** A. Evidence of type I or consistent findings from multiple studies of type II, III, or IV B. Evidence of type II, III, or IV, and findings generally consistent C. Evidence of type II, III, or IV, but findings inconsistent D. Little or no evidence, or type V evidence only	**Strength of Evidence** A. Scientific evidence provided by well-designed, well-conducted, controlled trials (randomized and nonrandomized) with statistically significant results that consistently support guideline recommendation B. Scientific evidence provided by observational studies or by controlled trials with less consistent results to support guideline recommendation C. Expert opinion that supports guideline recommendation because available scientific evidence did not present consistent results or because controlled trials were lacking **Type of Evidence** I. Evidence from systematic review or meta-analysis of all relevant randomized controlled trials (RCTs) or EBP clinical practice guidelines based on systematic reviews or RCTs II. Evidence from at least one well-designed RCT III. Evidence from well-designed controlled trials without randomization	**Quality of Evidence** I. Evidence obtained from at least one properly randomized controlled trial II-1. Evidence obtained from well-designed controlled trials without randomization II-2. Evidence obtained from well-designed cohort or case-control analytical studies, preferably from more than one center or research group II-3. Evidence obtained from multiple time series with or without intervention; dramatic results in uncontrolled experiments (such as results of introduction of penicillin treatment in 1940s) also could be regarded as this type of evidence III. Opinions of respected authorities, based on clinical experience; descriptive studies and case reports; or reports of expert committees **Category Rating Validity of Each Study** Good = Meets all criteria for that study design Fair = Does not meet all criteria for this study design, but has no fatal flaws that invalidate the results Poor = Study contains a fatal flaw **Recommendation Grades** A. Strongly recommends that clinicians routinely provide [the service] to eligible patients (found good evidence that [the service] improves important health outcomes and concludes that benefits substantially outweigh harms)

Continued

TABLE 19-3 **Summary of Evidence-Based Practice Rating Systems—cont'd**

Guideline for Management of Acute and Chronic Pain in Sickle-Cell Disease (APS, 1999b)	ACCP/AACVPR Pulmonary Rehabilitation Guideline Panel (ACCP/AACVPR, 1997)	U.S. Preventative Services Task Force (Harris et al., 2001)
	IV. Evidence from well-designed case-control and cohort studies V. Evidence from systematic reviews of descriptive and qualitative studies VI. Evidence from single descriptive or qualitative study VII. Evidence from opinion of authorities and/or reports of expert committees (Melnyk and Fineout-Overholt, 2005)	B. Recommends that clinicians routinely provide [the service] to eligible patients (found at least fair evidence that [the service] improves important health outcomes and concludes that benefits outweigh harm) C. Makes no recommendation for or against routine provision of [the service] (found at least fair evidence that [the service] can improve health outcomes but concludes that balance of benefits and harms is too close to justify general recommendation) D. Recommends against routinely providing [the service] to asymptomatic patients (found at least fair evidence that [the service] is ineffective or that harms outweigh benefits) E. Concludes that evidence is insufficient to recommend for or against routinely providing [the service] (evidence that [the service] is effective is lacking, of poor quality, or conflicted and balance of benefits and harms cannot be determined)

Nursing (http://www.awhonn.org); the Gerontological Nursing Interventions Research Center (http://www.nursing.uiowa.edu/gnirc); and the American Thoracic Society (http://www.thoracic.org). Current best evidence from specific studies of clinical problems can be found in an increasing number of electronic databases such as the Cochrane Library (http://www.update-software.com/publications/cochrane; www.updateusa.com), the Centers for Health Evidence (www.cche.net), and Best Evidence (www.acponline.org). Another electronic database, Evidence-Based Medicine Reviews (EBMR) from Ovid Technologies (http://www.ovid.com), combines several electronic databases including the Cochrane Database of Systematic Reviews, Best Evidence, Evidence-Based Mental Health, Evidence-Based Nursing, Cancerlit, Healthstar, Aidsline, Bioethicsline, and MEDLINE, plus links to over 200 full-text journals. EBMR links these databases to one another; if a study on a topic of interest is found on MEDLINE and also has been included in a systematic review in the Cochrane Library, then the review also can be readily and easily accessed. In using these sources, it is important to identify key search terms and to use the expertise of health science librarians in locating publications relevant to the project. Additional information about locating the evidence is in Chapter 4.

Once the literature is located, it is helpful to classify the articles as either conceptual (theory and clinical articles) or data-based (systematic research reviews, e.g., meta-analysis, research articles, and EBP guidelines) (see Chapter 4). Before reading and critiquing the research, it is useful to read theoretical and clinical articles to have a broad view of the nature of the topic and related concepts, and to then review existing EBP guidelines. It is helpful to read articles in the following order:

1. Clinical articles to understand the state of the practice
2. Theory articles to understand the various theoretical perspectives and concepts that may be encountered in critiquing studies
3. Systematic review articles to understand the state of the science (e.g., meta-analyses and other nonquantitative systematic reviews)
4. EBP guidelines and evidence reports
5. Research articles (e.g., individual randomized clinical trials, (RCTs)

 EVIDENCE-BASED PRACTICE TIP

The focused clinical question is used as a basis for searching the literature in order to identify relevant external evidence from research.

Schemas for Grading the Evidence

There is no consensus among professional organizations or across health care disciplines regarding the best system to use for denoting the type and quality of evidence, or the grading schemas to denote the strength of the body of evidence (West et al., 2002). As illustrated in Table 19-3, for example, The Joint ACCP/AACVPR Pulmonary Rehabilitation

Guidelines Panel (1997) used an A, B, C rating scale to reflect the quality of the studies, including study designs and the consistency of the results of the scientific evidence: A = scientific evidence provided by well-conducted, controlled trials (randomized and nonrandomized) with statistically significant results that consistently support the recommendation; B = scientific evidence provided by observational studies or by controlled trials with less consistent results; and C = expert opinion because available scientific evidence did not present consistent results or because controlled trials were lacking. In comparison, the U.S. Preventative Services Task Force classifies the hierarchy of research design, grades the quality of each study on a three-point scale (good, fair, poor), and then grades recommendations using one of five classifications (A, B, C, D, I) reflecting the strength of the evidence and magnitude of net benefit (Harris et al., 2001). Table 2-1, in Chapter 2, presents the hierarchy of evidence model used throughout this book for rating evidence. It also appears in Table 19-3.

In "grading the evidence" two important areas are essential to address: (1) the quality of the individual research; and (2) the strength of the body of evidence. Important domains and elements of any system used to rate quality of individual studies are listed in Box 19-3 by type of study. The important domains and elements to include in grading the strength of the evidence are defined in Table 19-4. The AHRQ technology report is necessary reading for those undertaking synthesis of evidence for practice and public policy; the scholars reviewed 121 systems (checklists, scales, guidance documents) as the basis of this report. From this set, 19 systems fully addressed the key domains for assessing study quality, and 7 systems fully addressed all 3 domains for grading the strength of the evidence.

Before critiquing research articles, reading relevant literature, and reviewing EBP guidelines, it is imperative that an organization or group responsible for the review agree on methods for noting the type of research, rating the quality of

> **BOX 19-3** IMPORTANT DOMAINS AND ELEMENTS FOR SYSTEMS TO RATE QUALITY OF INDIVIDUAL ARTICLES
>
> | **Systematic Reviews** | **Randomized Clinical Trials** | **Observational Studies** | **Diagnostic Test Studies** |
> |---|---|---|---|
> | • *Study question* | • *Study question* | • Study question | • *Study population* |
> | • *Search strategy* | • *Study population* | • Study population | • *Adequate description of test* |
> | • *Inclusion and exclusion criteria* | • *Randomization* | • *Comparability of subjects* | • *Appropriate reference standard* |
> | • Interventions | • *Blinding* | • *Exposure or intervention* | • *Blinded comparison of test and reference* |
> | • Outcomes | • *Interventions* | • *Outcome measurement* | • *Avoidance of verification bias* |
> | • *Data extraction* | • *Outcomes* | • *Statistical analysis* | |
> | • *Study quality and validity* | • *Statistical analysis* | • Results | |
> | • *Data synthesis and analysis* | • Results | • Discussion | |
> | • Results | • Discussion | • *Funding or sponsorship* | |
> | • Discussion | • *Funding or sponsorship* | | |
> | • *Funding or sponsorship* | | | |
>
> Key domains in *italics*.
> Adapted from Agency for Healthcare Research and Quality: *Systems to rate the strength of scientific evidence,* Evidence Report/Technology Assessment No. 47, Rockville, Md, 2002, Agency for Healthcare Research and Quality, U.S. Department of Health and Human Services, AHRQ Publication No. 02-E016.

TABLE **19-4** **Important Domains and Elements for Systems to Grade the Strength of Evidence**

Quality:	Aggregate of quality ratings for individual studies, predicated on extent to which bias was minimized
Quantity:	Magnitude of effect, numbers of studies, and sample size or power
Consistency:	For any given topic, extent to which similar findings are reported using similar and different study designs

Adapted from Agency for Healthcare Research and Quality: *Systems to rate the strength of scientific evidence,* Evidence Report/Technology Assessment No. 47, Rockville, Md, 2002, Agency for Healthcare Research and Quality, U.S. Department of Health and Human Services, AHRQ Publication No. 02-E016.

individual articles, and grading the strength of the body of evidence. Users will have to evaluate which systems are most appropriate for the task being undertaken, the length of time to complete each instrument, and its ease of use (West et al., 2002). It is also important to decide how the strength of the evidence will be reflected in the guideline. For example, the pulmonary rehabilitation guidelines set forth the practice recommendation and evidence grade, followed by a narrative summary of the research evidence, with reference citations, to support the recommendation. In a recently developed guideline for acute pain management in the elderly (Herr et al., 2000), the practice recommendation is followed by the reference citations in APA format and the evidence grade that reflects the strength of the body of evidence for the recommendation.

 EVIDENCE-BASED PRACTICE TIP

Both research evidence from systematic reviews and individual research studies are critically appraised for strength, quality, and consistency, which will influence their validity and generalizability.

Critique of Evidence-Based Practice Guidelines

As the number of EBP guidelines proliferate, it becomes increasingly important that nurses critique these guidelines with regard to the methods used for formulating them and consider how they might be used in their practice. Critical areas that should be assessed when critiquing EBP guidelines include the following: (1) date of publication or release; (2) authors of the guideline; (3) endorsement of the guideline; (4) a clear purpose of what the guideline covers and the patient groups for which it was designed; (5) types of evidence (research, nonresearch) used in formulating the guideline; (6) types of research included in formulating the guideline (e.g., "We considered only randomized and other prospective controlled trials in determining efficacy of therapeutic interventions . . ."); (7) a description of the methods used in grading the evidence; (8) search terms and retrieval methods used to acquire research and nonresearch evidence used in the guideline; (9) well-referenced statements regarding practice; (10) comprehensive reference list; (11) review of the guideline by experts; (12) explanation of whether the guideline has been used or tested in practice and, if so, with what types of patients and in what types of settings. Evidence-based guidelines that are formulated using rigorous methods provide a useful starting point for nurses to understand the evidence base of certain practices. However, more research may be available since the publication of the guideline and refinements may be needed. Although information in well-developed, national, EB guidelines is a helpful reference, it is usually necessary to localize the guideline using institution-specific EB policies, procedures, or standards before application within a specific setting. A useful tool for critiquing guidelines is the AGREE tool available at http://www.agreecollaboration.org/.

Critique of Research

Critique of each study should use the same methodology, and the critique process should be a shared responsibility. It is helpful, however, to have one individual provide leadership for the project and design strategies for completing critiques. A group approach to critiques is recommended because it distributes the workload, helps those responsible for implementing the changes to understand the scientific base for the change in practice, arms nurses with citations and research-based sound bites to use in effecting practice changes with peers and other disciplines, and provides novices an environment to learn critique and application of research findings. Methods to make the critique process fun and interesting include the following:

- Using a journal club to discuss critiques done by each member of the group
- Pairing a novice and expert to do critiques
- Eliciting assistance from students who may be interested in the topic and want experience doing critiques
- Assigning the critique process to graduate students interested in the topic
- Making a class project of critique and synthesis of research for a given topic
- Several resources available to assist with the critique process include the following:
- Evidence-Based Medicine: How to Practice and Teach EBM, and accompanying compact disc (Sackett et al., 2000)
- The Evidence-Based Practice Manual for Nurses (Craig and Smyth, 2002)
- *Evidence-Based Nursing: A Guide to Clinical Practice* (DiCenso et al., 2004)

As you may remember from Chapter 1, developing your competence as a research consumer who can access, appraise, and apply evidence to your practice is a major objective of this book. To accomplish this outcome, you have begun to build your critical appraisal, that is, critiquing skills through use of the critiquing criteria associated with each component of a research study that appear at the end of Chapters 3 to 16. Chapters 8 and 18 provide you with overall criteria for critiquing qualitative and quantitative research studies as well as examples of critiqued research studies. Chapter 20 will provide you with additional critical appraisal tools.

> **HELPFUL** H I N T
>
> Keep critique processes simple, and encourage participation by staff members who are providing direct patient care.

> **EVIDENCE-BASED PRACTICE TIP**
>
> Regardless of the type of study, you should always ask yourself whether the results of the study are valid: Is the way the study was designed and carried out likely to give a true result?

Synthesis of the Research

Once studies are critiqued, a decision is made regarding use of each study in the synthesis of the evidence for application in clinical practice. Factors that should be considered for inclusion of studies in the synthesis of findings are overall scientific merit of the study; type (e.g., age, gender, pathology) of subjects enrolled in the study and the similarity to the patient population to which the findings will be applied; and relevance of the study to the topic of question. For example, if the practice area is prevention of deep venous thrombosis in postoperative patients, a descriptive study using a heterogeneous population of medical patients is not appropriate for inclusion in the synthesis of findings.

To synthesize the findings from research critiques, it is helpful to use a summary table (see Chapters 8 and 18), in which critical information from studies can be documented. Essential information to include in such summary is the following:

- Study purpose
- Research questions/hypotheses
- The variables studied
- A description of the study sample and setting
- The type of research design
- The methods used to measure each variable
- Detailed description of the independent variable/intervention tested
- The study findings

An example of a summary form is illustrated in Table 19-5. An example of a written synthesis of evidence that might appear in a PICO report or in an EBP team proposal for a change in practice appears below:

Clinical Question: "What is the most effective approach to sedation management for patients on long-term mechanical ventilation?"

Research corroborates that long-term mechanical ventilation is associated with significant patient risks, such as ventilator-associated pneumonias, nosocomial infections, debilitation, and the need for a tracheostomy (Cohen, 2002; Brook et al., 1999; McGaffigan, 2002). Research also suggests that not using a sedation protocol in an intensive care unit is associated with prolonged sedation, longer ventilation times, longer hospital stays, and higher costs (Cohen, 2002; Brook et al., 1999; Jacobi et al., 2002). To compound the problem, patients that are intubated and mechanically ventilated experience a wide variety of noxious stimuli that lead to physical and psychological discomfort. Mechanically ventilated patients typically experience pain, anxiety, and discomforts that are often accompanied by agitation, sleep deprivation, and psychosis. Adequate treatment of these patients with opioids and/or sedative-hypnotics can help to minimize the psychological and adrenergic responses to such stimuli, which otherwise may lead to unwanted agitation and cardiopulmonary instability (Barr, 1995). Thus a systematic multidisciplinary approach to prevent pain, and under- or oversedation, produces both clinical and economic benefits, the main goal of this EBP project (Brook, 1999).

Evidence suggests that the use of protocol-directed sedation reduced the duration of mechanical ventilation for patients with acute respiratory failure compared with the practice of non–protocol-directed sedation (Cohen, 2000; Brook et al., 1999). Brook and colleagues confirm the presence of a statistically significant relationship between the duration of continuous intravenous sedation and the duration of mechanical ventilation. This finding suggests that the use of continuous intravenous sedation is, at least partially, a determinant of the duration of mechanical ventilation for

TABLE **19-5** **Example of a Summary Table for Research Critiques**

Citation	Purpose and Research Question	Research Design*	Sample	Independent Variables and Measures	Dependent Variables and Measures	Statistical Tests	Results	Implications	General Strengths	General Weaknesses	Overall Quality of Study†	Summary Statements for Practice

*Identify the level of evidence provided by the design using a consistent hierarchy of evidence model (e.g., Table 19-3 or Table 2-1).
†Use a consistent rating system (e.g., good, fair, poor).

patients with acute respiratory failure (Cohen, 2000; Brook et al., 1999; Jacobi et al., 2002; Izurieta and Rabatin, 2002).

 HELPFUL H I N T

Use of a summary form helps identify commonalities across several studies with regard to study findings and the types of patients to which study findings can be applied.

 EVIDENCE-BASED PRACTICE TIP

The written synthesis of the evidence highlights the strengths and weaknesses of the available evidence, which will guide you in making a decision about its applicability to practice for your patient population.

Setting Forth Evidence-Based Practice Recommendations

Based on the critique of EBP guidelines and synthesis of research, recommendations for practice are set forth. The type and strength of evidence used to support the practice needs to be clearly delineated. Box 19-4 is a useful tool to assist with this activity. The following are examples of practice recommendation statements:

- Older people who have recurrent falls should be offered long-term exercise and balance training (strength of recommendation = B) (American Geriatrics Society, British Geriatrics Society, American Academy of Orthopaedic Surgeons, and Panel on Falls Prevention, 2001).
- "Apply dressings that maintain a moist wound environment. Examples of moist dressings include, but are not limited to, hydrogels, hydrocolloids, saline-moistened gauze, transparent film dressings. The ulcer bed should be kept continuously moist (Evidence Grade = B) (Kurzuk-Howard et al., 1985; Saydak, 1990; Fowler and Goupil, 1984; Gorse and Messner, 1987; Sebern,

---

BOX 19-4 CONSISTENCY OF EVIDENCE FROM CRITIQUED RESEARCH, APPRAISALS OF EVIDENCE-BASED PRACTICE GUIDELINES, CRITIQUED SYSTEMATIC REVIEWS, AND NONRESEARCH LITERATURE

1. Is there replication of studies with consistent results?
2. Are the studies well designed?
3. Are recommendations consistent among systematic reviews, evidence-based practice guidelines, and critiqued research?
4. Are there identified risks to the patient by applying evidence-based practice recommendations?
5. Are there identified benefits to the patient?
6. Have cost analysis studies been conducted on the recommended action, intervention, or treatment?
7. Have recommendations about assessments, actions, and interventions/treatments from the research, systematic reviews, and evidence-based guidelines been summarized with an assigned evidence grade?

One Example of Grading the Evidence

A. Evidence from well-designed meta-analysis or other systematic reviews
B. Evidence from well-designed controlled trials, both randomized and nonrandomized, with results that consistently support a specific action (e.g., assessment, intervention, or treatment).
C. Evidence from observational studies (e.g., correlational descriptive studies) or controlled trials with inconsistent results
D. Evidence from expert opinion or multiple case studies

Adapted from Titler, 2002.

1986; Alm et al., 1989; Colwell et al., 1992; Neill et al., 1989; Oleske et al., 1986; Xakellis and Chrischilles, 1992)" (Folkedahl, Frantz, and Goode, 2002).

- Perform meatal care for patients with indwelling catheters using mild soap and water daily, or more often as needed. Encrustation can also be removed with mild soap and water (strength of recommendation = B)(Asci and Beyea, 1996; Winn, 1996).

Decision to Change Practice

After studies are critiqued and synthesized and EBPs are set forth, the next step is to decide if findings are appropriate for use in practice. Criteria to consider in making these decisions include the following:

- Relevance of evidence for practice
- Consistency in findings across studies and/or guidelines
- A significant number of studies and/or EBP guidelines with sample characteristics similar to those to which the findings will be used
- Consistency among evidence from research and other nonresearch evidence
- Feasibility for use in practice
- The risk/benefit ratio (risk of harm; potential benefit for the patient)

It is recommended that practice changes be based on knowledge/evidence derived from several sources (e.g., several research studies) that demonstrate consistent findings.

Synthesis of study findings and other evidence may result in supporting current practice, making minor practice modifications, undertaking major practice changes, or developing a new area of practice. For example, a project on gauze versus transparent dressings did not result in a practice change because the studies reviewed substantiated current practice (Pettit and Kraus, 1995). In comparison, a guideline for assessing return of bowel motility after abdominal surgery used a combination of research findings and expert consultation and resulted in a change in practice for assessing bowel motility in this adult inpatient population (Madsen et al., in review). This project resulted in (1) deleting bowel sound assessment as a marker of return of gastrointestinal motility and (2) using return of flatus, first bowel movement, and absence of abdominal distention as primary indicators of return of bowel motility following abdominal surgery in adults.

Development of Evidence-Based Practice

The next step is to put in writing the evidence base of the practice (Haber et al., 1994) using the grading schema that has been agreed upon. When results of the critique and synthesis of evidence support current practice or suggest a change in practice, a written evidence-based (EB) practice standard (e.g., policy, procedure, guideline) is warranted. This is necessary so that individuals in the setting know (1) the practices are based on evidence and (2) the type of evidence (e.g., randomized clinical trial, expert opinion) used in developing the EB standard. Several different formats can be used to document EBP changes. The format chosen is influenced by what and how the document will be used. Written EBPs should be part of the organizational policy and procedure manual and should include linkages to the references for the parts of the policy and procedure that are based upon research and other types of evidence. For example, two staff nurses participating in a pilot EBP program to develop unit-based research resource nurses (RRNs) formulated a clinical question related to the "best practice for management of an inwelling urinary catheter in hospitalized adults 65 years and older." The format used at their medical center was a process standard that is equivalent to an EBP policy or protocol. Clinicians (e.g., nurses, physicians, pharmacists) who adopt EBPs are influenced by the perceived participation they have had in developing and reviewing the protocol (Titler, 2004a). It is imperative that once the EBP standard is written, key stakeholders have an opportunity to review it and provide feedback to the individual(s) responsible for writing it. For example, initially the standard for management of indwelling urinary catheters was presented at the Nursing Practice Council and then to another important stakeholder, the Infection Control Committee, followed by the Medical Products Committee (for cost/benefit analysis), and finally the Information Systems Committee for modification of the electronic patient record (EPR) to include a 3-day post urinary catheter insertion prompt for nurses and physicians to evaluate discontinuation of the catheter (Haber, 2005).

Use of focus groups is a practical way to provide discussion about the EB standard and to identify key areas that may be potentially troublesome during the implementation phase. Key questions that can be used in the focus groups are in Box 19-5.

 EVIDENCE-BASED PRACTICE TIP

> Use a consistent approach to writing EBP standards and referencing the research and related literature.

Implementing the Practice Change

If a practice change is warranted, the next steps are to make the EB changes in practice. This goes beyond writing a policy or procedure that is evidence-based; it requires interaction among direct care providers to champion and foster evidence adoption, leadership support, and system changes. Rogers' seminal work on diffusion of innovations is extremely useful in selecting strategies for promoting adoption of EBPs. Other investigators describing barriers to and strategies for adoption of evidence-based practices have used Rogers' (2003a) model (Sackett et al., 2000). According to this model, adoption of innovations, such as EBPs, is influenced by the nature

---

BOX 19-5 KEY QUESTIONS FOR FOCUS GROUPS

1. What is needed by nurses/physicians to use the EBP with patients in units (specify unit)?
2. In your opinion, how will this standard improve patient care in your unit/practice?
3. What modifications would you suggest in the EBP standard before using it in your practice?
4. What content in the EBP standard is unclear? What needs revision?
5. What would you change about the format of the EBP standard?
6. What part of this EBP change do you view most challenging?
7. Do you have any other suggestions?

---

of the innovation (e.g., the type and strength of evidence; the clinical topic) and the manner in which it is communicated (disseminated) to members (nurses) of a social system (organization, nursing profession) (Rogers, 1995; Titler and Everett, 2001). Strategies for promoting adoption of EBPs must address these four areas within a context of participative, planned change (See Figure 19-4).

EVIDENCE-BASED PRACTICE TIP

> Remember how important effective communication is in marketing a proposed EBP change to key stakeholders in your organization.

Nature of the Innovation/EBP

Implementation processes that encourage practitioner adaptation/reinvention of guidelines for use in their local agency increase adherence to the guidelines (Schoenbaum et al., 1995a; Schoenbaum et al., 1995b; Titler and Everett, 2001). Studies funded by AHRQ (Farquhar et al., 2002) and others suggest that clinical systems, computerized decision support, and prompts that support practice (e.g., decision-making algorithms, equianalgesic chart) have a positive effect on aligning practices with the evidence-base (Oxman et al., 1995). To move evidence from the "book to the bedside," information from EBPs must have perceived benefits for patients, nurses, physicians, and administrators; be "reinvented" and integrated into daily patient care processes; impart evidence in a readily available format; and make EB practices observable for practitioners (Berwick, 2003; Rogers, 2003a). Those responsible for implementing the EBP standard need to consider use of practice prompts, decision support systems, and quick reference guides as part of the implementation process. An example of a quick reference guide is shown in Figure 19-5.

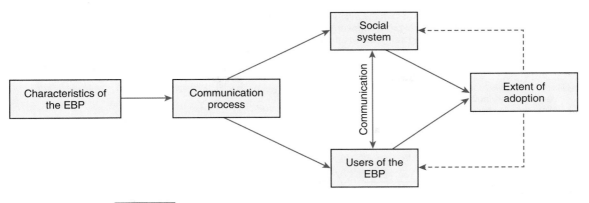

Figure 19-4. Implementation model. (Redrawn from Rogers, 1995; Titler and Everett, 2001.)

Methods of Communication

Methods of communicating the EBP standard to those delivering care affects adoption of the practice (Funk, Tornquist, and Champagne, 1995; Rogers, 1995). Education of staff; use of opinion leaders, change champions, and core groups; and consultation by experts in the content area (e.g., advanced practice nurses) are essential components of the implementation process. *Continuing education* alone does little to change practice behavior (Mazmanian et al., 1998; Oxman et al., 1995; Schneider and Eisenberg, 1998). Interactive education and didactic education, used in combination with other practice-reinforcing strategies, have more positive effects than education alone (Bookbinder et al., 1996; Elliott et al., 1997; Oxman et al., 1995; Schneider and Eisenberg, 1998).

It is important that staff know the scientific basis for the changes in practice, and improvements in quality of care anticipated by the change. Disseminating this information to staff needs to be done creatively using various educational strategies. A staff in-service may not be the most effective method or reach the majority of the staff. Although it is unrealistic for all staff to have participated in the critique process or to have read all studies used to develop the EBP, it is important that they know the myths and realities of the practice. Education of staff also must

include ensuring that they are competent in the skills necessary to carry out the new practice. For example, if a pain assessment tool is being implemented to assess pain in cognitively impaired elders in the long-term care (LTC) setting, it is essential that caregivers have the knowledge and skill to use the tool in their practice setting.

One method of communicating information to staff is through use of colorful posters that identify myths and realities or describe the essence of the change in practice (Titler et al., 2001). Visibly identifying those who have learned the information and are using the EBP (e.g., buttons, ribbons, pins) stimulates interest in others who may not have internalized the change. As a result, the "new" learner may begin asking questions about the practice and be more open to learning. Other educational strategies such as train-the-trainer programs, computer-assisted instruction, and competency testing are helpful in education of staff.

Several studies have demonstrated that opinion leaders are effective in changing behaviors of health care practitioners (Berner et al., 2003; Cullen, 2005; Locock et al., 2001a, 2001b; Oxman et al., 1995; Thomson O'Brien et al., 2002). *Opinion leaders (OLs)* are effective in changing behaviors of health care practitioners, especially in combination with (1) outreach or (2) performance feedback. OLs are from the local

Use this quick reference guide to help in the assessment of pain:
- Before patients undergo medical procedures or surgeries that can cause pain
- When patients are experiencing pain from recent surgeries, medical procedures, trauma or other acute illness

Words that appear in color signal you to additional information on the back of this reference guide.

General principles for assessing pain in older adults:
- Verify sensory ability (Can the person see you? Hear you?).
- Allow time to respond.
- Repeat questions/instructions as necessary.
- Use printed materials with large type and dark lines.

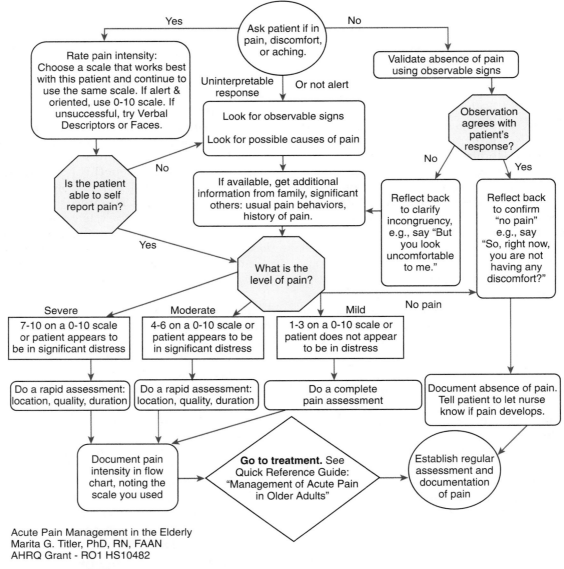

Acute Pain Management in the Elderly
Marita G. Titler, PhD, RN, FAAN
AHRQ Grant - RO1 HS10482

Figure 19-5. Quick reference guide: assessment of acute pain in older adults. (Redrawn from Herr et al., 2000.)

peer group and viewed as a respected source of influence, considered by associates as technically competent, and trusted to judge the fit between the EBP and the local situation. OLs use the EBG, influence peers, and alter group norms (Collins, Hawks, and Davis, 2000; Rogers, 2003a). The key characteristic of an opinion leader is that he or she is trusted to evaluate new information in the context of group norms. To do this, an opinion leader must be considered by associates as technically competent and a full and dedicated member of the local group (Oxman et al., 1995; Rogers, 2003a). Social interactions such as "hallway chats," one-on-one discussions, and addressing questions are important, yet often overlooked components of translation (Berwick, 2003; Rogers, 2003a). Thus having local OLs (early adopters) discuss the EBPs with members of their peer group is necessary to translate research into practice. If the EBP change that is being implemented is interdisciplinary in nature (e.g., pain management), it is recommended that an opinion leader be selected for each discipline (nursing, medicine, pharmacy). Role expectations of an opinion leader are illustrated in Box 19-6.

Change champions are necessary for implementing EBP changes in practice (Rogers, 2003a; Titler, 2004a). They are practitioners within the local group who are expert clinicians, passionate about the clinical topic, committed to improving quality of care, and have a positive working relationship with other health professionals (Harvey et al., 2002; Rogers, 2003a). They circulate information, encourage peers to align their practice with the best evidence, arrange demonstrations, and orient staff to the EBP (Shively et al., 1997; Titler, 2004a). The change champion believes in an idea, will not take "no" for an answer, is undaunted by insults and rebuffs, and, above all, persists. For potential research-based changes in practice to reach the bedside, it is imperative that one or two "change champions" be identified for each patient care unit or service where the change is being made (Titler, 2003). Staff nurses are some of the best change champions for EBP.

Using a "core group" in conjunction with change champions is also helpful for implementing the practice change (Titler et al., 2001). A core group is a select group of practitioners with the mutual goal of disseminating information regarding a practice change and facilitating the change in practice by other staff in their unit or peer group. Success of the core group approach requires that core group members work well with the change champion and represent various shifts, days of the week, and tenure in the practice setting. Core group members become knowledgeable about the scientific basis for the practice, assist with disseminating the EB information to other staff, and reinforce the practice change on a daily basis. The change champion educates the core group members and assists them in changing their practices. Each member of the core group, in turn, takes the responsibility for effecting the change in two to three of their peers. Core group members provide positive feedback to their assigned staff who are changing their practices and encourage those reluctant to change to try the new practice. Core group members also are able to assist the change champion in identifying the best way to teach staff about the practice change and to proactively solve issues that arise (Titler et al., 2001). Using a core group approach in conjunction with a

---

BOX 19-6 ROLE EXPECTATIONS OF AN OPINION LEADER

1. Be/become an expert in the evidence-based practice.
2. Provide organizational/unit leadership for adopting the evidence-based practice.
3. Implement various strategies to educate peers about the evidence-based practice.
4. Work with peers, other disciplines, and leadership staff to incorporate key information about the evidence-based practice into organizational/unit standards, policies, procedures, and documentation systems.
5. Promote initial and ongoing use of the evidence-based practice by peers.

From AHRQ funded study on acute pain management in the elderly (Titler PI; RO1 HS10482).

change champion results in a critical mass of practitioners promoting adoption of the EBP (Rogers, 2003a).

Outreach and consultation by an expert promote positive changes in practice behaviors of nurses and physicians (Thomson O'Brien et al., 2003b). *Outreach (academic detailing)* is done by an expert who meets one-on-one with practitioners in their setting to provide information about the EBP and to give feedback on provider performance; outreach can be accomplished either alone or in combination with others and results in positive changes in health care practices (Davis et al., 1995; Thomson O'Brien et al., 2003a, 2003b). Advanced practice nurses (APNs) can provide one-on-one consultation to staff regarding use of the EBP with specific patients, assist staff in troubleshooting issues in application of the practice, and provide feedback on provider performance regarding use of the EBPs. Studies have demonstrated that use of APNs as facilitators of change promotes adherence to the EBP.

 EVIDENCE-BASED PRACTICE TIP

Opinion leaders and change champions are essential to the success of implementing an EBP change. They are often found among the informal leaders of an organization.

Users of the Innovation/EBP

Members of a social system influence how quickly and widely EBPs are adopted (Rogers, 2003a). Audit and feedback, performance gap assessment (PGA), and use of the EBP are strategies that have been tested (Lomas et al., 1991; Rogers, 2003a; Titler et al., 1994, 2001). PGA and audit and feedback have consistently shown a positive effect on changing the practice behavior of providers (Fiore et al., 1996; Lomas et al., 1991; Thomson O'Brien et al., 2003a). PGA (baseline practice performance) informs members, at the *beginning* of change, about a practice performance and opportunities for improvement. Spe-

cific practice indicators selected for performance gap assessment are related to the practices that are the focus of change, such as pain assessment every 4 hours for acute pain management.

Audit and feedback is an ongoing auditing of performance indicators (e.g., pain assessment every 4 hours) throughout the implementation process, and includes discussing the findings with practitioners *during* the practice change (Jamtvedt et al., 2004; Titler, 2004a). This strategy helps staff know and see how their efforts to improve care and patient outcomes are progressing throughout the implementation process. Audit and feedback should be done at regular intervals throughout the implementation process (e.g., every 4 to 6 weeks) (Jamtvedt et al., 2004; Thomson O'Brien et al., 2003a). Performance gap assessment and audit and feedback data can be provided in run charts, statistical process control charts, or bar graphs (Carey, 2002) (see Figure 19-6).

Characteristics of users such as educational preparation, practice specialty, and views on innovativeness influence adoption of an innovation (Rogers, 2003a; Schneider and Eisenberg, 1998). Users of an innovation usually try it for a period of time before adopting it in their practice (Meyer and Goes, 1988; Rogers, 2003a). When "trying an EBP" (piloting the change) is incorporated as part of the implementation process, users have an opportunity to use it for a period of time, provide feedback to those in charge of implementation, and modify the practice if necessary. Piloting the EBP as part of implementation has a positive influence on the extent of adoption of the new practice (Rogers, 2003a; Titler, 2003; Titler et al., 2001).

 EVIDENCE-BASED PRACTICE TIP

Collecting baseline data before implementation of a new evidence-based practice, and at specified intervals thereafter, provides staff members with a concrete picture of how this evidence-based change in practice is contributing to improving patient outcomes.

Unit A: Fictitious Fall Rate

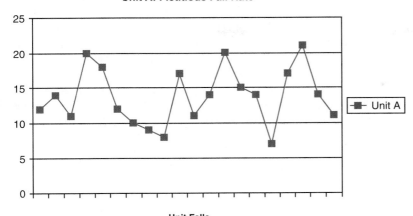

Unit Falls

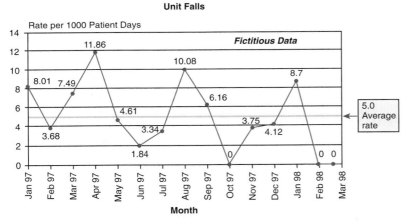

Figure 19-6. Examples of audit and feedback data.

Top Ten Units in Rate of Falls per 1000 Patient Days*

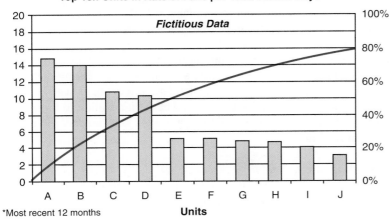

*Most recent 12 months

Social System

The social system (context) has a high degree of influence on adoption of an innovation (Foxcroft et al., 2002; Fraser, 2004a, 2004b; Institute of Medicine, 2001; Rogers, 2003a; Thompson, 2001; Vaughn et al., 2002). Leadership support is critical for promoting use of EBPs (Baggs and Mick, 2000; Berwick, 2003; Carr and Schott, 2002; Nagy et al., 2001; Retsas, 2000; Stetler, 2003) and is expressed verbally, by providing necessary resources, materials, and time to fulfill assigned responsibilities. Additional organizational variables that influence adoption include the following: (1) access to inventers/researchers; (2) authority to change practice; and (3) support from and collaboration with peers, other disciplines, and administrators to align practice with EBGs (Bach, 1995; Funk et al., 1995; Nutley and Davies, 2000; Thomson O'Brien et al., 2002; Tranmer et al., 1998; Walshe and Rundall, 2001). It is important that organizational and unit practice standards as well as documentation systems support use of the EBPs (Titler, 2004a).

The role of the nurse manager is critical in making EBP changes a reality for staff at the bedside. Nurse managers must expect that staff will participate in EBP activities, role-model the change in their practice, and provide written and verbal support for the practice change. When selecting a potential topic, it is important that the nurse manager values the idea and supports the potential changes.

APNs are critical to helping staff retrieve and critique the studies and other evidence on the selected topic. Although staff nurses are often willing to participate, the APN provides significant leadership in the process by facilitating synthesis of the research and other evidence, critically analyzing what practices should be changed, assisting staff to communicate these changes to their peers, and role-modeling changes in practice.

As part of the work of implementing the change, it is important that the social system—unit, service line, and/or clinic—ensure that policies, procedures, standards, clinical pathways, and documentation systems support the use of the EBPs. Documentation forms or clinical information systems may need revision to support changes in practice; documentation systems that fail to readily support the new practice impede change. For example, if staff members are expected to reassess and document pain intensity within 30 minutes following administration of an analgesic agent, then documentation forms must reflect this practice standard. It is the role of upper and middle level leadership to ensure that organizational documents and systems are flexible and supportive of the EBPs.

In summary, making an EB change in practice involves a series of steps and a process that is often nonlinear. Implementing the change will take several weeks to months, depending on the nature of the practice change. It is important that those leading the project are aware of change as a process and continue to encourage and teach peers about the change in practice. The new practice must be continually reinforced and sustained or the practice change will be intermittent and soon fade, allowing more traditional methods of care to return.

☀ EVIDENCE-BASED PRACTICE TIP

Obtaining "buy-in" from the nurse manager is essential since she/he needs to support the staff nurses working on the EBP project. This includes arranging for release time and coverage from patient care responsibilities to provide time to think about and formulate the clinical question, search the literature, appraise the evidence, and develop the EBP product (e.g., policy, standard, protocol), as well as present and market the innovation to the appropriate organization stakeholders.

Evaluation

Evaluation provides an opportunity to collect and analyze data with regard to use of a new EBP and then to modify the practice as necessary. It is important that the EB change is evaluated, both when in the pilot phase and when the practice change is implemented in additional patient care areas. The importance of the evaluation cannot be overemphasized; it not only provides information for performance gap assessment and audit and feedback but also provides information necessary to determine if the EBP should be retained, modified, or eliminated.

A desired outcome achieved in a more controlled environment, when a researcher is implementing a study protocol for a homogeneous group of patients (conduct of research), may not result in the same outcome when the practice is implemented in the natural clinical setting, by several caregivers, to a more heterogeneous patient population. Steps of the evaluation process are summarized in Box 19-7.

Evaluation should include both process and outcome measures (Lepper and Titler, 1999; Rosswurm and Larrabee, 1999). The process component focuses on how the EBP change is being implemented. It is important to know if staff are using the practice in care delivery and if they are implementing the practice as noted in the written EBP standard. Evaluation of the process also should note the following: (1) barriers that staff encounter in carrying out the practice (e.g., lack of information, skills, or necessary equipment); (2) differences in opinions among health care providers; and (3) difficulty in carrying out the steps of the practice as originally designed (e.g., shutting off tube feedings 1 hour before aspirating contents for checking placement of nasointestinal tubes). Process data can be collected from staff and/or patient self-reports, medical record audits, or observation of clinical practice. Examples of process and outcome questions are shown in Figure 19-7.

Outcome data are an equally important part of evaluation. The purpose of outcome evaluation is to assess whether the patient, staff, and/or fiscal outcomes expected are achieved. Therefore it is important that baseline data be used for a pre/post comparison (Cullen, 2005; Titler et al., 2001). The outcome variables measured should

---

BOX 19-7   STEPS OF EVALUATION FOR EVIDENCE-BASED PROJECTS

1. Identify process and outcome variables of interest.
   Example: Process variable—patients >65 years of age will have a Braden scale completed upon admission
   Outcome variable—presence/absence of nosocomial pressure ulcer; if present, determine stage as I, II, III, IV
2. Determine methods and frequency of data collection.
   Example: Process variable—chart audit of all patients >65 years old, 1 day a month
   Outcome variable—patient assessment of all patients >65 years old, 1 day a month
3. Determine baseline and follow-up sample sizes.
4. Design data-collection forms.
   Example: Process variable—chart audit abstraction form
   Outcome variable—pressure ulcer assessment form
5. Establish content validity of data-collection forms.
6. Train data collectors.
7. Assess interrater reliability of data collectors.
8. Collect data at specified intervals.
9. Provide "on-sight" feedback to staff regarding the progress in achieving the practice change.
10. Provide feedback of analyzed data to staff.
11. Use data to assist staff in modifying or integrating the evidence-based practice change.

---

be those that are projected to change as a result of changing practice (Rosswurm and Larrabee, 1999; Soukup, 2000). For example, research demonstrates that less restricted family visiting practices in critical care units result in improved satisfaction with care. Thus patient and family member satisfaction should be an outcome measure that is evaluated as part of changing visiting practices in adult critical care units. Outcome measures should be measured before the change in practice is implemented, after implementation, and every 6 to 12 months there-

EXAMPLE PROCESS QUESTIONS					
NURSES' SELF RATING	SD	D	NA/D	A	SA
1.` I feel well prepared to use the Braden Scale with older patients.	1	2	3	4	5
2. Malnutrition increases patient risk for pressure ulcer development	1	2	3	4	5

EXAMPLE OUTCOME QUESTION

PATIENT

1. On a scale of 0 (no pain) to 10 (worst possible pain), how much pain have you experienced over the past

   24 hours? _____
   　　　　　　　　(pain intensity)

SD, strongly disagree; *D*, disagree; *NA/D*, neither agree nor disagree; *A*, agree; *SA*, strongly agree

Figure 19-7. Examples of evaluation measures.

after. Findings must be provided to clinicians to reinforce the impact of the change in practice and to ensure that they are incorporated into quality improvement programs. For example, an organizational task force to institute EBPs for pain management included members from the Department of Nursing Quality Improvement Committee. Data collection focused on adequacy of pain control and patient satisfaction with pain management. Representatives from divisional quality improvement committees were responsible for collecting data from at least 20 patients per unit or clinical area. Results of the quality improvement monitor were distributed to each nursing unit, and staff were encouraged to use this information in identifying ways to improve pain management practices (JCAHO, 2001; Schmidt et al., 1996).

When collecting process and outcome data for evaluation of EBP change, it is important that the data-collection tools are user-friendly, short, concise, and easy to complete and have content validity. Focus must be on collecting the most essential data. Those responsible for collecting

evaluative data must be trained on the methods of data collection and be assessed for interrater reliability (see Chapter 14). It is our experience that those individuals who have participated in implementing the protocol can be very helpful in evaluation by collecting data, providing timely feedback to staff, and assisting staff to overcome barriers encountered when implementing the changes in practice.

One question that often arises is how much data are needed to evaluate this change. The preferred number of patients (*N*) is somewhat dependent on the size of the patient population affected by the practice change. For example, if the practice change is for families of critically ill adult patients and the organization has 1000 adult critical care patients annually, then 50 to 100 satisfaction responses preimplementation and 25 to 50 responses postimplementation, at 3 and 6 months, should be adequate to look for trends in satisfaction and possible areas that need to be addressed in continuing this practice (e.g., more bedside chairs in patient rooms). The rule of thumb is to keep the evaluation simple, because data often are collected by busy clinicians who may lose interest if the data collection, analysis, and feedback are too long and tedious.

The evaluation process includes planned feedback to staff who are making the change. The feedback includes verbal and/or written appreciation for the work and visual demonstration of progress in implementation and improvement in patient outcomes. The key to effective evaluation is to ensure that the EB change in practice is warranted (e.g., will improve quality of care) and that the intervention does not bring harm to patients (Lepper and Titler, 1999). For example, when instituting a change in practice for assessing return of bowel motility following abdominal surgery in adults, it was important to inform staff that using other markers for return of bowel motility, rather than bowel sound assessment, did not result in increased paralytic ileus or bowel obstruction (Madsen et al., in review).

 HELPFUL H I N T

Include patient outcome measures (e.g., pressure ulcer prevalence) and cost (e.g., cost savings, cost avoidance) in evaluation.

CREATING A CULTURE OF EVIDENCE-BASED PRACTICE

Use of research evidence to guide clinical and operational decisions is a necessity in health care delivery (Cullen, 2005). Chief nurse executives and their leadership staff set the stage and culture for evidence-based practice in their settings. How this is done varies, but essential components are necessary for evidence-based practices (both the process and the product) to be an integral part of the organization.

Providing this leadership is a continuous process that involves four major building blocks (see Figure 19-8):

- Incorporating evidence-based practice terminology into the mission, vision, strategic plan, and philosophy of care delivery
- Establishing explicit performance expectations about EBP for staff at all levels of the organization
- Integrating the work of EBP into the governance structure of nursing departments and the health care system
- Recognizing and rewarding evidence-based practice behaviors

The *first building block* is to assure that the mission and vision statements of the health care system and nursing services reflect a commitment to the provision of evidence-based health

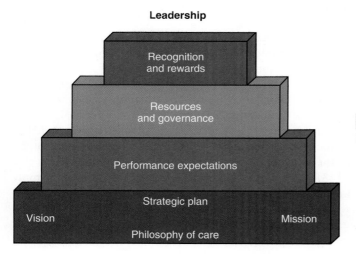

Figure 19-8. Four major building blocks. (Copyright © Marita Titler, PhD, RN, FAAN.)

care. Examples of statements that codify this commitment include the following: "The mission of the UI healthcare system is to provide evidence-based healthcare to consumers across settings and sites of care delivery." "The vision of the department of nursing services and patient care is to be an international exemplar of using evidence to guide clinical and operational decision-making." "Our mission is to provide high-quality patient care based on our strong commitments to practice, education, research, innovation, and collaboration" (UIHC Department of Nursing, 2004).

These lay the foundation for the integration of evidence-based practices throughout the organization. For evidence-based practices to be manifested in everyday work, it is necessary to incorporate specific action statements that promote and foster evidence-based practices into the organization's or department's strategic plan. Such actions might include offering an annual evidence-based practice staff nurse internship program; integrating educational content about EBP into orientation of new staff; monitoring and acting upon the results of key indicators for selected evidence-based practices (e.g., acute pain management, prevention of pressure ulcers, fall prevention); and initiating two to three new evidence-based practices per year that are triggered by operational and/or quality improvement data. For example, if quality improvement data suggest that fall rates are particularly high in selected sites of care delivery, using an evidence-based process to understand the nature of the problem as well as to determine possible solutions might be among the action statements of a strategic initiative regarding patient safety. Equally important to a mission and vision that embraces EBP is clarity about the following: (1) the definition and meaning of EBP (some departments actually adopt a definition); (2) the organizational process or model of EBP; and (3) a philosophy of care that embraces clinical inquiry and questioning of the status quo.

The *second building block* is developing and using performance expectations regarding evidence-based practices. For example, EBP performance expectations for staff nurses should include critical thinking, continual questioning of practice, participating in making EBP practice changes, serving as leaders of change in their site of care delivery, and participating in evaluating evidence-based changes in practice. The chief nurse executive sets the tone for EBP and explicates role expectations of other nurse leaders within the organization regarding the knowledge, skills, and behaviors necessary to promote adoption of evidence-based practices. Performance expectations for nurse managers include creating a culture that fosters interdisciplinary quality improvement based on evidence. Advanced practice nurses' performance expectations include leading a team, finding the evidence, and synthesizing the evidence for practice. Advanced practice nurses assist staff with focusing their clinical question about improving practice, finding and evaluating the research evidence, and maneuvering through the committee structures to implement and sustain changes in practice. The ability of an APN to meet these performance criteria is an essential part of their annual performance appraisals.

Similarly, nurse managers set the tone, value, and work culture for the microsystems they lead. Staff migrate to microsystems that foster professional growth, professional nursing practice, data-based decision-making, and innovative practices, all characteristics of cultures that promote adoption of evidence-based nursing practices. Nurse managers also foster evidence-based practices in their units by allocation of resources, an important element for staff nurse participation in new EBP projects. Consequently, associate directors of nursing, who hire, retain, and value, via performance appraisals, nurse managers and advanced practice nurses skilled in evidence-based practice, are more likely to observe development of clinical innovations and adoption of evidence-based practices in the multiple units and sites of care delivery for which they are responsible.

Enactment of evidence-based practice behaviors by the chief nurse executive (CNE) includes providing resources for EBP such as easy access to evidence-based practice web sites, retaining personnel with expertise in evidence-based practice, supporting programs that develop a critical mass of staff nurses with expertise in EBP (e.g., Evidence-Based Practice Staff Nurse Internship Program; Cullen and Titler, in press), and providing access to assistance with analysis of data and transforming data into information. CNEs also enact the value of EBP by using information from evaluations of existing and new clinical programs in operational decisions, and by rewarding and recognizing direct care providers who make evidence-based practice a reality in their daily work. Using evidence in administrative decisions is another behavior modeled by CNEs that value EBP.

Assessing the work culture of nurses that contribute to job satisfaction and retention and then using this information, along with research evidence, to create administrative interventions that decrease turnover is one example of an evidence-based administrative practice. As it is difficult to support multiple evidence-based practice changes simultaneously, CNEs committed to EBP lead discussion and decision-making regarding priority-setting for areas of evidence-based practice (e.g., skin care, pain). Lastly, but most importantly, it is the CNE's responsibility to assure that the mission, vision, philosophy of care, strategic plan, and performance criteria incorporate language about the value and commitment of the organization to evidence-based practice. Box 19-8 lists examples of performance expectations regarding evidence-based practice.

The *third building block* is integrating EBP into the governance of the health care system, and assuring that resources are available to assist staff with this work. I am frequently asked, "Where should the work of EBP reside?" The short answer is "everywhere," because evidence-based practice saves health care dollars and improves patient outcomes (Farquhar et al., 2002; Guyatt and Rennie, 2002; Rogers, 1995). More explicitly, to sustain a vision of providing evidence-based health care, the work and accountability for EBP must be integrated into the governance structure. This includes interdis-

ciplinary collaboration across departments and services as well as coordination within discipline-specific areas of practice. For example, in nursing the process and evaluation of evidence-based changes in practice should be coordinated with professional nursing practice, quality improvement, research, policy and procedure, and staff education committees. An evidence-based project may be "born" out of a quality improvement committee when process or outcome indicators illustrate an opportunity to improve practice. Similarly, a professional nursing practice committee may initiate an evidence-based practice change in response to information published in research journals, by AHRQ Evidence-Based Practice Centers, or professional organizations. Evidence-based changes in practice must be coordinated with professional policy and procedure committees in order for the evidence to be reflected in practice standards. Documentation systems, be they electronic or manual, must support the evidence-based practices through reminder systems, decision-support algorithms, and easy-to-use documentation forms. Too often, we expect those in direct care to change practices without full modification of the documentation systems that capture and reinforce the desired changes. Although the primary responsibility for tracking and promoting evidence-based practice may reside in a specific department or program (e.g., research, education, quality improvement), EBP must be viewed and valued as essential work at all levels of the organization, and within the committees/councils that govern the health care system. Examples of language reflecting EBP work in functions of committees and councils are found in Box 19-9.

The *fourth building block* is recognition and rewarding EBP behaviors. Such recognition can range from submitting staff projects and names to national and international professional organizations that have recognition programs for excellence in evidence-based practice (e.g., STTI), to recognizing specific staff members in their unit at the change of shift for the care they provide based on evidence. Other recognition

BOX 19-8 SAMPLE EBP PERFORMANCE CRITERIA FOR NURSING ROLES

Staff Nurse (RN)	Advanced Practice Nurse (APN)	Nurse Manager (NM)	Associate Director for Clinical Services	Chief Nurse Executive
Questions current practices	Serves as coach and mentor in EBP	Creates a microsystem that fosters critical thinking	Hires and retains NMs and APNs with knowledge and skills in EBP	Assures the governance reflects EBP if initiated in councils and committees
Participates in implementing changes in practice based on evidence	Facilitates locating evidence	Challenges staff to seek out evidence to resolve clinical issues and improve care	Provides learning environment for EBP	Assigns accountabilty for EBP
Participates as a member of an EBP project team	Synthesizes evidence for practice	Role-models EBP	Uses evidence in leadership decisions	Assures explicit articulation of organizational and department commitment to EBP
Reads evidence related to one's practice	Uses evidence to write/modify practice standards	Uses evidence to guide operations and management decisions	Sets strategic directions for EBP	Modifies mission and vision to include EBP language
Participates in QI initiatives	Role-models use of evidence in practice	Uses performance criteria about EBP in evaluation of staff	Provides resources for EBP	Provides resources to support EBPs by direct care providers
Suggests resolutions for clinical issues based on evidence	Facilitates system changes to support use of EBPs		Integrates EBP processes into division/service line governance	Articulates value of EBP to CEO and governing board
				Role-models EBP in administrative decision-making

activities include an annual recognition day with a display of posters of the EBP work occurring in each unit; recognition in a weekly or monthly internal communication; postings on web sites; and broadcasting the stellar accomplishments in the local, regional, and national media. Some organizations integrate evidence-based practice expectations into the clinical ladder system, and others provide staff release time from direct patient care to do the work of evidence-based practice. Recognition by peers as well as senior administrators is important.

Criteria for evaluating the success of integrating EBPs into an organization include a combination of traditional scientific criteria, effect on the organizational climate, and improvements in providing cost-effective quality care. These criteria are summarized in Box 19-10.

TRANSLATION SCIENCE

Although there are a myriad of initiatives aimed at increasing use of evidence in practice, there is little systematic evidence of the effectiveness of these initiatives (Nutley et al., 2003). **Translation science** is the investigation of methods, interventions, and variables that influence adoption of evidence-based practices (EBPs) by individu-

BOX

19-9 EXAMPLES OF EBP FUNCTIONS OF GOVERNANCE COMMITTEES

Nursing Quality Management Committee
- Develop mechanisms for using evidence-based practice to improve quality care.
- Assist nursing staff to interpret and use data from internal and external sources to improve care or resolve identified problems.
- Coordinate or conduct interdisciplinary performance improvement and use results of evidence- based practice projects that impact patient care delivery from multiple services.
- Promote a scientific approach to problem-solving in management and delivery of patient care services.
- Promote discussion and exchange of information regarding status of evidence-based practice and process-improvement projects.

Professional Nursing Practice Committee
- Develop, evaluate, review, and revise policies and procedures related to professional nursing practice. Ensure policies and procedures are evidence-based, incorporate research findings, and reflect interdisciplinary collaboration as appropriate.

Nursing Research Committee
- Encourage and support the conduct and dissemination of nursing research regionally, nationally, and internationally.
- Develop mechanisms forusing evidence-based practice to improve quality of care.
- Provide leadership for other evidence as an integral component of clinical practice and management decision-making.
- Promote discussion and exchange of information regarding status of evidence-based practice and process-improvement projects.
- Provide education and consultation to staff regarding the process and product of evidence-based practice projects.
- Maintain committee liaison and communication with the college of nursing to encourage collaborative research and joint evidence-based practice projects between staff, faculty, and students.
- Consult with process-improvement and evidence-based practice project teams about the critique of research and funding opportunities.
- Develop selected areas of interdisciplinary research and/or evidence-based practice that are strategically aligned with departmental and institutional goals.

Retention Committee
- Review the results of the National Database of Nursing Quality Indicators (NDNQI). Survey and identify opportunities to improve the work environment.
- Make evidence-based practice recommendations to improve nurse retention.
- Provide consultation for the use of research findings and use of research findings and other evidence as an integral component of management decision-making regarding nurse retention.

BOX 19-10 OUTCOMES OF INTEGRATING EVIDENCE-BASED PRACTICE INTO ORGANIZATIONAL CULTURE

SCIENTIFIC CRITERIA

1. The number of evidence-based practice projects
2. The number of evidence-based practice publications
3. The number of grants submitted and funded in which staff are investigators

ORGANIZATIONAL CLIMATE CRITERIA

1. Number of evidence-based practice standards used by staff
2. Number of staff participating in evidence-based practice activities
3. Climate of inquiry whereby staff question their practice
4. Increased number of professional nurses recruited and retained
5. Return of nurses to school for baccalaureate or higher degrees
6. National reputation, external consultations, and visits to the organization

COST AND QUALITY OF CARE

1. Decreased length of stay
2. Cost avoidance
3. Cost savings
4. Improved quality of care (e.g., decreased nosocomial urinary tract infections, improved pain management, decrease in nosocomial pressure ulcer development, increased satisfaction of families of critically ill patients).

als and organizations to improve clinical and operational decision-making in health care (Kovner, Elton, and Billings, 2000; Titler and Everett, 2001; Walshe and Rundall, 2001). This includes testing the effect of interventions on *promoting* and *sustaining* adoption of EBPs. Examples of translation studies include describing facilitators and barriers to knowledge uptake and use, organizational predictors of adherence to ambulatory care guidelines, and attitudes toward evidence-based practices, and defining the structure of the scientific field (Dykes, 2003; Estabrooks, 2004; Kirchhoff, 2004; Titler, 2004a).

Studies of evidence-based practice in a diversity of health care settings are beginning to build an empirical foundation of translation science (Morrison and Siu, 2000; Woolf et al., 1996). The Agency for Healthcare Research and Quality (AHRQ) has funded descriptive and intervention studies (TRIP I and TRIP II) to test methods for translating research findings into practice, and results of these studies are forthcoming (Dufault, 2004; Farquhar et al., 2002; Feldman and Kane, 2003; Jones et al., 2004a, 2004b). More recently, AHRQ has funded a series of demonstration projects—Partnerships for Quality—to improve quality of care through promoting use of evidence in health care practices (AHRQ Website 2/2003). The VA QUERI program is also investigating methods for integrating evidence into care delivery at VA health care agencies (Demakis et al., 2000; Pineros et al., 2004). These investigations and others (Dufault, 2001; O'Neill and Duffey, 2000) provide a beginning scientific knowledge for promoting use of evidence in practice. To advance knowledge regarding the best mechanisms for promoting and sustaining adoption of EBPs in health care, translation science needs more experimental studies that test translating research into practice interventions (Titler, 2004a; Titler and Everett, 2001). Partnership models, which encourage ongoing interaction between researchers and practitioners, may be the way to carry out such studies (Nutley et al., 2003). The state-of-the-science as well as the challenges, issues, methods, and instruments used in translation research are described elsewhere (Dawson, 2004; Donaldson, Rutledge, and Ashley, 2004; Dufault, 2004; Feldman and McDonald, 2004; Fraser, 2004a, 2004b; Kirchhoff, 2004; Pineros et al., 2004; Titler, 2004a, 2004b; Tripp-Reimer and Doebbeling, 2004; U.S. Invitational Conference, 2004; Watson, 2004; Williams, 2004). Nurse scientists are leaders in testing TRIP interventions and provide exemplars for others interested in the specialized area of science.

FUTURE DIRECTIONS

For organizations to take advantage of EBP projects from various sites throughout the country, a National Center for Evidence-Based Practice and Translation Science is needed. Such a center would encompass a computerized database of EBPs that includes the relevant policy and procedure or practice standard, the population to which it applies, the quality improvement indicators and data-collection forms used in evaluation, a list of references, suggested strategies for change, the type of institutions where the EBP has been implemented, contact people at each agency, and the EBP topic content expert. This information should be available online through electronic communications such as a dedicated list serve, the Virtual Hospital System, or some other form of electronic media. Such a center could facilitate networking among health care professionals working on similar EB topics and provide helpful consultants and educational materials. This center also would provide data regarding the interventions/strategies that have been tested to translate research into practice and provide a "tool kit" of these interventions for use by all types of health care agencies (QUERI,

2004; Registered Nurses Association of Ontario, 2004; Titler, 2002). For example, the tool kit on use of opinion leaders to translate research into practice might include a definition of opinion leader, characteristics of opinion leaders, how to select an opinion leader, the function of the opinion leader, in what types of settings and projects opinion leaders have been used effectively, and methods to evaluate the effect of using opinion leaders in promoting adoption of certain EBPs. Lastly, such a center would also conduct translational research and provide consultation regarding research methods and design specifically for translation science (Titler, 2004a).

Education of nurses must include knowledge and skills in the use of research evidence in practice. Nurses are increasingly being held accountable for practices based on scientific evidence. Thus we must communicate and integrate into our profession the expectation that it is the professional responsibility of every nurse to read and use research in their practice and to communicate with nurse scientists the many and varied clinical problems for which we do not yet have a scientific base.

Critical Thinking Challenges

- Discuss the difference between nursing research, research utilization, and evidence-based practice. Support your discussion with examples.
- Why would it be important to use an evidence-based practice model, such as the Iowa Model of Evidence-Based Practice, to guide a practice project? What part of this model can a consumer of research participate in effectively? Justify your response.
- Discuss the role of technology that can be used to implement the steps of an evidence-based practice model. Include in your discussion how computer electronic databases might help you; support your position with examples.
- You are a graduate nurse assigned to an adult cardiac unit; many of your nursing colleagues do not understand evidence-based practice. How would you implement evidenced-based practice in your new clinical setting?
- What barriers do you see in applying evidence-based practice in the clinical setting? Discuss strategies to use to overcome these barriers.

KEY POINTS

- *Evidence-based practice (EBP)* is a broad term that encompasses use of the best research evidence with clinical expertise and patient values/preferences in deciding the evidence-base for practice.
- There are two forms of evidence use: conceptual and decision-driven.
- There are several models of evidence-based practice. A key feature of all models is the judicious review and synthesis of research and other types of evidence to develop an evidenced-based practice standard.
- The steps of EBP using the Iowa Model of Evidence-Based Practice are as follows: selecting a topic, forming a team, retrieving the evidence, grading the evidence, developing an EBP standard, implementing the evidence-based practice, and evaluating the effect on staff, patient, and fiscal outcomes.
- Adoption of EBP standards requires education and dissemination to staff and use of change strategies such as opinion leaders or change champions, use of a core group, and use of consultants.
- It is important to evaluate the change. Evaluation provides data for performance gap assessment and audit and feedback, and provides information necessary to determine if the practice should be retained.
- Evaluation includes both process and outcome measures.
- It is important for organizations to create a culture of EBP. Creating this culture requires an interactive process. To implement this culture, organizations need to provide access to information, access to individuals who have skills necessary for EBP, and a written and verbal commitment to EB practice in the organization's operations.

REFERENCES

ACCP/AACVPR: Special report: pulmonary rehabilitation, joint ACCP/AACVPR evidence-based guidelines, *Chest* 112(5): 1363-1396, 1997.

Agency for Healthcare Research and Quality: Retrieved August 1, 2003, from http://www.ahrq.gov.

Alderson P, Green S, and Higgins JPT: *Cochrane Reviewers' Handbook* 4.2.1, 2003. Retrieved March 30, 2004, from http://www.cochrane.org/resources/handbook/handbook.pdf .

American Geriatrics Society, British Geriatrics Society, American Academy of Orthopaedic Surgeons, and Panel on Falls Prevention: Guideline for the prevention of falls in older persons, *J Am Geriatr Soc* 49(5): 664-672, 2001.

APS: *Guideline for the management of acute and chronic pain in sickle cell disease,* Glenview, Ill, 1999, American Pain Society.

Asci JA, Beyea SC: Urologic update: indwelling urinary catheters—An integrative review of the research, *Online J Knowledge Synth Nurs* 3(2): 1-6, 1996.

Bach DM, editor: *Implementation of the Agency for Health Care Policy and Research postoperative pain management guideline,* Vol 30, Philadelphia, 1995, WB Saunders.

Baggs JG, Mick DJ: Collaboration: a tool addressing ethical issues for elderly patients near the end of life in intensive care units, *J Gerontol Nurs* 26(9): 41-47, 2000.

Berner ES, Baker CS, Funkhouser E, Heudebert GR, Allison JJ, Fargason CA, Li Q, Person SD, and Kiefe CI: Do local opinion leaders augment hospital quality improvement efforts? A randomized trial to promote adherence to unstable angina guideline, *Med Care* 41(3): 420-431, 2003.

Berwick DM: Disseminating innovations in health care, *JAMA* 289(15): 1969-1975, 2003.

Bookbinder M, Coyle N, Kiss M, Goldstein ML, Holritz K, Thaler H, Gianella A, Derby S, Brown M, Racolin A, Nah M, and Portenoy RK: Implementing national standards for cancer pain management: program model and evaluation, *J Pain Symptom Management* 12(6): 334-347, 1996.

Carey RA: *Improving healthcare with control charts: basic and advanced SPC methods and case studies,* Milwaukee, Wisconsin, 2002, American Society for Quality.

Carr CA, Schott A: Differences in evidence-based care in midwifery practice and education, *J Nurs Scholarship* 34(2): 153-158, 2002.

Collins BA, Hawks JW, and Davis RL: From theory to practice: identifying authentic opinion leaders to improve care, *Managed Care* July: 56-62, 2000.

Cook D: Evidence-based critical care medicine: a potential tool for change, *New Horizons* 6(1): 20-25, 1998.

Craig JV, Smyth RL: *The evidence-based practice manual for nurses*, London, 2002, Churchill Livingstone.

Cullen L: Evidence-based practice: strategies for nursing leaders. In Huber D, editor: *Leadership and nursing care management*, ed 3, Philadelphia, 2005, Elsevier.

Cullen L, Titler MG: Promoting evidence-based practice: an internship for staff nurses, *Worldviews Evidence-Based Pract* (in press).

Dawson JD: Quantitative analytical methods in translation research, *Worldviews Evidence-Based Nurs* 1(suppl 1): S60-S64, 2004.

Demakis JG, McQueen L, Kizer KW, and Feussner JR: Quality Enhancement Research Initiative (QUERI): a collaboration between research and clinical practice, *Med Care* 38(6)(suppl 1): 17-25, 2000.

DiCenso A, Ciliska D, Cullum N, and Guyatt G: *Evidence-based nursing: a guide to clinical practice*, St Louis, 2004, Mosby.

Donaldson NE, Rutledge DN, and Ashley J: Outcomes of adoption: measuring evidence uptake by individuals and organizations, *Worldviews Evidence-Based Nurs* 1(suppl 1): S41-S51, 2004.

Dufault MA: A program of research evaluating the effects of collaborative research utilization model, *Online J Knowledge Synth Nurs* 8(3): 7, 2001.

Dufault MA: Testing a collaborative research utilization model to translate best practices in pain management, *Worldviews Evidence-Based Nurs* 1(suppl 1): S26-S32, 2004.

Dykes PC: Practice guidelines and measurement: state-of-the-science, *Nurs Outlook* 51: 65-69, 2003.

Eisenberg JM, Kamerow DB: The Agency for Healthcare Research and Quality and the U.S. Preventive Services Task Force: public support for translating evidence into prevention practice and policy, *Am J Prev Med* 20(3S): 1-2, 2001.

Estabrooks CA: Thoughts on evidence-based nursing and its science: a Canadian perspective, *Worldviews Evidence-Based Nurs* 1(2): 88-91, 2004.

Farquhar CM, Stryer D, and Slutsky J: Translating research into practice: the future ahead, *Int J Quality Health Care* 14(3): 233-249, 2002.

Feldman PH, Kane RL: Strengthening research to improve the practice and management of long-term care, *Milbank Quart* 81(2): 179-220, 2003.

Feldman PH, McDonald MV: Conducting translation research in the home care setting: lessons from a just-in-time reminder study, *Worldviews Evidence-Based Nurs* 1: 49-59, 2004.

Fiore MC, Bailey WC, and Cohen SJ, et al.: *Smoking cessation: information for specialists*, Rockville, Md. U.S. Department of Health and Human Services, Public Health Service, Agency for Health Care Policy and Research and Centers for Disease Control and Prevention, AHCPR Pub. No. 96-0694, April 1996.

Folkedahl B, Frantz R, and Goode C: *Evidence-based protocol: treatment of pressure ulcers* (Titler MG, series editor). Iowa City: Research Dissemination Core, Gerontological Nursing Interventions Research Center, 2002, University of Iowa College of Nursing (P30 NR03979; PI: T. Tripp-Reimer).

Foxcroft DR, Cole N, Fulbrook P, Johnston L, and Stevens K: Organisational infrastructures to promote evidence based nursing practice (protocol for a Cochrane Review), *Cochrane Library* 2, 2002.

Fraser I: Organizational research with impact: working backwards, *Worldviews Evidence-Based Nurs* 1(suppl 1): S52-S59, 2004a.

Fraser I: Translation research: where do we go from here, *Worldviews Evidence-Based Nurs* 1(S1): S78-S83, 2004b.

Funk SG, Tornquist EM, and Champagne MT: Barriers and facilitators of research utilization: an integrative review. In Titler M, Goode C, editors: *The Nursing Clinics of North America*, Vol 30, pp 395-408, Philadelphia, 1995, WB Saunders.

Gillbody S, Whitty P, Grimshaw J, and Thomas R: Educational and organizational interventions to improve the management of depression in primary care (A Systematic Review), *JAMA* 289(23): 3145-3151, 2003.

Guyatt GH, Rennie D: *Users' guide to the medical literature: essentials of evidence-based clinical practice*, Chicago, 2002, American Medical Association.

Haber J: Research resource nurse program, 2005 (personal communication).

Haber J, Feldman HR, Penney N, Carter E, Bidwell-Cerone S, and Hott JR: Shaping nursing practice through research-based protocols, *J NY State Nurses Assoc* 25(3): 4-12, 1994.

Haller KB, Reynolds MA, and Horsley JA: Developing research-based innovation protocols: process, criteria, and issues, *Res Nurs Health* 2: 45-51, 1979.

Harris RP, Helfan M, Woolf SH, Lohr KN, Mulrow CD, Teutsch SM, and Atkins D: Current methods of the U.S. Preventive Services Task Force: a review of the process, *Am J Prev Med* 20(3S): 21-35, 2001.

Harvey G, Loftus-Hills A, Rycroft-Malone J, Titchen A, Kitson A, McCormack B, and Seers K: Getting evidence into practice: the role and function of facilitation, *J Adv Nurs* 37(6): 577-588, 2002.

Health Grades Inc.: *Health grades quality study: patient safety in American hospitals*, Health Grades, Inc., 2004.

Herr K, Titler M, Sorofman B, Ardery G, Schmitt M, and Young D: *Evidence-based guideline: acute pain management in the elderly*, Iowa City, 2000, The University of Iowa. From *Book to bedside: acute pain management in the elderly*, 1 R01, HS10482-01.

Horsley JA, Crane J, Crabtree MK, and Wood DJ: *Using research to improve nursing practice: a guide*, New York, 1983, Grune and Stratton.

Institute of Medicine: *Crossing the quality chasm: a new health system for the 21st century*, Washington, DC, 2001, National Academy Press.

Institute of Medicine: *Priority areas for national action: transforming health care quality*, Washington, DC, 2003, National Academy Press.

Jamtvedt G, Young JM, Kristoffersen DT, Thomson O'Brien MA, and Oxman AD: Audit and feedback: effects on professional practice and health care outcomes (Cochrane Review), *The Cochrane Library, Issue 1*, Chichester, U.K., 2004, John Wiley and Sons, Ltd.

JCAHO: *Monograph: improving the quality of pain management through measurement and action*, Oakbrook Terrace, Ill, 2001, Joint Commission on Accreditation of Healthcare Organizations.

Jones J: Performance improvement through clinical research utilization: the linkage model, *J Nurs Care Qual* 15(1): 49-54, 2000.

Jones KR, Fink R, Vojir C, Pepper G, Hutt E, Clark L, Scott J, Martinez R, Vincent D, and Mellis BK: Translation research in long-term care: improving pain management in nursing homes, *Worldviews Evidence-Based Nurs* 1(suppl 1): S13-S20, 2004a.

Jones KR, Fink R, Pepper G, Hutt E, Vojir CP, Scott J, Clark L, and Mellis K: Improving nursing home staff knowledge and attitudes about pain, *Gerontologist* 44(4): 469-478, 2004b.

Katz DA, Muehlenbruch DR, Brown RB, Fiore MC, and Baker TB: Effectiveness of a clinic-based strategy for implementing the AHRQ Smoking Cessation Guideline in primary care, *Preventive Med* 35: 293-302, 2002.

Kirchhoff KT: State of the science of translational research: from demonstration projects to intervention testing, *Worldviews Evidence-Based Nurs* 1(suppl 1): S6-S12, 2004.

Kovner AR, Elton JJ, and Billings J: Evidence-based management, *Front Health Serv Manage* 16(4): 3-24, 2000.

Lavis JN, Robertson D, Woodside JM, McLeod CB, and Abelson J, Knowledge Transfer Study Group: How can research organizations more effectively transfer research knowledge to decision makers, *Milbank Quart* 81(2): 221-248, 2003.

Lepper HS, Titler MG: Program evaluation. In Mateo MA, Kirchhoff KT, editors: *Using and conducting nursing research in the clinical setting*, ed 2, pp 90-104, Philadelphia, 1999, WB Saunders.

Locock L, Dopson S, Chambers D, and Gabbay J: Implementation of evidence-based medicine: evaluation of the Promoting Action on Clinical Effectiveness program, *J Health Serv Res Policy* 6(1): 23-31, 2001a.

Locock L, Dopson S, Chambers D, and Gabbay J: Understanding the role of opinion leaders in improving clinical effectiveness, *Soc Sci Med* 53: 745-757, 2001b.

Lomas J, Enkin M, Anderson GM, Hannah WJ, Vayda E, and Singer J: Opinion leaders vs. audit and feedback to implement practice guidelines: delivery after previous cesarean section, *JAMA* 265: 2202-2207, 1991.

Madsen D, Sebolt T, Cullen L, Folkedahl B, Mueller T, Richardson C, and Titler M: Why listen to bowel sounds? Report of an evidence-based practice project, *Am J Nurs* (in review).

Mazmanian PE, Daffron SR, Johnson RE, Davis DA, and Kantrowitz MP: Information about barriers to planned change: a randomized controlled trial involving continuing medical education lectures and commitment to change, *Acad Med* 73(8): 882-886, 1998.

Meyer AD, Goes JB: Organizational assimilation of innovations: a multilevel contextual analysis, *Acad Management J* 31: 897-923, 1988.

Morrison RS, Siu AL: A comparison of pain and its treatment in advanced dementia and cognitively intact patients with hip fracture, *J Pain Sympt Manage* 19(4): 240-248, 2000.

Nagy S, Lumby J, McKinley S, and Macfarlane C: Nurses' beliefs about the conditions that hinder or support evidence-based nursing, *Int J Nurs Pract* 7(5): 314-321, 2001.

Nightingale F: *Notes on matters affecting the health, efficiency, and hospital administration of the British Army,* London, 1858, Harrison and Sons.

Nightingale F: *A contribution to the sanitary history of the British Army during the late war with Russia,* London, 1859, John W. Parker and Sons.

Nightingale F: *Notes on hospitals,* London, 1863a, Longman, Green, Roberts, and Green.

Nightingale F: *Observation on the evidence contained in the statistical reports submitted by her to the Royal Commission on the Sanitary State of the Army in India,* London, 1863b, Edward Stanford.

Nutley S and Davies HTO: Making a reality of evidence-based practice: some lessons from the diffusion of innovations, *Public Money Manage* October-December: 35-42, 2000.

Nutley S, Davies H, and Walter I: *Evidence based policy and practice: cross sector lessons from the UK,* Wellington, New Zealand, 2003, Keynote paper for the Social Policy Research and Evaluation Conference.

Olade RA: Evidence-based practice and research utilization activities among rural nurses, *J Nurs Schol* 36(3): 220-225, 2004.

O'Neill AL, Duffey MA: Communication of research and practice knowledge in nursing literature, *Nurs Res* 49(4): 224-230, 2000.

Oxman AD, Thomson MA, Davis DA, and Haynes RB: No magic bullets: a systematic review of 102 trials of interventions to improve professional practice, *Can Med Assoc J* 153(10): 1423-1431, 1995.

Pettit DM, Kraus V: The use of gauze versus transparent dressings for peripheral intravenous catheter sites. In Titler MG, Goode CJ, editors: *Nursing Clinics of North America,* Philadelphia, 1995, WB Saunders.

Pineros SL, Sales AE, Yu-Fang L, and Sharp ND: Improving care to patients with ischemic heart disease: experiences in a single network of the Veterans Health Administration, *Worldviews Evidence-Based Nurs* 1(suppl 1): S33-S40, 2004.

QUERI: Retrieved November 30, 2004, from http://www.hsrd.research.va.gov/queri/implementation/section_2/default.cfm.

Redfern S, Christian S: Achieving change in health care practice, *J Eval Clin Pract* 9(2): 225-238, 2003.

Registered Nurses Association of Ontario: *Implementation of clinical practice guidelines,* Retrieved November 30, 2004, from http://www.rnao.org/bestpractices/completed_guidelines/BPG_Guide_C1_Toolkit.asp.

Retsas A: Barriers to using research evidence in nursing practice, *J Adv Nurs* 31(3): 599-606, 2000.

Rogers EM: *Diffusion of innovations,* New York, 1995, The Free Press.

Rogers EM: *Diffusion of innovations,* ed 5, New York, 2003a, The Free Press.

Rogers EM: Innovation in organizations. In Rogers EM, editor: *Diffusion of innovations,* ed 5, New York, 2003b, The Free Press.

Rosswurm MA, Larrabee JH: A model for change to evidence-based practice, *Image: J Nurs Schol* 31(4): 317-322, 1999.

Rycroft-Malone J, Kitson A, Harvey G, McCormack B, Seers K, Titchen A, and Estabrooks CA: Ingredients for change: revisiting a conceptual framework, *Quality Safety Health Care* 11: 174-180, 2002.

Sackett D, Rosenberg W, Gray J, Haynes R, and Richardson W: Evidence based medicine: what it is and what it isn't, *BMJ* 312: 71-72, 1996.

Sackett DL, Straus SE, Richardson WS, Rosenberg W, and Haynes RB: *Evidence-based medicine: how to practice and teach EBM,* London, 2000, Churchill Livingstone.

Schneider EC, Eisenberg JM: Strategies and methods for aligning current and best medical practices: the role of information technologies, *West J Med* 168(5): 311-318, 1998.

Schoenbaum SC, Sundwall DN, Bergman D, Buckle JM, Chernov A, George J, Havighurst C, Jurkiewicz MJ, Kelly JT, Metzler S, Miaskowski C, Romeo SJW, Schyve PM, Simmons B, Spath P, Stevic M, Winslow C, and Zatz S: *Using clinical practice guidelines to evaluate quality of care, Volume 1: Issues,* Rockville, Md, 1995a, U.S. Department of Health and Human Services, Public Health Service, Agency for Health Care Policy and Research, AHCPR Pub. No. 95-0045.

Schoenbaum SC, Sundwall DN, Bergman D, Buckle JM, Chernov A, George J, Havighurst C, Jurkiewicz MJ, Kelly JT, Metzler S, Miaskowski C, Romeo SJW, Schyve PM, Simmons B, Spath P, Stevic M, Winslow C, and Zatz S: *Using clinical practice guidelines to evaluate quality of care, Volume 2: Methods,* Rockville, Md, 1995b, U.S. Department of Health and Human Services, Public Health Service, Agency for Health Care Policy and Research.

Soukup SM: The center for advanced nursing practice evidence-based practice model, *Nurs Clin North Am* 35(2): 301-309, 2000.

Stetler CB: Role of the organization in translating research into evidence-based practice, *Outcomes Manage* 7(3): 97-105, 2003.

Thompson CJ: The meaning of research utilization: a preliminary typology, *Crit Care Nurs Clin North Am* 13(4): 475-485, 2001.

Thomson O'Brien MA, Oxman AD, Haynes RB, Davis DA, Freemantle N, and Harvey EL: Local opinion leaders: effects on professional practice and health care outcomes (Cochrane Review), *The Cochrane Library,* Issue 2, Oxford, 2002, Update Software.

Thomson O'Brien MA, Oxman AD, Davis DA, Haynes RB, Freemantle N, and Harvey EL: Audit and feedback versus alternative strategies: effects on professional practice and health care outcomes, *The Cochrane Library,* Issue 2, Oxford, 2003a, Update Software.

Thomson O'Brien MA, Oxman AD, Davis DA, Haynes RB, Freemantle N, and Harvey EL: Educational outreach visits: effects on professional practice and health care outcomes, *The Cochrane Library,* Issue 2, Oxford, 2003b, Update Software.

Titler MG: *Toolkit for promoting evidence-based practice,* Iowa City, 2002, Department of Nursing Services and Patient Care, University of Iowa Hospitals and Clinics.

Titler M: *TRIP intervention saves healthcare dollars and improves quality of care (abstract/poster),* July 22-24, 2003. Paper presented at the Translating Research Into Practice: What's Working? What's Missing? What's Next?, Sponsored by the Agency for Healthcare Research and Quality, Washington, DC.

Titler MG: Methods in translation science, *Worldviews Evidence-Based Nurs* 1: 38-48, 2004a.

Titler MG: Overview of the U.S. Invitational Conference "Advancing Quality Care Through Translation Research," *Worldviews Evidence-Based Nurs* 1(suppl 1): S1-S5, 2004b.

Titler MG, Everett LQ: Translating research into practice: considerations for critical care investigators, *Crit Care Nurs Clin North Am* 13(4): 587-604, 2001.

Titler MG, Kleiber C, Steelman V, Goode C, Rakel B, Barry-Walker J, Small S, and Buckwalter KC: Infusing research into practice to promote quality care, *Nurs Res* 43(5): 307-313, 1994.

Titler MG, Kleiber C, Steelman VJ, Rakel BA, Budreau G, Buckwalter KC, Tripp-Reimer T, and Goode CJ: The Iowa model of evidence-based practice to promote quality care, *Crit Care Nurs Clin North Am* 13(4): 497-509, 2001.

Titler MG, Herr K, Schilling ML, Marsh JL, Xie X, Ardery G, Clarke WR, and Everett LQ: Acute pain treatment for older adults hospitalized with hip fracture: current nursing practices and perceived barriers, *Appl Nurs Res* 16(4): 211-227, 2003.

Tranmer JE, Coulson K, Holtom D, Lively T, and Maloney R: The emergence of a culture that promotes evidence-based clinical decision making within an acute care setting, *Can J Nurs Admin* 11(2): 36-58, 1998.

Tripp-Reimer T, Doebbeling BN: Qualitative perspectives in translational research, *Worldviews Evidence-Based Nurs* 1(suppl 1): S65-S72, 2004.

UIHC Department of Nursing: http://www.uihealthcare.com/depts/nursing/about/index.html, 2004.

University of Illinois at Chicago: *Evidence based medicine. Finding the best literature,* 2003. Accessed March 2004 from http://www.uic.edu/depts/lib/lhsp/resources/pico.shtml).

U.S. Invitational Conference: *Advancing quality care through translation research,* set of two CD-ROMs, Conference Proceedings, 2004.

Wagner EH, Austin BT, Davis C, Hindmarsh M, Schaefer J, and Bonomi A: Improving chronic illness care: translating evidence into action, *Health Affairs (Millwood)* 20: 64-78, 2001.

Walshe K, Rundall TG: Evidence-based management: from theory to practice in health care, *Milbank Quart* 79(3): 429-457, 2001.

Watson NM: Advancing quality of urinary incontinence evaluation and treatment in nursing homes through translation research, *Worldviews Evidence-Based Nurs* 1(suppl 2): S21-S25, 2004.

West S, King V, Carey TS, Lohr KN, McKoy N, Sutton SF, and Lux L: *Systems to rate the strength of scientific evidence.* Evidence Report/Technology Assessment No. 47 (Prepared by the Research Triangle Institute-University of North Carolina Evidence-Based Practice Center under Contract No. 290-97-0011), AHRQ Publication No. 02-E016, Rockville, Md, 2002, Agency for Healthcare Research and Quality.

Williams CA: Preparing the next generation of scientists in translation research, *Worldviews Evidence-Based Nurs* 1(suppl 1): S73-S77, 2004.

Winn J: Basing catheter care on research principles, *Nurs Standard* 10(18): 38-40, 1996.

Woolf SH, Diguiseppi CG, Atkins D, and Kamerow DB: Developing evidence-based clinical practice guidelines: lessons learned by the U.S. Preventive Services Task Force, *Annu Rev Public Health* 17: 511-538, 1996.

FOR FURTHER STUDY...

🌐 Go to your Companion CD for review activities for this chapter.

evolve Go to Evolve at http://evolve.elsevier.com/LoBiondo/ for WebLinks, Content Updates, and additional research articles, for practice in reviewing and critiquing.

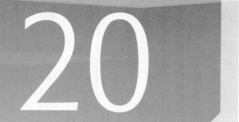

CARL KIRTON

Tools for Applying Evidence to Practice

LEARNING OUTCOMES

After reading this chapter, the student should be able to do the following:
- Identify the key elements of a focused clinical question.
- Discuss the use of databases to search the literature.
- Learn how to screen an article for relevance and credibility.
- Evaluate study results and apply the findings to individual patients.
- Learn how to make clinical decisions based on evidence from the literature.

STUDY RESOURCES

Go to your Companion CD for review activities for this chapter.

evolve Go to Evolve at http://evolve.elsevier.com/LoBiondo/ for Weblinks, Content Updates, and additional research articles for practice in reviewing and critiquing.

n today's environment of knowledge explosion, new investigations are published at a frequency with which even seasoned practitioners have a hard time keeping pace. With so much new information, maintaining a clinical practice that is based on new evidence in the literature can be challenging. However, the development of evidence-based nursing practice is contingent on applying new and important evidence to clinical practice. A few simple techniques will help you move to a practice that is evidence-oriented. This chapter will assist you in becoming a more efficient and effective reader of the professional literature. Through a few important tools and a crisp understanding of the important components of a study, you will be able to use an evidence-base to determine the merits of a study for your practice and for your patients.

Consider the following case of a nurse who uses evidence from the literature to support her practice:

Jasmine Sanchez is a registered nurse who works in an asthma and allergy practice. As part of her work in this clinic, Jasmine teaches patients how to decrease allergens in the environment to reduce exacerbations of wheezing and asthma attacks. One of Jasmine's patients is particularly allergic to dust mites, and Jasmine recommends both physical and chemical methods to eliminate them. The patient asks Jasmine, "Of the methods described which one is best at eliminating mites?" Unaware of the answer to this question, Jasmine tells the patient she has asked a very good question, one to which she does not know the answer, but will find out. They agree to discuss this again at their next visit.

EVIDENCE-BASED TOOL #1: ASKING A FOCUSED CLINICAL QUESTION

Developing a focused clinical question will help Jasmine to focus on the relevant issue and prepare her for subsequent steps in the evidenced-based practice (EBP) process (see Chapters 3 and 19). A focused clinical question is developed by answering the following four questions:

1. What is the population I am interested in?
2. What is the intervention I am interested in?
3. What will this intervention be compared to? (Note: depending on the study design, this step may or may not apply.)
4. How will I know if the intervention makes things better or worse (identify an outcome that is measurable)?

As you recall from Chapter 19, most evidence-based practitioners use the simple mnemonic called PICO to help them recall all of the requirements for a well-designed clinical question (see Table 20-1).

Because Jasmine is familiar with the evidence-based practice approach for developing clinical questions, she identifies the four important components and develops the following clinical question: In patients with bronchial asthma which method of mite control, chemical or physical, is most effective in improving allergy symptoms?

Once a clinical question has been framed, it can be organized into one of four types of clinical categories used by clinicians:

1. **Therapy category:** When a nurse wants to answer a question about the effectiveness of a particular treatment or intervention, she or he will select studies that have the following characteristics:
   - Experimental or quasiexperimental study design (see Chapter 10)
   - Outcome known or of probable clinical importance observed over a clinically significant period of time

TABLE 20-1 **Using PICO to Formulate Clinical Questions**

Patient population	What group do you want information on?	Adults with bronchial asthma
Intervention (or exposure)	What event do you want to study the effect of?	Chemical mite control methods
Comparison	Compared to what? Better or worse than no intervention at all, or than another intervention?	Physical mite control methods
Outcomes	What is the effect of the intervention?	Improvement in allergy symptoms

When studies are in this category, the nurse uses a therapy appraisal tool to evaluate the article. A therapy tool can be accessed at http://www. phru.nhs.uk/casp/rct.pdf.

2. **Diagnosis category:** When a nurse wants to answer a question about the usefulness, accuracy, selection, or interpretation of a particular measurement instrument or laboratory test, he or she will select studies that have the following characteristics:

   - Cross-sectional study design (see Chapter 11) with people suspected to have the condition of interest
   - Administration to the patient of both the new instrument or diagnostic test and the accepted "gold standard" measure
   - Comparison of the results of the new instrument or test and the "gold standard"

When studies are in this category, the nurse uses a diagnostic test appraisal tool to evaluate the article. A diagnostic tool can be accessed at http://www.phru.nhs.uk/casp/diagtest.htm.

3. **Prognosis category:** When the nurse wants to answer a question about a patient's likely course for a particular disease state or identify factors that may alter the patient's prognosis, she or he will select studies that have the following characteristics:

   - Nonexperimental, usually longitudinal study of a particular group for a particular outcome or disease (see Chapter 11)
   - Follow-up for a clinically relevant period of time (time is the exposure)
   - Determination of factors in those who do and do not develop a particular outcome

When studies are in this category, the nurse uses a prognosis (sometimes called a cohort tool) appraisal tool to evaluate the article. A prognosis tool can be accessed at http://www.phru.nhs.uk/casp/cohort/2012/20questions.pdf.

4. **Etiology/Causation/Harm category:** When the nurse wants to determine whether or not one thing is related to or caused by another, he or she will select studies that have the following characteristics:

   - Nonexperimental, usually longitudinal or retrospective (ex post facto) study designs over a clinically relevant period of time (see Chapter 11)
   - Assessment of whether or not the patient has been exposed to the independent variable

When studies are in this category, the nurse uses a harm (sometimes called a case-control tool) appraisal tool to evaluate the article. A etiology/causation/harm tool can be accessed at http://www.phru.nhs.uk/casp/case_control_studies.htm.

There are two important reasons for applying clinical categories to the professional literature. First, knowing to which category a clinical question belongs helps you search the literature efficiently (see Chapter 4). Second, structured tools exist that can be used to systematically appraise the strength and quality of evidence provided in research articles (see http://www.phru.nhs.uk/casp/appraisa.htm).

EVIDENCE-BASED TOOL #2: SEARCHING THE LITERATURE

All the skills that Jasmine needs to consult the literature and answer a clinical question are conceptually defined as **information literacy** (Jacobs, Rosenfeld, and Haber, 2003). Your librarian is the best person to help you develop the necessary skills to become information literate. Part of being information literate is having the skills necessary to search the professional literature to obtain the best evidence for answering your clinical question. To assist nurses and other health professionals with accessing theoretical, clinical, and research articles, these publications are organized into electronic indexes or databases. Generally speaking, you can access these databases free through your health care organization or university library. Most clinical agencies recognize the importance of clinicians having immediate access to the most current health care information and thus provide access to electronic databases at the point of care.

Chapter 4 discusses the differences among databases and how nurses use these databases to search the literature. One or two sessions with a librarian will help you focus your search to your clinical question and structure your search to yield articles that are most likely to answer your question. You can learn how to effectively search databases through a 90-minute tutorial located athttp://www.shef.ac.uk/scharr/reswce/reswce3.htm.

Using the PubMed database, Jasmine uses the clinical category filter and selects the therapy option (which will only yield articles that use an experimental study design). She enters the term "dust mites." Her search yields 118 individual articles with a controlled study design. A careful perusal of the list of articles and a well-designed clinical question will help Jasmine to narrow her search to a few key articles.

 EVIDENCE-BASED PRACTICE TIP

Prefiltered sources of evidence can be found in journal format and electronic format. Prefiltered evidence is evidence in which an editorial team has already read and summarized articles on a topic and discussed its relevance to clinical care. Prefiltered sources include *Clinical Evidence,* available online at http://clinicalevidence.com/ceweb/conditions/index.jsp and in print; *Evidence-Based Nursing* is available online at http://ebn.bmjjournals.com/ and in print.

EVIDENCE-BASED TOOL #3: SCREENING YOUR FINDINGS

Once you have searched and selected potential article(s), how do you know which article is appropriate to answer your clinical question? This is accomplished by screening the article(s) for relevance and credibility by answering the following three questions (Miser, 1999):

1. Is this article from a peer-reviewed journal? Articles published in a peer-reviewed journal have had an extensive review and editing process.
2. Are the setting and sample of the study similar to mine so that results, if valid, would apply to my practice or to my patient population?
3. Is the study sponsored by an organization that may influence the study or the design or results?

Your responses to these screening questions help you decide to what extent you want to appraise an individual article. For example, if the study population is markedly different from the one to which you will apply the results, you may want to consider selecting a more appropriate study. If the article is worth evaluating, you should use the category-specific tool URLs identified in Evidence-Based Tool #1 to critically appraise the article.

Jasmine reviews a variety of articles and selects the following article: "House dust mite control measures in the management of asthma: Meta-analysis." This study was published in the Medical Journal in 1998 (Gøtzsche, Hammarquist, and Burr, 1998), a peer-reviewed journal. This is a study that combines the results of several individual studies (a meta-analysis; see Chapters 4, 11, and 19). The studies analyzed were from RCTs of both children and adults; however, Jasmine does not think that the inclusion of pediatric articles in the meta-analysis significantly reduces generalizability to her adult practice. There were no funding or conflict of interest issues noted. Jasmine decides that this study is worth evaluating.

 HELPFUL H I N T

When evaluating studies obtained in a search, consider both positive studies (treatment is better) and negative studies (treatment is worse or there is no difference). Negative studies are more difficult to find but are equally important.

EVIDENCE-BASED TOOL #4: APPRAISE EACH ARTICLE'S FINDINGS

Applying study results to individual patients or to a specific patient population and communicating study findings to patients in a meaningful way are the hallmark of evidence-based practice. Common EBP conventions that researchers and research consumers use to appraise and report study results in clinical practice are identified by four different types of clinical categories: therapy, diagnosis (sensitivity and specificity), prognosis, and harm. The language common to meta-analysis, which is a special type of method, will also be discussed. Familiarity with these EBP clinical categories will help Jasmine, as well as you, to search for, screen, select, and appraise articles appropriate for answering clinical questions.

Therapy Category

In articles that belong to the therapy category (sometimes called individual studies, experimental design studies, randomized controlled trials [RCTs], interventions studies), investigators attempt to determine if a difference exists between two or more treatments. The evidence-based language used in a therapy article depends on whether the variables studied are *continuous* (degree of change) or *dichotomous* (proportion who experience or do not experience an event) variables (see Table 20-2; see Chapter16). When investigators undertake a study to determine whether or not a change has occurred in a par-

ticular variable, the variable is first measured at baseline and then the intervention is applied, and finally the variable is measured again (see Chapter 10). When researchers are interested in the degree of change in the variable of interest, they generally present their results as measures of central tendency (see Chapter 16). For example, in the study by Van Cleve and colleagues (2004) on the pain experience of children with leukemia (Appendix B), the degree of change in several continuous variables is measured (e.g., pain intensity and pain quality). Several tools used for data collection measure the experience of pain at seven different points in time. The mean pain intensity scores, before and after pain management strategies, are indicated in Table 2, p. 000, of Appendix B for two different age groups. In contrast, in experimental studies with dichotomous variables, researchers are interested in determining the proportion of patients who either experience or do not experience an event (i.e., it either happened or did not happen). For example, McCorkle and colleagues (2000) conducted an RCT involving older cancer patients; they were interested in determining if a specialized home care intervention, provided by advanced practice nurses, compared to standard home care, improved the survival of older cancer patients. In this study, survival was identified as the main outcome. Survival is a dichotomous outcome because at the study end point the researchers determined if the patient was either dead or alive.

TABLE **20-2** **Difference between Continuous and Dichotomous Variables**

Variable	Example	Outcome Measure
CONTINUOUS VARIABLES		
Researcher is interested in degree of change after exposure to an intervention	Pain quality, levels of psychological distress, blood pressure, weight	Measures of central tendency
DICHOTOMOUS VARIABLES		
Researcher is interested in whether or not an "event" occurred or did not occur	Death, diarrhea, pressure ulcer, pregnancy	Measures of effect and association

In therapy studies using dichotomous variables (also called outcomes), researchers generally present their results as measures of association as illustrated in Table 20-3. Understanding these measures is challenging but particularly important because they are used by nurses and other health care providers to communicate to patients the risks and benefits or lack of benefits of a treatment(s). They are particularly useful to nurses because they inform decision making that validates current practice or provides evidence that supports the need for change in clinical practice.

For example, insertion of intravenous catheters is a common nursing procedure. A variety of nurse factors and patient factors can make this relatively common procedure difficult and time consuming (e.g., overused veins and sympathetic nervous system stimulation). A variety of techniques are used by nurses to facilitate insertion of an intravenous cannula into a difficult vein (e.g., tapping the vein over the insertion site, clenching the hand, or warming the insertion site). Lenhardt and colleagues (2002) attempted to answer the following clinical question: "Does local warming of the insertion site result in successful cannulation?" These investigators tested the use of a warming device and measured the first-attempt cannulation success rates in those that had active warming (device on) compared to those that had passive warming (device off). The results of this randomized controlled trial are described in Table 20-4 followed by a description of the different ways in which authors can present study results. Because the study was undertaken to determine if an experimental treatment (the warming device) increases the probability of a good outcome (successful cannulation), the nurse is interested in examining if there is a relative benefit increase (RBI) or an absolute benefit increase (ABI) (Table 20-3). Using the data contained in the article, the nurse calculates (see Table 20-4) the RBI and finds that the warming device increases the benefit of successful cannulation by 30% more than would occur if they did not use the warming mitt.

When a study, such as the Lenhardt (2002) study that compared the effectiveness of a warming vs. a nonwarming device, is carried out, researchers are interested in seeing how well the results would apply to a certain population. Because it is not feasible to study all members of a certain population, a random sample of individuals who are reflective of the population of interest is selected for inclusion in the study (see Chapter 12). Statistical tests, such as confidence intervals, are commonly found in therapy articles; confidence intervals allow nurses to make inferences about how realistically the results about the effectiveness of an intervention can be generalized to a population of patients with similar characteristics.

A **confidence interval (CI)** is a range of values, based on a random sample, that often accompanies measures of central tendency and measures of association and provides the nurse with a measure of precision or uncertainty about the sample findings. Typically investigators record their CI results as a 95% degree of certainty; at times you may also see the degree of certainty recorded as 99%. Today professional journals often require investigators to include confidence intervals as one of the statistical methods used to interpret study findings. Even when confidence intervals are not reported, they can be easily calculated from study data. The method for performing these calculations is widely available in statistical texts.

Returning to the Lenhardt (2002) study, it was learned that the warming device increases the benefit of successful cannulation by 30% more than would occur if they did not use the warming mitt. Lenhardt and colleagues did not present confidence intervals for the RBI and the number needed to treat (NNT), but the CI is calculated for you and presented as results in Table 20-5. The CI helps us to place the study results in context for all patients similar to those in the study (generalization).

TABLE 20-3 **Measures of Association for Trials that Report Dichotomous Outcomes**

Measure of Association	Definition	Comment
Control event rate (CER)	Proportion of patients in control group in which an event is observed	This event rate is found by dividing the number of patients who experienced the outcome of interest by the total number of patients in the control group.
Experimental event rate (EER)	Proportion of patients in control and experimental treatment groups in which an event is observed	This event rate is found by dividing the number of patients who experienced the outcome of interest by the total number of patients in the experimental group.
Relative risk (RR), also called risk ratio	Risk of event after experimental treatment as a percentage of original risk	If CER and EER have the same effect, RR = 1.0 (this means there is no difference between the treatment and control group outcomes). If the risk of the event is reduced in EER compared with CER, then RR < 1.0. If the risk of an event is greater in EER compared with CER, RR > 1.0.

A NOTE REGARDING RISK: *It is important to note that the identification of a risk of an event does not imply that there is a causal relationship between the factor and the condition. However, the higher a relative risk is, the more likely it becomes that the risk of the event is causal and not due to chance.*

When the experimental treatment *reduces* the probability of a *bad outcome* (e.g., death), the following terms are used:

Absolute risk reduction (ARR), also called risk difference or attributable risk reduction	This value tells us the reduction in absolute terms. The ARR is considered the "real" reduction because it is the difference between the risk observed in those who did and did not experience the event.	Arithmetic difference in risk of outcome between patients who have had the therapy and those who have not had the therapy Calculated as $|EER - CER|$
Relative risk reduction (RRR)	This value tells us the reduction in risk in relative terms. The relative risk reduction is an estimate of the percentage of baseline risk that is removed as a result of the therapy; it is calculated as the ARR between the treatment and control groups divided by the absolute risk among patients in the control group.	Percent reduction in risk that is removed after considering the percent of risk that would occur anyway (the control group's risk) Calculated as $|EER - CER|/CER$
Number needed to treat (NNT)	The number needed to treat (NNT) is a useful way of reporting the results of randomized controlled trials. In a trial comparing a new treatment with a standard one, the number needed to treat is the estimated number of patients who need to be treated with the new treatment rather than the standard treatment for one additional patient to benefit. It can be obtained for any trial that has reported a dichotomous outcome.	Calculated as $1/ARR$

Measure of Association	Definition	Comment

When the experimental treatment *increases* the probability of a *good outcome* (satisfactory hemoglobin A1c levels), the following terms are used:

Measure of Association	Definition	Comment
Absolute benefit increase (ABI)	This value tell us about the proportional increases in rates of good outcomes between experimental and control patients in a trial.	Calculated as |EER − CER|
Relative benefit increase (RBI)	This is the absolute arithmetic difference in rates of good outcomes between experimental and control patients in a trial.	Calculated as |EER − CER|/CER

When the experimental treatment *increases* the probability of a *bad outcome* (e.g., rash), the following terms are used:

Measure of Association	Definition	Comment
Absolute risk increase (ARI)	This value is the absolute arithmetic difference in rates of bad outcomes between experimental and control patients in a trial.	Arithmetic difference in risk of outcome between patients who have had the therapy and those who have not had the therapy Calculated as |EER − CER|
Relative risk increase (ARI)	This is the proportional increase in rates of bad outcomes between experimental and control patients in a trial.	Percent increase in risk that is added after considering the percent of risk that would occur anyway (the control group's risk) Calculated as |EER − CER|/CER
Number needed to harm (NNH)	The number needed to treat (NNH) is a useful way of reporting the results of randomized controlled trials. In a trial comparing a new treatment with a standard one, the number needed to harm is the estimated number of patients who need to be treated with the new treatment rather than the standard treatment for one additional patient to be harmed or have a bad outcome. It can be obtained for any trial that has reported a dichotomous outcome.	Calculated as 1/ARI

Reporting events in terms of the probability of it occurring (good or bad):

Measure of Association	Definition	Comment
Odds ratio	Instead of looking at the risk of an event, we could estimate the odds of an event occurring. The OR is usually the measure of choice in the analysis of nonexperimental design studies. It is the ratio of the odds of treated or exposed patients to the odds of untreated or nonexposed patients (where the odds are the ratio of the probability of a given event occurring to the probability of the event not occurring).	

TABLE **20-4 Interpretation of Measures of Association**

Clinical question: Does local warming of the hand and lower arm facilitate insertion of peripheral venous cannulas?

Treatment	Total Number of Patients	Insertion Success Rate	Insertion Failure
Active warming (Thermamed warming mitt heated to 52° C)	50	44	3
Passive warming (mitt not heated)	50	36	14

CALCULATIONS MADE FROM STUDY RESULTS

Experimental event rate	44/50 = 0.94 or 94%
	Interpretation: Actively warming the hand for 15 min with a Thermamed mitt heated to 52° C resulted in successful cannulation 94% of the time.
Control event rate	36/50 = 0.72 or 72%
	Interpretation: Actively warming the hand for 15 min with an unheated Thermamed mitt resulted in successful cannulation 72% of the time.
Relative benefit increase	100((0.94 − 0.72)/0.72) = 30%
	Interpretation: Actively warming the hand for 15 min with a Thermamed mitt heated to 52° C increased the rate of successful cannulation by 30% more than would occur using an unheated mitt.
Absolute benefit increase	94% − 72% = 22%
	Interpretation: Actively warming the hand for 15 min with a Thermamed mitt heated to 52° C increased the rate of successful cannulation by 22%.
NNT (100/ARR)	100/0.22 = 4.5 or 5
	Interpretation: Using the Thermamed mitt heated to 52° C for 15 min will prevent 1 in 5 patients from experiencing an unsuccessful cannulation.

TABLE **20-5 Active Warming vs. Passive Warming before Insertion of Peripheral Venous Cannulas in Neurosurgical Patients**

Outcome	Active Warming	Passive Warming	RBI (95% CI)	NNT (CI)
Successful insertions on first attempt	94%	72%	30% (10 to 62)	5 (3 to 13)

Data from Lenhardt R, Seybold T, Kimberger O, Stoiser R, and Sessler D: Local warming and insertion of peripheral venous cannulas: single-blinded, prospective randomized controlled trial and and single-blinded crossover trial, *Brit J Med* 325: 409–412, 2002.

As a result of the calculated CI for the Lenhardt et al. study, it can be stated that in neurosurgical patients (the study population) we can be 95% certain that when a Thermamed hand warmer is used, the nurse will have a successful insertion on the first attempt anywhere from 10% to 62% of the time. You will note that the NNT also has a calculated confidence interval. By observing the CI, we can state that using the Thermamed hand warmer the nurse will successfully cannulate anywhere between 1 in 3 or between 1 in 15 neurosurgical patients. Knowing these ranges helps you to make important decisions about implementing change in practice or applying an intervention to a patient (clinical significance of the study results). We might think differently about changing or adopting a new intervention if our confidence interval is large, for example, CI = 2 to 170. What this tells us is that the relative benefit (in the case of a good outcome) or reduction in risk (in the case of a bad outcome) is anywhere from 2% to 170%. With such large numbers the clinical significance is widely variable and depending on the experiment may or may not be worth the effort, expense, or uncertainty. From a statistical standpoint such a large CI indicates that the study was not sufficiently powered; that is, the study did not enroll enough study patients to provide meaningful results (see Chapter 12). As the number of patients enrolled in a study increases, the CI narrows.

A unique feature of the confidence interval is that it can tell us whether or not the study results are statistically significant. When an experimental value is obtained that indicates there is no difference between the treatment and control groups, we label that value "the value of no effect" or the **null value.** The value of no effect varies according to the outcome measure. When examining a CI, if the interval does not include the value of no effect the effect is said to be statistically significant. When the CI does contain the null value, the results are said to be nonsignificant because the null value represents the value of no difference; that is, there is no difference between the treatment and control groups. In studies of equivalence this is a desired finding, but in studies of superiority or inferiority this is not the case. The null value varies depending on the outcome measure. For relative risk, relative risk reduction, and absolute risk reduction, the null value is equal to zero.

Investigators were interested in answering the following clinical question: "Does the effect of digoxin therapy differ in men and women with heart failure (HF) and depressed left ventricular systolic function?" In a study by Rathore, Wang, and Krumholz (2002), a large number of men and women ($n = 6800$) with heart failure were randomized to receive digoxin (a treatment for heart failure) or a placebo. The main study outcome was death due to any cause ("all cause mortality"). Secondary outcomes such as hospital admission, worsening heart failure, and cardiovascular death were also studied and are presented in Table 20-6. Examining the "all cause mortality" row in the table and the columns

TABLE 20-6 **Digoxin vs. Placebo for Heart Failure (HF) in Men and Women**

Outcomes at ≤48 months	Sex	Digitalis	Placebo	Adjusted RRR (95% CI)	Adjusted NNT (CI)
All cause mortality	**Men**	35.2%	36.9%	6% (−2 to 12)	Not significant
Cardiovascular death		30.5%	31.1%	3% (−5 to 11)	Not significant
Death from worsening HF		11.4%	13.6%	20% (7 to 30)	38 (25 to 99)
Hospital admission for worsening HF		25.8%	34.7%	29% (23 to 35)	10 (9 to 13)
Hospital admission for other causes		39.9%	35.0%	13% (6 to 21)	22 (14 to 52)
All cause mortality	**Women**	33.1%	28.9%	19% (2 to 36)	19 (10 to 207)
Cardiovascular death		27.8%	24.1%	20% (2 to 42)	21 (10 to 240)
Death from worsening HF		12.4%	11.9%	16% (−12 to 51)	Not significant
Hospital admission for other causes		35.9%	32.2%	12% (−2 to 28)	Not significant
Hospital admission for worsening HF		30.2%	34.4%	11% (−3 to 24)	Not significant

Data from: Rathore SS, Wang Y, and Krumholz HM: Sex-based differences in the effect of digoxin for the treatment of heart failure, *N Engl J Med* 347: 1403–1411, 2002.

labeled "digitalis" (the experimental group) and "placebo" (the control group), the nurse can observe that at 48 months the percentage of deaths was slightly less in the digoxin group (35.2%) compared to the placebo group (36.9%) for men. However, for women the percentage of deaths in the digoxin group (33.1%) was increased compared to the placebo group (28.9%). If you also examine for secondary outcomes, you will see that for "cardiovascular deaths" more women who received digoxin died compared to the women's placebo group. The same is not true for men. One conclusion to be drawn from this study is that digoxin leads to an increased risk of "all cause mortality" and "cardiovascular deaths" in women but not in men. But how precise is this finding? This question can be answered by examining the confidence intervals. By examining the adjusted RRR column (the risk reduction is adjusted because there were differences between the men and women at baseline), we see that the RRR is accompanied by a

CI. Examine the CI that accompanies the RRR in the "all cause mortality" row. As stated previously, for relative risk, relative risk reduction, and absolute risk reduction, the null value is equal to zero. For men the CI includes the null value of zero (−2 to 12), and thus the finding that digoxin reduces the risk of death in men compared to those who do not take digoxin is not a statistically significant finding for men. Examine "all cause mortality" for women; because the CI does not include the null value (10 to 207), this finding is statistically significant for women. Similarly if we examine the confidence interval for women's cardiovascular death, we also find that this is a statistically significant event (10 to 240) (see Figure 20-1). While the study results are interesting and the reason for the difference between men and women cannot be explained by any one variable, it does point to the importance of considering sex-based differences in treatment (Rathore, Wang, and Krumholz, 2002). Further research is needed to warrant a change in prac-

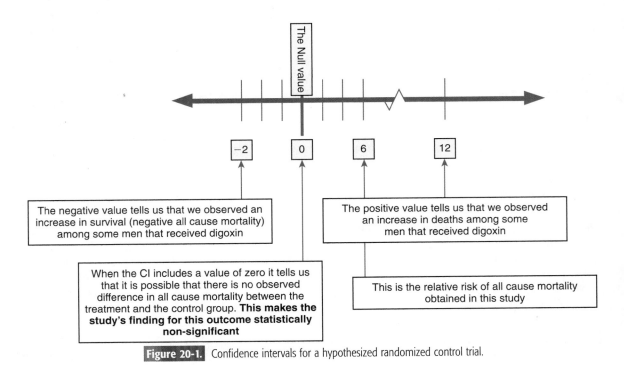

Figure 20-1. Confidence intervals for a hypothesized randomized control trial.

tice, but the nurse should note the study results and the implications for women with heart failure who are receiving digoxin.

Diagnosis Articles

In articles that answer clinical questions of diagnosis, investigators study the ability of screening or diagnostic tests, tools, or components of the clinical examination to detect (or not detect) disease when the patient has (or does not have) the particular disease of interest. The accuracy of a test, technique, or tool is measured by its sensitivity and specificity (see Table 20-7). **Sensitivity** is the proportion of those with disease who test positive; that is, sensitivity is a measure of how well the test detects disease when it is really there; a sensitive test has few false negatives. **Specificity** is the proportion of those without disease who test negative. It measures how well the test rules out disease when it is really absent; a specific test has few false positives. Sensitivity and specificity have some deficiencies in clinical use, primarily because sensitivity and specificity are merely characteristics of the test.

Describing diagnostic tests in this way tells us how good the test is, but what is more useful is how well the test performs in a particular population with a particular prevalence of a disease. This is important because in a population in which a disease is quite prevalent, there are fewer incorrect test results (false positives), as compared with populations with low disease prevalence, for which a positive test may truly be a false positive. Predictive values are a measure of accuracy that accounts for the prevalence of a disease. As illustrated in Table 20-7, a **positive predictive value expresses** (PPV) the proportion of those with positive test results who truly have disease, and a **negative predictive value expresses** the proportion of those with negative test results who truly do not have disease. Let us observe how these characteristics of diagnostic tests are used in nursing practice.

A study was conducted to evaluate a new method of on-site evaluation of bacteriuria in incontinent nursing home adult patients. Researchers compared a new method of pressing a urine dipstick into a wet incontinence pad and compared this method with the gold standard of sending a clean-catch specimen to a laboratory for culture. The investigators compared and contrasted the new method with the gold standard using several different data combinations. The measures of accuracy using the dipstick/pad method and the result of nitrite alone are listed in Table 20-8 (Midthun et al., 2003). The test characteristics in Table 20-8 show that the dipstick/pad method has a sensitivity of 70% and a specificity of 97%. This method compares well with the laboratory method of detecting nitrates in the urine, which has a sensitivity of 66.7% and a specificity of 98.6%. Recall that sensitivity and specificity apply to the diagnostic test alone and do not change even as the disease prevalence changes in the population. In a population in which a disease is very prevalent, a positive test is more meaningful compared with a positive test in a population in which the disease is very rare.

From Table 20-8 we learn that the prevalence of bacteriuria in an elderly, primarily female population is 28%. Combining this information with sensitivity and specificity, we find that the PPV is 90%; this means that 90% of primarily elderly female nursing home residents with a positive dipstick/pad method will have bacteriuria.

LIKELIHOOD RATIOS IN CLINIC PRACTICE

Likelihood ratios provide nurses with information about the accuracy of a diagnostic test and can also help nurses be more efficient decision makers by allowing quantification of the probability of disease for any individual patient. As illustrated in Table 20-9, a test with a large positive likelihood ratio (e.g., > 10), when applied, provides the clinician with a high degree of certainty that the patient has the suspected disorder. Conversely, tests with a very low positive likelihood ratio (e.g., < 2), when applied, provide the clinician with little to no changes in the degree

TABLE 20-7 **Measures of Accuracy**

Reporting the Outcome Results of Diagnostic Trials		
Measure of Accuracy	**Definition**	**Comments**
Sensitivity	A characteristic of a diagnostic test. It is the ability of the test to detect the proportion of people with the disease or disorder of interest. For a test to be useful in ruling out a disease, it must have a high sensitivity.	Formula for sensitivity: TP/(TP + FN), where TP and FN are number of true positive and false negative results, respectively
Specificity	A characteristic of a diagnostic test. It is the ability of the test to detect the proportion of people without the disease or disorder of interest. For a test to be useful at confirming a disease, it must have a high specificity.	Formula for sensitivity: TN/(TN + FP), where TN and FP are number of true negative and false positive results, respectively
Positive predictive value (PPV) and negative predictive value (NPV) are closely related to sensitivity and specificity (how well the test performs) but differ in that sensitivity and specificity are fixed characteristics of a diagnostic test whereas PPV and NPV consider how well the test performs and how frequent or infrequent the target disorder occurs in the tested population.		
Positive predictive value	This is the proportion of people with a positive test who have the target disorder.	Formula for positive predictive value: PPV = TP/(TP + FP)
Negative predictive value	This is the proportion of people with a negative test who do not have the target disorder.	Formula for negative predictive value: NPV = TN/(TN + FN)
Likelihood ratio (LR): A likelihood ratio is a measure that a given test result would be expected in a patient with the target disorder compared to the likelihood that the same result would be expected in a patient without the target disorder. It measures the power of a test to change the pretest into the posttest probability of a disease being present.		
Positive likelihood ratio	The LR of a positive test tells us how well a positive test result does by comparing its performance when the disease is present to that when it is absent. The best test to use for ruling in a disease is the one with the largest likelihood ratio of a positive test.	Formula for positive likelihood ratio: sensitivity/(1 − specificity)
Negative likelihood ratio	The LR of a negative test tells us how well a negative test result does by comparing its performance when the disease is absent to that when it is present. The better test to use to rule out disease is the one with the smaller likelihood ratio of a negative test.	Formula for negative likelihood ratio: (1 − sensitivity)/specificity

of certainty that the client has the suspected disorder (see Table 20-9). When a test has a likelihood ratio of 1, the null value, the test will not contribute to decision making in any meaningful way and should not be used. More and more journal articles require authors to provide test likelihood ratios; they may also be available in secondary sources.

TABLE 20-8 **Nitrite Results Indicative for Bacteriuria Using the Dipstick/Pad Method**

| | | (Gold Standard) Culture Results | | |
		Positive	Negative	Totals
Dispstick/pad	Positive	**19**	**2**	21
(New Test)		(a)	(b)	
	Negative	**8**	**69**	77
		(c)	(d)	
Totals		**27**	**71**	98

CALCULATIONS MADE FROM STUDY RESULTS

Sensitivity = a/(a + c)
19/27 = .70 or 70%
Interpretation: The dipstick/pad method is 70% accurate in detecting the proportion of patients with positive tests as having bacteriuria.

Specificity = d/(b + d)
69/71 = .972 or 97%
Interpretation: The dipstick/pad method is 97% accurate in detecting the proportion of patients with negative test as not having bacteriuria.

Prevalence of bacteriuria in this population (elderly, primarily female nursing home residents) = (a + c)/total population
27/98 = .275
Interpretation: The prevalence of bacteriuria in an elderly female population is 28%.

Positive predictive value = a/(a + b)
19/21 = .70 or 90%
Interpretation: 90% of primarily elderly female nursing home residents with a positive dipstick/pad method will have bacteriuria. 10% will not have bacteriuria.

Negative predictive value = d/(c + d)
69/77 = .896 or 90%
Interpretation: 90% of primarily elderly female nursing home residents with a negative dipstick/pad method will not have bacteriuria. 10% will have bacteriuria.

Likelihood ratio (LR+) = sensitivity/(1 − specificity)
.70/(1 − .972) = .70/0.028 = 25
Interpretation: A large LR+. A positive dipstick/pad method test will dramatically change the posttest odds of the patients having bacteriuira.

Likelihood ratio (LR−) = (1 − sensitivity)/specificity
1 − 0.72/.97 = .29
Interpretation: A large LR−. A negative dipstick/pad method test will dramatically change the posttest odds of the patients not having bacteriuria.

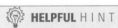
HELPFUL H I N T

When evaluating whether or not you should spend time reviewing an article, examine the article's table. The information you need to answer your clinical question should be contained in one or more of the tables.

TABLE 20-9 **How Much do LRs Change Disease Likelihood?**

LRs > 10 or < 0.1	Cause large changes
LRs 5-10 or 0.1-0.2	Cause moderate changes
LRs 2-5 or 0.2-0.5	Cause small changes
LRs < 2 or > 0.5	Cause tiny changes
LRs = 1.0	Cause no change at all

Prognosis Articles

In articles that answer clinical questions of prognosis, investigators conduct studies in which they want to determine the outcome of a particular disease or condition. Prognosis studies can often be identified by their longitudinal design (see Chapter 11). At the conclusion of a longitudinal study, investigators statistically analyze data to determine which factors are strongly associated with the study outcomes. Because researchers are interested in demonstrating the occurrence of events at specific points in time, one way of presenting data is to present measures of association (see Table 20-3) for a variety of data points or several different points in time. A more efficient manner of presenting this type of data is in survival curves. A **survival curve** is a graph that shows the probability that a patient "survives" in a given state for at least a specified time (or longer). Although survival curves were originally developed to study how long a patient survived symptom- or disease-free periods, almost any dichotomous data can be plotted on a curve, e.g., how long a patient stayed on a medication or in a nurse-managed program. When analyzing survival curves, investigators often report the study outcomes in terms of hazard ratios. A **hazard ratio** is essentially a weighted relative risk based on the analysis of survival curves over the whole course of the study period. The hazard is the slope of the survival curve—a measure of how rapidly subjects are dying (or some other outcome). The hazard ratio compares the slope between two groups. If the hazard ratio is 2.0, then the rate of deaths in one treatment group is twice the rate in the other group. Let us see how hazard ratios are used in a longitudinal study of elderly persons.

A prospective, longitudinal study was carried out for 12 years to identify predictors of institutionalization in elderly patients based on a variety of factors measured at baseline and then every 2 years (Bharucha et al., 2004). The study outcomes after 12 years are presented in Table 20-10, with their respective confidence intervals.

In this table you will find the hazard ratios used as a measure of association. The interpretation of hazard ratios is similar to and interpreted in the same way as the risk ratio (see Table 20-3). The major difference is the interpretation of the CI. With the risk ratio the null value is equal to zero, and with hazard ratios the null value is equal to 1. Thus any hazard ratio CI interval that contains a null value of 1 is not a significant finding. This is further demonstrated by the nonsignificant p values that accompany all of the CI intervals in Table 20-10 that contain the null value. This table further illustrates that p values are not necessary to report when CI, the preferred method of reporting certainty, is given.

A review of Table 20-10 indicates that for this group, the strongest predictor of institutionalism was dementia (hazard ratio [HR] 5.09; CI 2.92 to 8.84). This means that individuals with dementia were 5 times more likely to be institutionalized; because the confidence interval does not include the null value, it is statistically significant. Weak indicators for institutionalism, but nonetheless statistically significant findings, are advancing age, greater functional disability, greater number of prescription medications, and worse/less social support.

Using prognostic information with an evidence-based lens helps the nurse and patient focus on reducing factors that may lead to disease or disability. It also helps the nurse provide education and information to patients and their families regarding the course of the condition.

Harm Articles

In articles that answer clinical questions of harm, investigators want to determine if an individual has been harmed by being exposed to a particular event. Harm studies can be identified by their case-control design (see Chapter 11). In this type of study, investigators select the outcome they are interested in (e.g., pressure ulcers), and they examine if any one factor explains those who have and do not have the outcome of interest.

TABLE 20-10 **Predictors of Institutionalization (N = 1147)**

Potential Predictor	Hazard Ratio	95% Confidence Interval	p Value
Age*	1.06	1.03-1.10	<0.001
Sex (male vs. female)	0.94	0.64-1.38	0.753
Education (<high school vs. ≥high school)	0.84	0.61-1.12	0.843
Cognitive functioning (Mini-Mental State Examination score)*	1.05	0.97-1.13	0.205
Living arrangement (not living alone vs. living alone)	1.15	0.70-1.87	0.588
Marital status (currently married vs. not married)	1.08	0.65-1.79	0.774
Social support (social support score)*	1.27	1.10-1.46	0.001
Functional disability (instrumental activities of daily living score)*	1.31	1.15-1.50	<0.001
Depression (<5 symptoms vs. ≥5)	0.80	0.48-1.34	0.404
History of hospitalization in past year (no vs. yes)	1.32	0.93-1.88	0.314
Number of prescription drugs*	1.21	1.11-1.32	<0.001
Dementia	5.09	2.92-8.84	<0.001
Dementia and number of prescription drugs (interaction)	0.81	0.70-0.95	0.001

*Continuous variable.
Source: Bharucha AJ, Pandav R, Shen C, Dodge HH, and Ganguli M: Predictors of nursing facility admission: a 12-year epidemiological study in the United States, *J Am Geriatr Soc* 52: 434–439, 2004.

The measure of association that best describes the analyzed data in case-control studies is the odds ratio (OR). The **odds ratio (OR)** communicates the probability of an event. An OR is calculated by dividing the odds in the treated or exposed group by the odds in the control group. Investigators present OR of factors in study tables, and thus calculation of odds ratio is rarely necessary. The interpretation of odds ratio is straightforward and presented in Table 20-11. Note that the null value for the odds ratio is equal to 1.

The use of the odds ratio to describe the probability of an event is illustrated by a study in which investigators sought to determine risk factors for the death of full-term, postneonatal, healthy infants born to young mothers (Phipps, Blume, and DeMonner, 2002). The study authors used a large data set (*n* = 1,830,350) of mothers 12 to 29 years of age who delivered healthy babies. The investigators wanted to determine if death of the infant occurred within the first year after birth to young mothers as compared with infants born to older mothers. The result of the study's main outcome stratified by age is described in Table 20-12. For both unadjusted and adjusted odds, it is easy to see that as the mother's age declines, the probability of death of an infant in the postneonatal period increases (the OR gets larger). Healthy, full-term infants born to mothers less than 15 years of age are 3 to 4 times more likely to die within their first year compared to infants born to mothers 23 to 29 years of age. The study was not designed to determine which factors are associated with death. However, the authors did indicate that unmeasured social factors could have a potential association; further studies are needed to test the validity of this association. With this evidence the nurse could justify the need for increased home-care visits to younger mothers in the immediate postpartum period. Another nurse can use this evidence to start a nurse-managed support group for babies born to younger mothers. Similarly,

TABLE **20-11** **Interpretation of Odds Ratios**

	Type of Outcome	
Odds ratio	Adverse outcome, e.g., myocardial infarction	Beneficial outcome, e.g., adherence
Less than 1, e.g., 0.375	Intervention better	Intervention worse
Equal to 1	Intervention no better/worse	Intervention no better/worse
More than 1, e.g., 4.0	Intervention worse	Intervention better

TABLE **20-12** **Odds Ratios for Postneonatal Mortality Associated With Maternal Age Groups**

Maternal Age (y)	Crude OR	Adjusted OR*
≤15	4.1 (3.4, 4.8)	3.0 (2.5, 3.6)
16-17	3.1 (2.8, 3.5)	2.4 (2.1, 2.7)
18-19	2.5 (2.3, 2.8)	2.0 (1.8, 2.3)
20-22	1.8 (1.6, 2.0)	1.5 (1.4, 1.7)
23-29	1.0	1.0

OR = odds ratio.
Data are given an OR (95% confidence interval).
*Adjusted for material raco'ethnology, adequacy of prenatal care utilization, and marital status.
Source: Phipps M, Blume J, and DeMonner S: Young maternal age associated with increased risk of postneonatal death, *Obstetr Gynecol* 100: 481–486, 2002.

the RCT conducted by Koniak-Griffin and colleagues (2003) that appears in Appendix A tested the effectiveness of an early intervention program (EIP) on maternal and infant outcomes in a sample of young mothers. The findings reported the benefits of this program in contrast to a traditional public health nursing program.

Harm data with its measure of probabilities help the nurse to identify factors that may or may not contribute to an adverse or beneficial outcome. This information will be useful for the nursing plan of care, program planning, or patient and family education.

> *Jasmine's search yielded a large number of controlled and noncontrolled trials relevant to her clinical question. She selected a meta-analysis to answer her clinical question because she knows*

that a meta-analysis is a special type of method that statistically combines the results of many studies on a particular topic. A meta-analysis provides Level I evidence, the highest level of evidence on any evidence hierarchy rating model (see Chapters 2 and 19).

Meta-Analysis

Meta-analysis is not a type of study design but a research method that statistically combines the results of multiple studies (usually RCTs) to answer focused clinical questions through an objective appraisal of carefully synthesized research evidence (see Chapter 11). When talking about a meta-analysis, people sometimes use this term and systematic review interchangeably. In reality, a meta-analysis is a quantitative approach to a systematic review. Systematic review is the process whereby the investigators find all relevant studies, published and unpublished, on the topic or question. Then at least two members of the review team independently assess the quality of each study, include or exclude studies based on preestablished criteria, statistically combine the results of individual studies, and present a balanced and impartial evidence summary of the findings that represents a "state of the science" conclusion about the evidence supporting benefits and risks of a given health care practice (Stevens, 2001). Each meta-analysis is a complex project and, as such, is conducted by a multidisciplinary team of clinicians, health scientists, clinical epidemiologists, meta-analytic statisticians, EBP librarians, and informatics specialists.

In the evidence-based hierarchy, the findings of a meta-analysis are considered to provide the strongest evidence available to the clinician because they summarize large amounts of information derived from multiple experimental studies investigating the effect of the same intervention. A methodologically sound meta-analysis is more likely than an individual study in identifying the true effect of an intervention because it limits bias.

In a **systematic review**, the meta-analysis quantitatively combines the data from the selected experimental studies by using their measures of association (Table 20-3). An odds ratio is the statistic of choice for use in a meta-analysis. The same interpretation of odds ratio described in Table 20-11 applies to the odds ratios seen in a meta-analysis.

The usual manner of displaying data from a meta-analysis is by a pictorial representation known as a blobbogram, accompanied by a summary measure of effect size in odds ratio. Before we examine the meta-analysis described in the case study, let us see how blobbograms and odds ratios are used to summarize the studies in a systematic review by practicing with the data in Figure 20-2. In this meta-analysis, the investiga-

tors were interested in comparing the efficacy of a beta-agonist given by a metered-dose inhaler with a chamber versus a nebulizer on hospital admission in children under 5 years of age (Castro-Rodriquez and Rodrigo, 2004). The investigators searched the literature for RCTs that treated children under 5 in the emergency department (ED) with acute asthma who were randomized to receive either a metered-dose inhaler with a chamber or a nebulizer. The investigators found six trials that met this criterion, and they are listed in Figure 20-2. The study groups are represented by a fraction; for example, in the trial published by Close, 4/17 children in the metered-dose inhaler with a chamber group were admitted to the hospital and 4/17 children in the nebulizer group were admitted to the hospital. In the center of the table, you see that each trial in the analysis is represented by a horizontal line. The findings from each individual study are represented as a blob or square (the measured effect) on the vertical line. The size of the blob or square (sometimes just a small vertical line) may vary to reflect the amount of information in that individual study. The width of the horizontal line represents the 95% confidence interval. A vertical line is the line

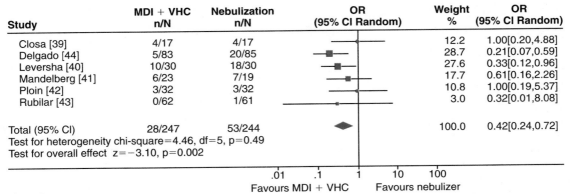

Study	MDI + VHC n/N	Nebulization n/N	OR (95% CI Random)	Weight %	OR (95% CI Random)
Closa [39]	4/17	4/17		12.2	1.00[0.20,4.88]
Delgado [44]	5/83	20/85		28.7	0.21[0.07,0.59]
Leversha [40]	10/30	18/30		27.6	0.33[0.12,0.96]
Mandelberg [41]	6/23	7/19		17.7	0.61[0.16,2.26]
Ploin [42]	3/32	3/32		10.8	1.00[0.19,5.37]
Rubilar [43]	0/62	1/61		3.0	0.32[0.01,8.08]
Total (95% CI)	28/247	53/244		100.0	0.42[0.24,0.72]

Test for heterogeneity chi-square=4.46, df=5, p=0.49
Test for overall effect z=−3.10, p=0.002

.01   .1   1   10   100
Favours MDI + VHC   Favours nebulizer

Figure 20-2. Systematic review with meta-analysis data showing the efficacy of a beta-agonist given by metered-dose inhaler with a valved holding chamber (MDI+VHC) vs. nebulizer in children under 5 years of age with acute exacerbation of wheezing or asthma in the emergency department on hospitalization. (From Castro-Rodriquez J, and Rodrigo G: Beta-agonists through metered-dose inhaler with valved holding chamber versus nebulizer for acute exacerbation of wheezing or asthma in children under 5 years of age: a systematic review with meta-analysis, *J Pediatr* 145(2): 172-177, 2004.)

of no effect (odds ratio = 1). When the confidence interval of the result (horizontal line) crosses the line of no effect (vertical line), then the differences in the effect of the treatment are not statistically significant. If the confidence interval does not cross the vertical line, then the study results are statistically significant.

In examining the blobbograms in Figure 20-2, it is clear that only two of the six studies do not cross the line of no effect—study 2 published by Delgado and study 3 published by Leversha. Because the analysis line does not cross the line of no effect, these studies have statistically significant findings. In columns 4 and 5 of this table, the investigators have also provided the numerical equivalent of each blobbogram. You will also notice other important information and additional statistical analysis that may accompany the blobbogram table such as a test to determine how well the results of each of the individual trials are mathematically compatible (heterogeneity). The reader is referred to a book of advanced research methods for discussion.

The summary odds ratio for all of the studies combined is represented by a diamond. In this case, after statistically pooling the results of each of the controlled trials, it shows that these studies, statistically combined, favor the metered-dose inhaler with a chamber for preventing hospitalization of children under 5 years of age and that this option is statistically significant. If this were a methodologically sound meta-analysis, it would support the clinical practice of providing children under 5 years of age with asthma exacerbation with a metered-dose inhaler with a chamber to prevent hospitalization. A simple tool to help the nurse determine whether or not a systematic review is methodologically sound can be found at http://www.phru.nhs.uk/casp/reviews.pdf.

EVIDENCE-BASED TOOL #5: APPLYING THE FINDINGS

Sackett and colleagues (1996) stated that evidence-based practice is about integrating indi-

 EVIDENCE-BASED PRACTICE TIP

When answering a clinical question check to see if a Cochrane review has been performed. This will save you time searching the literature. A Cochrane review is a systematic review that primarily uses meta-analysis to investigate the effects of interventions for prevention, treatment, and rehabilitation in a health care setting or on health-related disorders. Most Cochrane reviews are based on RCTs, but other types of evidence may also be taken into account, if appropriate. If the data collected in a review are of sufficient quality and similar enough, they are summarized statistically in a meta-analysis. The nurse should always check the Cochrane website, http://www. cochrane. org/index0.htm, to see if a review has been published on their topic of interest.

vidual clinical expertise and patient preferences with the best external evidence to guide clinical decision making. With a few simple tools (see www links described above) and some practice, your day-to-day practice can be more evidence-based. More and more studies are being conducted that actually demonstrate whether or not a practice that is rooted in evidence actually improves the quality of care. We know that using evidence in clinical decision making by nurses and all other health care professionals interested in matters associated with the care of individuals, communities, and health systems is increasingly important to achieving quality patient outcomes and cannot be ignored. Let us see how Jasmine, our allergy and asthma nurse, uses evidence to make a clinically effective decision and perhaps make a practice change.

Jasmine reviews the following article:"House dust mite control measures in the management of asthma: meta-analysis." The article summarizes data in three different ways (three different blobbograms). Jasmine selects Figure 1 from the article because she feels that it is most appropriate to

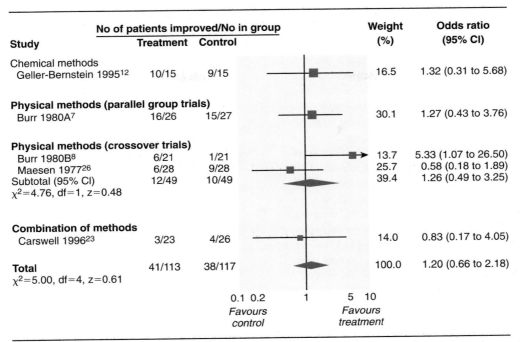

Study	No of patients improved/No in group		Weight (%)	Odds ratio (95% CI)
	Treatment	Control		
Chemical methods				
Geller-Bernstein 1995[12]	10/15	9/15	16.5	1.32 (0.31 to 5.68)
Physical methods (parallel group trials)				
Burr 1980A[7]	16/26	15/27	30.1	1.27 (0.43 to 3.76)
Physical methods (crossover trials)				
Burr 1980B[8]	6/21	1/21	13.7	5.33 (1.07 to 26.50)
Maesen 1977[26]	6/28	9/28	25.7	0.58 (0.18 to 1.89)
Subtotal (95% CI)	12/49	10/49	39.4	1.26 (0.49 to 3.25)
$\chi^2=4.76$, df$=1$, z$=0.48$				
Combination of methods				
Carswell 1996[23]	3/23	4/26	14.0	0.83 (0.17 to 4.05)
Total	41/113	38/117	100.0	1.20 (0.66 to 2.18)
$\chi^2=5.00$, df$=4$, z$=0.61$				

0.1 0.2   1   5   10
Favours control   Favours treatment

Figure 20-3. Odds ratios (95% confidence interval) of number of asthma patients whose symptoms improved after the use of either chemical or physical methods to reduce exposure to house dust mites. (From Gøtzsche PC, Hammarquist C, and Burr M: House dust mite control measures in the management of asthma: meta-analysis, *Brit Med J* 317: 1105-1110, 1998.)

answer her clinical question (see Figure 20-3). Jasmine quickly learns, from viewing the blobbogram, that all but one of the studies reviewed, the Burr study conducted in 1980, cross the vertical line of no effect (null value = 1). She also reviews the CI intervals for each of the studies and knows that for odds ratio, a CI that includes the null value (null value = 1) represents nonsignificant findings. The Burr study does not cross the value of no effect but is weighted low relative to all of the other studies. Jasmine examines the CI interval for this study and finds that the CI is wide. She knows that a wide confidence interval may be statistically significant but indicates a wide variation in the effect of treatment, sometimes so wide that its clinical importance may be reduced. She also knows that a wide CI is a sign that too few patients were enrolled in the study and thus the significance of the effect of the treatment was

based on too few patients, again introducing a degree of uncertainty. The summary odds ratios cross the vertical line and the CI intervals contain the null value. This suggests that neither physical methods nor chemical methods of eliminating mites were effective in improving symptoms. She examines another table (not shown) and finds the same data for the effectiveness of physical and chemical methods to improve the peak expiratory flow rate in the morning.

As a result of this review of the literature, Jasmine has learned that in a meta-analysis of 23 studies of methods to reduce the exposure of asthma patients to mites the investigators failed to find a clinical benefit from any of the measures and believe that current chemical and physical methods cannot be recommended as prophylactic treatment for asthma patients who are sensitive to mites.

These findings are informative because they begin to challenge the widely held belief that chemical and physical methods are highly effective and these methods should be used by patients with asthma to reduce their exposure to dust mites. Jasmine will also share this information with her patient and her professional practice group. Because chemical methods can be costly, she will discontinue recommending this as a method. Because the meta-analysis did not detail the type of physical methods used in each of the studies, she is interested in knowing which methods have been tested. Physical methods are less costly, and Jasmine also knows that successful controlled trials have used physical measures, such as bed covers, washing bedding in hot water, and carpet removal, rather than chemical treatment to control mites. Jasmine decides to return to the literature at a later date and continue to explore the evidence in this area.

When Jasmine sees the patient at the next office visit, she informs the patient that her research found that neither method she described at their last visit has been shown to be particularly effective in controlling asthma-related symptoms in individuals particularly sensitive to mites and, as such, no one particular method can be identified as being better than the other. Although this study did not find that any particular physical or chemical method improves symptoms, there are particular environmental conditions that will support the proliferation of mites. Jasmine recommends that she and the patient continue to test and implement different control measures, such as washing bed covers and reducing humidity. It is only through the right combination of methods that they will they be effective in controlling her symptoms.

Critical Thinking Challenges

- You are asked to identify a patient and clinical problem and develop a clinical question.
- Discuss the process of developing an answerable clinical question useful to evidence-based practice.
- As a student, you have researched many papers for class. Compare and contrast the steps used in evidence-based practice to those used to write a standard research paper. Give examples.
- Why is the level of evidence from a meta-analysis about the effectiveness of an intervention higher than the level of evidence provided by a single randomized clinical trial about the effectiveness of an intervention?
- How would you use the PICO approach to answer a clinical question? Provide a clinical example.
- How do you think the concept of evidence-based practice has changed research utilization (RU) models? Do you think that the review of the literature is the same for developing a research proposal as it is for developing an evidence-based practice protocol? Support your position.

KEY POINTS

- Asking a focused clinical question using the PICO approach is an important EBP tool.
- Four types of EBP clinical categories used by nurses and other clinicians are the following: therapy, diagnosis, prognosis, and harm. These categories focus development of the clinical question, the literature search, and critical appraisal of research studies.
- An efficient and effective literature search, using information literacy skills, is critical in locating evidence to answer the clinical question.
- Sources of evidence (e.g., articles, EBP guidelines, EBP protocols) must be screened for relevance and credibility.
- Critiquing the evidence generated by research studies using an evidence rating model and accepted critiquing criteria is essential in determining the strength, quality, and consistency of evidence offered by a quantitative or qualitative research study.
- Articles that belong to the therapy category are designed to determine if a difference exists between two or more treatments.
- Articles that belong to the diagnosis category are designed to investigate the ability of screening or diagnostic tests, tools, or components of the clinical examination to detect whether or not the patient has a particular disease using sensitivity and specificity tests.
- Articles in the prognosis category are designed to determine the outcomes of a particular disease or condition.
- Articles in the harm category are designed to determine if an individual has been harmed by being exposed to a particular event.
- Meta-analysis is a research method that statistically combines the results of multiple studies (usually RCTs) and is designed to answer a focused clinical question through objective appraisal of synthesized evidence.

REFERENCES

Altman D: Confidence intervals for the number needed to treat, *Brit Med J* 317: 309-312, 1998.

Bharucha AJ, Pandav R, Shen C, Dodge HH, and Ganguli M: Predictors of nursing facility admission: a 12-year epidemiological study in the United States, *J Am Geriatr Soc* 52: 434-439, 2004.

Castro-Rodriquez J and Rodrigo G: Beta-agonists through metered-dose inhaler with valved holding chamber versus nebulizer for acute exacerbation of wheezing or asthma in children under 5 years of age: a systematic review with meta-analysis, *J Pediatr* 145(2): 172-177, 2004.

Gøtzsche PC, Hammarquist C, and Burr M: House dust mite control measures in the management of asthma: meta-analysis, *Brit Med J* 317: 1105-1110, 1998.

Jacobs SK, Rosenfeld P, and Haber J: Information literacy as the foundation for evidence-based practice in graduate nursing education: a curriculum-integrated approach, *J Profess Nurs* 19(5): 320-328, 2003.

Koniak-Griffin D, Verzemniecks IL, Anderson NLR, Brecht ML, Lesser J, Kim S, and Turner-Pluta C: Nurse visitation for adolescent mothers: two year infant and maternal outcomes, *Nurs Res* 52(2): 127-136, 2003.

Lenhardt R, Seybold T, Kimberger O, Stoiser R, and Sessler D: Local warming and insertion of peripheral venous cannulas: single blinded prospective randomised controlled trial and single blinded randomized crossover trial, *Brit J Med* 325: 409-412, 2002.

McCorkle R, Strumpf N, Nuamah I, Adler D, Cooley M, Jepson C, Lusk E, and Torosian M: A randomized clinical trial of a specialized home care intervention on survival among elderly post-surgical cancer patients, *J Am Geriatr Soc* 48: 1707-1713, 2000.

Midthun SJ, Paur RA, Lindseth G, and Von Duvillard SP: Bacteriuria detection with a urine dipstick applied to incontinence pads of nursing home residents, *Geriatr Nurs* 24(4): 206-209, 2003.

Miser WF: Critical appraisal of the literature, *J Am Board Family Pract* 12: 315-333. 1999.

Phipps M, Blume J, DeMonner S: Young maternal age associated with increased risk of postneonatal death, *Obstetr Gynecol* 100: 481-486, 2002.

Rathore SS, Wang Y, and Krumholz HM: Sex-based differences in the effect of digoxin for the treatment of heart failure, *New Engl J Med* 347: 1403-1411, 2002.

Sackett DL, Rosenberg WMC, Gray JAM, Haynes RB, and Richardson WS: Evidence based medicine: what it is and what it isn't, *Brit Med J* 312: 71-72, 1996.

Stevens K: Systematic reviews: the heart of evidence-based practice, *AACN Clin Issues: Adv Pract Acute Crit Care* 12(4): 529-538, 2001.

Van Cleve L, Bossert E, Beecroft P, Adlard K, Alvarez O, and Savedra MC: The pain experience of children with leukemia during the first year after diagnosis, *Nurs Res* 53(1): 1-10, 2004.

FOR FURTHER STUDY

Go to your Companion CD for review activities for this chapter.

evolve Go to Evolve at http://evolve.elsevier.com/LoBiondo/ for WebLinks, Content Updates, and additional research articles, for practice in reviewing and critiquing.

DEBORAH KONIAK-GRIFFIN,

INESE L. VERZEMNIEKS, NANCY L. R. ANDERSON,

MARY-LYNN BRECHT, JANNA LESSER,

SUE KIM, CARMEN TURNER-PLUTA

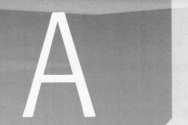

Nurse Visitation for Adolescent Mothers Two-Year Infant Health and Maternal Outcomes

▶ **Background:** Children of adolescent mothers have higher rates of morbidity and unintentional injuries and hospitalizations during the first 5 years of life than do children of adult mothers.

▶ **Objective:** The purpose of this study was to evaluate the 2-year postbirth infant health and maternal outcomes of an early intervention program (EIP) of home visitation by public health nurses (PHNs).

▶ **Methods:** In a randomized controlled trial, a sample of predominantly Latina and African American adolescent mothers was followed from pregnancy through 2 years postpartum. The experimental group (EIP, $n = 56$) received preparation-for-motherhood classes plus intense home visitation by PHNs from pregnancy through 1 year postbirth; the control group (TPHNC, $n = 45$) received traditional public health nursing care (TPHNC). Health outcomes were determined based on medical record data; other measures evaluated selected maternal behaviors, social competence, and mother-child interactions.

▶ **Results:** The total days of non-birth-related infant hospitalizations during the first 24 months was significantly lower in the EIP (143 days) than the TPHNC group (211 days) and episodes of hospitalization were fewer; more EIP than

THHNC infants were never seen in the emergency room. The EIP mothers had 15% fewer repeat pregnancies in the first 2 years postbirth than TPHNC mothers. The TPHNC mothers significantly increased marijuana use over time, whereas EIP mothers did not.

▶ **Conclusions:** The EIP improved in selected areas of infant and maternal health, and these

Deborah Koniak-Griffin, EdD, RN, FAAN, is Professor and Director of the Center for Vulnerable Populations Research at the UCLA School of Nursing, Los Angeles, California.

Inese L. Verzemnieks, PhD, RN, was a Postdoctoral Fellow with the Vulnerable Populations Training Grant at the UCLA School of Nursing, Los Angeles, California.

Nancy L. R. Anderson, PhD, RN, is Professor Emeritus at the UCLA School of Nursing, Los Angeles, California.

Mary-Lynn Brecht, PhD, was Principal Statistician at the UCLA School of Nursing and is Director of the Research Support Core of the Center for Vulnerable Populations Research, UCLA School of Nursing, Los Angeles, California.

Janna Lesser, PhD, RN, CS, was formerly Adjunct Assistant Professor at the UCLA School of Nursing; she is now Assistant Professor at Florida State University, Tallahassee.

Sue Kim, PhD, RN, was a doctoral student at the UCLA School of Nursing; she is now Assistant Professor and Theresa A. Thomas Faculty at the University of Virginia School of Nursing, Charlottesville.

Carmen Turner-Pluta, BMus, is an Administrative Analyst at the UCLA School of Nursing, Los Angeles, California.

improvements were sustained for a period of 1 year following program termination. These findings have important implications for healthcare services.

▶ *Key Words:* adolescent mothers • infant hospitalization • nurse home visitation • repeat pregnancy

Although teen birth rates have declined sharply in recent years by 22% from 1991 to 2000 (Martin, Hamilton, Ventura, Menacker, & Park, 2002), Hispanic and Black adolescents continue to have a much higher birth rate than non-Hispanic Whites. Early childbearing impacts the nation's healthcare system, and social and economic functioning; hence, community-based nursing intervention programs are needed to improve health and social outcomes for teen mothers and their children.

Adolescent mothers and their children may benefit from home visitation, as they often lack the resources needed to maintain health and reduce risk factors in their lives. Many of these women live in poverty, have low educational attainment, and lack adequate social support (Alan Guttmacher Institute, 1994). Furthermore, their children have higher rates of morbidity and unintentional injuries leading to emergency room (ER) visits and hospitalizations during the first 5 years of life, as compared to children of adult mothers (Alan Guttmacher Institute, 1994; McClure-Martinez & Cohn, 1996).

In order to reduce risks associated with early child-bearing, a variety of programs have been implemented. An important consideration in evaluation of health promotion interventions for adolescent mothers and their children is whether the effects are maintained beyond the treatment period. Positive outcomes for some programs last only during or for a short time after the intervention, while others produce long-term, sustained effects (Olds et al., 1997; Olds, Henderson, & Kitzman, 1994). Some studies have reported additonal positive outcomes not evident until a year or more following program termination

(Barnard & Bee, 1983; Olds et al., 1999). This article describes the research of a randomized clinical trial designed to determine the effects of an early intervention program (EIP) provided through home visits by public health nurses (PHNs) to culturally diverse adolescent mothers and their children on infant health and maternal outcomes at 24 months.

REVIEW OF LITERATURE

Home visitation can provide early intervention services to improve prenatal care, offer instruction in parenting skills and family planning, and counsel adolescent mothers on ways to improve their own life course and that of their children. Notable among nurse home visitation programs that have demonstrated improvement in both maternal and child outcomes is the series of randomized clinical trials by Olds and associates (Olds et al., 1999). Their longitudinal intervention programs use a model in which nurse visits begin during pregnancy and continue until the child's 2nd birthday. In the first of these studies, a predominantly White sample of mothers visited by nurse ($N = 400$) decreased smoking, improved diet, reported greater informal and formal social support, and had fewer kidney infections and instances of pregnancy-induced hypertension than a control group. Premature births to women who smoked were 75% fewer in the nurse-visited group, while birth weights of infants born to mothers under 17 years of age at intake were higher (Olds, Henderson, Tatelbaum, & Chamberlin, 1986). During their 2nd year, children of low-income, unmarried teens who received nurse visits had 32% fewer ER visits for injuries and accidents than their counterparts (Olds et al., 1986). At the 4-year follow-up these children had reduced rates of injuries and ingestions possibly associated with child abuse and neglect (Olds et al., 1994). Findings of the 15-

---

Adolescent mothers often lack the resources needed to maintain health and reduce risk factors.

year follow-up showed further benefits in terms of (a) improved maternal life course, with fewer and deferred subsequent pregnancies, (b) increased employment rates, and (c) fewer months on welfare (Olds et al., 1997).

In a second trail, with a sample ($N = 1,139$) of primarily African American, low-income, unmarried adolescents, nurse-visited women were found to have lower rates of morbidity for selected prenatal health conditions than a comparison group (Kitzman et al., 1997). However, positive effects on birth weights and premature birth rates were not replicated, possibly attributable to a lower smoking rate. During their first 2 years, nurse-visited children had fewer healthcare encounters and hospitalization days related to injuries and ingestions; however, these benefits were concentrated among children of mothers identified as having "low psychological resources." Nurse-visited mothers had homes rated as more conducive to children's development. Repeat pregnancy rates were reduced for the intervention group in both studies.

Less comprehensive home visiting programs by PHNs have (a) decreased incidence of low birth weight (LBW) infants (Norbeck, DeJoseph, & Smith, 1996); (b) improved mother-child interactions and maternal educational attainment (Booth, Barnard, Mitchell, & Spieker, 1987); (c) reduced rates of school dropout and repeat pregnancy; and (d) improved immunization rates (O'Sullivan & Jacobsen, 1992).

Earlier findings laid important groundwork for the 2-year postbirth outcomes reported here from a longitudinal study on the effects of a PHN EIP for adolescent mothers. This randomized clinical trial compared effects of intense home visitation EIP vs. traditional PHN care (TPHNC). Findings revealed that infants in the EIP had significantly fewer total days of birth-related hospitalization and re-hospitalization in the 1st year of life, and higher immunization rates than TPHNC infants (Koniak-Griffin et al., 2002; Koniak-Griffin, Anderson, Verzemnieks, & Brecht, 2000). Only seven infants were premature; none with very LBW. The EIP mothers demonstrated significantly more positive educational achievement at 6 weeks postpartum; at 1 year this difference only approached significance. It was hypothesized that at 2 years postbirth, participants in the EIP would demonstrate improved infant health and maternal outcomes in comparison to those in the TPHNC group.

Theoretical Framework

The EIP was designed to help the young mother achieve program objectives as a result of improved social competence. The construct of social competence was conceived to have two facets: internal and external. The young mother's internal competence (ability to handle her inner world) was proposed to be increased through training in self-management skills, including self-care, life planning and decision making, handling emotions, and coping with stress and depression. At the same time, her external competence (ability to interact effectively with partners, family, peers, and social agencies) was anticipated to improve through training in communication and social skills. Previous investigators have proposed that competence in adolescents entails both an emotional component and social skills (Clausen, 1991). The theoretical approach used in the EIP was supported by research findings demonstrating that stress, depression, resource deficits (i.e., economic, educational, and social), and lack of adequate communication and social skills to access available community resources have a negative effect on both maternal and child outcomes (Olds et al., 1999).

METHODS

Setting and Sample

Adolescents were recruited from referrals to the Community Health Services Division of the County Health Department in San Bernardino, California. They were eligible if they were: (a) 14-19 years of age; (b) at 26 weeks gestation or less; (c) having their first child; and (d) planning to keep the infant. Excluded were those dependent on narcotic or injection drugs, or having a documented serious medical or obstetric problem. Recruitment continued until the sample reached a target number ($N = 144$) based on power analysis ($\alpha = .05$, power $= .80$, and a moderate effect size of approximately .47) using pilot data available for a measure of maternal-child interaction. Because of attrition the sample size ($n = 101$) available for analysis of 24-month outcomes, adjusting for unequal n, was adequate to detect a moderate effect size of $d = .57$ in group differences on outcomes.

Procedure

After securing written informed consent in accordance with the university Internal Review Board requirements for pregnant minors, adolescents were randomly assigned, using a computer-based program, into the EIP or TPHNC group, based on specific criteria (maternal age, ethnicity, language, gestation age, geographic region of residence). To avoid contamination of treatment conditions, each PHN provided individualized care on a one-to-one basis to adolescents in only one group. The initial training for EIP PHNs was approximately 60 hours, followed by periodic booster sessions.

The Early Intervention Program (EIP)

All adolescents in the EIP ($n = 56$) received care by PHNs, using a case management approach with one nurse providing continuous care to her assigned adolescent from pregnancy through 1 year postpartum. The EIP was designed to (a) improve maternal health behaviors during and after pregnancy; (b) improve birth outcomes, and mother and infant health; (c) build maternal caretaking skills and improve the quality of mother-child interaction; (d) prevent rapid repeat pregnancy; (e) increase educational achievement; and (f) build social competence. Protocols were developed for interventions to ensure uniformity of care in five major areas: health, sexuality and family planning, maternal role, life skills, and social support. A series of four

"preparation-for-motherhood" classes focused on behaviors to promote health during pregnancy, parent-child communication, and the transition to motherhood. Following childbirth, PHNs demonstrated selected components of the Neonatal Behavioral Assessment Scale (NBAS) (Brazelton, 1984) and provided videotape instruction and feedback to improve parenting behaviors (Koniak-Griffin, Verzemnieks, & Cahill, 1992). Teaching and counseling were directed towards health promotion, life planning, building problem-solving skills, and securing needed resources (e.g., social support, child care, and health services). The EIP was designed to include a maximum of 17 home visits: 2 prenatal, and 15 postpartum (1.5 to 2 hours each); however, the number of visits varied among families depending on the mother's availability. The mean number of visits completed by the nurses in the prenatal period was 2.13 ($SD = .77$), and in the postnatal period, 10.35 ($SD = 3.04$). Fidelity of the intervention was documented by use of antepartum and postpartum flowsheets in which nurses used a coding system to indicate components of care provided. In addition, an onsite PHN supervisor from the agency and the project director oversaw the nurses' implementation of study protocols. Review of these flowsheets and the nurses' healthcare records revealed that the greatest challenge for implementation was videotherapy. A variety of factors contributed to their difficulties, including (a) mothers not being available for scheduled visits; (b) infants being asleep during the home visit; and (c) refusal by mothers to be videotaped.

Traditional Public Health Nursing Care

The TPHNC mothers ($n = 45$) received services comparable to those often available in county health departments lacking special funding for adolescent programs. One prenatal home visit was made shortly after the participant's entry into the study, and a second during the 3rd trimester. These visits focused on (a) assessment and counseling related to prenatal healthcare (source and adequacy), (b) self-care, (c) preparation for childbirth, (d) education planning, and (e) well-baby care, including immunizations. Within 6 weeks postpartum, the PHN made an additional home visit to provide the mother with general information about child care, postpartum recovery, maternal and infant nutrition, home safety, community resources, and family planning. The mean number of home visits actually made was 1.02 ($SD = .26$) in the prenatal period and 1.09 ($SD = .42$) in the postpartum period.

Adolescents in both groups were provided services by baccalaureate-prepared, California-certified, experienced PHNs. These nurses worked under subcontract with the university conducting the research; consequently, they carried a mixed caseload of study participants and other clients. Protocols called for telephone calls by PHNs to participants in both groups, at specified intervals, to prevent attrition and to arrange and confirm home visits.

Measures

Data on infant and maternal outcomes were collected through a variety of measures, administered at six time points: intake, 6 weeks after the birth, and 6, 12, 18, and 24 months postpartum. These included medical records, written questionnaires, observation scales, and structured interviews by the nurse. Except for the HOME scale, all of the interview questions and instruments measuring outcome variables were administered at each of the data points.

Interviews

All interviews were conducted by evaluator PHNs who were not involved in the intervention and were blind to group assignment. Interviewers assessed health-related behaviors, use of healthcare services, complications of pregnancy and birth, maternal and infant health, history of childhood physical/sexual abuse, community resource use, and educational and employment status. The interview questions were validated for content (by a panel of four nurses with expertise in research methods and adolescent develop-

ment) and assessed by a field test for both meaning and language appropriateness.

Infant Health

Data collected on infant health included hospitalizations (i.e., length in days, number of episodes, diagnoses) and ER visits during the 24 months following birth. This information, initially collected via maternal reports, was subsequently verified by medical records whenever possible. Medical record data were available for 80% of the reported hospitalization episodes and 61% of the ER episodes. All maternal reports of episodes of hospitalization were found to be accurate (100%), with few and minor variations in length of stay. When discrepancies existed in the duration of hospitalization, the medical record data were employed. Of the total number of episodes of ER visits, 22% were based on hospital data that had not been reported by mothers. The distribution of missing infant health data was higher for participants receiving TPHNC than those in the EIP group. Data on infant immunizations were confirmed by medical records or by review of immunization cards issued by the county health department or direct care provider, as verified by the evaluator nurse. Immunizations were considered *adequate* if four or more doses of diptheria-tetanus-pertussis vaccine, three or more doses of poliovirus vaccine, and one or more doses of measles-containing vaccine were received by 24 months of age, as recommended by the Centers for Disease Control and Prevention (CDC) (1995). These immunizations were selected based upon criteria established by the California Department of Health Services, Immunization Branch (2000) for a similar cohort.

Instruments

Selected data on background factors (e.g., age, ethnicity, marital status, acculturation), sexual history, past and current substance use, educational goals, and social competence were collected via a self-administered questionnaire covering several topics. This data collection method was selected based upon methodological research indicating that people are more likely to report sensitive behaviors in self-administered questionnaires than in face-to-face inter-views (Catania, McDermott, & Pollack, 1986).

Substance use items included frequency-of-use categories (e.g., 0, 1-2, 3-9, 10-19, 20+ times) during the past 30 days, 12 months, and lifetime use for tobacco, alcohol, marijuana, cocaine, hallucinogens, and heroin. For the descriptive analyses in this article, categories were collapsed to "not used"/"used" because of the complexities of disentangling intensity of use from frequency.

The *Shortened Acculturation Scale* (Marín & Marín, 1991), a 5-item measure, addresses the language (a) used for reading, speaking, and thinking; (b) spoken at home and with friends; and (c) used during childhood. The instrument has shown good psychometric characteristics and correlates highly with validity criteria such as respondents' generation and length of residence in the US (Marín & Marín, 1991). Possible scores range from 1 to 5 (low to high acculturation).

The *Nursing Child Assessment Teaching Scale (NCATS)*, a 73-item, binary scale, measures maternal and child contributions to dyadic inter-active quality. Items are summed to yield a mother score and a child score. Adequate relia-bility and validity of the NCATS as a predictor of later parent-child interactions and child cogni-tive outcomes have been established with African American, Hispanic, and White samples, as well as with adolescent mothers. Internal consistency is estimated at 0.87 for the mother score, 0.81 for the child score, and 0.87 for the total NCATS (Sumner & Spietz, 1994). The Cronbach alpha measure of internal consistency for this sample was .77 (mother score), .80 (total score), and .71 (child score). Videotapes of mothers and infants interacting in a structured play episode were made at each data point and were scored at 6 weeks and at 12 and 24 months postpartum using the NCATS, by an NCAST-trained evaluator.

The *HOME scale* was used at 12 and 24 months postpartum to measure the overall quality of the child's home environment (e.g., physical structure, play materials, amount of stimulation) (Caldwell & Bradley, 1978). This widely used 45-item measure has been found to correlate significantly with child development and has an internal consistency coefficient of .89 for the total score (Elardo, Bradley, & Caldwell, 1977). The Cronbach alpha for the study sample was .71.

Social competence measures were composites derived from the following established instru-ments with adequate psychometric qualities, believed to represent key variables in the theo-retical framework based upon the literature: (a) the Rosenberg Self-Esteem Inventory (Rosenberg, 1965); (b) Pearlin's Sense of Mastery Scale (Pearlin & Schooler, 1978); (c) the Center for Epidemiological Studies Depression Scale (Radloff, 1977); (d) the Perceived Stress Scale (Cohen, Kamarck, & Mermelstein, 1983); (e) the Community Life Skills Scale (CLSS) (Barnard, 1988); and (f) the Social Skills Inventory (SSI) (Booth et al., 1987).

Using composite scores enabled the interre-lated components of the social competence con-struct in the theoretical model to be presented in a more parsimonious way. Factor analysis with varimax rotation of six total scores for measures of (a) self-esteem, (b) sense of mastery, (c) depression, (d) perceived stress, (e) community life skills, and (f) social skills supported the model of two factors representing internal and external social competence. Factor loadings showed that four psychological measures (a-f above) comprise internal social competence, with the factor explaining 48% and 44% of the variance at intake and 6 weeks postpartum, respectively.

Two additional measures, the CLSS and the SSI, comprise external social competence; this factor explains 19% and 23% of the variance at the two time periods. Composite measures of the two conceptual factors were formed by first stan-dardizing each measure to a 0-100 scale with higher numbers representing higher skills, then averaging the relevant translated scores.

Statistical Analyses

Comparisons of groups were made using statistical tests appropriate for level of measurement and distributional characteristics of the specific outcome measure. For total days of hospitalization, groups were compared using a goodness-of-fit chi-square to text whether the totals were in the same proportion as the number of participants in the two groups (Zar, 1984). Group totals of ER visits were treated in the same way. Totals rather than averages across subjects were compared, because many subjects had no hospitalizations or ER visits, thus data were non-normally distributed. Groups were compared on immunization, educational, and repeat pregnancy status using chi-square statistics. Time from initial birth to repeat pregnancy was examined using survival analysis with Cox Regression technique. Differences between groups in their change in substance use (alcohol, smoking, and marijuana) patterns over time were tested using Wald chi-square statistics comparing marginal homogeneity across groups. In a repeated measures analysis with categorical outcomes (using a linear multinomial model), marginal homogeneity is a specific contrast which tests whether the distribution of responses on an outcome measure is the same at two time periods (Woodward, Bonett, & Brecht, 1990). GANOVA/GENLOG software was used to calculate Wald chi-square values (Brecht & Woodward, 1989). Changes in other outcome measures were compared using repeated measures ANOVA to examine effects for group, time and group by time interactions.

RESULTS

Comparison of sociodemographic characteristics (i.e., age, ethnicity/race, socioeconomic status [Hollinghead, 1975], marital status, educational level, maternal acculturation [if Latina], abuse history, length of gestation, and infant birth-weight) and baseline dependent variables between dropouts ($n = 43$) and study completers ($n = 101$) revealed no significant group differences. All infants admitted to the NICU following birth because of prematurity or illness remained in the study. Similarly, no significant group difference was found in the subject attrition rate between the EIP and TPHNC groups.

Participants had a mean age of 16.70 (SD = 1.13) and were predominantly poor, unmarried, and from ethnic groups of color (Table 1). Of the young women who described themselves as Latina, 43 (the majority) were born in the United States (US), 17 in Mexico, and 3 in Central America. The average score on the Short Acculturation Scale (Marín & Marín, 1991), administered to Latinas who identified themselves as either "Spanish-speaking only" or "bilingual in Spanish and English" ($n = 40$), was 3.46 (SD = .81), representing a moderate degree of acculturation. At intake nearly half of the adolescents were enrolled and attending school; however, more than 25% had dropped out. Histories of childhood physical abuse ($n = 58$, 57%), ranging from being slapped to being threatened with a weapon, and sexual abuse ($n = 25$, 25%) of varying degrees of severity (e.g., fondling to forced sexual intercourse) were reported. Twelve participants (12%) reported one or more suicide attempts within the previous year.

Child Health Outcomes

Infant Hospitalizations

The total days for non-birth-related infant hospitalizations during the first 24 months of life was significantly lower in the EIP (143 days) than the TPHNC group (211 days) ($\chi^2 = 32.48$, $p < .001$) (Table 2). Twenty-eight children were hospitalized, 16 in the TPHNC and 12 in the EIP. The actual number of episodes of hospitalization was significantly higher for the TPHNC ($n = 36$) than for the EIP ($n = 19$; $\chi^2 = 9.73$, $p = .002$). Similarly, the mean number of episodes of hospitalization per hospitalized child was higher in the TPHNC ($M = 2.19$, $\pm = 2.46$) than in the EIP

TABLE 1 **Sociodemographic Characteristics of Sample at Baseline**

	Early Intervention Program (n = 56)	Traditional Public Health Nursing (n = 45)	Total (N = 101)	p Value for Test of Group Differences[a]
	M (SD)			
Age (years)	16.75 (1.24)	16.84 (1.00)	16.79 (1.13)	.68
Gestational age (weeks)	20.67 (5.92)	20.25 (5.12)	20.48 (5.54)	.71
Hollingshead 4-Factor Index of Socioeconomic Status	24.43 (10.12)	20.98 (10.19)	22.90 (10.24)	.10
Acculturation	3.40 (.75)	3.51 (.89)	3.46 (.81)	.68
	n (%)			
Ethnic/racial background				.91
Latina	36 (64)	27 (60)	63 (62)	
African-American	6 (11)	7 (16)	13 (13)	
Non-Hispanic White	10 (18)	8 (18)	18 (18)	
Other (mixed ethnicity)	3 (5)	1 (2)	4 (4)	
Marital status				.17
Single	54 (96)	39 (87)	93 (92)	
Married	2 (4)	5 (11)	7 (7)	
Divorced	0 (0)	1 (2)	1 (1)	
Educational status				.43
Enrolled, attending high school	27 (48)	23 (51)	50 (49)	
Enrolled, not attending	10 (18)	3 (7)	13 (13)	
Dropped out	13 (23)	14 (31)	27 (27)	
Graduated high school/GED	5 (9)	3 (7)	8 (8)	
Other	1 (2)	2 (4)	3 (3)	

[a]Group comparisons t-texts for interval data, and χ^2 for nominal data.
Note: GED = graduate equivalency degree.

$(M = 1.58, \pm = 1.44)$. The most common diagnostic categories accounting for episodes of hospitalization were respiratory problems (e.g., bronchitis, pneumonia, asthma, RSV, laryngotrachitis, croup), followed by fever/rule-our sepsis, and gastrointestinal disorders (e.g., diarrhea, vomiting, dehydration). Less common reasons included seizures, meningitis, failure to thrive, and urinary tract infection.

Infant Emergency Room Visits

Although there were no significant group differences for total number of ER visits in the first 24 months of life, a significantly greater number of EIP mothers ($n = 20$, 36%) never used the ER for child health problems, as compared to THPNC mothers ($n = 5$, 11%) ($\chi^2 = 8.11$, $p = .004$). The large majority of ER visits were for illnesses; only eight children were treated for injuries and accidents (e.g., falls, burns, a near-drowning, ingestion). Both ER use and hospitalization were reported for 12 (21%) children in the EIP group compared to 16 (36%) in the TPHNC group. All adolescent mothers who reported at least one hospitalization of their child, also reported at least one ER visit.

TABLE 2 **Infant Health Outcomes and Repeat Childbearing During the First 24 Months Postpartum**

Measure	Early Intervention Program (n = 56)	Traditional Public Health Nursing Care (n = 45)	Total (N = 101)
Infant hospitalizations (excludes birth-related)			
days hospitalized[a],***	143	211	354
Episodes of hospitalization**	19	36	55
Children hospitalized	12 (21%)	16 (36%)	28 (28%)
Emergency room visits			
Total number of ER visits	149	118	267
Number of children with ER visits	36 (64%)	40 (89%)	76 (75%)
Number of children with no ER visits			
within first 24 months*	20 (36%)	5 (11%)	25 (25%)
Immunization status			
Children adequately immunized	77%	87%	82%
		n (%)	
Pregnancies and births within 24 months postpartum			
None	38 (68)	24 (53)	62 (61)
Second birth	6 (11)	4 (9)	10 (10)
Currently pregnant	9 (16)	13 (29)	22 (23)
Conception	18 (32)	21 (47)	39 (40)

*$p < .05$; **$p < .01$; ***$p < .001$

Note: ER = Emergency room; EIP = early intervention program; TPHNC = traditional public health nursing care.

Infant Immunization Rates at 24 Months of Age

Results of chi-square analyses revealed no significant difference for adequacy of immunization rates between infants in the EIP (77%) and those in the TPHNC (87%) group.

Maternal Outcomes

Substance Use

Wald χ^2 statistics were computed to test for differences between groups for change in maternal substance use from intake to 2 years postpartum (i.e., comparing marginal homogeneity across groups) (Woodward et al., 1990). There was a significant difference between groups for marijuana use (Wald $\chi^2 = 6.61$, $p < .01$). Adolescents who received TPHNC reported an increase in marijuana use over time, from 0% at intake to 14% at 2 years postbirth. Use in the EIP group remained more stable with 6% at intake and 4% at the 2-year follow-up. A statistically significant pattern of increase for alcohol and tobacco consumption from intake to 24 months postpartum was found for both groups (Figure 1). At intake (while pregnant), only 2% of adolescents reported alcohol use in the past 30 days, vs. 38% at 2 years postbirth (Wald $\chi^2 = 48.16$, $p < .001$). Smoking increased from 7% to 29% (Wald $\chi^2 = 25.20$, $p < .001$).

Education

At 24 months postpartum, no significant differences were found in educational outcomes between the EIP and TPHNC groups ($\chi^2 = .60$, $p > .05$); 64% of EIP and 59% of TPHNC mothers had a positive educational status

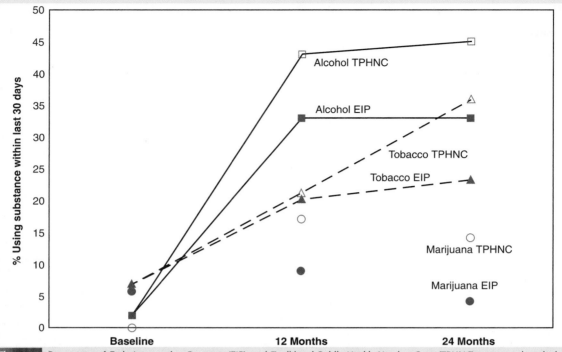

Figure 1. Percentage of Early Intervention Program (EIP) and Traditional Public Health Nursing Care (TPHNC) groups using alcohol, tobacco, and marijuana in previous 30 days at baseline, 12 months, and 24 months.

(enrolled and attending high school, graduated high school, or attending college).

Repeat Pregnancies

Chi-square analyses showed no significant group differences in repeat pregnancy or birth rates. By 24 months postpartum, 10 (10%) repeat births had occurred, 22 (22%) young women were pregnant, and 7 (7%) adolescents reported a miscarriage or therapeutic abortion. The overall rate of subsequent conceptions (including pregnancies, spontaneous and therapeutic abortions, and births) was 15% higher in the TPHNC ($n = 21$, 47%) than in the EIP ($n = 18$, 32%). The results of a survival analysis using Cox regression again showed no significant group difference in the time from initial birth to repeat pregnancy, Exp (B) = 1.66, Wald $\chi^2 = 2.39$, $p > .10$.

Social Competence

Results of repeated measures analysis of variance (ANOVA) with all data collection points approached significance for group by time interaction for the internal social competence measure ($F[1, 5] = 2.17$, $p = .057$). Although scores of both groups increased, adolescents receiving the EIP showed a slightly greater gain over time in internal social competence. No significant group differences in change over time were found for the external social competence measure, but a significant time effect was observed, with scores increasing from intake to 2-year follow-up in both groups ($F[1,5] = 20.74$, $p < .001$).

NCATS and HOME

Results of repeated measures ANOVA revealed no significant group differences in the change in

NCATS mother, child, or total scores over time. However, significant time effects were found for all three measures from 6 weeks to 24 months postpartum (total scale: $F[2,66] = 102.72$, $p < .001$; mother scores: $F[2,66] = 72.27$, $p < .001$; child score: $F[2,66] = 66.14$, $p < .001$). For both groups, the scores markedly increased from birth to 12 months and then showed little change in the 2nd year of life. Similarly, a main effect for time was found for the total HOME scores, without significant differences between groups in the pattern of change ($F[1,91] = 10.47$, $p < .01$). Scores increased for both groups from 1 to 2 years postpartum.

DISCUSSION

The findings of this study demonstrate that the early intervention program of home visitation by PHNs achieved three of its most important goals: (a) improving child health outcomes, and enhancing (b) selected aspects of maternal health and (c) life-course competence of adolescent mothers. Infants in the EIP experienced decreased morbidity as evidenced by total hospitalization days and number of hospitalization episodes. This result was observed within 6 weeks of birth and sustained for a 24-month period that included the year following termination of the intervention.

The nature and content of the EIP and the greater opportunity for communication with the PHN about children's illnesses before seeking care may have contributed to the dramatic differences seen in total hospitalization days.

Although the rates of adequate infant immunizations at 24 months did not significantly differ between the EIP and TPHNC groups, the sample as a whole had an 81% immunization rate higher than a comparable state cohort (California Department of Health Services, 2000). Anticipatory guidance about immunization is a core component of public health nursing care of pregnant women and new mothers.

Maternal outcomes improved in selected areas. A significant group difference was found between groups for change in marijuana use. The rise in substance use observed in this investigation has been noted in other longitudinal studies of adolescents' substance use behavior from pregnancy through the postpartum (Flanagan & Kokotailo, 1999; Gilchrist, Hussey, Gillmore, Lohr, & Morrison, 1996).

Adolescents in the EIP and TPHNC groups experienced significant increases in their internal and external social competence scores from baseline to the 24-month evaluation. These scores reflect improvements in ability to manage emotions (internal component) and to communicate and use effective social interaction skills (external component) that may be due in part to maturational changes in adolescence as well as benefits from PHN visitation of varying intensities. While group differences for internal social competence approached but did not achieve statistical significance, the finding has clinical relevance. Improved emotional well-being may have positively affected other maternal outcomes of EIP adolescents, such as seeking early treatment for child illnesses; however, causal inferences should not be made.

The lower repeat pregnancy rate in adolescent mothers who received home visitation, although not statistically significant, is clinically important because of the negative impact short-interval births may have on the life course of these mothers and their children.

In interpreting the findings of this study, consideration must be given to its limitations. The complexities of obtaining medical records from multiple sources and providers made collection of these data very difficult. As a result, a small portion of the infant health data were collected by maternal report only. The nature of the data collected does not permit associations to be made between specific episodes of hospitalizations and exact ER visits. Evaluation of substance use was based on retrospective recall without use of biochemical verification procedures. More intense and direct supervision of the PHNs may have provided a stronger measure of the fidelity with which the intervention was delivered and increased the actual number of home visits provided to selected young mothers. While the benefits of this program at 24 months postpartum are evident, additional effects may take longer to become apparent.

Research findings suggest that maximum benefit for parents at social and economic risk can be achieved when programs use nurses who follow comprehensive program models and whose sole responsibility is to implement services as intended by those models (Olds, Hill, Robinson, Song, & Little, 2000). In this study the PHNs were employees of the country health department and worked on the study part-time under subcontract with the university. At times the nurses struggled to deliver EIP services while balancing their caseloads with other responsibilities. In an attempt to minimize participant attrition, the PHNs maintained regular telephone contact with adolescents in both groups throughout the 1st year postpartum. These interactions may have unintentionally served as an intervention. Findings from other studies suggest that telephone contact may, in itself, constitute an effective intervention (Moore et al., 1998).

The findings contribute to the research literature demonstrating the benefits of home visitation by nurses, and thus have implications for healthcare services. Our sample was comprised predominantly of Latina adolescents, who received home visits by PHNs plus preparation-for-motherhood classes. Several elements of the EIP are believed to have contributed to the program's accomplishments: (a) the time of service delivery (from pregnancy through the 1st year postpartum); (b) use of a case management approach with individualized care by specially trained PHNs; (c) inclusion of first-time mothers only; and (d) the comprehensive nature of services (e.g., health counseling and teaching, with an added focus on parent education). These elements have been identified as critical factors in programs for adolescent mothers and their children (Perrone Hoyer, 1998). However, the EIP did not meet another specific condition

identified for program success, as the home visitation ended at 1-year postpartum rather than extending through the 2nd year. Furthermore, less frequent home visitation was provided during pregnancy and the 1st-year postpartum than that offered by Olds and associates. ▼

Accepted for publication December 3, 2002.

This study was supported by grants from the National Institute of Nursing Research (NINR) (1-R01 NR02325 and NR02325-S1) and the Office of Research on Women's Health (NR02325-S2). Financial support for the second author was also provided by the NINR (5-T32-NR7077).

The authors thank Anne Ivey, RN, MS, Chief (now retired) and Susan Willis, RN, Supervising Public Health Nurse, of the Division of Community Health Services, San Bernardino County Department of Public Health, for their administrative support in implementation of the project. We also thank Lorraine O. Walker, RN, PhD, FAAN, Luci B. Johnson Professor of Nursing, University of Texas at Austin; and Ramona T. Mercer, RN, PhD, FAAN, Professor Emeritus, University of California, San Francisco School of Nursing for expert research consultation. Finally, we thank the many public health nurses who provided care to the study participants, and the young mothers who welcomed us into their lives.

Correspondence to: Deborah Koniak-Griffin, EdD RN, FAAN, UCLA School of Nursing, Box 956919, Los Angeles, CA 900095-6919 (e-mail: dkoniak@sonnet.ucla.edu).

REFERENCES

Alan Guttmacher Institute. (1994). *Sex and America's teenagers.* New York: Alan Guttmacher Institute.

Barnard KE (1988). *Community life skills scale.* Nursing Child Assessment Satellite Training: Seattle, WA: University of Washington.

Barnard KE, and Bee HL (1983). The impact of temporally patterned stimulation on the development of preterm infants. *Child Development,* 54: 1156-1167.

Booth CL, Barnard KE, Mitchell SK, and Spieker SJ (1987). Successful intervention with multi-problem mothers: Effects on the mother-infant relationship. *Infant Mental Health Journal*, 8: 288-306.

Brazelton TB (1984). *Neonatal behavioral assessment scale*. Philadelphia: Lippincott.

Brecht ML, and Woodward JA 1989. *GANOVA: Microcomputer software for general univariate and multivariate analysis of variance* (users manual and software). Los Angeles, CA.

Caldwell BM, and Bradley R (1978). *Home observation for measurement of the environment*. Little Rock: University of Arkansas at Little Rock.

California Department of Health Services, Immunization Branch (2000, August 15). *2000 Kindergarten Retrospective Results*. Retrieved December 4, 2002 from http://www.dhs.ca.gov/ps/dcdc/izgroup/levels.htm

Catania JA, McDermott LJ, and Pollack LM (1986). Questionnaire response bias and face-to-face interview sample bias in sexuality research. *Journal of Sex Research*, 22: 52-72.

Centers for Disease Control and Prevention. (1995, June 16). Recommended childhood immunization schedule—United States, 1995. *Morbidity and Mortality Weekly Report*, 44 (RR-5), 1-9.

Centers for Disease Control and Prevention. (1998). Youth risk behavior surveillance—United States, 1997. *Morbidity and Mortality Weekly Report, CDC Surveillance Summary*, 17: 1-89.

Clausen JA (1991). Adolescent competence and the life course, or why one social psychologist needed a concept of personality. *Social Psychology Quarterly*, 54: 4-14.

Cohen S, Kamarck T, and Mermelstein R (1983). A global measure of perceived stress. *Journal of Health & Social Behavior*, 24: 385-396.

Elardo R, Bradley R, and Caldwell B (1977). A longitudinal study of the infants' home environment to language development at age three. *Child Development*, 49: 593-603.

Flanagan P, and Kokotailo P (1999). Adolescent pregnancy and substance use. *Clinical Perinatology*, 26: 185-200.

Gilchrist LD, Hussey JM, Gillmore MR, Lohr MD, and Morrison DM (1996). Drug use among adolescent mothers: Prepregnancy to 18 months postpartum. *Journal of Adolescent Health*, 19: 337-344.

Hollingshead AB (1975). *Four factor index of social status*. Department of Sociology, Yale University. New Haven, CT.

Kitzman H, Olds DL, Henderson CR, Jr., Hanks C, Cole R, Tatelbaum R et al. (1997). Effect of prenatal and infancy home visitation by nurses on pregnancy outcomes, childhood injuries, and repeated childbearing: A randomized clinical trial. *Journal of the American Medical Association*, 278: 644-652.

Koniak-Griffin D, Anderson NLR, Brecht M-L, Verzemnieks, I., Lesser, J., & Kim, S. (2002). Public health nursing care for adolescent mothers: Impact on infant health and selected maternal outcomes at 1 year postbirth. *Journal of Adolescent Health*, 30: 44-54.

Koniak-Griffin D, Anderson NLR, Verzemnieks I, and Brecht ML (2000). A public health nursing early intervention program for adolescent mothers: Outcomes from pregnancy through 6 weeks postpartum. *Nursing Research*, 49: 130-138.

Koniak-Griffin D, Verzemnieks I, and Cahill D (1992). Using videotape instruction and feedback to improve adolescents' mothering behaviors. *Journal of Adolescent Health*, 13: 570-575.

Marín G, and Marín, BV (1991). *Research with Hispanic populations* (Vol. 23). Applied Social Research Methods Series. Newbury Park, CA: Sage.

Martin JA, Hamilton BE, Ventura SJ, Menacker F, and Park MM (2002). *Births: Final data for 2000*. National Vital Statistics Reports, Vol. 50, No. 5. Hyattsville, MD: National Center for Health Statistics.

Maynard R, and Rangarajan A (1994). Contraceptive use and repeat pregnancies among welfare-dependent teenage mothers. *Family Planning Perspectives*, 26: 198-205.

McClure-Martinez K, and Cohn L (1996). Adolescent and adult mothers' perceptions of hazardous situations for their children. *Journal of Adolescent Health*, 18: 227-231.

Moore ML, Meis PJ, Ernest JM, Well HB, Zaccaro DJ, and Terrell T (1998). A randomized trial of nurse intervention to reduce preterm and low birth weight births. *Obstetrics and Gynecology*, 91: 656-661.

Norbeck JS, DeJoseph JF, and Smith RT (1996). A randomized trial of an empirically-derived social support intervention to prevent low birthweight among African American women. *Social Science and Medicine*, 43: 947-954.

Olds DL, Eckenrode J, Henderson CR, Kitzman H, Powers J, Cole R et al. (1997). Long-term effects of home visitation on maternal life course and child abuse and neglect: Fifteen-year follow-up of a randomized trial. *Journal of the American Medical Association*, 278: 637-643.

Olds DL, Henderson CR, and Kitzman H (1994). Does prenatal and infancy nurse home visitation have enduring effects on qualities of parental caregiving and child health at 25 to 50 months of life? *Pediatrics*, 93: 89-98.

Olds DL, Henderson CR, Kitzman HJ, Eckenrode JJ, Cole RE, and Tatelbaum RC (1999). Prenatal and infancy home visitation by nurses: Recent findings. *Future of Children: Home Visiting: Recent Program Evaluations*, 9: 44-65.

LOIS VAN CLEVE, ELIZABETH BOSSERT
PAULINE BEECROFT, KATHLEEN ADLARD
OFELIA ALVAREZ, MARILYN C. SAVEDRA

The Pain Experience of Children with Leukemia During the First Year after Diagnosis

▶ **Background:** Children with cancer experience pain related to the disease process, the treatment, and the associated procedures. For children with leukemia, the pain experienced after diagnosis has received scant attention.

▶ **Objective:** To examine the pain experience, management strategies, and outcomes during the first year after the diagnosis of acute leukemia.

▶ **Methods:** A longitudinal descriptive approach was used to collect data at seven data points from 95 English- and Spanish-speaking children, ages 4 to 17 years, receiving care in one of three southern California hospitals, and from their English- and Spanish-speaking parents. Age-appropriate instruments were used to examine the variables of pain intensity, location, pattern over time, and quality, as well as strategies for managing pain, perceived effectiveness of management strategies, and functional status.

▶ **Results:** All the children reported pain over the course of the year. Pain intensity scores incorporated the full range of possible responses. For the children 4 to 7 years old, the highest and lowest mean scores, respectively, were 2 and 1.6 (scale, 0-4). For the children 8 to 17 years old, the highest and lowest mean scores, respectively, were 50.1 and 39.5 (scale, 0-100). The most common location of pain was the legs (26.5%) in all seven interviews. Other frequently noted sites were the abdomen (16.6%), head/neck (16.6%), and back (14.2%). The words used most frequently by the older English- and Spanish-speaking children to describe pain were "uncomfortable" (incómodo) and "annoying" (molesto). According to the interviews, the most frequently used strategy for pain management was stressor modification (e.g., medication, sleep, hot/cold, and massage). The most common coping strategies according to a Likert scale rating were "watch TV" (n = 426), "lie down" (n = 421), "wish for it to go away" (n = 417), and "tell my mother or father" (n = 416). The pain intensity scores after pain management were significantly lower for the younger children in three of the seven interviews and for the older children in all seven interviews. For both the younger and older children, functional status (i.e., the ability to engage in

Lois Van Cleve, PhD, RN, FAAN, is Professor, Loma Linda University School of Nursing, California.

Elizabeth Bossert, DNS, RN, is Professor, Loma Linda University School of Nursing, California.

Pauline Beecroft, PhD, RN, FAAN, is Nurse Research, Childrens Hospital Los Angeles, California.

Kathleen Adlard, MN, RN, is Oncology Clinical Nurse Specialist, Children's Hospital Orange County, California.

Ofelia Alvarez, MD, is Assistant Professor, University of Miami School of Medicine, Florida.

Marilyn C. Savedra, DNS, RN, FAAN, is Professor Emeritus, University of California San Francisco.

routine activities) was above the median score at the seven interviews.

▶ **Conclusions:** Children with leukemia experience pain throughout the first year of treatment. In this study, the pain was responsive to the management strategies used by the parents and children.

▶ *Key Words:* children · leukemia · pain

Children with cancer, including those with leukemia, experience pain from the disease process, the treatment, and the diagnostic procedures (Ljungman, Gordh, Sorensen, & Krueger, 1999, 2000; Miser, Dothage, Wesley, & Miser, 1987; Miser & Miser, 1989; Patterson, 1992). Yet knowledge of pain over time as reported by children is limited. There is a significant lack of knowledge about Latino children and how they experience and report pain.

BACKGROUND LITERATURE REVIEW

Leukemia is diagnosed for approximately 3,000 children each year in the United States (American Cancer Society, 2002). Acute lymphocytic leukemia (ALL) is the most common form of childhood cancer, accounting for nearly three fourths of childhood leukemia cases, and it represents 31.5% of cancer in children younger than 15 years.

The 5-year relative survival rate for children younger than 15 years with cancer has increased over the past three decades. The largest increase in survival rate was for children with acute lymphocytic leukemia. More than one half survived the disease in 1973-1995, and currently almost three in four survive (Ries, Kosary, Hankey, Miller, & Edwards, 1998). Aggressive treatment protocols have increased survival rates greatly for most types of childhood cancer, but drug toxicity often results in painful conditions including mucositis, infection, and peripheral neuropathy (Agency for Health Care Policy and Research, 1994).

Cancer pain research with children has focused almost exclusively on procedure-related pain, with an emphasis on the effectiveness of nonpharmacologic strategies for managing pain (e.g., Hamner & Miles, 1988; Hockenberry, 1988; Woodgate & McClement, 1998). Six reports with direct relevance for this study were found. Three of these studies (Ljungman & McGrath, 2003; Ljungman et al. 1999; Miser, McCalla, Dothage, Wesley, & Miser, 1987) reported that pain was a presenting symptom at diagnosis in 74%, 33%, and 78% of the children, respectively, with pain intensity ranging from mild to severe (Ljungman & McGrath, 2003). Pain during treatment ranged from moderate to severe (Cornaglia et al., 1984). Procedure and treatment-related pain dominated during treatment (Ljungman et al., 1996, 1999), although procedure pain gradually diminished (Ljungman et al., 1999). The four persisting treatment problems were mucositis, abdominal pain, and neuropathic pain in the legs and pain related to infection pain (Ljungman et al., 1999, 2000). Chronic pain, persisting more that 1 year after eradication of all known tumor, was reported occasionally (Miser, McCalla, et al., 1987). Retrospective chart and cross-sectional analyses have documented the presence of pain, yet have provided minimal data on dimensions of the pain experience and the effectiveness of management strategies.

THEORETICAL FRAMEWORK

The Symptom Management Model of the University of California, San Francisco (UCSF) School of Nursing Symptom Management Faculty Group (1994) with its three interrelated dimensions guided this study. The symptom experience dimension included elements of perception, evaluation, and response. The symptom management strategies dimension included the perspective of patient, healthcare system, health-

---

Leukemia (ALL) is diagnosed for approximately 3,000 children each year in the United States

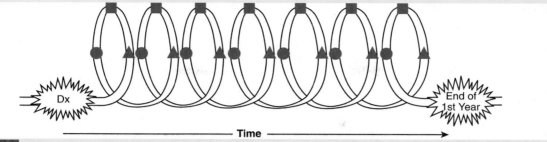

Figure 1. Adaptation of conceptual model of pain management for children with leukemia: pain, management, and outcome. ▲ = pain experience; ■ = pain management strategies; ● = pain outcomes.

care provider, and family, whereas the symptom outcomes dimension included areas such as functional status, quality of life, morbidity/comorbidity, and health service utilization. This model, adapted for the current study, provided direction for evaluating the pain experience of children and adolescents on the basis of their perception (Figure 1).

The three dimensions from the original model, depicted within a spiral, represent episodes over time rather than a single episode. The specific aims of the study, based on the model, were to describe the children's pain for 1 year after their diagnosis of acute lymphocytic leukemia, to describe strategies used by children and their families to manage pain associated with acute lymphocytic leukemia, and to examine the outcomes of management effectiveness and functional status.

METHODS

The study used a longitudinal, descriptive design. The sample was obtained from the pediatric oncology populations of three facilities in southern California, all using the Children's Cancer Group (now Children's Oncology Group) protocols. Children were interviewed either in the clinic or the hospital. On the basis of the inclusion criteria, children were invited to participate if they were 4- to 17-year-olds with acute lymphocytic leukemia, within 1 month of diagnosis,

and either English or Spanish speaking. The exclusion criteria specified another chronic illness associated with pain, a fulminating disease, known cognitive disability, or inability to cope with the burden of research tasks as determined by the primary nurse.

Pain, management, and outcomes were assessed. Self-report was used to measure pain intensity and determine location. Children 8 to 17 years of age self-reported all remaining pain experiences and coping measures. Parents completed the pain pattern and management measures for the children 4 to 7 years of age and the functional status measure for all the children. Attention was given to subject burden relating to time for completion. All the instruments were available in both English and Spanish.

Instruments

The Poker Chip Tool

The Poker Chip Tool is a self-report measure of pain intensity for children 4-13 years of age. The child chooses one to four red chips ("pieces of hurt"). One chip represents a "little bit" of pain, and four chips represent the most pain the child can have. Evidence supports strong **convergent and discriminate validity** for this tool (Hester, Foster, & Kristensen, 1989, 1990).

Acute lymphocytic leukemia represents 31.5% of cancer in children younger than 15 years

Preschool Body Outline

This self-report instrument is a gender-neutral outline of a preschool child's body. The child is given a red pencil or pen and asked to draw where it hurts. An overlay grid depicting 43 distinct body areas is used to tally the child's responses. Validity was established with 4- to 7-year-old hospitalized children (Van Cleve & Savedra, 1993).

Adolescent Pediatric Pain Tool

The Adolescent Pediatric Pain Tool (APPT) (Savedra, Tesler, Holzemer, & Ward, 1989) is a self-report measure for 8- to 17-year-olds. It has three components: (a) a body outline with overlay grid of 43 areas, (b) a word graphic intensity scale using a 100-mm line with pain intensity increasing from left to right, and a word list of 67 adjectives describing pain. Psychometric properties were established for each component of the APPT including alternate forms validity of 94%, 91%, and 83%, respectively (Savedra et al., 1989), test-retest reliability indicated by an *r* of 0.78 to 0.96 (Wilkie et al., 1990), and **construct validity** between child report and chart (Savedra, Tesler, Holzemer, Wilkie, & Ward, 1990; Savedra et al., 1989). All three components of the APPT were translated into Spanish for this study (Van Cleve, Muñoz, Bossert, & Savedra, 2001).

Dot Matrix

The Dot Matrix is a self-report measure of the pain pattern daily and weekly for children older than 8 years. The y-axis represents increasing pain intensity from no pain to worst pain, and the x-axis represents time. Six basic patterns of pain have been identified. Concurrent validity for the Dot Matrix has been established by comparison with other measures of intensity and location of pain (Savedra, Tesler, Holzemer, & Brokaw, 1995). The parents completed the Dot Matrix for children 4 to 7 years of age, whereas older children self-reported for this measure.

Two instruments were used to assess management. An open-ended question in the interview asked the child, followed by supplemental input from the parent, about the strategies used to manage pain. This was tape-recorded, transcribed, and translated as needed. Content analysis as described by Krippendorff (1980), Weber (1985) as well as Ryan-Wenger's (1992) taxonomy was used for analysis.

Pediatric Pain Coping Inventory

The Pediatric Pain Coping Inventory (PPCI) is a 41-item, 3-point Likert tool with a possible score of 0 to 82. Higher scores indicate better coping. The PPCI has three versions: a parent version (for 4- to 7-year-olds), a child version (for 8- to 11-year-olds), and an adolescent version (for 12- to 16-year-olds). All three versions contain identical information phrased in developmentally appropriate language. The demonstrated internal consistency of the PPCI is .85. The PPCI was normed with a group of chronically ill children 5 to 16 years of age (Varni et al., 1996).

Perception of Management Effectiveness

Perception of management effectiveness was determined by a 100-mm word graphic rating scale, measured from the left, with the higher scores indicating greater effectiveness. Parental report was used for the younger group (4- to 7-year-olds) because of the children's developmental level. The older children (ages 8-17 years) self-reported for this measure.

Functional Status II

Functional Status II (Revised) (Stein & Jessop, 1990) is a parental (caregiver) report tool developed for use with healthy and chronically ill children 0 to 16 years of age. The 14-item version with a 3-point Likert type scale was used for this study. Part 1 asks whether the child exhibits a specific behavior (e.g., "eats well" or "sleeps well" "never of rarely," "some of the time," or "almost always"). The possible scores range from 0 to 28, with the higher scores indicating better functioning. The internal consistency for all versions of Functional Status II is indicated by a Cronbach alpha exceeding .80, with no differences in reliability attributable to age groups. Discriminant and concurrent validity also have been demonstrated (Stein & Jessop, 1990).

Data Collection Procedure

Approval was obtained from the institutional review board of each facility. Permission was obtained from parents, and assent was obtained from the children. Demographic data were obtained from the parent, and the specific treatment protocol was noted from the record. Data were collected within 2 weeks of diagnosis and at the end of the following treatment phases during the first year: induction, consolidation, maintenance I, intensification I, maintenance II, and intensification II (a total of seven data collection points).

The child and parents participated in the interview schedule, which was audiotaped for transcription. The questions were directed to the child, with supplemental responses from the parent. During the interview, instruments were administered as appropriate for moving from the symptom experience to management and outcomes. Data collection, requiring 20 to 30 minutes, took place in the hospital or clinic, depending on where the child was at the time of the scheduled interview. Tokens of appreciation such as stickers and pencils were given to the child after data collection.

The interviews were read by two of three research associates, with one associate consistently involved in each session. The interrater reliability for the process was determined to be 99%. Disagreements were resolved by discussion and brought to the research team meeting if any question remained.

Data Analysis

Data were entered using double data entry to check for accuracy. Using SPSS, the data were analyzed via descriptive and **inferential statistics**, *t*-test, and analysis of variance (ANOVA). All the children interviewed four or more times were included in the analysis. Missing data were managed using mean substitution by subject.

The acceptance level for significance was set at an alpha of .05 or less.

RESULTS

The analyses indicated no differences between facility samples in terms of age, gender, or type of leukemia. One facility reported fewer Latino children than the others, resulting in a significant difference (<.01) in ethnicity between facilities. However there were no statistical differences in the reported dimensions of pain between Latinos and Whites. There were 48 Latino subjects, 32 of whom were Spanish speaking. The remaining 16 chose to respond in English. The data reflected the demographics of the three counties in which the facilities were located. Therefore, data from the three sites were merged for further analyses. All potential participants were willing to participate. Follow-up evaluation on one subject was not possible because of inconsistent attendance at the clinic.

The sample consisted of 95 children from the three facilities with a broad representation of age groups, genders, ethnic groups, and treatment protocols (Table 1).

Pain Experience

The presence or absence of pain was established at the beginning of the interview. Most of the children reported pain at all the interviews (Figure 2). According to the McNemar nonparametric test, there was a significant difference in pain presence between interviews 1 and 2 ($p = .012$), 1 and 3 ($p = .012$), 1 and 6 ($p = .021$), and 1 and 7($p = .21$) for the younger children, and between interviews 1 and 6 ($p = .16$) and 1 and 7 ($p = .12$) for the older children. For the children experiencing pain, the following dimensions were assessed at all the data points: intensity, location, pattern over time, and quality.

The mean intensities of pain for both age groups at all the interviews are reported in Table 2. The Poker Chip Tool, with its choice range of 0 to 4, was used by children 4 to 7 years of age to measure pain intensity. Before management, the

TABLE 1 **Demographic Characteristics by Site (*n* = 95)**

	Site 1 *n* (% at site)	Site 2 *n* (% at site)	Site 3 *n* (% at site)	Total *n* (%)
Number	30	42	23	95
Sex				
Female	16 (53.3)	17 (40.0)	7 (30.0)	40 (42.1)
Male	14 (46.7)	25 (60.0)	16 (70.0)	55 (57.9)
Age (years)				
4-7	20 (66.7)	25 (59.5)	12 (52.2)	57 (60.0)
8-17	10 (33.3)	17 (40.5)	11 (47.8)	38 (40.0)
Ethnicity				
African American	2 (6.7)	0 (.0)	0 (.0)	2 (2.1)
Asian	0 (0.0)	5 (11.9)	1 (4.3)	6 (6.3)
Latino	17 (56.7)	25 (59.6)	6 (26.1)	48 (50.5)
White	6 (20.0)	10 (23.8)	14 (60.9)	30 (31.6)
Other	5 (16.7)	2 (4.7)	2 (8.7)	9 (9.5)
Language				
English	22 (73.3)	24 (57.1)	17 (73.9)	63 (66.3)
Spanish	8 (26.7)	18 (42.9)	6 (26.1)	32 (33.7)
Treatment protocol				
CCG 1952	12 (40.0)	18 (42.9)	14 (60.9)	44 (46.3)
CCG 1961	15 (50.0)	11 (26.2)	7 (30.4)	33 (34.7)
Other ALL	3 (10.0)	13 (30.9)	2 (8.7)	18 (19.0)

CCG = Children Cancer Group

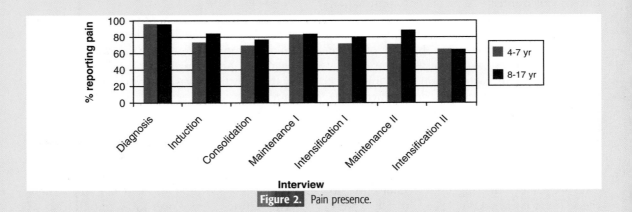

Figure 2. Pain presence.

TABLE 2 **Intensity Before and After Management and Coping Difference in Pain**

Age/Interview	Before $\overline{X}$ (SD)	After $\overline{X}$ (SD)	% change	t	p
4-7-year-olds (Poker Chip Tool, possible 0-4)					
Interview 1 (n = 36)	1.86 (1.22)	1.33 (0.99)	13.25	−2.574	.014*
Interview 2 (n = 30)	1.60 (1.48)	1.03 (1.13)	14.25	−1.979	.057
Interview 3 (n = 26)	1.62 (1.39)	1.46 (1.33)	4.0	−0.537	.596
Interview 4 (n = 25)	2.16 (1.43)	1.16 (1.11)	25.0	−2.887	.008**
Interview 5 (n = 27)	1.93 (1.38)	1.37 (1.18)	14.0	−1.922	.066
Interview 6 (n = 22)	1.91 (1.48)	.91 (0.92)	25.0	−2.925	.008**
Interview 7 (n = 23)	1.91 (1.59)	1.26 (1.21)	16.25	−1.845	.079
8-17-year-olds (Word Graphic Rating Scale, possible 0-100)					
Interview 1 (n = 16)	56.31 (22.24)	32.13 (18.05)	24.18	−3.599	.003**
Interview 2 (n = 17)	45.59 (25.09)	25.06 (24.32)	20.53	−2.946	.009*
Interview 3 (n = 15)	42.33 (27.72)	16.80 (12.24)	25.53	−3.590	.003**
Interview 4 (n = 20)	38.35 (25.60)	22.00 (21.67)	16.35	−2.914	.009**
Interview 5 (n = 14)	42.57 (30.30)	19.57 (17.01)	23.0	−3.726	.003**
Interview 6 (n = 15)	47.33 (30.35)	21.47 (26.01)	25.86	−3.263	.006**
Interview 7 (n = 16)	43.50 (24.78)	14.31 (15.56)	29.19	−5.473	.000**

*p < .05; **p < .01; ***p < .001

highest mean pain score occurred at interview 4 and the lowest at interview 2. After management, the highest mean pain score occurred at interview 3 and the lowest at interview 6.

Children 8 to 17 years of age used the 100-mm word graphic rating scale from the APPT. Before management, the highest mean pain score occurred at interview 1 and the lowest at the interview 4. After management, the highest mean pain score occurred at interview 1 and the lowest at interview 7.

The most commonly identified locations of pain for all ages and all interviews combined, involving 1,516 separately identified locations, were the legs, abdomen, head and neck, and back (Table 3). The legs were identified as the most common pain location in all seven interviews.

Two patterns of pain were selected to describe pain over the course of a day and during a week at all the interviews. The pattern of pain selected most frequently for the day and for the week was pain starting high and decreasing lin-

TABLE 3 **Pain Location (n = 1, 516)**

	4-7 years n (%)	8-17 years n (%)	Total Sample n (%)
Legs	240 (29.1)	159 (23.4)	399 (26.4)
Abdomen	149 (18.0)	106 (15.6)	255 (16.6)
Head/Neck	102 (12.4)	147 (20.6)	249 (16.4)
Back	116 (14.1)	104 (15.3)	220 (14.5)

Note: Only the 4 most frequently selected locations are given.

early to a low level. The second most frequently selected pattern involved pain starting low and increasing linearly to a high level. These patterns were selected by both the 8- to 17-year-olds and the parents of the 4- 7-year-olds. The remaining four patterns were selected in 9% of the cases or less.

The quality of the pain was examined in the 8- to 17-year-old age group using the word list from the APPT (Savedra et al., 1989). This was administered only to the older group because qualitative word lists are not available for younger children. Although there was some variation across the interview data points, the words marked most frequently were: "annoying" (n = 89), "uncomfortable" (n = 84), "comes and goes" (n = 70), "sore" (n = 62), "aching" (n = 59), and "hurting" (n = 52). The Latino children selected the Spanish words for "annoying" (molesto) (n = 44) and "uncomfortable" (incómodo) (n = 40) most frequently.

Pain Management

In the assessment of analgesics use, the older children and the parents of the younger children were asked the frequency of use for Tylenol, Tylenol with codeine, or other pain medications. The use of analgesics over time is illustrated in Figure 3. Analgesics specifically identified but reported less frequently than 1% of the time were Ben-Gay, Demerol, EMLA, fentanyl, ketamine, morphine, Motrin, Versed, and Vicodin.

The five most frequently selected coping strategies on the PPCI (Varni et al., 1996) were "watch TV" (n = 407), "lie down" (n = 406), "tell my parents" (n = 406), "wish for it to go away" (n = 403), and "go to bed" (n = 400). The first two were consistently used in the self-report of the older groups and by the parents of the younger children. There was a significant difference by age group (t = −5.905; p = .001) in the number of strategies used. The parents reported greater numbers of coping strategies for children ages 4 to 7 years than the children ages 8 to 17 years self-reported. There was no difference by gender in the number of strategies used by the younger

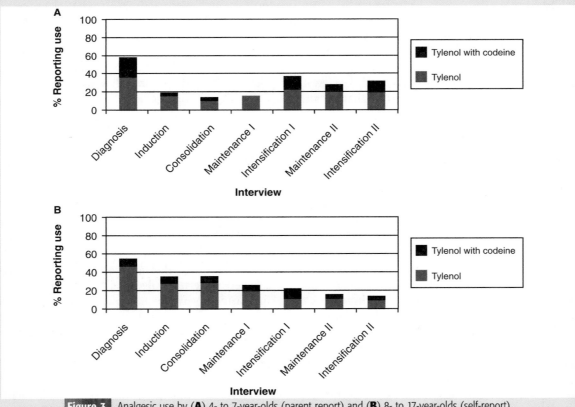

Figure 3. Analgesic use by (**A**) 4- to 7-year-olds (parent report) and (**B**) 8- to 17-year-olds (self-report).

group ($t = .439$, not significant), but for the older group there was a significant difference ($t = -2.707$; $p = .007$), with the females reporting more strategies than the males. There was no significant difference in the number of coping strategies selected over the seven interviews for the younger group ($F = .360$, not significant) or for the older children ($F = .834$, not significant).

Pain management strategies ($n = 957$) reported by the children during the seven interviews were analyzed using content analysis and Ryan-Wengers' (1992) taxonomy of children's coping. The most frequently used category was stressor modification ($n = 721$). Because of the many responses, the following subcategories were identified: use of medications ($n = 268$), sleep/rest ($n = 108$), and hot/cold ($n = 96$), and rub/massage/stretch ($n = 93$). Other major categories were social support ($n = 85$), distrac-

tion/behavioral/cognitive ($n = 61$), and eat/drink ($n = 56$). The next most frequent category was identified fewer than 20 times.

Pain Outcomes

Measures of outcomes were change in pain intensity before and after management, perception of management effectiveness, and functional status. Pain intensity scores before and after management were compared for each age group of children and found to be significantly lower after management for the younger children in interviews 1, 4, and 6 (Table 2 and Figure 4). Pain intensity scores were significantly lower in all seven interviews of the older children. When Latino children (both English and Spanish speaking) were examined as a group, there were no significant changes after management except for interview 4 ($t = -3.045$; $p = .01$) in the

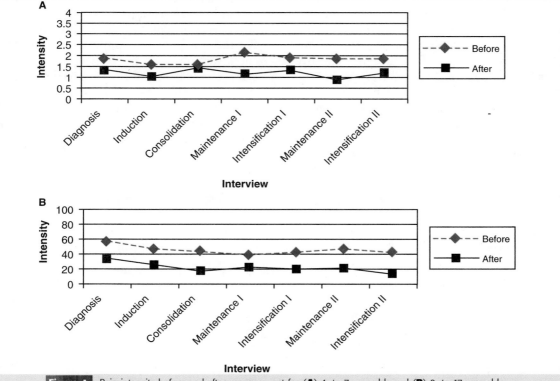

Figure 4. Pain intensity before and after management for (**A**) 4- to 7-year-olds and (**B**) 8- to 17-year-olds.

younger group. For the older children, there were significant changes at interviews 1 ($t = -2.784$; $p = .032$), 4 ($t = -2.944$; $p = .019$), and 7 ($t = -3.046$; $p = .029$).

The perception of management effectiveness ("how much it helped"), assessed using a word graphic rating scale, indicated that for the 4- to 7-year-old group (parent report), the mean effectiveness score across the seven interviews was between 63.21 and 71.92, with a minimum of 0 for three interviews and a maximum of 100 for one interview. For the 8- to 17-year-old group (self-report), the mean effectiveness score across the seven interviews was between 47.96 and 71.21, with a minimum of 0 for five interviews and a maximum of 100 for one interview (Table 4). There was a significant difference (independent $t = 3.796$; $p < .001$) in the perception of management effectiveness when combined scores were examined by age groups, with the higher scores recorded for the younger children (parent report). When the possible effect of ethnicity by age group was examined, no significant differences were found between the Latino and White children in perception of management effectiveness (Mann-Whitney $U < 8$ years; $Z = -.519$, not significant; $=8$ years; $Z = -.729$, not significant). Other ethnic groups were not large enough for statistical analysis.

The relations between the pain intensity scores after management and the management effectiveness scores were examined. The older children (self-report) showed a significant relation between pain intensity and management effectiveness in interviews 2 ($r = -.651$; $p = .009$), 5 ($r = -.574$; $p = .025$), and 7 ($r = -.656$; $p = .008$), indicating that pain decreased as management effectiveness increased. For the younger children (self-report for pain and parental report for management effectiveness), there was no significant relation between management effectiveness and pain intensity afterward.

Functional status, a measure of the child's ability to engage in routine activities as reported by the parents, had a possible range of 0 to 28. For both the younger and older children, the mean score at all seven interviews was above the median score (Figure 5). The lowest mean score for both groups was 18 for the 4- to 7-year-olds and 17.9 for the 8- to 17-year-olds, as reported at the first interview. To test for differences between functional status scores across all the interviews, a significance level of .002 was determined to be appropriate in controlling for multiple testing. For the younger children, the significant differences were between interviews 1 and 2 ($t = -4.235$; $p = .000$), 1 and 3 ($t = -4.335$; $p = .001$), 1 and 5 ($t = -4.621$; $p < .001$), 1 and 6 ($t = -3.713$; $p = .001$), 1 and 7 ($t = -4.712$; $p < .001$). For the older children, the significant differences were between interviews 1 and 3 ($t = -3.326$; $p = .002$), 1 and 5 ($t = -3.959$; $p < .001$), 1 and 6 ($t = -4.432$;

TABLE 4 **Perception of Management Effectiveness: Descriptive Statistics over 7 Interviews**

Age Interview	4-7 years		8-17 years	
	X̄ (SD)	Range	X̄ (SD)	Range
1	64.19 (27.15)	14-99	53.23 (26.44)	5-99
2	71.89 (25.44)	16-99	55.89 (26.76)	3-99
3	63.21 (33.93)	0-99	55.16 (30.65)	0-99
4	63.37 (28.58)	0-99	59.65 (24.91)	0-99
5	69.45 (24.39)	2-99	55.35 (30.58)	0-99
6	71.92 (27.54)	0-9	47.96 (32.59)	0-99
7	69.59 (27.48)	3-100	71.21 (26.72)	0-100

Note: Possible 0-100.

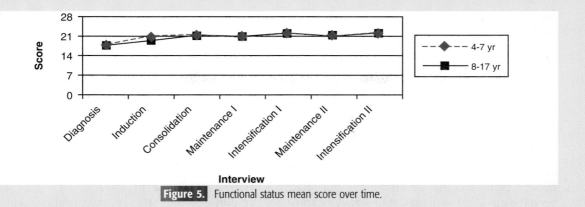

Figure 5. Functional status mean score over time.

$p < .001$), 1 and 7 ($t = -4.346$; $p < .001$). For the Latino children (all ages combined because of the lower number), the significant differences were between interviews 1 and 2 ($t = -3.58$; $p = .001$), 1 and 3 ($t = -3.891$; $p < .001$), 1 and 5 ($t = -4.473$; $p < .001$), 1 and 7 ($t = -4.459$; $p < .001$).

DISCUSSION

Most of the participants reported either current or recent pain at the date points throughout the year, although some of the children reported "no pain" at one or more data points. There are several possible explanations for the variability in pain presence: there are individual differences in pain threshold, tolerance, and sensitivity (Chen, Craske, Katz, Schwartz, & Zeltzer, 2000); earlier life experiences with pain differ among children and result in different interpretations of the pain experiences; and one method of coping with pain is avoidance, which is manifested by not thinking or talking about the pain.

The pain intensity mean scores remained at about the midpoint in both the younger and older age groups throughout the seven data points across the year. This assessment pertained to pain from all sources. The pain level did not significantly change across the seven interviews. The highest mean pain score for the older children was recorded at the first interview, and this may have been related directly to the additive effect of the disease process, the diagnostic pro-

cedures, and individual variations in the psychosocial response to the experience.

These findings confirm the results of previous studies. In a retrospective chart study, Cornaglia et al. (1984) reported that half of the children reported moderate to severe pain. In their studies, Miser, Dothage et al. (1987) and Miser, McCalla et al. (1987) reported pain intensity as moderate to severe, and Ljungman et al. (2000) found that cancer-related pain experienced by children at diagnosis fluctuated throughout the course of treatment.

Specifics on the location of pain as involving the legs, head/neck, abdomen, and back are supported by the findings of Ljungman and McGrath (2003), who also identified the first three locations as the most common pain locations. The locations identified by the children are consistent with the potential sources of pain such as the disease process, chemotherapy side effects, or lumbar and bone marrow aspiration. Miser, Dothage, et al. (1987), identifying the etiology of pain in children with cancer, not specifically leukemia, alluded to pain location in their references to "peripheral neuropathy," "postlumbar headache," and "abdominal pain from protracted chemotherapy-inducted vomiting" (pp. 77-78). Although the Miser sample included all types of cancer instead of focusing on leukemia, the similarity is striking. The children with leukemia frequently commented that the leg pain occurred about 2 days after they had received chemotherapy, sometimes mentioning vincristine specifically. A known side effect of this drug is neuritic pain (Wilson, Shannon, & Stang, 1999).

Similarly, the source of the headaches may have been related to several of the chemotherapy medications included in the various treatment protocols (e.g. cytarabine, dexamethasone, hydrocortisone, prednisone, methotrexate, or vincristine), or they may have resulted from a lumbar puncture, as in the Miser study. Asparaginase, dexamethasone, or vincristine may have been the direct cause of abdominal pain for some of the children, or the pain may have resulted indirectly from repeated vomiting.

The children's responses indicated that pain peaked at the beginning of the day and then decreased gradually during the day. This suggests that pain management decreases overnight, resulting in greater pain in the morning. Alternately, it is possible that early in the morning the pain level seems more intense because distraction and activity at that time of day is less than later in the day. A similar pattern of decreasing pain over a week may reflect the effect of time on the resolution of neuritic pain, lumbar puncture, headache, or abdominal pain from decreasing emesis.

"Aching" was one of the primary words used by the children in the current study to describe pain, which is similar to the results reported by Fowler-Kerry (1990) in an ethnoscience study examining oncology survivors' memory of pain. In the Fowler-Kerry (1990) study, words were self-generated, whereas in the current study, they were selected from a list. "Uncomfortable" (incómodo) and "annoying" (molesto) also overlap in two of the three most frequently used words from both English- and Spanish-speaking children. This gives some indication that these children describe pain similarly in both languages. The third most frequently selected word group, "come and goes," is reflective of the most frequently selected pattern of pain, which moved from a high to low intensity over the course of a day or week. This demonstrates congruence of the pain experience between the words used to describe the pain and the patterned diagram of the pain as described by the children.

The identification of many strategies used to take care of the pain in this study is paralleled by the qualitative work of Boyd and Hunsberger (1998), who found that chronically ill children (10 to 13 years of age) use a repertoire of coping strategies. Categorization of the children's responses according to the taxonomy proposed by Ryan-Wenger (1992) provided an organization matrix that fit all responses. The high response in the stressor modification category makes sense because the typical human response to pain is to try to stop or decrease it. The most frequent response, analgesics for the pain, is a logical first response when the use of medication is available and appropriate. Notably, analgesic used decreased over the course of the year. Sleep or rest serves to avoid aggravating the source of pain, possibly preventing increased pain. Thermal modalities such as heat and cold are used, as well as rubbing, massaging, or stretching of the painful area to effect the sensation. Ryan-Wenger (1992) in the development of their taxonomy noted that social support and distraction, the two most commonly used categories after stressor modification, were commonly used by children as coping strategies.

The most frequent management behaviors selected from among the closed option choices of the PPCI provide a picture of the children's coping similar to that derived from the categories developed from the open-ended question on coping. Although the order of frequency is different, "watching TV" parallels distraction, "lie down" is similar to resting, "telling my mother or father" fits the social support category, and "know that I can ask for something that will make the pain or hurt feel better" reflects the use of medication. Only "wish for it to go away" was not represented in the spontaneous coping responses given by the children. Perhaps this did not fit with the structure of the original inquiry of "What do you do to take care of the pain?" Yet in the structured response format, the child recognized this as a common response to the pain events.

Both the younger and older children tended to report significantly less pain intensity after pain management. However, this finding was not substantiated in the comparison of Latino and White children. The Latinos reported a perception of less effective pain management. This underscores the importance of managing and reassessing pain in a timely manner after intervention to ascertain its efficacy.

The reported functional status of children is noteworthy. For both the 4- to 7-year-olds and the 8- to 17-year-olds, as well as the Latino group, functional status increased significantly after treatment began. The mean scores for both age groups at all the interviews were consistently above the median point of the scale. This appears to indicate that most children were able to continue the normal activities of daily life during the first year of leukemia treatment.

The major limitation of this study was missing data that resulted when some children reported no pain at the time of interview and thus provided no data at that scheduled interview, and when missed interviews were missed because of varying circumstances, such as inability to make contact during that treatment phase or transfer of the child to another facility for a transplant. This resulted in insufficient numbers for appropriate use of repeated measure ANOVA, examination of the possible predictors of pain outcome, or assessment of changes and trends over time. Despite numerous strategies for maintaining data consistency, this was a challenging aspect of the current study. An additional limitation was the focus on leukemia, precluding **generalization** of the findings to other types of childhood cancer.

This study demonstrated the usefulness of the Symptom Management Model (UCSF, 1994) for examining the multidimensional pain experience. All the children experienced pain over the course of the first year after their diagnosis of leukemia. The experiences of Latino and White children were similar. The outcome of functional status remained above average despite the experience of pain. The findings provide reassurance to healthcare professionals and families that self-care strategies for managing pain are effective.

Accepted for publication October 7, 2003.

The authors thank the pediatric oncologists Antranik Bedros, MD, Violet Shen, MD, Stuart E. Siegel, MD and their colleagues, who granted access to the children and their parents, and to our research assistants, who participated in all phases of the study.

Supported by grant #NR04201, National Institute of Nursing Research.

Corresponding author: Lois Van Cleve, phD, RN, FAAN, Loma Linda University School of Nursing, Loma Linda, CA 92450 (e-mail: lvancleve@sn.llu.edu).

REFERENCES

Agency for Health Care Policy and Research (AHCPR) (1994). *Management of cancer pain: Clinical Practice Guideline No. 9.* AHCPR Publication No. 94-0592. Rockville, MD: Agency of Health Care Policy and Research, U.S. Department of Health and Human Services, Public Health Service.

American Cancer Society (2002). *Cancer facts and figures 2002.* Retrieved October 14, 2002 from http://www.cancer.org.

Boyd, J. R., & Hunsberger, M. (1998). Chronically ill children coping with repeated hospitalizations: Their perceptions and suggested interventions. *Journal of Pediatric Nursing, 13*(6), 330-342.

Chen, E., Craske, M. B., Katz, E. R., Schwartz, E., & Zeltzer, L. K. (2000). Pain-sensitive temperament: Does it predict procedural distress and response to psychological treatment among children with cancer? *Journal of Pediatric Psychology, 25*(4), 269-278.

Cornaglia, C., Massimo, L., Haupt, R., Melodia, A., Sizemore, W., & Benedetti, C. (1984). Incidence of pain in children with neoplastic diseases. *Pain,* Suppl. S28.

Fowler-Kerry, S. (1990). Adolescent oncology survivors' recollection of pain. *Advances in Pain Research Therapy, 15,* 265-370.

Hamner, S. B., & Miles, M. S. (1988). Coping strategies in children undergoing bone marrow aspirations. *Journal of Association of Pediatric Oncology Nursing, 5*(3), 11-15.

Hester, N. O., Foster, R. I., & Kristensen, K. (1989). *Sensitivity, convergent and discriminant validity of the pain ladder and the poker chip tool.* Paper presented at the Third International Nursing Research Symposium, Clinical Care of the Child and Family, Montreal, Canada.

Hester, N. O., Foster, R. I., & Kristensen, K. (1990). Measurement of pain in children: Generalizability and validity of the pain ladder and the poker chip tool, in D. C. Tyler & E. J. Krane (Eds), *Advances in pain research and therapy: Vol 15: Pediatric pain.* New York: Raven Press.

Hockenberry, M. J. (1988). Relaxation techniques in children with cancer: The nurse's role. *Journal of the Association of Pediatric Oncology Nursing, 5*(1,2), 7-11.

Krippendorff, L. (1980). *Content analysis: An introduction to its methodology.* Newbury Park, CA: Sage.

Ljungman, G., Gordh, T., Sorensen, S., & Kreuger, A. (1999). Pain in paediatric oncology: Interviews with children, adolescents, and their parents. *Acta Paediatrica, 88,* 623-630.

Ljungman, G., Gordh, T., Sorensen, S., & Kreuger, A. (2000). Pain variations during cancer treatment in children: A descriptive survey. *Pediatric Hematology and Oncology, 17,* 221-221.

Ljungman, G., Kreuger, A., Gordh, T., Berg, T., Sorensen, S., & Rawal, N. (1996). Treatment of pain in pediatric oncology: A Swedish nationwide survey. *Pain, 68*(2-3), 385-394.

Ljungman, G., & McGrath, P. J. (2003). *The prevalence of pain in children with cancer: An epidemiological study in an impatient setting* [Abstract]. Pain in Childhood: The Big Questions: 6th International Symposium on Paediatric Pain, Sydney, Australia, *6,* 114.

Miser, A. W., Dothage, J. A., Wesley, R. A., & Miser, J. S. (1987). The prevalence of pain in a pediatric and young adult cancer population. *Pain, 29*(1), 73-83.

Miser, A. W., McCalla, J., Dothage, J. A., Wesley, M., & Miser, J. S. (1987). Pain as a presenting symptom in children and young adults with newly diagnosed malignancy. *Pain, 29*(1), 85-90.

Miser, A. W., & Miser, J. S. (1989). The treatment of cancer pain in children. *Pediatric Clinics of North America, 36*(4), 979-999.

Patterson, K. L. (1992). Pain in the pediatric oncology patient. *Journal of Pediatric Oncology Nursing, 9*(3), 119-130.

Ries, L. A. G., Kosary, C. L., Hankey, B. F., Miller, B. A., & Edwards, B. K. (Eds). (1998). *SEER Cancer Statistics Review, 1973-1995.* Bethesda, MD: National Cancer Institute.

Ryan-Wenger, N. M. (1992). A taxonomy of children's coping strategies: A step toward theory development. *American Journal of Orthopsychiatry, 62*(2), 256-263.

Savedra, M. C., Tesler, M. D., Holzemer, W. L., & Brokaw, P. (1995). A strategy to assess the temporal dimension of pain in children and adolescents. *Nursing Research, 44,* 272-276.

Savedra, M. C., Tesler, M. D., Holzemer, W. L., & Ward, J. A. (1989). *Adolescent pediatric pain tool (APPT preliminary users manual).* San Francisco: University of California, San Francisco, School of Nursing.

Savedra, M. C., Tesler, M. D., Holzemer, W. L., Wilkie, D. J., & Ward, J. A. (1990). Testing a tool to access postoperative pediatric and adolescent pain. *Advances in Pain Research Therapy, 15,* 33-41.

Stein, R. E. K., & Jessop, D. J. (1990). A measure of child health status. *Medical Care, 28*(11), 1041-1055.

University of California, San Francisco (UCSF) School of Nursing Symptom Management Faculty Group. (1994). A model for symptom management. *Image: Journal of Nursing Scholarship, 26*(4), 272-276.

Van Cleve, L., Muñoz, C., Bossert, E. A., & Savedra, M. C. (2001). Children's and adolescents' pain language in Spanish: Translation of a measure. *Pain Management Nursing, 2*(3), 110-118.

Van Cleve, L., & Savedra, M. (1993). Pain location, validity, and reliability of body outline markings by hospitalized 4-7 year-old children. *Pediatric Nursing, 19*(3), 217-220.

Varni, J. W., Ealdorn, S. A., Gragg, R. A., Rapoff, M. A., Bernstein, B. H., Lindsley, C. B., et al. (1996). Development of the Waldron/Varni Pediatric Pain Coping Inventory. *Pain, 67*(1), 141-150.

Weber, R. P. (1985). *Basic content analysis.* Beverly Hills, CA: Sage.

Wilkie, D. J., Holzemer, W. L., Tesler, M. D., Ward, J. A., Paul, S. M., & Savedra, M. C. (1990). Measuring pain quality: Validity and reliability of children's and adolescents' pain language. *Pain, 41,* 151-159.

Wilson, B. A., Shannon, M. T., & Stang, C. L. (1999). *Nurses Drug Guide.* Stamford, CT: Appleton & Lange.

Woodgate, R., & McClement, S. (1998). Symptom distress in children with cancer: The need to adopt a meaning-centered approach. *Journal of Pediatric Oncology Nursing, 15*(1), 3-12.

SANDRA K. PLACH
PATRICIA E. STEVENS
VICKI A. MOSS

Social Role Experiences of Women Living with Rheumatoid Arthritis

*This study was designed as the **qualitative** arm of a larger quantitative study (N = 156) of the relationships among social role quality, physical health, and psychological well-being of women living with rheumatoid arthritis (RA). A subset of 20 midlife and late-life women from this larger sample participated in semistructured interviews with the specific aims of investigating how fulfilling they found social roles to be, including their spouse, mother, worker, and homemaker roles, while contending with RA, and what circumstances made social role experiences more positive. The results of the current follow-up qualitative study illustrate how difficult it can be to fulfill social roles during exacerbations of the illness in their formative adult years. The circumstance that best facilitated their positive experience in social roles was the unburdening of social role obligations as they grew older. Implications for nursing practice are discussed.*

Keywords: *women; social roles; arthritis; chronic disease*

Of the more than 2.1 million Americans diagnosed with rheumatoid arthritis (RA), most are midlife and older women (National Institute of Arthritis and Musculoskeletal and Skin Diseases, 2003). RA-related symptoms, such as pain, joint stiffness, and fatigue, and associated disability, have a signifi-cant impact on everyday tasks, family relationships, and social activities (Fyrand, Moum, Finset, & Glennas, 2001; Gornisiewicz & Moreland, 2001; Katz & Yelin, 1995). Despite advances in drug therapy, progressive functional impairment remains a common problem. The majority of individuals with RA must alter their lifestyles, and almost 32% are too disabled to work 10 years after disease onset (Wolfe & Hawley, 1998).

The burden of RA bears on emotional as well as physical health. Fears of helplessness and uncertainty about the future are heightened by unpredictable disease flare-ups and subsequent physical deformities (Mahat, 1997; Read, McEachern, & Mitchell, 2001). Altered functional ability gives rise to feelings of disablement, uselessness, and apprehension about premature aging (Griffith & Carr, 2001; Kamwendo, Askenbom, & Wahlgren, 1999; McPherson, Brander, Taylor, & McNaughton, 2001). Progressive inability to perform valued activities and

SANDRA K. PLACH, PHD, RN, CCRN, College of Nursing, University of Wisconsin–Milwaukee and Froedtert Hospital, Milwaukee, Wisconsin
PATRICIA E. STEVENS, PHD, RN, FAAN, College of Nursing, University of Wisconsin–Milwaukee
VICKI A. MOSS, DNSC, RN, College of Nursing, University of Wisconsin–Oshkosh

sustain family and social roles brings about depressive symptoms and feelings of stress (Katz & Yelin, 2001; van Lankveld, Naring, van't Pad Bosch, & van de Putte, 2000). When physical decline precludes a woman's ability to meet household and nurturing activities, the onus of RA extends to the entire family as members shift roles to maintain family functioning (Medeiros, Ferraz, & Quaresma, 2000; Revenson & Gibofsky, 1995). The effect of RA on social roles and responsibilities appears to be more problematic for women than for men. Women with RA have greater difficulty maintaining paid employment and tending to family and household obligations than do men, and women also report less satisfaction with sexual relations, and more emotional distress (Dowdy, Dwyer, Smith, & Wallston, 1996; Lapsley et al., 2002; Majerovitz & Revenson, 1994; Yelin, 1992).

In summary, discomforts and progressive disability appear to limit Women's ability to carry out social, occupational, and leisure activities in the face of RA and, therefore, increase their vulnerability for impaired well-being. Given these morbidity problems, it is important to learn more about women with RA and their experience in social roles so that appropriate and effective interventions might be planned. With this in mind, a large quantitative study ($N = 156$) was undertaken to examine relationships among social role quality, physical health, and psychological well-being in midlife and late-life women diagnosed with RA (M age = 59, $SD = 11$, range = 39 to 87). Results from this larger study are reported elsewhere (Plach, Heidrich, & Waite, 2003). The conclusion reached from this larger study was that women with RA who had positive social role experiences had less depression and

more purpose in life, despite physical difficulties, than those who did not have positive social role experiences. Given these promising results, a qualitative follow-up study was designed to explore in greater depth the nature of social role experiences for women living with RA. A subset of 20 women from the original sample of 156 was purposively selected to participate in semistructured interviews with the specific aim of investigating their insider views on how fulfilling they found particular roles to be, including spouse, mother, worker, and homemaker, while contending with RA. A second specific aim was to better understand what circumstances made social role experiences more positive for women living with RA. The results of this follow-up qualitative study are reported here.

METHOD

The setting for the larger quantitative study of women living with RA included several metropolitan communities in a Midwestern state. The convenience sample of 156 participants was recruited from private physician offices, health clinics, and community newsletters. Inclusion criteria were that participants be female, carry a diagnosis of RA, and be able to read and write English so that they could complete written survey instruments about social role quality, physical health, and psychological well-being. The purposive sample of 20 participants who took part in this qualitative follow-up study consisted of women who had previously participated in the quantitative study and had given their permission to be contacted again for any subsequent investigations. (Of the original sample, 85% gave permission to be contacted again.) The purposive sample was chosen using two criteria: length of time since diagnosis and age. We wanted to include women in the qualitative study who had enough years since their diagnosis with RA to have a long-lasting subjective experience of the illness that they could tell us about. Because the first couple of years of an illness such as RA involve adjusting to the diagnosis and initial

This research was funded in party by a grant from the University of Wisconsin–Oshkosh Faculty Development Program awarded to Drs. Plach and Moss.
Address all correspondence to Sandra K. Plach, PhD, RN, CCRN, Assistant Professor, College of Nursing, University of Wisconsin–Milwaukee, Cunningham Hall, PO Box 413, Milwaukee, WI 53201; e-mail:placs@uwm.edu.

treatment regimens, women who had lived with a diagnosis of RA for 3 years or longer were selected. Because results of the larger study had indicated a difference in the level of depression between midlife and late-life women living with RA, we also wanted to ensure similar numbers of midlife and late-life women in the qualitative study.

The 20 participants ranged in age from 39 to 86 years ($M = 61$), all but one was White. More than one half were married, reported a yearly household income of at least U.S.$30,000, and had lived with RA for more than 10 years (Table 1). Eight women had children who were still living at home. Nine worked outside the home, 10 were retired, and two categorized themselves as disabled.

Semistructured interviews were conducted in private, conveniently located places, mostly in participants' homes. The interview guide con-

sisted of **open-ended** questions about what it was like to live with RA and what it was like to carry out their social roles. Interviews varied in length from 45 min to 90 min and were audiotaped and transcribed verbatim. Institutional Review Board approval was obtained for all study procedures.

We used qualitative **content analysis** (Lofland & Lofland, 1995) to find common patterns and themes within participants' characterizations of their social role experiences. In the initial coding, the researchers divided the data according to the social roles discussed: spouse, mother, worker, and so on. Labels were then assigned to units of meaning. The second level of coding involved reading all the labeled descriptions of what it was like being a spouse, and then identifying the context and circumstances of positive spouse role experiences. This second level of coding was repeated for each social role.

Then, as we sorted, aggregated, and synthesized the data further, we looked for themes that represented the relationships among codes. The last analytic step was to identify major categories of experience that represented the relationships among the themes. In the process, each woman's experience was systematically compared and contrasted with experiences of the other participants. Analytic memos and diagrams were created to show how initial codes related to one another, how themes fit together, and what major categories began to emerge (Miles & Huberman, 1994). Trustworthiness and rigor were strengthened throughout the analysis as the three researchers met at regular intervals to compare and discuss coding and reach consensus on what was represented in the data. Our findings are presented with ample verbatim excerpts from the women's interviews for readers to judge their veracity.

TABLE 1 **Demographic Characteristics of Participants (_N_ = 20)**

Characteristic	*n*	*%*
Age		
39 to 65 years	11	55
66 to 86 years	9	45
Ethnicity/Race		
White	19	95
Hispanic	1	5
Marital status		
Married	12	60
Widowed	4	20
Divorced	3	15
Single (never married)	1	5
Yearly household income		
Less than U.S.$10,000	1	5
$10,000 to $30,000	7	35
More than $30,000	12	60
Length of time since RA diagnosis		
3 to 5 years	5	25
6 to 10 years	4	20
More than 10 years	11	55

Note: *RA* = rheumatoid arthritis

RESULTS

No Roles Left Untouched by RA

Our data indicated that as women with RA moved through adulthood they struggled to balance multiple roles as spouse, mother, worker, and homemaker, while at the same time contending with fatigue, pain, and disability imposed by RA. No roles were left untouched. The midlife women in the sample were embroiled in social role dilemmas as they raised school-aged children, worked full-time jobs outside the home, tried to have satisfying relationships with their husbands, and did all in their power to keep the house clean and the family well fed. The late-life women in the sample recalled such dilemmas from earlier in their lives and recounted them in their interviews; however, they spoke from a standpoint wherein adult children were no longer dependent on them, they were retired, conflicted marriages had either ended or settled into a tolerable routine, and their households were calmer. When reflecting on their formative adult years living with the disease, however, these late-life women told stories very similar to the younger participants.

When illness-related symptoms precluded women's capacity to meet family expectations and social role norms, they felt frustrated and disappointed. Although most described a tremendous capacity to cope with the symptoms of RA and strive to maintain as much normalcy in their lives as they could, they still experienced guilt and lowered self-esteem when family expectations exceeded what their illness allowed them to do. They were determined to fulfill their roles and maintain relationships as expected, yet they lacked the energy to take care of themselves as they focused on doing right by others.

Stories from all the women in the study illustrate these social role dilemmas. The midlife women talked about what it was currently like, and the late-life women talked about what it used to be like being spouse, mother, worker, and homemaker.

For instance, in their role as spouse, many of the women had felt inadequate at times due to the RA:

> I remember coming home from work and being exhausted and laying down and resting, which was what I was supposed to do. And I remember my ex-husband coming in and slamming pots and pans around because he thought I should be up cooking his dinner. I pushed and pushed myself. I figured maybe I wasn't doing all that I should be doing. I thought maybe I was lazy. Maybe just because I have rheumatoid arthritis doesn't mean that I should be allowed to lay down. I lived with that a long time. I kept trying to be everything—go to work all day, come home and clean, have his food ready, be his sex kitten at night.
>
> As far as the wife part of it, that was difficult because I really couldn't be a wife with all the pain and everything that I had. My husband tried to be as supportive as possible, but he admitted to me that he resented my sickness. He resented that I could not do all the things that I used to do.
>
> I think the fatigue probably does more to a relationship than the immobility. Because sometimes I just don't have the energy to be in a relationship. I just don't have the energy to listen to his concerns or deal with his emotions. I get through the day. I don't have anything else to give.

Women's role as a mother with RA was no less troublesome:

> My kids had a hard time dealing with my pain, and they didn't understand what it was. They tell me now that when they were little they just remember me screaming a lot with pain and being in bed. I feel bad. That's not much of a childhood. It makes me feel bad that they feel that's what their childhood was all about.
>
> I tried to do the mother things even when I was sick. I tried to be there for the kids when they came home from school. Even though I was in bed, they still felt comfortable coming after school or after dates to sit and talk with me. But, one of my daughters, who was a teenager at the time I was most sick, has never really gotten over going from the closeness we had to all of a sudden my not being available to her the way she really wanted me to be.

My kids have always seen me with arthritis. Sometimes I wish they knew me before I had rheumatoid arthritis. I'm very grateful they help me when I need it, but it makes me feel sometimes like I'm not a full mom like I want to be. Because instead of me caring for them, they're caring for me.

Because of the RA, women suffered losses in their role as worker, too.

Let me tell you what I lost—I lost my profession. I loved it. I was a beautician, and I can't even do my own hair today. When I had to quit my job, I was already starting to lose my speed and my dexterity, and I was dropping things a lot. I was dropping my combs, dropping my brushes.

They compensated as best they could at their jobs.

I have a tendency to do much more than I should at work, because I want to make sure they know I can do my job even though I have rheumatoid arthritis. I sometimes have trouble setting limits when I think people expect too much of me as an employee. Then, I don't have the energy to keep up my volunteer work at the church.

Their work role in the household as a homemaker was affected as well.

I've always been in charge in my home, and everything was just a certain way. Now that I am fighting with this disease and trying to cope with everything, I keep going as much as I can. It's what everyone expects. But, I get really tired and sometimes I lay down on the couch. Then my family says I'm lazy. I also feel guilty about not cooking much anymore.

It's frustrating because I can't keep the house the way I would like it to be kept. And I read booklets from the Arthritis Foundation. There are so many platitudes: "Let it go. Don't worry about it. Just relax." It sounds so easy, but it's difficult in reality to watch dust pile up, dirt pile up. It's very difficult. It makes me angry when healthy people tell afflicted people how they should feel.

Women felt badly that their families were so deeply affected by their illness over the years.

My rheumatoid arthritis affects my whole family. Everybody is pulled in. That compounds it, and I feel worse, because I don't want to see them held back by me. It gives me a sense of guilt over something I can't control, and that bothers me very much.

I get frustrated because I tell my family over and over, "I can't do this. I can't do this." And it's like they don't hear me. It's like they don't get it. And to have to keep repeating your limitations, you feel like you're whining or you're being a victim. And I don't like taking that role.

The emotional and physical effects of the RA tended to isolate them from friends as well.

With rheumatoid arthritis, there's just no avenue to let out your feelings. It all just stays inside. It makes me lonely and isolated. I isolated myself a lot from people. I did not have the energy, and people didn't understand. I stopped going out. I lost a lot of friends.

In general, these data suggest that dealing with the ramifications of RA during midlife negatively affected the quality of women's social roles. The impact of RA on women's lives seemed to have a domino effect. Discomfort and dysfunction affected their ability to perform in social roles. Their self-image of who they were in relation to others became shaken. Family dynamics changed as roles shifted and realigned to accommodate the intrusion of RA. Relationships became strained and altered. Some social roles, such as being a professional in the workplace, an active church member, or a dependable friend, were lost.

Benefits of Growing Older and Wiser With RA

There was evidence of positive social role experiences in the data as well. Most of these stories came from the late-life women in the sample who had discovered that growing older helped them better balance the restrictions of RA and find meaning and strength in their daily lives. For the older women in this study, RA seemed to be less problematic as their lives were less referenced by the needs of growing families and demanding careers. The busyness of younger years that had often rendered them physically and emotionally exhausted was now behind them, and they contended with fewer daily hassles and pressures. Although they were not free from the pain and limitations that accompanied the disease, many appraised their lives positively. As one participant put it, "I have rheumatoid arthritis, it doesn't have me."

As the following quote illustrates, many of the older women in the study were able to set aside multiple social role responsibilities to focus on the one role that gave them the most pleasure.

> My house doesn't look like it did 10 years ago. I clean it a lot less now—too many aches and pains. There are some things I can't get done, like I used to decorate for every season. Well, I don't do that anymore, and nobody misses it except me. Oh, there are uncomfortable moments, and the fact that I can't do some things, that does bother me. But, on the whole, my husband and I are able to do a lot, go out to eat, visit friends. We traveled to Florida last year. It is easier now that the kids are grown, and I don't have to struggle with work anymore.

RA seemed less overwhelming than it had been earlier in life because they could slow down and adjust plans to accommodate discomforts, unlike in their younger years when everyday responsibilities dictated that they carry on despite severe fatigue and pain.

> Now that I'm older, I feel like I don't have to work so hard to please everyone, to do everything no matter how sore I am. I get to do what I want to do. If I want to get dressed and go out shopping, I'll do that. Some days I really hurt, so I just stay home. I don't like any demands, anybody saying, "Wednesday we'll go here," or

"Thursday, you gotta do that." I had people telling me what to do for years, but not anymore.

At their age, these late-life women with RA were freed from juggling family and work responsibilities, and they had more time to reflect on their lives and negotiate around their health problems. They resisted self-pity and found new meaning and purpose in their life circumstances:

> I don't mind getting older. I think I know myself better. I'm more creative. I'm more productive, maybe not physically, but spiritually and psychologically. RA makes me slow down, and I'm able to be in the moment and appreciate it. When I was younger, I was always trying to get to the next moment, the next thing, taking care of everybody and everything: the kids, my husband, my employer. Now I'm reclaiming myself. I wouldn't wish RA on anyone, but it has changed me—and not really for the worse.
>
> Rheumatoid arthritis has changed my lifestyle, but I think there is more quality. Instead of all the physical things, I read, write, and pray more. It has brought out a different side of me and helped me to find other gifts.

Some were even able to identify a positive legacy they were leaving as a result of having RA:

> A plus with this is that my children don't feel awkward around people who are disabled. Most people grow up never knowing how to deal with somebody who is disabled. My children grew up learning how to do for me, and that's good.
>
> My granddaughter told her mother, "Mama, if you ever get sick, I'll take care of you like you take care of Grandma." It's good for kids to see that sometimes people need help that way.

One woman reflected back on her life, not discounting the difficulties posed by the illness, but finding serenity in her role accomplishments:

> I am 73. I had my first serious bout with rheumatoid arthritis at the age of 9, when I was completely immobile. At age 35, another bout

with it lasted years. But I kept moving, raised the kids and all. Now at 73, I consider myself in remission, although there are still problems. I have had a total hip replacement, a total knee replacement, and all my joints are lumpy and stiff. But, I'm very thankful to the Lord for all the blessings I've received and for helping me through my problems. So, what I do is volunteer for the Rheumatoid Arthritis Foundation when they do their fund drive every year. It makes me feel like I'm contributing.

DISCUSSION

Similar to other research, findings from this study highlight the deleterious effects a chronic, debilitating illness such as rheumatoid arthritis can have on social role activities and psychological health for women (Brown & Williams, 1995; DeVillis, Patterson, Blalock, Renner, & DeVellis, 1997; Katz & Yelin, 1995; Plach & Heidrich, 2002; Plach & Stevens, 2001; Walsh, Blanchard, Kremer, & Blanchard, 1999). No role was left untouched by RA. When limited in their ability to perform their spouse, mother, worker, and homemaker roles, women in the current study felt angry, sad, and sometimes useless. During active exacerbations of their illness in their formative adult years, the social roles women with RA tried to fulfill became even more difficult, and they were exhausted. According to these data from midlife and late-life women, the circumstance that best facilitated their positive experience in social roles was the unburdening of social role obligations as they grew older. Achieving older age helped women in the current study to shed a portion of the contentious social role responsibilities they had earlier in life and gain wisdom about their illness and its effects on their lives and the lives of their families. They seemed better able to balance the constraints of RA without the multiple role obligations of earlier years. Late-life women with RA had the time and energy to negotiate around their health problems, pursue more of their own interests, and contribute to their own well-being and that of

their families and society in ways that gave meaning and purpose to their lives.

These findings bear some similarity to findings by Dildy (1996), Neill (2002), and Shaul (1997), in that they seem to indicate that women with RA go through a process of adaptation over time in which they learn to balance resources and demands, and that they are able through a process of personal transformation to achieve success in managing their lives despite their limitations. The turning point, however, seems to be the unburdening of social role obligations that are at conflict with women's RA-related pain, fatigue, and disablement. For these participants, that turning point, which pointed the way to more positive role experiences, came with advancement in age. The clinical implication in these findings lies in pursuing ways to help women with RA to reach a positive plane in their social role experiences while they are still in their formative adult years. The ordinary arrangements of family and work life are often characterized by inequity that consistently disadvantages women (Robinson, 1998), so any work in this area must address this broader social concern.

It may be that experiencing RA at one developmental stage in life's trajectory is more problematic for emotional well-being than it is at a different developmental stage. For example, experiencing physical limitations from RA may be perceived by late-life women as somewhat consistent with their same-age peers whose activities have slowed because of the aging process. Whereas, experiencing these same physical limitations at midlife may make women feel dissimilar from same-age peers whom they perceive as boundlessly energetic and achievement oriented. In the larger quantitative study of women with RA ($N = 156$), we found these kinds of differences between late-life and midlife women. Despite significantly more health problems, late-life women fared better than their younger counterparts from a psychosocial perspective, reporting more role satisfaction and less depression (Plach, Napholz, & Kelber, 2003a). We found similar differences in a previous quantitative study with women with heart disease ($N = 157$). Regardless of the extent of physical health problems, late-life women had less anxiety and depression, and more positive well-being and role satisfaction than midlife women (Plach & Heidrich, 2002; Plach, Napholz, & Kelber, 2003b).

Feminist researchers suggest that women use a process of repatterning to juggle competing family, work, and personal demands. With this process, they reorganize activities to reduce or overcome the negative effects of role demands (Wuest, 2000). Perhaps nurses could help women with RA mitigate the effect of RA on social role expectations by providing education about repatterning strategies, such as relinquishing and replenishing (Wuest, 2000). Relinquishing is the process of consciously deciding which activities to give up, giving women a sense of control that helps to offset stressors associated with uncontrolled losses. For example, a woman might choose to stop hosting major family events. With replenishing, women learn to pay attention to themselves, attending to their physical, emotional, intellectual, and social needs. In this instance, a woman might choose to join a book club to develop new knowledge and increase her social network.

Such strategies hold little potential for success unless women and their families are involved in intervention. Family dynamics play a major part in whether women with RA feel fulfilled and satisfied in their social roles (Nyman & Lutzen, 1999). Often family members are not present for education sessions in the physician office or clinic setting, and an opportunity is missed to teach the family how they can best give physical and emotional support to their loved ones. By encouraging patients to bring a family member with them to clinic appointements or by scheduling in-hospital education at times when family members are available, nurses can provide family-centered education about the effects of RA on functional ability and help family members plan strategies to realign role responsibilities and expectations. By working with the family to determine realistic and flexible role expectations and modifications, nurses can help keep a woman's important roles intact. Family-centered education may help to maintain family balance and optimize women's emotional well-being. Such interventions need to be tested.

A support network or support group of peers could help women living with RA feel safe expressing and responding to the emotional and physical turmoil imposed by the presence of RA in their everyday lives as spouses, mothers, workers, and homemakers. Participating in a support group provides an opportunity to share illness experiences with like-minded women contending with similar challenges to their well-being (Ruffing-Rahal, 1998). One outcome may be to help women with RA move toward accepting fewer responsibilities and feeling less guilt about not attending as closely to the needs of others (Charmaz, 2002). Support groups can also provide education, and when facilitated by a community health or rheumatology advanced practice nurse, participants can receive consultation and self-care information, ask health-related questions, and learn about other health and community resources (Ruffing-Rahal, 1998). According to latest recommendations for our nation's health, evidence-based arthritis education should be an integral part of an individual's management of their arthritis (Office of Disease and Health Promotion, 2001). A viable strategy to meet this objective would be the development of multidimensional support groups facilitated by advanced practice nurses. Clinic and office nurses could refer and encourage women's participation in support groups.

Caution is warranted in generalizing from the findings of the current qualitative study. The experiences of these predominately White women cannot be taken as representative of women from other ethnic/racial groups. Further research about women with RA would benefit from a sampling strategy that optimizes ethnic/racial diversity so that similarities and differences in women's experiences with RA could be explored and the design of future interventions made culturally competent. Although the findings cannot be generalized to all women with RA or similar illnesses, the information derived from naturalistic studies such as this one may be transferable to other women in similar situations (Lincoln & Guba, 1985). For example, there may be some applicability to other women living with chronic illnesses that are debilitating, have pain and fatigue associated with them, and have a clinical course that involves exacerbations and remissions. Larger studies involving women with varying diagnoses, as well as longitudinal designs, might allow for examination of the varied day-to-day circumstances of women's social roles with changes in disease trajectory over time.

In summary, women with RA contend with many challenges in their social roles as they live with RA. Findings from the current study help to shed light on women's everyday experiences with the negative psychological and social sequelae of RA. This elucidation of qualitative data about the social context of women's lives provides a fuller appreciation of women's experiences of illness and adds information about the impact of chronic, disabling illness. A challenge for nurses is to incorporate insights provided through women's accounts of social role experiences into care plans and clinical practice (Brown & Williams, 1995) so that women can be helped to engineer the best possible everyday well-being.

REFERENCES

Brown, S., & Williams, A. (1995). Women's experience of rheumatoid arthritis. *Journal of Advanced Nursing, 21,* 695-701.

Charmaz, K. (2002). The self as habit: The reconstruction of self in chronic illness. *Occupational Therapy Journal of Research, 22*(Suppl), 31S-41S.

DeVellis, R. F., Patterson, C. C., Blalock, S. J., Renner, B. R., & DeVellis, B. M. (1997). Do people with rheumatoid arthritis develop illness-related schemas? *Arthritis Care and Research, 10,* 78-88.

Dildy, S. P. (1996). Suffering in people with rheumatoid arthritis. *Applied Nursing Research, 9,* 177-183.

Dowdy, S. W., Dwyer, K. A., Smith C. A., & Wallston, K. A. (1996). Gender and psychological well-being of persons with rheumatoid arthritis. *Arthritis Care and Research, 9,* 449-456.

Fyrand, L., Moum, T., Finset, A., & Glennas, A. (2001). The impact of disability and disease duration on social support of women with rheumatoid arthritis. *Journal of Behavioral Medicine, 25*(3), 251-268.

Gornisiewicz, M., & Moreland, L. W. (2001). Rheumatoid arthritis. In L. Robbins, C. S. Burkhardt, M. T. Hannan, & R. J. DeHoratius (Eds.), *Clinical care in the rheumatic diseases* (2nd ed., pp. 89-96). Atlanta, GA: Association of Rheumatology Health Professionals.

Griffith, J., & Carr, A. (2001). What is the impact of early rheumatoid arthritis on the individual? *Best Practice and Research Clinical Rheumatology, 15*(1), 77-90.

Kamwendo, K., Askenbom, M., & Wahlgren, C. (1999). Physical activity in the life of the patient with rheumatoid arthritis. *Physiotherapy Research International, 4,* 278-292.

Katz, P. P., & Yelin, E. H. (1995). The development of depressive symptoms among women with rheumatoid arthritis: The role of function. *Arthritis and Rheumatism, 38,* 49-56.

Katz, P. P., & Yelin, E. H. (2001). Activity loss and the onset of depressive symptoms. *Arthritis and Rheumatism, 44,* 1194-1202.

Lapsley, H. M., March, L. M., Tribe, K. L., Cross, M. J., Courtenay, B. G., & Brooks, P. M. (2002). Living with rheumatoid arthritis: Expenditures, health status, and social impact on patients. *Annals of the Rheumatic Diseases, 61,* 818-821.

Lincoln, Y. S., & Guba, E. G. (1985). *Naturalistic inquiry.* Beverly Hills, CA: Sage.

Lofland, J., & Lofland, L. (1995). *Analyzing social settings: A guide to qualitative observation and analysis* (3rd ed.). Belmont, CA: Wadsworth.

Mahat, G. (1997). Perceived stressors and coping strategies among individuals with rheumatoid arthritis. *Journal of Advanced Nursing, 25,* 1144-1150.

Majerovitz, S. D., & Revenson, T. A. (1994). Sexuality and rheumatic disease: The significance of gender. *Arthritis Care and Research, 7,* 29-34.

McPherson, K. M., Brander, P., Taylor, W. J., & McNaughton, H. K. (2001). Living with arthritis— What is important? *Disability and Rehabilitation, 23,* 706-721.

Medeiros, M. M. C., Ferraz, M. B., & Quaresma, M. R. (2000). The effect of rheumatoid arthritis on the quality of life of primary caregivers. *Journal of Rheumatology, 27,* 76-83.

Miles, M. B., & Huberman, A. M. (1994). *Qualitative data analysis: An expanded sourcebook* (2nd ed.). Newbury Park, CA: Sage.

National Institute of Arthritis and Musculoskeletal and Skin Diseases. (2003). *Handout on health: Rheumatoid arthritis.* Retrieved May 22, 2003, from http://niams. nih.gov/hi/topics/arthritis/rahandout.htm

Neill, J. (2002). Transcendence and transformation in the life patterns of women living with rheumatoid arthritis. *Advances in Nursing Science, 24*(4), 27-47.

Nyman, C. S., & Lutzen, K. (1999). Caring needs of patients with rheumatoid arthritis. *Nursing Science Quarterly, 12*(2), 164-169.

Office of Disease and Health Promotion. (2001). *Healthy people 2010.* Available from http://www. healthypeople.gov/

Plach, S. K., & Heidrich, S. M. (2002). Social role quality, physical health, and psychological well-being in women after heart surgery. *Research in Nursing & Health, 25,* 189-202.

Plach, S. K., Heidrich, S. M., & Waite, R. M. (2003). Relationship of social role quality to psychological well-being in women with rheumatoid arthritis. *Research in Nursing and Health, 26,* 190-202.

Plach, S. K., Napholz, L., & Kelber, S. T. (2003a). Depression during early recovery from heart surgery among early middle-age, midlife, and elderly women. *Health Care for Women International, 24,* 327-339.

Plach, S. K., Napholz, L., & Kelber, S. T. (2003b). *Developmental, social, and health factors associated with depressive disorders among women with rheumatoid arthritis.* Manuscript submitted for publication.

Plach, S. K., & Stevens, P. E. (2001). Midlife women's experiences living with heart disease. *Applied Nursing Research, 14,* 201-209.

Read, E., McEachern, C., & Mitchell, T. (2001). Psychological well-being of patients with rheumatoid arthritis. *British Journal of Nursing, 10,* 1385-1391.

Revenson, T. A., & Gibofsky, A. (1995). Marriage, social support, and adjustment to rheumatic disease. *Bulletin on the Rheumatic Diseases, 44*(3), 5-8.

Robinson, C. A. (1998). Women, families, chronic illness, and nursing interventions: From burden to balance. *Journal of Family Nursing, 4*(3), 271-290.

Ruffing-Ruhal, M. A. (1998). Well-being and its shadow: Health promotion implications for older women. *Health Care for Women International, 19,* 457-465.

Shaul, M. P. (1997). Transitions in chronic illness: Rheumatoid arthritis in women. *Rehabilitation Nursing, 22,* 199-205.

van Lankveld, W., Naring, G., van't Pad Bosch, P., & van de Putte, L. (2000). The negative effect of decreasing the level of activity in coping with pain in rheumatoid arthritis: An increases in psychological distress and disease impact. *Journal of Behavioral Medicine, 23*(4), 377-391.

Walsh, J. D., Blanchard, E. B., Kremer, J. M., & Blanchard, C. G. (1999). The psychosocial effects of rheumatoid arthritis on the patient and the well partner. *Behavior Research and Therapy, 37,* 259-271.

Wolfe, F., & Hawley, D. J. (1998). The long-term outcomes of rheumatoid arthritis: Work disability: A prospective 18-year study of 832 patients. *Journal of Rheumatology, 25,* 2108-2117.

Wuest, J. (2000). Repatterning care: Women's proactive management of family caregiving demands. *Health Care for Women International, 21,* 393-411.

Yelin, E. (1992). Arthritis: The cumulative impact of a common chronic condition. *Arthritis and Rheumatism, 35,* 489-497.

Sandra K. Plach, PhD, RN, CCRN, is an assistant professor at the University of Wisconsin–Milwaukee College of Nursing. Her research interest is the impact of chronic illness on women's social roles and the contribution of women's social roles to psychological well-being in the context of a chronic illness. She is particularly interested in women with heart disease, women with rheumatoid arthritis, and women with HIV/AIDS. In addition to her faculty role, she is the coordinator of Nursing Research at Froedtert Hospital, Milwaukee, Wisconsin. In this role, she provides research consultation, facilitates nursing research, and promotes evidence-based nursing practice. Her recent publications include (with L Napholz & ST Kelber) "Depression During Early Recovery From Heart Surgery Among Early Middle-Age, Midlife and Elderly Women" in Health Care for Women International *(2003) and (with SM Heidrich & RM Waite) "Relationship of Social Role Quality to Psychological Well-Being in Women With Rheumatoid Arthritis" in* Research in Nursing and Health *(2003).*

Patricia E. Stevens, PhD, RN, FAAN, is a professor at the University of Wisconsin–Milwaukee College of Nursing. She is currently primary investigator on the National Institutes of Health-funded study In-Depth Longitudinal Study of HIV-Infected Women *(#R01 NR04840) in which she and her coinvestigators are developing innovative narrative analyses of women's experiences of the impact of HIV/AIDS, their struggles with symptoms, their efforts to adhere to medical regimens, their actions in reducing sexual and drug-using risks, and their access to health care and social services. Her recent publications include (with PK Pletsch) "Ethical Issues of Informed Consent: Mothers' Experiences Enrolling Their Children in Bone Marrow Transplantation Research" in* Cancer Nursing: An International Journal for Cancer Care *(2002) and (with PK Pletsch) "Informed Consent and the History of Inclusion of Women in Clinical Research" in* Health Care for Women International *(2002).*

Vicki A. Moss, DNSc, RN, is an associate professor at the University of Wisconsin–Oshkosh College of Nursing. Her research interests are women's issues and chronic illness. She has done research with women and domestic violence, women and rheumatoid arthritis, and families of persons with dementia. She is also interested in natural/alternative/complementary (NAC) therapies and is faculty for a postmasters NAC certificate program. Her recent publications include (with B Nesbitt) "Making Research Real: An Experiential Approach" in Nurse Educator *(2003) and (with C Rogers, L Halstead, & J Campbell) "The Experience of Terminating an Abusive Relationship From an Anglo and African American Perspective: A Qualitative Descriptive Study" in* Issues in Mental Health Nursing *(1997).*

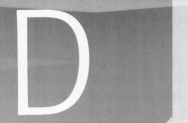

B. JOYCE DAVISON
S. LARRY GOLDENBERG
MARTIN E. GLEAVE
LESLEY F. DEGNER

Provision of Individualized Information to Men and Their Partners to Facilitate Treatment Decision Making in Prostate Cancer

Purpose/Objectives: To determine if providing individualized information to men who are newly diagnosed with prostate cancer and their partners would lower their levels of psychological distress and enable them to become more active participants in treatment decision making.

Design: Quasiexperimental, one group, pretest/post-test.

Setting: The Prostate Centre at Vancouver General Hospital in British Columbia, Canada.

Sample: Convenience sample of 74 couples. 73 men had early-stage prostate cancer. Mean age of the men was 62.2 years, and mean age of the partners was 58.1 years. The majority (>50%) had received their high school diplomas.

Methods: Respondents completed measures of decision preferences and psychological distress at the time of diagnosis and four months later. All participants used a computer to identify their information and decision preferences. Computer-generated, graphic printouts were used to guide the information counseling session.

Findings: Patients reported assuming a more active role in medical decision making than originally intended, partners assumed a more passive role in decision making than originally intended, and all participants had lower levels of psychological distress at four months.

Conclusions: Evidence supports the need to provide informational support to couples at the prostate cancer diagnosis to facilitate treatment decision making and lower levels of psychological distress. Future research is needed to evaluate this type of approach in the context of a randomized clinical trial design.

Implications for Nursing: The personalized, computer-graphic printouts can provide clini-

B. Joyce Davison, RN, PhD, is a nurse scientist, *S. Larry Goldenberg, MD, FRCSC, FACS,* is the director of the Prostate Centre, and *Martin E. Gleave, MD, FRCSC, FACS,* is director of clinical trials, all at the Prostate Centre at Vancouver General Hospital in British Columbia, Canada, and faculty of medicine at the University of British Columbia. *Lesley F. Degner, RN, PhD,* is a professor with the faculty of nursing at the University of Manitoba in Winnipeg.
This research was supported by the Prostate Cancer Research Initiative, the National Cancer Institute of Canada, and a Scholar Award to the first author from Vancouver General Hospital. (Submitted February 2002. Accepted for publication May 15, 2002.) (Mention of specific products and opinions related to those products do not indicate or imply endorsement by the Oncology Nursing Forum *or the Oncology Nursing Society.)*

cians with an innovative method of guiding information counseling and providing decisional support to men with prostate cancer and their partners.

KEY POINTS

- The Patient Information Program computer program provides clinicians with a method of assessing and providing information to men who are newly diagnosed with prostate cancer and their partners.
- Evidence indicates that such an individualized information decision support intervention assists men in becoming more active participants in treatment decision making.
- Provision of individualized information at the time of diagnosis lessens the psychological distress of couples after a definitive treatment decision has been made.
- Further research is needed to explore how partners use information and how satisfied they are with their reported level of involvement in treatment decision making at the time of diagnosis.

Prostate cancer poses a significant health concern for men and their families. Currently, prostate cancer is the most commonly diagnosed nonskin malignancy and second most common cause of male cancer-related deaths in North America (Jemal, Thomas, Murray, & Thun, 2002; National Cancer Institute of Canada, 2002). Etiology remains unknown, optimal treatment is controversial, survival rates vary, and all prostate cancer therapies have an impact on quality of life (Brawley & Barnes, 2001; McPherson, Swenson, & Kjellberg, 2001; O'Rourke, 2001). The diagnosis often is unexpected and particularly stressful for men and their partners as they first adjust to the cancer diagnosis and try to make sense of the various treatment options. Although the majority of oncology healthcare professionals believe that patients with cancer should be involved in making informed treatment choices, a significant number of men are presenting to physician offices for treatment

discussions with little to no knowledge of the disease or potential treatment options (Onel et al., 1998). Treatment choices often are made as a response to lay information or a result of a bias toward surgery as a cure (O'Rourke & Germino, 1998). Informal sources such as family, friends, and men with prostate cancer remain the most frequently cited sources of information used by men and their partners (Davison & Degner, 1997; Davison, Degner, & Morgan, 1995).

Men with prostate cancer have been shown to prefer to participate in treatment decision making with their physicians (Davison & Degner, 1997; Wong et al., 2000), but the extent to which partners wish to participate in treatment decisions and the influence they have on the final treatment decision currently is unknown. Data exist to indicate that older female spouses tend to ask more questions than their partners and assume a more active role in medical encounters (Beisecker & Moore, 1994). However, information is limited regarding how younger or same-sex partners wish to be involved in medical decision making. Investigators have demonstrated that providing information to men who are newly diagnosed with prostate cancer does result in benefits such as increased participation in treatment decision making, decreased levels of anxiety, and improved communication of illness-related information to family (Davison & Degner, 1997). The benefits of providing information to partners are unknown.

LITERATURE REVIEW

Davison and Degner (1997) measured the effect of providing self-efficacy information to a group of men who were newly diagnosed with prostate cancer and measured an assumed-decisional role as the primary patient outcome. Men received either a written information package or an intervention that consisted of a written information package with discussion, a list of questions they could ask their physicians, and an opportunity to have their medical consultations audiotaped. Because the majority of men were married, they were encouraged to have their partners present during the treatment discussion with their physicians. The intervention resulted in lowering men's levels of state anxiety at six weeks following the treatment decision and men assuming more active roles in treatment decision making than originally preferred. Men reported that all three parts of the intervention were important. Married men from both groups reported that their wives read all or most of the information package. This information intervention was shown to be effective in helping men to assume a more active role in treatment decision making. The authors suggested that further efforts be made to include spouses in all treatment-related information sessions and to study how partners wished to be involved in the treatment decisions with their spouses.

Men with prostate cancer and their partners experience a variety of stressful events at the time of diagnosis that could place them at risk for poor psychological and emotional adjustment. Fear of cancer contributes to anxiety, helplessness, and loss of control. In a literature review by Northouse and Peters-Golden (1993) about the impact of cancer on spouses, three specific concerns were identified as universal to spouses of patients with cancer: dealing with the fear and threat associated with a cancer diagnosis, helping partners to deal with the emotional repercussions of the cancer, and managing changes and disruptions of daily life brought on by disease. Additional concerns included lack of information, obstacles encountered when seeking information to make a treatment decision, perceived lack of time physicians spent explaining treatment options, difficulties getting second opinions from physicians other than urologists, and lack of information at the time of discharge to deal with symptoms (Heyman & Rosner, 1996; Oberst & James, 1985; Oberst & Scott, 1988; O'Rourke & Germino, 1998).

The immediate postoperative period has been identified as the most stressful for men with prostate cancer and their families (Moore & Estey, 1999). Spouses and family members have been identified as the two most important and available sources of support. However, spouses should not automatically be regarded as the natural support system because evidence suggests that a mutuality of psychological response between patients with cancer and their family members exists (Baider, Ever-Hadani, & De-Nour, 1995; Cassileth et al., 1985). The degree of psychological distress also has been shown to vary throughout the course of the illness. The crisis of a cancer diagnosis and treatment is not resolved for patients or their spouses, even at three to six months postdischarge (Oberst & Scott, 1988). In fact, the crisis has been shown to worsen at the time of treatment and in the palliative care phase (Cassileth et al., 1985). Oberst and Scott reported that all surgically treated patients with cancer in their study reported severe distress at 10 days postdischarge, with spouses' levels of anxiety being significantly higher than patients' during hospitalization and the predischarge period. In addition, Oberst and James (1985) reported that the incidence of spouses reporting illnesses and somatic complaints was increased 30–90 days after discharge, as concerns shifted to their own health and the impact of cancer on their life. Costello and Kiernan (1993) also identified admission for surgery and time of discharge as extremely anxiety provoking for men with prostate cancer. Currently, research is unclear as to whether assessing and providing information to patients with cancer and their partners at the time of diagnosis will lessen psychological distress.

Certain sociodemographic and disease-related variables have been reported to be associated with levels of psychological distress experienced by patients with cancer and their partners. Edlund and Sneed (1989) reported that although the youngest group (<50 years of age) experienced the most distress in learning of their diagnosis, the oldest group (>70 years of age) experienced significantly less psychological distress than all other age groups. Baider et al. (1995) indicated that male patients and their partners reported minimal amounts of distress and appeared to be better adjusted than couples where the patients were female. Stage of illness also has been reported to be correlated significantly with adaptation among patients' significant others, with spouses being more distressed by the frequency of physical symptoms and role limitations (Ell, Nishimoto, Mantell, & Hamovitch, 1988). More specifically, partners of men with prostate cancer have been reported to have significantly greater levels of psychological distress when their husbands' disease was more advanced (Kornblith, Herr, Ofman, Scher, & Holland, 1994). In contrast, Cassileth et al. (1985) reported that variables such as age, sex, time since diagnosis, and clinical factors did not have an influence on levels of anxiety, mood disturbance, or global mental health of patients with cancer.

CONCEPTUAL FRAMEWORK

Lazarus' Transactional Model of Stress and Coping (Lazarus & Folkman, 1984) provided a framework to explain how men and their partners cope with the stress and uncertainty of a prostate cancer diagnosis. Individuals use cognitive appraisal to (a) evaluate how such an event affects their well-being (primary appraisal or stress), (b) assess available resources or options to deal with or mediate the situation (secondary appraisal or coping), (c) evaluate how effective specific actions have been (reappraisal or modifications), and (d) subsequently adjust to the stimulus-stressor (adaptation or outcome). Information seeking is identified as the most frequent method individuals use to cope with and maintain control over a stressful life event (Cohen & Lazarus, 1979). Information is conceptualized as a form of cognitive control because it provides individuals with a way to interpret events and take action to lessen the threat or impact of the event. The model is transactional because individuals constantly are interacting with their environment and making decisions based on personal and situational factors. Study hypotheses empirically tested how

providing individuals with the type of information they preferred would help them to cope with the stress of a prostate cancer diagnosis (as indicated by levels of psychological distress) and the extent to which they chose to assume control in making a treatment decision. Lazarus and Folkman (1984) suggested that to adequately measure coping, individuals must be assessed at several points over time. Empirical testing of how such an information intervention affects reappraisal and adaptation will be tested in a future longitudinal study.

STUDY PURPOSE AND HYPOTHESES

The purpose of the current study was to determine whether providing individualized information to men who were newly diagnosed with prostate cancer and their partners would lower their levels of psychological distress and enable them to be more actively involved in treatment decision making. Researchers hypothesized that at four months following the individualized information counseling session, patients and their partners would report lower levels of state anxiety and depression, patients would report they had assumed a more active role in medical decision making than they originally had preferred to play, and partners would report that they had assumed a more active role in their spouses' treatment choice than they originally had preferred to play.

METHODS

Participants

A consecutive sample of 80 couples referred to the Prostate Centre at Vancouver General Hospital was recruited for the study. Several urologists practicing in greater Vancouver currently refer patients to the center at the time of diagnosis to access informational resources. Criteria for study participation included patients who were aware of their diagnosis, had their initial treatment consultation, were able to read and speak

English, showed no evidence of mental confusion, and were in an ongoing relationship. "Ongoing relationship" was defined as men who were married, living with common-law partners, or living in same-sex relationships. Partners also were required to speak and read English.

Instruments

The **Patient Information Program (PIP)** is a computer program that was developed to measure information and decision preferences of men with prostate cancer and their partners. This was the first time PIP was used with patients and their partners. PIP consists of two tools previously used to measure decision and information preferences of men newly diagnosed with prostate cancer (Davison & Degner, 1997; Davison et al., 1995). A detailed description of the analytic procedures involved in the development of PIP recently has been published (Davison et al., 2002).

The first part of PIP uses a computerized version of the **Control Preferences Scale (CPS)**, a card sort developed by Degner and Sloan (1992) to elicit patients' preferences for control over treatment decision making. The tool consists of five statements about different roles that individuals can assume in treatment decision making. The five statements are presented in fixed-order pairs to participants who are asked to select their preferred choice. Previous use of CPS demonstrated that 82% of the decisional preferences of men who were newly diagnosed with prostate cancer fell into the psychological dimension of a preference about keeping, sharing, or giving away control of treatment decision making to their physicians (Davison & Degner, 1997). Statements used to measure partners' preferred roles in decision making were derived from the original CPS statements (Figure 1). All statements were changed to the past tense, and a "pick one" methodology was used to measure the roles patients and their partners reported they had assumed in the treatment decision-making process. For example, the statement "I prefer to leave all decisions regarding my treat-

Active
- I prefer to make the final treatment decision.
- I prefer to make the final treatment decision after seriously considering my doctor's (partner's) opinion.

Collaborative
- I prefer that my doctor (partner) and I share responsibility for deciding which treatment is best.

Passive
- I prefer that my doctor (partner) makes the final treatment decision but seriously considers my opinion.
- I prefer to leave all treatment decisions to my doctor (partner).

Figure 1. Statements in Control Preferences Scale for Patients and Partners

ment to my doctor (partner)," now read "I left all decisions regarding my treatment to my doctor (partner)."

The second part of PIP consists of a computerized version of a paper-and-pencil **survey questionnaire** previously developed and used by Davison et al. (1995) to assess the information needs of a group of men who were newly diagnosed with prostate cancer. The nine categories and descriptive statements include prognosis (likelihood of cure), stage of disease (spread and extent of cancer), side effects (possible side effects of treatment), treatment options (treatments available), social activities (impact on work, daily activities, and social life), family risk (hereditary risks of prostate cancer), home self-care (healthcare needs during and following treatment), impact on family (helping family members deal with cancer diagnosis), and sexuality (treatment options and counseling for sexual concerns). The information categories were presented in pairs using a Thurstone methodology (Thurstone, 1974) and in a fixed order using Ross's matrix of optimal ordering (Ross, 1974). Participants selected the one information category from each pair that was most important that day. Davison et al. (1995) previously had reported that this questionnaire demonstrated moderate agreement among profiles of men who were newly diagnosed with prostate cancer as indicated by Kendall's coefficient of agreement ($W = 0.248$).

The **Spielberger State Anxiety Inventory (STAI-Y Form),** a 20-item self-report (Spielberger, Gorsuch, & Lushene, 1970), was used to measure how participants were feeling "at that moment." **Reliability coefficients** in the alpha coefficient range of 0.83-0.94 have been reported in studies conducted with surgically treated patients with cancer (Oberst & Scott, 1988), patients newly diagnosed with prostate cancer (Davison & Degner, 1997), and patients being asked about their prostate cancer screening preferences (Davison, Kirk, Degner, & Hassard, 1999). Mean state anxiety scores for working male and female subjects between the ages of 50-69 years have been reported as 35.72 (SD = 10.34) and 32.2 (SD = 8.67), respectively (Spielberger et al., 1970).

The **Center for Epidemiologic Studies Depression Scale (CES-D),** a 20-item self-report, was used to measure levels of depression. Originally developed to measure depressive symptoms in the general population, CES-D has been used in research on the psychosocial health of patients with cancer. Each item is scored on a four-point scale (0-3), with higher scores indicating more severe symptoms. The total score can range from 0-60. Radloff (1977) recommended that respondents scoring more than 16 should be screened for a diagnosis of major depression. An internal consistency **reliability** of 0.87 was reported in a 1998 study that was conducted to examine the psychometric properties of this scale in patients newly diagnosed with cancer (Beeber, Shea, & McCorkle, 1998). A sociodemographic questionnaire was used to gather personal data and record disease-related information.

Procedure

The present study used a one-arm, quasi-experimental, pretest/post-test design. Data collection commenced following ethical approval of the study protocol by the appropriate institutional review committees. The first author provided an explanation of the purpose of the study and obtained written consent from each participant who had made an appointment at the Prostate Centre to access information. The first author conducted all interviews. Two couples who met the study criteria refused to participate in this study. Six of the original 80 participating couples dropped out of the study. This article reports on data from 74 couples who completed interviews at the time of diagnosis and again at four months.

At the first interview, each participant completed the sociodemographic questionnaire, STAI, and CES-D measures and was assisted in using the computer program. Patients completed one arm of the computer program that included measurement of preferred role in making a treatment decision with their doctors, preferred role in making a treatment decision, with their partners, and information preferences. Partners completed another arm of the computer program that included two sections: preferred role in making a treatment decision with patients and information preferences. Although couples completed the paper questionnaires and computer program in the same room, every effort was made to ensure all participants completed the study protocol without input from their spouse or partner. For example, while patients completed questionnaires, their partners used the computer program.

Graphic printouts of each part of the computer program were used to guide the individualized information counseling session with each couple. For example, patients received a graphic printout of the role they wished to play in making a treatment decision with their physicians, the role they wished to play in making a treatment decision with their partners, and a hierarchical profile of the information categories they considered most important to discuss that day. Partners received graphic printouts displaying the role they wished to play in patients' treatment decision and a hierarchical profile of information categories they thought were most important to them that day. Different roles patients could play in making a treatment decision with physicians were discussed in the context of patients' preferred role. Preferred role expectations of each member of the couple also was discussed.

Information categories identified by each participant as being the most important were identified, compared, and confirmed. The type and amount of information provided in the counseling session differed according to individual couples' information profiles. Information was discussed within the context of each patient's specific disease characteristics. The physician referral information included treatments recommended, prostate-specific antigen (PSA) blood test result at the time of diagnosis, histologic grade of cancer (Gleason score), clinical stage of disease, and biopsy results. For example, if side effects was chosen as a main information category, side effects associated with each of the physician-recommended treatment options were identified, described, and discussed within the context of how each would affect patients' and their partners' future lifestyles. All participants also were asked to identify other methods they wished to use to access additional information. Method choices included written information and videos, as well as lists of suggested Internet sites, questions to ask physicians, and local prostate support groups. These supplemental resources were provided to couples at the end of the counseling session. Participants were encouraged to call their physicians to discuss specific questions relating to their disease and treatment.

All couples were telephoned by the first author approximately three months following the initial interview to arrange second interviews at the center. At the second interview, participants completed the STAI. CES-D, and CPS (pick one statement) measures.

Data Analysis

SPSS 9.0® (SPSS Inc., Chicago, IL) was used to analyze the data. The study's directional hypotheses were tested on a one-tailed basis. Thurstone scaling data analysis was conducted using the Statistical Analysis System® (SAS Institute, Inc., Cary, NC). A 0.05 critical value of alpha was used to determine statistical significance.

Coombs' (1976) unfolding theory was used to confirm that patients and their partners did perceive their decision preferences along a single dimension. This scaling method is based on the theory of preferential choice. Participants were asked to rank the statements in terms of their proximity to their personal preference. Individual preference orders were unfolded to determine whether they were consistent with the existence of an underlying psychological dimension, providing a direct test of the hypothesis that participants do have systematic preferences about the degree of control they want in treatment decision making, ranging from no control to complete control. Preference orders fell on the dimension if they were in a sequence that captured the hypothetical rank order of the decisional roles and the midpoints between them. The combination of the five decisional roles and their midpoints produced a dimension with 12 possible sets of 11 response patterns each. Coombs set the criterion for accepting the dimensionality of any particular scale at 50% plus one of observed preference orders having unfolded onto the dimension. Several articles have been published to provide a detailed description of the analytic methods (Degner, Sloan, & Venkatesh, 1997; McIver & Carmines, 1991).

Men's preferred roles with physicians and partner's preferred roles with patients were found to be valid (according to Coombs' [1976] criterion) at 62% and 81%, respectively. However, only 45% of men's preferred roles with partners were found to be valid. When an invalid sequence was identified on the computer printout, participants were presented with a list of the five statements of the CPS, and they were asked to pick the role they preferred. This choice was the same as the computer-generated first choice in the majority of preferred role selections; patients with physician (86%), patients with partners (88%), and partners with patients (100%). For example, 36 of the 43 invalid "patients' preferred role with partners" were the same as the statement selected from the CPS.

Preferred and assumed decisional categories were collapsed into active (A, B), collaborative (C), and passive (D, E) for analysis. Chi-square tests were used to measure differences between patients' and partners' preferred and assumed roles. Chi-square tests also were used to identify differences in decision preferences (assuming a less active role than originally preferred, the same role, or a more active role than originally preferred) according to study demographic variables (age, education, stage of disease, and treatment status).

Two measures of reliability were used in the analysis of the computerized version of the information preferences questionnaire (Davison et al., 2002). Kendall's coefficient of agreement demonstrated moderate agreement among profiles of men (W = 0.31) and partners (W = 0.29) in their paired comparative judgments. However, participants' individual responses, as measured by the Gulliksen and Tukey reliability measure, indicated high reliability for men ($R^2 = 0.938$) and partners ($R^2 = 0.946$).

The STAI and CES-D are unidimensional scales and were considered to have interval levels of data. The internal consistency values of these scales, as measured by Cronbach's alpha were as follows: (a) STAI-pretest (patients = 0.934, partners = 0.931), post-test (patients = 0.859, partners = 0.902), (b) CES-D pretest (patients = 0.881, partners = 0.911), post-test (patients = 0.923, partners = 0.94). Student-paired t tests were used to identify differences between the pre- and post-test scores of men and their partners. One-way analysis of variance statistical procedures were used to measure differences in levels of anxiety and depression according to participants who assumed a less active role than originally preferred, the same role, or a more active role than originally preferred.

RESULTS

Patient Characteristics

Seventy-four of the original 80 couples who agreed to participate in this study completed

TABLE 1 **Participant Characteristics**

Variable	Men (N = 74)		Partners (N = 74)	
	n	%	n	%
Age (years)				
X̄	62.2		58.1	
SD	6.9		8.8	
40-49	2	3	12	16
50-59	23	31	27	37
60-69	41	55	29	39
70-79	8	11	6	8
Education				
< Hight school	14	19	8	11
High school	20	27	22	30
> High school	40	54	44	60
Employment Status				
Full-time	34	46	15	20
Part-time	4	5	14	19
Retired	36	49	31	42
Unemployed	–	–	14	19
Residence				
Urban	56	76	–	–
Rural	18	24	–	–

Note: Because of rounding. not all percentages total 100.

both sets of questionnaires (Table 1). The second set of questionnaires was mailed in a self-addressed envelope to 20 couples who were unable to travel to the center. One of the six couples that withdrew from the study had a marriage breakup, and the other five did not return calls or questionnaires. Couples that withdrew were not remarkably different from the other couples.

The mean age of patients was 62.2 years (SD = 6.9) with a range of 41-79 years. Fifty-four percent of patients had more than a high school diploma, and 51% were employed on a full-time or part-time basis. Partners ranged in age from 29-76 years with a mean age of 58.1 years (SD = 8.8), and 60% had greater than a high school diploma. The majority (61%) of partners were not working outside the home. Ninety percent of couples were married, and 10% were cohabiting. The sample included one same-sex couple.

Seventy-three patients had clinical stage T1 or T2 prostate cancer, 70% had Gleason scores of 6 or 7, and 70% had PSA scores of less than 10. Radical prostatectomy was the treatment of choice for approximately three-quarters of patients. Fifty-one percent of patients had received definitive treatment at the time of the second interview. Range of time to second interviews was 3.5-5 months.

Preferred and Assumed Roles in Treatment Decision Making

Patients with physicians: The majority of patients had a preference to play either an active (51%) or collaborative (42%) role in decision making with their physician. However, a significantly higher proportion of patients reported assuming a more active role in making their treatment decision than originally intended (x^2 [2, n = 74] = 15.02, p < 0.001) (see Table 2). Age (<60 years versus ≥60 years) (x^2 [2, n = 74] = 2.30, p > 0.1), level of education (≤ grade 12 versus > grade 12) (x^2 [2, n = 74] = 4.84, p > 0.1), and status of definitive treatment at time of second measurement (completed versus not completed) (x^2 [2, n = 74] = 1.15, p = 0.56) were not found to be predictive of assuming a more or less active role in treatment decision making than originally intended.

Patients with Partners

Forty-seven percent of patients wanted to either make the treatment decision alone (10%) or after seriously considering their partners' opinions (37%), and 54% wanted to share the decision making with their partner. The roles that patients preferred their partners to play in their treatment choice and the roles they thought their partners had played were not significantly different from one another (x^2 [2, n = 74] = 2.76) (see Table 2). Definitive treatment status (completed versus not completed at time of second interview) (x^2 [2, n = 74] = 0.56, p = 0.76) and level of education (≤ grade 12 versus > grade 12) (x^2 [2, n = 74] = 1.03, p > 0.1) were not shown to have an influ-

TABLE 2 **Preferred and Assumed Roles in Treatment Decision Making**

Control Preferences Scale Statement[a]	Active		Collaborative		Passive	
	n	%	n	%	n	%
Patient with doctor						
Preferred	38	51	31	42	5	7
Assumed	58	78	10	14	6	8
Patient with partner						
Preferred	34	46	40	54	–	–
Assumed	44	60	30	41	–	–
Partner with patient						
Preferred	2	3	41	55	31	42
Assumed	–	–	12	16	62	84

N = 74
[a] See Figure 1.

ence on the roles patients assumed versus the role they originally preferred to play with their partner. The impact of patients' ages was not able to be determined because of the small sample size. However, a trend was identified for men who were older than 60 to have a preference for their partners to be more active in the treatment decision-making process.

Partners with Patients

Partners had a preference to play either a collaborative (55%) or passive (42%) role in the treatment decision making. In the passive group (n = 31), 23 partners wanted the patient to made the decision after considering their opinion and 8 partners wanted the patient to make the decision himself. Only two women wanted to make the decision for their husband. A significantly higher proportion of the partners reported assuming a more passive role in the treatment decision than originally preferred (x^2 [1, n = 74] = 29.42, p < 0.0001) (Table 2). Of the 62 partners who reported assuming a passive role in the treatment decision making, 52 reported that the patients had made the decision after considering their opinion, and 10 partners reported that patients had made the treatment decision themselves.

Levels of Psychological Distress

Compared to the time of the first interview, all participants reported significantly lower levers of state anxiety and depression at the time of completing the second set of questionnaires. Partners' levels of state anxiety were slightly higher than previously reported values of employed female subjects at the time of both interviews (Table 3). Patients' state anxiety scores were within the reported normal limits by the time of the second interview. All participants reported depression scores that were within normal limits at both interviews.

Patients' levels of psychological distress did not have a significant influence on the roles they reported assuming versus the roles they originally had preferred to play with either their physician anxiety (F [2, 70] = 1.03, p = 0.36) and depression (F [2, 70] = 0.48, p = 0.62) or partner anxiety (F [2, 70] = 1.27, p = 0.29) and depression (F [2, 70] = 1.50, p = 0.23). Similarly, partners' levels of anxiety (F [2, 70] = 0.28, p = 0.76) and depression (F [2, 70] = 0.32, p = 0.73) were not found to have a significant effect on the role they preferred to play with patients in treatment decision making versus the role they actually assumed.

DISCUSSION

Results of this study supported the hypotheses that providing individualized information to these patients and their partners at the time of diagnosis does have potential beneficial effects, such as lowering couples' levels of psychological distress and enabling patients to participate more actively a medical decision making. The hypothesis that partners would assume a more active role in decision making than originally intended following the provision of an individualized information counseling session was not supported.

Patients in this study did report that they had assumed a more active role than originally intended. Several possible explanations could account for this finding, but the most plausible explanation is that providing information in the contend of a counseling session lowered their levels of psychological distress; this enabled them to assume more control in the decision-making process. Steginga et al. (2001) also reported on the importance men with prostate cancer attach to information resources and counseling services, especially at the time of diagnosis. Similar results were reported in two randomized clinical trials conducted with men newly diagnosed with prostate cancer (Davison & Degner, 1997) and men making a prostate cancer screening decision (Davison et al., 1999). Men in these studies reported assuming more active roles in making medical decisions than originally preferred fol-

TABLE **3 Levels of State Anxiety and Depression**

Characteristic	$\overline{X}$	SD	t test[a]	p
Men (N = 73)				
State anxiety				
● Pretest	41.92	12.03	5.03	0.000
● Post-test	35.58	10.82	–	–
Depression				
● Pretest	11.49	8.21	2.42	0.018
● Post-test	9.21	7.93	–	–
Partners (N = 73)				
State anxiety				
● Pretest	45.10	12.23	4.60	0.000
● Post-test	38.32	12.14	–	–
Depression				
● Pretest	15.15	10.94	3.27	0.002
● Post-test	11.04	9.58	–	–

[a] Student-paired t test. One couple did not complete second set of questionnaires. Mean state anxiety scores for working male and female subjects between the ages of 50-69 have been reported as 35.72 (SD = 10.34) and 32.2 (SD = 8.67), respectively (Spielberger et al., 1970). Depression scores greater than 16 were considered clinically relevant (Radloff, 1977).

lowing a coaching type of information intervention. Although the finding from the current study is that the patients and their partners chose to be proactive, other factors may provide a reasonable explanation for their actions, because patients receive information from multiple sources and the uncontrolled design of this study cannot confirm this conclusion.

Approximately half of the partners in this study had a preference to play a collaborative role with their spouses in choosing a definitive treatment for prostate cancer. However, the majority of partners in this study reported that they had assumed a supportive role. Most partners reported that patients "made the final treatment decision after seriously considering their opinions." The most frequent rationale given by partners for assuming this role was that it was not their body so the final choice had to be made by their spouses, as they would have to live with the consequences of the treatment chosen. Similarly, O' Rourke (1997, 1999) and O'Rourke and Germino (1998) reported that partners deferred treatment decisions to their husbands and denied having an influence on the definitive treatment choice. One explanation for this finding is that the additional information partners received made them aware of the high degree of uncertainty surrounding each treatment choice and that this knowledge resulted in them not wanting to assume responsibility for the potential consequences of such a decision. Perhaps these partners should have been asked about how they used the information to help them make sense of the treatments that are available for prostate cancer. Still another reason is that partners' levels of anxiety precluded them from assuming more control in the decision-making process.

Partners' levels of state anxiety were lower at the time of the second interview, but still higher than working women in the general population. This finding was not surprising because almost half of the patients were recovering from surgery and many of the partners reported that they were assuming more household and daily responsibil-

ities. At the time of the second interview, partners also expressed concerns about helping their husbands deal with the impending treatment or side effects of treatments and concealing fears of recurrence. Oberst and Scott (1988) also reported that spouses of patients with cancer had higher levels of distress from one to three months following surgery when the spouses' concerns started to shift from the patient's health to how the illness was going to affect their life. Perhaps another session may have been required specifically for partners to discuss their concerns and address more practical issues such as home self-care and usual timing of medical follow-up appointments. Because the current study only had one same-sex couple, making any conclusions regarding differences in how male and female partners cope with a prostate cancer diagnosis was not possible. Providing pertinent treatment-related homecare information and emotional support to partners is certainly an area that requires further study.

Limitations

Study design, sample recruitment, and generalizability to other patient populations were identified as major limitations of this study. Without a control group, investigators cannot conclude with certainty that the benefits reported were actually the result of the information counseling session. Recruitment procedures also were **biased** because urologists only referred patients they thought would be interested in accessing information and willing to participate in such a study. The inclusion of all men at the time of diagnosis from a variety of community urology practices would have been valuable, but only men who wanted more information than was already provided by their urologist came to the center. In addition, the demographic profile of couples attending this metropolitan, university-affiliated center may not be generalizable to other community urology practices. Cultural issues also were not addressed because only patients who spoke and understood English were asked to participate in the study.

NURSING IMPLICATIONS

Evidence exists to demonstrate the need to provide information to patients who are newly diagnosed with prostate cancer and their partners at the time of diagnosis to facilitate treatment decision making. The PIP computer program used in this study proved useful in focusing the information counseling session and addressing questions and concerns pertaining to information priorities and related concerns on that particular day. Using this categorical approach to guide the delivery of information was found to be a reasonable and time-effective means of providing decisional support in an outpatient setting. This methodology also was able to address the variation between what information healthcare providers believe patients should receive versus what patients actually want to learn. For example, some patients ranked sexuality as the most important information need and wanted all information provided within the context of how treatment choice would affect this aspect of their lives. Additional information resources also were found to assist individuals in addressing questions or concerns that arose following the counseling session. Physicians and other oncology healthcare professionals could use this computer program to guide treatment-related discussions. The efficacy of using this approach with other newly diagnosed patients with cancer requires further study.

SUMMARY

In conclusion, results of this study suggest that assisting men and their partners in identifying and discussing the information they consider important at the time of diagnosis is beneficial. Counseling couples at the time of diagnosis using this type of approach enables couples to access information that is both timely and relevant. A research study currently is under way to evaluate this approach within the context of a randomized clinical trial design.

The authors acknowledge the following urologists in recruitment of patients for this study in Vancouver: K. Carlson, MD, V. Chow, MD, H. Fenster, MD. M. McLoughlin, MD, M. Nigro, MD, W. Taylor, MD, and J. Wright, MD.

Author Contact: B. Joyce Davison, RN, PhD, can be reached at jdavison@vanhosp.bc.ca, with copy to editor at rose_mary@earthlink.net.

REFERENCES

Baider, L., Ever-Hadani, P., & De-Nour, A.K. (1995). The impact of culture on perception of patient-physician satisfaction. *Israel Journal of Medical Science, 31*, 179-185.

Beeber, L.S., Shea, J., & McCorkle, R. (1998). The Center for Epidemiologic Studies Depression Scale as a measure of depressive symptoms in newly diagnosed patients. *Journal of Psychosocial Oncology, 16*(1), 1-20.

Beisecker, A.E., & Moore, W.P. (1994). Oncologists' perceptions of the effects of cancer patients' companions on physician-patient interactions. *Journal of Psychosocial Oncology, 12*(1/2), 23-39.

Brawley, O.W., & Barnes, S. (2001). The epidemiology of prostate cancer in the United States. *Seminars in Oncology Nursing, 17*, 72-77.

Cassileth, B.R., Lusk, E.J., Strouse, T.B., Miller, D.S., Brown, L.L., & Cross, P.A. (1985). A psychological analysis of cancer patients and their next-of-kin. *Cancer, 55*, 72-76.

Cohen, F., & Lazarus, R.D. (1979). Coping with stress of illness. In G.C. Stone, F. Cohen, & N.E. Adler (Eds.), *Health psychology* (pp. 217-224). San Francisco: Jossey-Bass.

Coombs, C.H. (1976). *A theory of data.* Ann Arbor, MI: Mathesis Press.

Costello, D., & Kiernan, M. (1993). Patients with radical prostatectomy: Postdischarge telephone calls. *Urologic Nursing, 13*(2), 55-57.

Davison, B.J., & Degner, L.F. (1997). Empowerment of men newly diagnosed with prostate cancer. *Cancer Nursing, 20*, 187-196.

Davison, B.J., Degner, L.F., & Morgan, T.R. (1995). Information and decision-making preferences of men with prostate cancer. *Oncology Nursing Forum, 22,* 1401-1408.

Davison, B.J., Gleave, M.E., Goldenberg, S.L., Degner, L.F., Hoffart, D., & Berkowitz, J. (2002). Assessing information and decision preferences of men with prostate cancer and their partners. *Cancer Nursing, 25,* 42-49.

Davison, B.J., Kirk, P., Degner, L.F., & Hassard, T.H. (1999). Information and patient participation in screening for prostate cancer. *Patient Education and Counseling, 37,* 255-263.

Degner, L.F., & Sloan, J.A. (1992). Decision-making during serious illness: What role do patients really want to play? *Journal of Clinical Epidemiology, 45,* 941-950.

Degner, L.F., Sloan, J.A., & Venkatesh, P. (1997). The control preferences scale. *Canadian Journal of Nursing Research, 29*(3), 21-43.

Edlund, B., & Sneed, N.V. (1989). Emotional responses to the diagnosis of cancer: Age-related comparisons. *Oncology Nursing Forum, 16,* 691-697.

Ell, O., Nishimoto, R.H., Mantell, J.E., & Hamovitch, H.B. (1988). Psychological adaptation to cancer: A comparison among patients, spouses, and non-spouses. *Family Systems Medicine, 6,* 335-348.

Heyman, E.N., & Rosner, T.T. (1996). Prostate cancer: An intimate view from patients and wives. *Urologic Nursing, 16*(2), 37-44.

Jemal, A., Thomas, A., Murray, T., & Thun, M. (2002). Cancer statistics 2002. *CA: A Cancer Journal for Clinicians, 52,* 23-47.

Kornblith, A.B., Herr, H.W., Ofman, U.S., Scher, H.I., & Holland, J.C. (1994). Quality of life of patients with prostate cancer and their spouses: The value of a database in clinical care. *Cancer, 73,* 2791-2802.

Lazarus, R.S., & Folkman, S. (1984). *Stress, appraisal and coping.* New York: Springer.

McIver, J.P., & Carmines, E.G. (1991). *Unidimensional scaling.* Thousand Oaks. CA: Sage.

McPherson, C.P., Swenson, K.K., & Kjellberg, J. (2001). Quality of life in patients with prostate cancer. *Seminars in Oncology Nursing, 17,* 138-146.

Moore, K.N., & Estey, A. (1999). The early post-operative concerns of men after radical prostatectomy. *Journal of Advanced Nursing, 29,* 1121-1129.

National Cancer Institute of Canada. (2002). *Canadian cancer statistics 2002.* Toronto, Canada: Author.

Northouse, L.L., & Peters-Golden, H. (1993). Cancer and the family: Strategies to assist spouses. *Seminars in Oncology Nursing, 9,* 74-82.

Oberst, M.T., & James, R.H. (1985). Going home: Patient and spouse adjustment following cancer surgery. *Topics in Clinical Nursing, 7*(1), 46-57.

Oberst, M.T., & Scott, D.W. (1988). Post-discharge distress in surgically treated cancer patients and their spouses. *Research in Nursing and Health, 11,* 223-233.

Onel, E., Hamond, C., Wasson. J.H., Berlin, B.B., Ely, M.G., Laudone, V.P., et al. (1998). Assessment of the feasibility and impact of shared decision making in prostate cancer. *Urology, 51,* 63-66.

O'Rourke, M.E. (1997). *Prostate cancer treatment selection: The family decision process.* Unpublished doctoral dissertation, University of North Carolina. Chapel Hill, NC.

O'Rourke, M.E. (1999). Narrowing the options: The process of deciding on prostate cancer treatment. *Cancer Investigation, 17,* 349-359.

O'Rourke, M.E. (2001). Decision making and prostate cancer treatment selection: A review. *Seminars in Oncology Nursing, 17,* 108-117.

O'Rourke, M.E., & Germino, B.B. (1998). Prostate cancer treatment decisions: A focus group exploration. *Oncology Nursing Forum, 25,* 97-104.

Radloff, L.S. (1997). The CES-D scale: A self-report depression scale for research in the general population. *Applied Psychological Measurement, 1,* 385-401.

Ross, R.T. (1974). Optimal orders in the method of paired comparisons. In G.M. Maranell (Ed.). *Scaling: A sourcebook for behavioral scientists* (pp. 106-109). Chicago: Aldine.

Spielberger, C.D., Gorsuch, R.L., & Lushene. R.L. (1970). *STAI manual.* Palo Alto. CA: Consulting Psychologists Press.

Steginga, S.K., Occhipinti, S., Dunn, J., Gardiner, R.A., Heathcote, P., & Yaxley, J. (2001). The supportive care needs of men with prostate cancer (2000). *Psycho-Oncology, 10,* 66-75.

Thurstone, L.L. (1974). A law of comparative judgment. In G.M. Maranell (Ed.). *Scaling: A sourcebook for behavioral scientists* (pp. 81-92). Chicago: Aldine.

Wong, F., Stewart, D.E., Dancey, J., Meana, M., McAndrews, M.P., Bunston, T., et al. (2000). Men with prostate cancer: Influence of psychological factors on informational needs and decision making. *Journal of Psychosomatic Research, 49*, 13-19.

FOR MORE INFORMATION . . .

- CaP Cure—Association for the Cure of Cancer of the Prostate
  www.capcure.org
- MEDLINEplus: Prostate Cancer
  www.nlm.nih.gov/medlineplus/
  prostatecancer.html
- Prostate Cancer Information
  www.prostateinfo.com

*Links can be found using ONS
Online at www.ons.org.*

Example Glossary

A

a priori From Latin: the former; before the study or analysis.

abstract A brief, comprehensive summary of a study.

Example: See Van Cleve et al. (2004, Appendix B). A brief description of the study is located at the beginning of the report.

accessible population A population that meets the population criteria and is available.

Example: See Koniak-Griffin et al. (2004, Appendix A). The accessible population was teens referred from the County Health Department in San Bernardino, California.

after-only design An experimental design with two randomly assigned groups—a treatment group and a control group. This design differs from the true experiment in that both groups are measured only after the experimental treatment.

after-only nonequivalent control group design A quasi-experimental design similar to the after-only experimental design, but subjects are not randomly assigned to the treatment or control groups.

alternate form reliability Two or more alternate forms of a measure are administered to the same subjects at different times. The scores of the two tests determine the degree of relationship between the measures.

Example: See Hoskins (1988, Chapter 15, p.17). Two forms of the Partner Relationship Inventory were used.

analysis of covariance (ANCOVA) A statistic that measures differences among group means and uses a statistical technique to equate the groups under study in relation to an important variable.

analysis of variance (ANOVA) A statistic that tests whether group means differ from each other, rather than testing each pair of means separately. ANOVA considers the variation among all groups.

Example: See Koniak-Griffin et al. (2003, Appendix A). These researchers used ANOVA to examine effects for group, time, and group by time interactions.

animal rights Guidelines used to protect the rights of animals in the conduct of research.

anonymity A research participant's protection in a study so that no one, not even the researcher, can link the subject with the information given.

antecedent variable A variable that affects the dependent variable but occurs before the introduction of the independent variable.

Example: See Koniak-Griffin et al. (2003, Appendix A). Age, educational level, and marital status are antecedent variables.

assent An aspect of informed consent that pertains to protecting the rights of children as research subjects.

Example: See Van Cleve et al. (2004, Appendix B). Parents were asked for their permission, and children in the study were asked for their assent.

assumption A basic principle assumed to be true without the need for scientific proof.

auditability The researcher's development of the research process in a qualitative study that allows a researcher or reader to follow the thinking or conclusions of the researcher.

axial coding A data-analysis strategy using the grounded theory method. It requires intense coding around a single theme.

B

beneficence An obligation to act to benefit others and to maximize possible benefits.

Example: See the Ivory Coast, Africa, AIDS/AZT study (1994, Table 13-1) for a violation of the ethical principle of beneficence.

benefit Potential positive outcomes of participation in a research study.

Example: See Koniak-Griffin et al. (2004, Appendix A). The benefits to adolescent mothers and their infants were the potential for improved maternal and infant health, improved mother-child interaction, and increased education and social competency.

bias A distortion in the data-analysis results.

Example: See Davison et al. (2003, Appendix D). Bias was involved when deciding who should be included in the study.

bracketed A process during which the researcher identifies personal biases about the phenomenon of interest to clarify how personal experience and beliefs may color what is heard and reported.

C

case studies The study of a selected phenomenon that provides an in-depth description of its dimensions and processes.

case study method The study of a selected contemporary phenomenon over time to provide an in-depth description of essential dimensions and processes of the phenomenon.

chance error Attributable to fluctuations in subject characteristics that occur at a specific point in time and are often beyond the awareness and control of the examiner. Also called random error.

Example: See Van Cleve et al. (2004, Appendix B). The researchers were missing some data because some children missed interviews.

chi-square (x^2) A nonparametric statistic that is used to determine whether the frequency found in each category is different from the frequency that would be expected by chance.

Example: See Koniak-Griffin et al. (2004, Appendix A). Chi-square is used to determine whether the differences between groups for their change in substance abuse (alcohol, smoking, and marijuana) were due to the intervention or to chance.

close-ended item Question that the respondent may answer with only one of a fixed number of choices.

Example: See Van Cleve et al. (2004, Appendix B). In The Pediatric Pain Coping Inventory for assessing children's pain, the child chooses from three responses: When I feel hurt or pain, I tell myself to be brave:

Not at all   Sometimes   A lot

cluster sampling A probability sampling strategy that involves a successive random sampling of units. The units sampled progress from large to small. Also known as multistage sampling.

cohort The subjects of a specific group that are being studied.

Example: See Davison et al. (2004, Appendix D). The cohort was men newly diagnosed with prostate cancer and their partners who participated in the study.

community-based participatory research Qualitative method that systematically accesses the voice of a community to plan context-appropriate action.

computer database Print database that is put on software programs that can be accessed online or on CD-ROM via the computer.

concealment Refers to whether the subjects know that they are being observed.

concept An image or symbolic representation of an abstract idea.

conceptual definition General meaning of a concept.

conceptual framework A structure of concepts and/or theories pulled together as a map for the study.

conceptual literature Published and unpublished non–data-based material, such as reports of theories, concepts, synthesis of research on concepts, or professional issues, some of which underlie reported research, as well as other nonresearch material.

conceptual model A set of interrelated concepts that symbolically represents a phenomenon.

concurrent validity The degree of correlation of two measures of the same concept that are administered at the same time.

conduct of research The analysis of data collected from a homogeneous group of subjects who meet study inclusion and exclusion criteria for the purpose of answering specific research questions or testing specified hypotheses.

confidence interval Quantifies the uncertainty of a statistic or the probably value range within which a population parameter is expected to lie.

Example: See Wang and Krumholz (2002, Figure 20-1). The confidence interval demonstrates that women's cardiovascular death is a statistically significant event.

confidentiality Assurance that a research participant's identity cannot be linked to the information that was provided to the researcher.

consent See *informed consent.*

consistency Data are collected from each subject in the study in exactly the same way or as close to the same way as possible.

Example: See Van Cleve et al. (2004, Appendix B). The investigators used one research associate consistently to ensure that all the interviews would be interpreted similarly.

constancy Methods and procedures of data collection are the same for all subjects.

constant comparative method A process of continuously comparing data as they are acquired during research with the grounded theory method.

Example: See Plach et al. (2004, Appendix C). The researchers compared and contrasted each woman's experience of rheumatoid arthritis with the experiences of the other study participants.

construct An abstraction that is adapted for scientific purpose.

construct replication The use of original methods, such as sampling techniques, instruments, or research design, to study a problem that has been investigated previously.

construct validity The extent to which an instrument is said to measure a theoretical construct or trait.

Example: See Van Cleve et al. (2004, Appendix B). The Adolescent Pediatric Pain Tool (APPT) has been shown to measure pain.

consumer One who actively uses and applies research findings in nursing practice.

content analysis A technique for the objective, systematic, and quantitative description of communications and documentary evidence.

Example: See Plach et al. (2004, Appendix C). The researchers examined and organized information obtained in the interviews of women with rheumatoid arthritis to identify themes.

content validity The degree to which the content of the measure represents the universe of content, or the domain of a given behavior.

Example: See Koniak-Griffin et al. (2003, Appendix A). The Shortened Acculturation Scale has content validity.

context Environment where event(s) occur(s).

contrasted-group approach A method used to assess construct validity. A researcher identifies two groups of individuals who are suspected to have an extremely high or low score on a characteristic. Scores from the groups are obtained and examined for sensitivity to the differences. Also called known-group approaches.

control Measures used to hold uniform or constant the conditions under which an investigation occurs.

control group The group in an experimental investigation that does not receive an intervention or treatment; the comparison group.

Example: See Koniak-Griffin et al. (2003, Appendix A). Mothers that received the Traditional Public Health Nursing Care were the control group. This group did not receive the Early Intervention Program.

convenience sampling A nonprobability sampling strategy that uses the most readily accessible persons or objects as subjects in a study.

Example: See Davison et al. (2003, Appendix D). The couples in the study were a convenience sample.

convergent validity A strategy for assessing construct validity in which two or more tools that theoretically measure the same construct are administered to subjects. If the measures are positively correlated, convergent validity is said to be supported.

Example: See Van Cleve et al. (2004, Appendix B). The Poker Chip Tool.

correlation The degree of association between two variables.

Example: See Koniak-Griffin et al. (2003, Appendix A). The HOME scale, a measure of the quality of the child's home environment, correlates highly with child development.

correlational study A type of nonexperimental research design that examines the relationship between two or more variables.

credibility Steps in qualitative research to ensure accuracy, validity, or soundness of data.

criterion-related validity Indicates the degree of relationship between performance on the measure and actual behavior either in the present (concurrent) or in the future (predictive).

critical reading An active interpretation and objective assessment of an article during which the reader is looking for key concepts, ideas, and justifications.

critical thinking The rational examination of ideas, inferences, principles, and conclusions.

critique The process of objectively and critically evaluating a research report's content for scientific merit and application to practice, theory, or education.

critiquing criteria The criteria used for objectively and critically evaluating a research article.

Cronbach's alpha Test of internal consistency that simultaneously compares each item in a scale to all others.

Example: See Koniak-Griffin et al. (2003, Appendix A). Cronbach's alpha was calculated for The Nursing Child Assessment Teaching Scale (NCATS).

cross-sectional study A nonexperimental research design that looks at data at one point in time, that is, in the immediate present.

culture The system of knowledge and linguistic expressions used by social groups that allows the researcher to interpret or make sense of the world.

Cumulative Index to Nursing and Allied Health Literature (CINAHL) A print or computerized database; computerized CINAHL is available on CD-ROM and online.

D

data Information systematically collected in the course of a study; the plural of datum.

database A compilation of information about a topic organized in a systematic way.

data-based literature Reports of completed research.

data saturation A point when data collection can cease. It occurs when the information being shared with the researcher becomes repetitive. Ideas conveyed by the participant have been shared before by other participants; inclusion of additional participants does not result in new ideas.

Example: See Plach et al. (2004, Appendix C). Data were collected from 20 participants using open-ended interviews. The reader could assume that data saturation had occurred by the time 20 interviews were completed.

debriefing The opportunity for researchers to discuss the study with the participants and for participants to refuse to have their data included in the study.

deductive reasoning A logical thought process in which hypotheses are derived from theory; reasoning moves from the general to the particular.

degrees of freedom The number of quantities that are unknown minus the number of independent equations linking these unknowns; a function of the number in the sample.

delimitations Those characteristics that restrict the population to a homogeneous group of subjects.

Delphi technique The technique of gaining expert opinion on a subject. It uses rounds or multiple stages of data collection, with each round using data from the previous round.

dependent variable In experimental studies, the presumed effect of the independent or experimental variable on the outcome.

Example: See Koniak-Griffin et al. (2003, Appendix A). Dependent variables were infant and maternal outcomes, such as infant emergency room visits and maternal substance abuse.

descriptive statistics Statistical methods used to describe and summarize sample data.

design The plan or blueprint for conduct of a study.

developmental study A type of nonexperimental research design that is concerned not only with the existing status and interrelationship of phenomena but also with changes that take place as a function of time.

diffusion The strategy for promoting adoption of evidence-based practices.

direct observation A method for measuring psychological and physiological behaviors for the purpose of evaluating change and facilitating recovery.

directional hypothesis Hypothesis that specifies the expected direction of the relationship between the independent and dependent variables.

Example: See Davison et al. (2003, Appendix D). Levels of psychological stress would be lower by providing individualized information to men who are newly diagnosed with prostate cancer and their partners.

dissemination The communication of research findings.

divergent validity A strategy for assessing construct validity in which two or more tools that theoretically measure the opposite of the construct are administered to subjects. If the measures are negatively correlated, divergent validity is said to be supported.

domains Symbolic categories that include the smaller categories of an ethnographic study.

downlink A receiver for programs beamed from other agencies that allows a person to participate in telecommunication conferences.

E

electronic database/electronic index The electronic means by which journal sources (periodicals) of data-based and conceptual articles on a variety of topics (e.g., doctoral dissertations) are found, as well as the publications of professional organizations and various governmental agencies.

element The most basic unit about which information is collected.

eligibility criteria Those characteristics that restrict the population to a homogeneous group of subjects.
Example: See Van Cleve et al. (2004, Appendix B). Children were invited to participate in the study if they were ages 4 to 17 years with acute lymphocytic leukemia (ALL), within 1 month of diagnosis, and either English or Spanish speaking. Also called inclusion criteria.

emic view The natives' or insiders' view of the world.

empirical The obtaining of evidence or objective data.

empirical analytical A general label for quantitative research approaches that test hypotheses.

empirical literature A synonym for data-based literature; see *data-based literature*.

Epistemology The theory of knowledge; the branch of philosophy that concerns how people know what they know.

equivalence Consistency or agreement among observers using the same measurement tool or agreement among alternate forms of a tool.

error variance The extent to which the variance in test scores is attributable to error rather than a true measure of the behaviors.

ethics The theory or discipline dealing with principles of moral values and moral conduct.

ethnographic method A method that scientifically describes cultural groups. The goal of the ethnographer is to understand the natives' view of their world.

ethnographic research See *ethnography*.

ethnography A qualitative research approach designed to produce cultural theory.

etic view An outsider's view of another's world.

evaluation research The use of scientific research methods and procedures to evaluate a program, treatment, practice, or policy outcomes; analytical means are used to document the worth of an activity.

evaluative research The use of scientific research methods and procedures for the purpose of making an evaluation.

evidence-based practice The conscious and judicious use of the current "best" evidence in the care of patients and delivery of health care services.
Example: See Titler et al. (2001, Figure 19-2). The Iowa Model of Evidence-Based Practice to Promote Quality Care.

evidence-based guidelines A set of guidelines that allow the researcher to better understand the evidence base of certain practices.

ex post facto study A type of nonexperimental research design that examines the relationships among the variables after the variations have occurred.

experiment A scientific investigation in which observations are made and data are collected by means of the characteristics of control, randomization, and manipulation.

experimental design A research design that has the following properties: randomization, control, and manipulation.
Example: See Koniak-Griffin et al. (2003, Appendix A). The subjects were place in random groups; there was a control group and the experimental group was manipulated when they received the Early Intervention Program (EIP).

experimental group The group in an experimental investigation that receives an intervention or treatment.

exploratory survey A type of nonexperimental research design that collects descriptions of existing phenomena for the purpose of using the data to justify or assess current conditions or to make plans for improvement of conditions.

external criticism A process used to judge the authenticity of historical data.

external validity The degree to which findings of a study can be generalized to other populations or environments.
Example: See Plach et al. (2004, Appendix C). The experiences of these predominantly white women with rheumatoid arthritis cannot be generalized to other racial or ethnic groups.

extraneous variable Variable that interferes with the operations of the phenomena being studied. Also called mediating variable.

Example: See Koniak-Griffin et al. (2003, Appendix A). The homogeneity of the sample was based on age and demographics. The homogeneity of the sample controls extraneous variables.

F

face validity A type of content validity that uses an expert's opinion to judge the accuracy of an instrument. (Some would say that face validity verifies that the instrument gives the subject or expert the appearance of measuring the concept.)

factor analysis A type of validity that uses a statistical procedure for determining the underlying dimensions or components of a variable.

Example: See Gary and Yarandi (2004, Chapter 15, p. 13, Table 15-2). The researchers carried out a factor analysis to determine the factor structure of the Beck Depression Inventory II (BDI-II) for African-American women.

findings Statistical results of a study.

Fisher's exact probability test A test used to compare frequencies when samples are small and expected frequencies are less than six in each cell.

fittingness Answers the questions: Are the findings applicable outside the study situation? Are the results meaningful to the individuals not involved in the research?

frequency distribution Descriptive statistical method for summarizing the occurrences of events under study.

G

generalizability (generalize) The inferences that the data are representative of similar phenomena in a population beyond the studied sample.

Example: See Van Cleve et al. (2004, Appendix B). The results of the study are generalizable only to children with leukemia.

grand theory All-inclusive conceptual structures that tend to include views on person, health, and environment to create a perspective of nursing.

grounded theory Theory that is constructed inductively from a base of observations of the world as it is lived by a selected group of people.

Example: See Calvin (2004, Chapter 7, p.15). The researcher uses interviews of dialysis patients to formulate a theory about personal preservation.

grounded theory method An inductive approach that uses a systematic set of procedures to arrive at theory about basic social processes.

H

hazard ratio A weighted relative risk based on the analysis of survival curves over the whole course of the study period.

historical research method The systematic compilation of data resulting from evaluation and interpretation of facts regarding people, events, and occurrences of the past.

history The internal validity threat that refers to events outside of the experimental setting that may affect the dependent variable.

Example: See Bull et al. (2000, Chapter 9, p. 15, Table 9-2). The study lasted for 27 months and took place in two hospitals. After the first year, both hospitals implemented strategies to decrease the length of hospital stay. The implementation of new polices may have affected patient reports of satisfaction with discharge planning.

homogeneity Similarity of conditions. Also called internal consistency.

hypothesis A prediction about the relationship between two or more variables.

hypothesis-testing validity A strategy for assessing construct validity in which the theory or concept underlying a measurement instrument's design is used to develop hypotheses that are tested. Inferences are made based on the findings about whether the rationale underlying the instrument's construction is adequate to explain the findings.

I

independent variable The antecedent or the variable that has the presumed effect on the dependent variable.

Example: See Koniak-Griffin et al. (2003, Appendix A). The independent variable was the Early Intervention Program (EIP).

inductive reasoning A logical thought process in which generalizations are developed from specific observations; reasoning moves from particular to general.

inferential statistics Procedures that combine mathematical processes and logic to test hypotheses about a population with the help of sample data.

Example: See Van Cleve et al. (2004, Appendix B). ANOVA and t test were examples of inferential statistics used in this study.

information literacy The skills needed to consult the literature and answer a clinical question.

informed consent An ethical principle that requires a researcher to obtain the voluntary participation of subjects after informing them of potential benefits and risks.

Example: See Van Cleve et al. (2004, Appendix B). Parents were asked for their permission, and children in the study were asked for their assent.

innovation diffusion Process by which an innovation or research findings are communicated through various channels over time among the members of a profession.

institutional review boards (IRBs) Boards established in agencies to review biomedical and behavioral research involving human subjects within the agency or in programs sponsored by the agency.

instrumental case study Research that is done when the researcher pursues insight into an issue or wants to challenge a generalization.

instrumentation Changes in the measurement of the variables that may account for changes in the obtained measurement.

integrative research review Synthesis review of the literature on a specific concept or topic.

internal consistency The extent to which items within a scale reflect or measure the same concept.

internal criticism A process of judging the reliability or consistency of information within a historical document.

internal validity The degree to which it can be inferred that the experimental treatment, rather than an uncontrolled condition, resulted in the observed effects.

Example: See Koniak-Griffin et al. (2003, Appendix A). Both groups demonstrated significant improvement in social competence. Was the improvement a result of the Early Intervention Program or maturation of the teen mothers? Growing up was a threat to the internal validity.

Internet The global electronic network that links a cadre of participating networks (e.g., commercial, educational, and governmental agencies).

interrater reliability The consistency of observations between two or more observers; often expressed as a percentage of agreement between raters or observers or a coefficient of agreement that takes into account the element of chance. This usually is used with the direct observation method.

Example: See Van Cleve et al. (2004, Appendix B). The investigators used one research associate consistently to ensure that all the interviews would be interpreted similarly. Interrater reliability was 99%.

interrelationship/difference studies The classification of a nonexperimental research design that attempts to trace relationships among variables. The four types are correlational, ex post facto, prediction, and developmental.

interval The level of measurement that provides different levels or gradations in response. The differences or intervals between responses are assumed to be approximately equal.

interval measurement Level used to show rankings of events or objects on a scale with equal intervals between numbers but with an arbitrary zero (e.g., centigrade temperature).

intervening variable A variable that occurs during an experimental or quasiexperimental study that affects the dependent variable.

Example: See Koniak-Griffin et al. (2003, Appendix A). Telephone interactions between the teen mothers and the nurses may have served as an unintentional intervention.

intervention Deals with whether or not the observer provokes actions from those who are being observed.

intervention fidelity Adherence and competent delivery of an intervention as detailed in a research proposal.

interviews A method of data collection in which a data collector questions a subject verbally. Interviews may be face-to-face or performed over the telephone, and they may consist of open-ended or close-ended questions.

intrinsic case study Research that is undertaken to have a better understanding of the essential nature of the case.

item to total correlation The relationship between each of the items on a scale and the total scale.

J

justice Human subjects should be treated fairly.

K

Kappa Expresses the level of agreement that is observed beyond the level that would be expected by chance alone. K > .08 is generally taken to indicate good reliability. K < .08 allows tentative conclusions to be drawn at times lower levels are accepted.

key informants Individuals who have special knowledge, status, or communication skills and who are willing to teach the ethnographer about the phenomenon.

knowledge-focused triggers Ideas that are generated when staff read research, listen to scientific papers at research conferences, or encounter evidence-based practice guidelines published by federal agencies or specialty organizations.

Kuder-Richardson (KR-20) coefficient The estimate of homogeneity used for instruments that use a dichotomous response pattern.

kurtosis The relative peakness or flatness of a distribution.

L

level of significance (alpha level) The risk of making a type I error, set by the researcher before the study begins.

levels of measurement Categorization of the precision with which an event can be measured (nominal, ordinal, interval, and ratio).

life context The matrix of human-human-environment relationships emerging over the course of one's life.

Likert-type scales Lists of statements for which respondents indicate whether they "strongly agree," "agree," "disagree," or "strongly disagree."

likelihood ratios Provide the nurse with information about the accuracy of a diagnostic test and can also help the nurse to be a more efficient decision maker by allowing the clinician to quantify the probability of disease for any individual patient.

limitation Weakness of a study.

linear structural relationships (LISREL) A computer program developed to analyze covariance and the testing of complex causal models.

literature Print and nonprint sources such as books, chapters of books, journal articles, critique reviews, abstracts published in conference proceedings, professional and governmental reports, and unpublished doctoral dissertations.

lived experience In phenomenological research a term used to refer to the focus on living through events and circumstances (prelingual) rather than thinking about these events and circumstances (conceptualized experience).

Example: See Plach et al. (2004, Appendix C). The researchers explored what it was like for these women to live with rheumatoid arthritis.

longitudinal study A nonexperimental research design in which a researcher collects data from the same group at different points in time.

Example: See Van Cleve et al. (2004, Appendix B). Data were collected on a total of seven occasions over a period of a year.

M

manipulation The provision of some experimental treatment, in one or varying degrees, to some of the subjects in the study.

matching A special sampling strategy used to construct an equivalent comparison sample group by filling it with subjects who are similar to each subject in another sample group in relation to preestablished variables, such as age and gender.

Example: See Koniak-Griffin et al. (2003, Appendix A). The teen mothers were randomly placed into the intervention group or the control group based upon maternal age, ethnicity, language, gestation age, and geographic region of residence.

maturation Developmental, biological, or psychological processes that operate within an individual as a function of time and are external to the events of the investigation.

Example: See Koniak-Griffin et al. (2003, Appendix A). Both groups demonstrated significant improvement in social competence, which may have been due to the maturation of the teen mothers.

mean A measure of central tendency; the arithmetic average of all scores.

measurement The assignment of numbers to objects or events according to rules.

measurement effects Administration of a pretest in a study that affects the generalizability of the findings to other populations.

measures of central tendency Descriptive statistical procedure that describes the average member of a sample (mean, median, and mode).

Example: See Van Cleve et al. (2004, Appendix B). The mean pain intensity scores as indicated in Table 2, p. 5, for two different age groups.

measures of variability Descriptive statistical procedure that describes how much dispersion there is in sample data.

Example: See Van Cleve et al. (2004, Appendix B). The standard deviations (SD), a measure of variability, for the mean pain intensity scores are included in Table 2, p. 5.

median A measure of central tendency; the middle score.

mediating variable A variable that is between or occurs between an independent and dependent variable and can produce an indirect effect of the independent variable on the dependent variable. Also called extraneous variable.

Example: See Koniak-Griffin et al. (2003, Appendix A). The homogeneity of the sample was based on age and demographics. The homogeneity of the sample controls mediating variables.

MEDLINE The print or computerized database of standard medical literature analysis and retrieval system online; it is also available on CD-ROM.

meta-analysis A research method that takes the results of multiple studies in a specific area and synthesizes the findings to make conclusions regarding the area of focus.

Example: See Edwards et al. (2004, Chapter 11, p. 19). The authors reviewed and combined the data of psychological interventions, with women who had metastic breast cancer, to determine if these studies demonstrated improved survival and psychological outcomes.

metasynthesis Integrates qualitative research findings on a topic and is based on comparative analysis and interpretative synthesis.

methodological research The controlled investigation and measurement of the means of gathering and analyzing data.

Example: See Barnason et al. (2002, Chapter 11, p. 17). These authors used methodological research to develop a tool to measure self-efficacy.

microrange theory The linking of concrete concepts into a statement that can be examined in practice and research.

midrange theory A focused conceptual structure that synthesizes practice-research into ideas central to the discipline.

modal percentage A measure of variability; percent of cases in the mode.

modality The number of peaks in a frequency distribution.

mode A measure of central tendency; most frequent score or result.

model A symbolic representation of a set of concepts that is created to depict relationships.

mortality The loss of subjects from time 1 data collection to time 2 data collection.

Example: See Koniak-Griffin et al. (2003, Appendix A). The sample size decreased from 144 to 101 over the 24 months of the study due to subjects dropping out of the study.

multiple analysis of variance (MANOVA) A test used to determine differences in group means; used when there is more than one dependent variable.

multiple regression Measure of the relationship between one interval level dependent variable and several independent variables. Canonical correlation is used when there is more than one dependent variable.

Example: See Zalon (2004, Chapter 16, p. 28). Pain, depression, and fatigue were variables that explained significant and different amounts of the variation in functional status and self-perception of older adults after abdominal surgery.

multistage sampling (cluster sampling) Involves a successive random sampling of units (clusters) that programs from large to small and meets sample eligibility criteria.

multitrait-multimethod approach A type of validity that uses more than one method to assess the accuracy of an instrument (e.g., observation and interview of anxiety).

N

naturalistic research A general label for qualitative research methods that involve the researcher going to a natural setting, that is, to where the phenomenon being studied is taking place.

negative predictive value Expresses the proportion of those with negative test results who truly do not have the disease.

network sampling (snowball effect sample) A strategy used for locating samples that are difficult to locate. It uses social networks and the fact that friends tend to have characteristics in common; subjects who meet the eligibility criteria are asked for assistance in getting in touch with others who meet the same criteria.

Example: See Brown (2004, Chapter 12, p. 23). Study participants were recruited at churches, cultural events, community organizations, beauty salons, and barber shops, via the Internet and newspaper ads, as well as by word-of-mouth referrals by interview participants.

nominal The level of measurement that simply assigns data into categories that are mutually exclusive.

nominal measurement Level used to classify objects or events into categories without any relative ranking (e.g., gender, hair color).

Example: See Koniak-Griffin et al. (2003, Appendix A). Ethnicity, race, and marital status are examples of nominal measurement.

nondirectional hypothesis One that indicates the existence of a relationship between the variables but does not specify the anticipated direction of the relationship.

nonequivalent control group design A quasiexperimental design that is similar to the true experiment, but subjects are not randomly assigned to the treatment or control groups.

nonexperimental research design Research design in which an investigator observes a phenomenon without manipulating the independent variable(s).

nonparametric statistics Statistics that are usually used when variables are measured at the nominal or ordinal level because they do not estimate population parameters and involve less restrictive assumptions about the underlying distribution.

nonparametric tests of significance Inferential statistics that make no assumptions about the population distribution.

nonprobability sampling A procedure in which elements are chosen by nonrandom methods.

normal curve A curve that is symmetrical about the mean and unimodal.

null hypothesis A statement that there is no relationship between the variables and that any relationship observed is a function of chance or fluctuations in sampling.

Example: See Davison et al. (2003 Chapter 16, p. 14). The hypothesis was tested by assuming that the intervention would have no effect as evidenced by no change from the pretest to the posttest.

null value In an experiment, when a value is obtained that indicates that there is no difference between the treatment and control groups.

O

objective Data that are not influenced by anyone who collects the information.

objectivity The use of facts without distortion by personal feelings or bias.

observed score The actual score obtained in a measurement.

odds ratio (OR) An estimate of relative risk used in logistic regression as a measure of association; describes the probability of an event.

Example: See Phipps et al. (2002, Chapter 20, p. 15). The probability of death of an infant in the postneonatal period increases as the mother's age declines; the OR gets larger.

ontology The study of being, of existence, and its relationship to nonexistence.

open-ended item Question that the respondent may answer in his or her own words.

Example: See Plach et al. (2004, Appendix C). Open-ended questions were used as a guide for the interviews of women with rheumatoid arthritis.

operational definition The measurements used to observe or measure a variable; delineates the procedures or operations required to measure a concept.

operationalization The process of translating concepts into observable, measurable phenomena.

Example: See Davison et al. (2003, Appendix D). The concept of "psychological distress" was defined as levels of anxiety and depression as measured by the Spielberger State Anxiety Inventory and the Center for Epidemiologic Studies Depression Scale.

ordinal The level of measurement that systematically categorizes data in an ordered or ranked manner. Ordinal measures do not permit a high level of differentiation among subjects.

ordinal measurement Level used to show rankings of events or objects; numbers are not equidistant, and zero is arbitrary (e.g., class ranking).

Example: See New York Heart Association Classification (Chapter 16, p. 6). Individuals with cardiac failure can be assigned to one of four classifications: I to IV.

P

paradigm From the Greek word meaning "pattern"; it has been applied to science to describe the way people in society think about the world.

parallel form reliability See *alternate form reliability*.

parameter A characteristic of a population.

parametric statistics Inferential statistics that involve the estimation of at least one parameter, require measurement at the interval level or above, and involve assumptions about the variables being studied. These assumptions usually include the fact that the variable is normally distributed.

path analysis A statistical technique in which the researcher hypothesizes how variables are related and in what order and then tests how strong those relationships or paths are.

Pearson correlation coefficient (Pearson *r*) A statistic that is calculated to reflect the degree of relationship between two interval level variables. Also called Pearson product moment correlation coefficient.

percentile A measure of rank; percentage of cases a given score exceeds.

phenomenological method A process of learning and constructing the meaning of human experience through intensive dialogue with persons who are living the experience.

Example: See Plach et al. (2004, Appendix C). Extensive interviews were conducted with study participants to assist the researchers in understanding what it was like to live with rheumatoid arthritis.

phenomenological research Phenomenological research is based on phenomenological philosophy and is research aimed at obtaining a description of an experience as it is lived in order to understand the meaning of that experience for those who have it.

phenomenology A qualitative research approach that aims to describe experience as it is lived through, before it is conceptualized.

philosophical beliefs The system of motivating values, concepts, principles, and the nature of human knowledge of an individual, group, or culture.

philosophical research Based on the investigation of the truths and principles of existence, knowledge, and conduct.

physiological measurement The use of specialized equipment to determine physical and biological status of subjects.

Example: See Giuliano et al. (2003, Chapter 14, p. 6). The researchers measured cardiac output and blood pressure in critically ill adults.

pilot study A small, simple study conducted as a prelude to a larger-scale study that is often called the "parent study."

Example: See Carfoot et al. (2004, Chapter 9, p. 7). The researchers used this pilot study to test an intervention and to assess their ideas in order to plan a larger study.

population A well-defined set that has certain specified properties.

Example: See Van Cleve et al. (2004, Appendix B). The population in this study is 4- to 17-year-old children with leukemia who speak either English or Spanish and are receiving care in one of three southern California hospitals.

population validity Generalization of results to other populations.

positive predictive value Expresses the proportion of those with positive test results who truly have disease.

prediction study A type of nonexperimental research design that attempts to make a forecast or prediction derived from particular phenomena.

predictive validity The degree of correlation between the measure of the concept and some future measure of the same concept.

Example: See Knauth et al. (2004, Chapter 15, p. 8). These authors evaluated the usefulness of the Differentiation of Self Inventory for Adolescents in predicting an individual's ability to differentiate between emotional and intellectual functioning.

primary source Scholarly literature that is written by person(s) who developed the theory or conducted the research. Primary sources include eyewitness accounts of historic events, provided by original documents, films, letters, diaries, records, artifacts, periodicals, or tapes.

Example: See Appendixes A, B, C, and D. All four of these studies are primary sources. See Chapter 4, p. 8, Table 4-4, for a comparison of primary and secondary sources.

print databases Indexes, card catalogues, and abstract reviews. Print indexes are used to find journal sources (periodicals) of data-based and conceptual articles on a variety of topics, as well as publications of professional organizations and various governmental agencies.

print index See *print databases*.

probability The probability of an event is the event's long-run relative frequency in repeated trials under similar conditions.

probability sampling A procedure that uses some form of random selection when the sample units are chosen.

problem statement An interrogative sentence or statement about the relationship between two or more variables.

Example: See Van Cleve et al. (2004, Appendix B). What are childrens' pain experiences, management strategies, and outcomes during the first year after the diagnosis of acute lymphocytic leukemia (ALL)?

problem-focused triggers Those that are identified by staff through quality improvement, risk surveillance, benchmarking data, financial data, or recurrent clinical problems.

process consent In qualitative research, the ongoing negotiation with subjects for their participation in a study.

product testing Testing of medical devices.

program A list of instructions in a machine-readable language written so that a computer's hardware can carry out an operation; software.

propositions The linkage of concepts that lays a foundation for the development of methods that test relationships.

prospective study Nonexperimental study that begins with an exploration of assumed causes and then moves forward in time to the presumed effect.

psychometrics The theory and development of measurement instruments.

purposive sampling A nonprobability sampling strategy in which the researcher selects subjects who are considered to be typical of the population.

Example: See Burns (2004, Chapter 12, p. 12). The researchers wanted to study the problems and coping strategies of African-Americans on hemodialysis. The 102 African-American patients who were over the age of 18 and had a confirmed diagnosis of end-stage renal disease (ESRD) requiring hemodialysis were a purposive sample.

Q

qualitative measurement The items or observed behaviors are assigned to mutually exclusive categories that are representative of the kinds of behavior exhibited by the subjects.

qualitative research The study of research questions about human experiences. It is often conducted in natural settings, and uses data that are words or text rather than numerical in order to describe the experiences that are being studied.

Example: See Plach et al. (2004, Appendix C). Extensive interviews were conducted with study participants to collect data to describe what it was like to live with rheumatoid arthritis.

quantitative measurement The assignment of items or behaviors to categories that represent the amount of a possessed characteristic.

quantitative research The process of testing relationships, differences, and cause and effect interactions among and between variables. These processes are tested with either hypotheses and/or research questions.

Example: See Appendixes A, B, and D. These three studies ask research questions and/or describe hypotheses that test relationships, assess differences, and seek to explain cause and effect interactions between variables and tests for intervention effectiveness. The numeric data are summarized and analyzed using statistics.

quasiexperiment Research designs in which the researcher initiates an experimental treatment but some characteristic of a true experiment is lacking.

quasiexperimental design A study design in which random assignment is not used but the independent variable is manipulated and certain mechanisms of control are used.

Example: See Davison et al. (2003, Appendix D). There was no control group in this study so it was not a true experiment.

questionnaires Paper and pencil instruments designed to gather data from individuals.

quota sampling A nonprobability sampling strategy that identifies the strata of the population and proportionately represents the strata in the sample.

Example: See McConnell et al. (2003, Chapter 12, p. 11). The researchers stratified nursing home residents into seven groups according to their level of cognitive impairment on admission.

R

random access memory (RAM) A computer's memory that the user can read or change.

random selection A selection process in which each element of the population has an equal and independent chance of being included in the sample.

randomization A sampling selection procedure in which each person or element in a population has an equal chance of being selected to either the experimental group or the control group.

Example: See Koniak-Griffin et al. (2003, Appendix A). Adolescent mothers were randomly assigned to be in either the control group or the experimental group.

range A measure of variability; difference between the highest and lowest scores in a set of sample data.

ratio The highest level of measurement that possesses the characteristics of categorizing, ordering, and ranking and also has an absolute or natural zero that has empirical meaning.

ratio measurement Level that ranks the order of events or objects and that has equal intervals and an absolute zero (e.g., height, weight).

reactivity The distortion created when those who are being observed change their behavior because they know that they are being observed.

Example: See Western Electric Corporation's Hawthorne Plant study (Chapter 9, p. 20). In a study of working conditions, researchers found that no matter what intervention was used workers' productivity increased. They concluded that production increased as a result of the workers' knowing that they were being studied rather than the interventions themselves. This is known as the Hawthorne effect.

recommendation Application of a study to practice, theory, and future research.

records or available data Information that is collected from existing materials, such as hospital records, historical documents, or videotapes.

refereed journal or peer-reviewed journal A scholarly journal that has a panel of external and internal reviewers or editors; the panel reviews submitted manuscripts for possible publication. The review panels use the same set of scholarly criteria to judge if the manuscripts are worthy of publication.

Example: See Chapter 4, p. 8, Box 4-3: Examples of Nursing Journals for Literature Reviews.

relationship/difference studies Studies that trace the relationships or differences between variables that can provide a deeper insight into a phenomenon.

reliability The consistency or constancy of a measuring instrument.

Example: See Davison et al. (2003, Appendix D). The Center for Epidemiologic Depression Scale (CES-D) has an internal reliability of 0.87.

reliability coefficient A number between 0 and 1 that expresses the relationship between the error variance, the true variance, and the observed score. A zero correlation indicates no relationship. The closer to 1 the coefficient is, the more reliable the tool.

Example: See Davison et al. (2003, Appendix D). The Spielberger State Anxiety Inventory (STAI-Y Form) has reliability coefficients of 0.83 to 0.94.

replication The repetition of a study that uses different samples and is conducted in different settings.

representative sample A sample whose key characteristics closely approximate those of the population.

research The systematic, logical, and empirical inquiry into the possible relationships among particular phenomena to produce verifiable knowledge.

research base The accumulated knowledge gained from several studies that investigate a similar problem.

research-based practice Nursing practice that is based on research studies, that is, supported by research findings.

research-based protocols Practice standards that are formulated from findings of several studies.

research hypothesis A statement about the expected relationship between the variables; also known as a scientific hypothesis.

research literature A synonym for data-based literature.

research problem Presents the question that is to be asked in a research study.

research question A key preliminary step wherein the foundation for a study is developed from the research problem and results in the research hypothesis.

Example: See Koniak-Griffin et al. (2003, Appendix A). The researchers question if the effect of an Early Intervention Program will last after the intervention has ended.

research utilization A systematic method of implementing sound research-based innovations in clinical practice, evaluating the outcome, and sharing the knowledge through the process of research dissemination.

respect for persons People have the right to self-determination and to treatment as autonomous agents; that is, they have the freedom to participate or not participate in research.

retrospective data Data that have been manifested, such as scores on a standard examination.

retrospective study A nonexperimental research design that begins with the phenomenon of interest (dependent variable) in the present and examines its relationship to another variable (independent variable) in the past.

Example: See Kearney et al. (2004, Chapter 11, p. 12). Data on the variables were abstracted from the medical records of 1,969 women after they had been screened for domestic abuse during pregnancy.

review of the literature An extensive, systematic, and critical review of the most important published scholarly literature on a particular topic. In most cases it is not considered exhaustive.

Example: See Davison et al. (2003, Appendix D). The researchers include an extensive literature review.

risk Potential negative outcome(s) of participation in research study.

risk-benefit ratio The extent to which the benefits of the study are maximized and the risks are minimized such that the subjects are protected from harm during the study.

S

sample A subset of sampling units from a population.

sampling A process in which representative units of a population are selected for study in a research investigation.

sampling error The tendency for statistics to fluctuate from one sample to another.

sampling frame A list of all units of the population.

Example: See Tolle et al. (2000, Chapter 12, p. 15). A sampling frame of n = 24,074 was used in this study.

sampling interval The standard distance between the elements chosen for the sample.

sampling unit The element or set of elements used for selecting the sample.

saturation See *data saturation*.

scale A self-report inventory that provides a set of response symbols for each item. A rating or score is assigned to each response.

scholarly literature Refers to published and unpublished data-based and conceptual literature materials found in print and nonprint forms.

scientific approach A logical, orderly, and objective means of generating and testing ideas.

scientific hypothesis The researcher's expectation about the outcome of a study; also known as the research hypothesis.

scientific literature A synonym for data-based literature; see *data-based literature*.

scientific merit The degree of validity of a study or group of studies.

scientific observation Collecting data about the environment and subjects. Data collection has specific objectives to guide it, is systematically planned and recorded, is checked and controlled, and is related to scientific concepts and theories.

secondary analysis A form of research in which the researcher takes previously collected and analyzed data from one study and reanalyzes the data for a secondary purpose.

Example: See Gift (2003, Chapter 11, p. 21). The researcher used the data from an earlier study on lung cancer to explore other research questions such as: "Are the severity of the cluster symptoms predictive of death?"

secondary source Scholarly material written by person(s) other than the individual who developed the theory or conducted the research. Most are usually published. Often a secondary source represents a response to or a summary and critique of a theorist's or researcher's work. Examples are documents, films, letters, diaries, records, artifacts, periodicals, or tapes that provide a view of the phenomenon from another's perspective.

Example: See Haber (2004, Chapter 11, p. 20). The author's published comment on the disappointing results of a meta-analysis she reviewed is a secondary source. See Chapter 4, p. 8, Table 4-4, for a comparison of primary and secondary sources.

selection The generalizability of the results to other populations.

selection bias The internal validity threat that arises when pretreatment differences between the experimental group and the control group are present.

Example: See Davison et al. (2003, Appendix D). Urologists selected study participants who they thought would be interested in accessing information and were willing to participate.

semiquartile range A measure of variability; range of the middle 50% of the scores. Also known as semiinterquartile range.

sensitivity The proportion of those with disease who test positive.

simple random sampling A probability sampling strategy in which the population is defined, a sampling frame is listed, and a subset from which the sample will be chosen is selected; members randomly selected.

Example: See Treat-Jacobson et al. (2004, Chapter 12, p. 15). All individuals, 21 years of age and older, scheduled for CABG surgery were identified and randomly selected for recruitment to the Post CABG Biobehavioral study.

skew Measure of the asymmetry of a set of scores.

snowball effect sampling (network sampling) A strategy used for locating samples difficult to locate. It uses the social network and the fact that friends tend to have characteristics in common; subjects who meet the eligibility criteria are asked for assistance in getting in touch with others who meet the same criteria.

social desirability The occasion when a subject responds in a manner that he or she believes will please the researcher rather than in an honest manner.

Example: See Tang et al. (2004, Chapter 18, p. 14). The interviewers read questions to the subjects, and this may have prompted the subjects to answer in a way that they thought would please the interviewer.

Solomon four-group design An experimental design with four randomly assigned groups—the pretest-posttest intervention group, the pretest-posttest control group, a treatment or intervention group with only posttest measurement, and a control group with only posttest measurement.

specificity The proportion of those without disease who test negative. It measures how well the test rules out disease when it is really absent; a specific test has few false positives.

split-half reliability An index of the comparison between the scores on one half of a test with those on the other half to determine the consistency in response to items that reflect specific content.

stability An instrument's ability to produce the same results with repeated testing.

standard deviation (SD) A measure of variability; measure of average deviation of scores from the mean.

standard error of the mean The standard deviation of a theoretical distribution of sample means. It indicates the average error in the estimation of the population mean.

statistical hypothesis States that there is no relationship between the independent and dependent variables. The statistical hypothesis also is known as the null hypothesis.

statistical reliability An index of the interval consistency of responses to all items of a single form of measure that is administered at one time.

stratified random sampling A probability sampling strategy in which the population is divided into strata or subgroups. An appropriate number of elements from each subgroup are randomly selected based on their proportion in the population.

Example: See Bezanson et al. (2004, Chapter 12, p. 18). Study participants were stratified into two groups: group 1 (early extubation) and group 2 (late extubation).

survey studies Descriptive, exploratory, or comparative studies that collect detailed descriptions of existing variables and use the data to justify and assess current conditions and practices, or to make more plans for improving health care practices.

survival curve A graph that shows the probability that a patient "survives" in a given state for at least a specified time (or longer).

symbolic interaction A theoretical perspective that holds that the relationship between self and society is an ongoing process of symbolic communication whereby individuals create a social reality.

systematic Data collection carried out in the same manner with all subjects.

systematic error Attributable to lasting characteristics of the subject that do not tend to fluctuate from one time to another. Also called constant error.

systematic sampling A probability sampling strategy that involves the selection of subjects randomly drawn from a population list at fixed intervals.

Example: See Lowry et al. (1998, Chapter 12, p. 22). Every sixth patient chart was selected, and the data were included in the study.

systematic review Process where investigators find all relevant studies, published and unpublished, on the topic or question, at least two members of the review team independently assess the quality of each study, include or exclude studies based on preestablished criteria, statistically combine the results of individual studies, and present a balanced and impartial evidence summary of the findings that represents a "state of the science" conclusion about the evidence supporting benefits and risks of a given health care practice.

T

t **statistic** Commonly used in nursing research; it tests whether two group means are more different than would be expected by chance. Groups may be related or independent.

Example: See Davison et al. (2003, Appendix D). The t test was used to determine if there was a difference between the anxiety and depression scores.

target population A population or group of individuals that meet the sampling criteria.

test A self-report inventory that provides for one response to each item that the examiner assigns a rating or score. Inferences are made from the total score about the degree to which a subject possesses whatever trait, emotion, attitude, or behavior the test is supposed to measure.

testable Variables of proposed study that lend themselves to observation, measurement, and analysis.

testing The effects of taking a pretest on the scores of a posttest.

test-retest reliability Administration of the same instrument twice to the same subjects under the same conditions within a prescribed time interval, with a comparison of the paired scores to determine the stability of the measure.

Example: See Shin et al. (2001, Chapter 15, p. 16). A Korean translation of the Exercise Self-Efficacy Scale was assessed for use in a Korean population. The test-retest interval was 2 weeks, and the test-retest reliability measure had a correlation coefficient of .77.

text Data in a contextual form, that is, narrative or words that are written and transcribed.

theoretical framework Theoretical rationale for the development of hypotheses.

Example: See Van Cleve et al. (2004, Appendix B). The section labeled "Theoretical Framework" discusses how the authors used theory to develop a research question.

theoretical literature A synonym for conceptual literature; see *conceptual literature.*

theoretical sampling Used to select experiences that will help the researcher test ideas and gather complete information about developing concepts when using the grounded theory method.

Example: See Keating-Lefler et al. (2004, Chapter 8, p. 9). The mothers chosen to be in the study were selected based upon emerging themes, as the study progressed, to ensure representation of important ideas.

theory Set of interrelated concepts, definitions, and propositions that present a systematic view of phenomena for the purpose of explaining and making predictions about those phenomena.

time series design A quasiexperimental design used to determine trends before and after an experimental treatment. Measurements are taken several times before the introduction of the experimental treatment, the treatment is introduced, and measurements are taken again at specified times afterward.

time-sharing Several users working on one mainframe via terminals at the same time.

triangulation The expansion of research methods in a single study or multiple studies to enhance diversity, enrich understanding, and accomplish specific goals.

Example: See Plach et al. (2004, Appendix C). These authors first conducted a quantitative study of women with rheumatoid arthritis. They then chose to interview 20 women from this first study for a qualitative study to help better understand the effect of rheumatoid arthritis on social roles.

true experiment Also known as the pretest-posttest control group design. In this design, subjects are randomly assigned to an experimental or control group, pretest measurements are performed, an intervention or treatment occurs in the experimental group, and posttest measurements are performed.

type I error The rejection of a null hypothesis that is actually true.

type II error The acceptance of a null hypothesis that is actually false.

U

uplink The ability to broadcast conferences so that they can be attended from a distance.

V

validation sample The sample that provides the initial data for determining the reliability and validity of a measurement tool.

validity Determination of whether a measurement instrument actually measures what it is purported to measure.

variable A defined concept.

W

Web browser Software program used to connect or "read" the World Wide Web (www).

World Wide Web (www) A conceptual group of servers on the Internet. The Web is multiple hypertext linked together in an Internet network that criss-crosses the whole Internet like a spider web.

worldview Another label for paradigm; the way people in society think about the world.

Z

Z score Used to compare measurements in standard units; examines the relative distance of the scores from the mean.

Index

Entries followed by *"b"* indicate boxes; *"f"* figures; *and "t"* tables.